OPERATIVE TECHNIQUES IN SPINE SURGERY

OPERATIVE TECHNIQUES IN SPINE SURGERY

EDITORS

John M. Rhee, MD
Associate Professor of Orthopaedic Surgery
Emory University School of Medicine
Atlanta, Georgia

Scott D. Boden, MD
Professor of Orthopaedic Surgery
Director, Emory Orthopaedics & Spine Center
The Emory Clinic
Staff Physician, Atlanta VA Medical Center
Atlanta, Georgia

John M. Flynn, MD
Associate Chief of Orthopaedic Surgery
The Children's Hospital of Philadelphia
Associate Professor of Orthopaedic Surgery
University of Pennsylvania School of Medicine
Philadelphia, Pennsylvania

EDITOR-IN-CHIEF

Sam W. Wiesel, MD
Professor and Chair of Orthopaedic Surgery
Georgetown University Medical School
Washington, DC

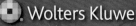 Wolters Kluwer | Lippincott Williams & Wilkins
Health
Philadelphia · Baltimore · New York · London
Buenos Aires · Hong Kong · Sydney · Tokyo

Acquisitions Editor: Brian Brown
Product Manager: Dave Murphy
Marketing Manager: Lisa Lawrence
Manufacturing Manager: Ben Rivera
Design Manager: Doug Smock
Compositor: Absolute Service, Inc.

© 2013 by LIPPINCOTT WILLIAMS & WILKINS, a WOLTERS KLUWER business
Two Commerce Square
2001 Market Street
Philadelphia, PA 19103

Operative techniques in spine surgery / editors, John M. Rhee, Scott D. Boden, John M. Flynn ; editor-in-chief, Sam W. Wiesel.
    p. ; cm. – (Operative techniques)
Includes bibliographical references and index.
ISBN 978-1-4511-2769-0
I. Rhee, John M. II. Wiesel, Sam W. III. Series: Operative techniques.
[DNLM: 1. Spine–surgery–Atlases. 2. Orthopedic Procedures–methods–Atlases. 3. Spinal Diseases–surgery–Atlases. WE 17]
617.5'6059–dc23
                        2012029686

Care has been taken to confirm the accuracy of the information presented and to describe generally accepted practices. However, the authors, editors, and publisher are not responsible for errors or omissions or for any consequences from application of the information in this book and make no warranty, expressed or implied, with respect to the currency, completeness, or accuracy of the contents of the publication. Application of the information in a particular situation remains the professional responsibility of the practitioner.

The authors, editors, and publisher have exerted every effort to ensure that drug selection and dosage set forth in this text are in accordance with current recommendations and practice at the time of publication. However, in view of ongoing research, changes in government regulations, and the constant flow of information relating to drug therapy and drug reactions, the reader is urged to check the package insert for each drug for any change in indications and dosage and for added warnings and precautions. This is particularly important when the recommended agent is a new or infrequently employed drug.

Some drugs and medical devices presented in the publication have Food and Drug Administration (FDA) clearance for limited use in restricted research settings. It is the responsibility of the health care provider to ascertain the FDA status of each drug or device planned for use in their clinical practice.

To purchase additional copies of this book, call our customer service department at (800) 638-3030 or fax orders to (301) 223-2320. International customers should call (301) 223-2300.

Visit Lippincott Williams & Wilkins on the Internet at LWW.com. Lippincott Williams & Wilkins customer service representatives are available from 8:30 a.m. to 6 p.m., EST.

10 9 8 7 6 5 4 3 2 1

Dedication

To my Lord and Savior, Jesus Christ, for His infinite blessings in my life. To Marcia, the most amazing wife I could ever imagine, for her treasured love, support, and encouragement. To my children, Julia and James, of whom I am so very proud. To my parents, Yoo and Cho Rhee, and Huen Cook, for their sacrifices in providing for me. To my Spine and Orthopaedic mentors at Wash U and UCSF, for training me and freely imparting their wisdom. To my partners at Emory, for defining excellence. To my patients, for entrusting themselves to me and also teaching me something new every day.

With sincere gratitude, JMR.

CONTENTS

vii

CONTRIBUTORS

Todd J. Albert, MD
Richard H. Rothman Professor
  and Chairman
Department of Orthopaedic Surgery
Professor of Neurosurgery
Thomas Jefferson University Hospital
Rothman Institute
Philadelphia, Pennsylvania

Behrooz Akbarnia, MD
Clinical Professor
University of California, San Diego
La Jolla, California

David Greg Anderson, MD
Professor of Orthopaedic Surgery and
  Neurological Surgery
Thomas Jefferson University and
  Rothman Institute
Clinical Director, Spine Section of the
  Orthopaedic Research Laboratory
Philadelphia, Pennsylvania

Paul A. Anderson, MD
Professor of Orthopedics & Rehabilitation
University of Wisconsin
Madison, Wisconsin

Casey C. Bachison, MD
Carlton-Harrison Orthopedic Clinic
Ogden, Utah

Kelley Banagan, MD
Assistant Professor of Orthopaedics
University of Maryland School of Medicine
Spine Surgeon
University of Maryland Medical Center
Baltimore, Maryland

Maneesh Bawa, MD
Department of Orthopaedics
Emory University School of Medicine
Atlanta, Georgia

Gordon R. Bell, MD
Head of Spinal Surgery
Vice-Chairman of Orthopaedic Surgery
The Cleveland Clinic
Cleveland, Ohio

Keith H. Bridwell, MD
J. Albert Key Distinguished Professor of
  Orthopaedic Surgery
Professor of Neurological Surgery
Founder and Codirector, Pediatric/Adult
  Spinal Deformity Service
Founder and Director, Washington
  University Spine Fellowship
Washington University School of Medicine
St. Louis, Missouri

Jacob M. Buchowski, MD, MS
Assistant Professor of Orthopaedic and
  Neurological Surgery
Washington University in St. Louis
St. Louis, Missouri

Patrick Cahill, MD
Staff Surgeon
Shriners Hospital for Children
Philadelphia, Pennsylvania

Gilbert Chan, MD
Clinical Fellow
Division of Orthopaedics
The Children's Hospital of Philadelphia
Philadelphia, Pennsylvania

Charles C. Chang, MD
Department of Orthopaedic Surgery
University of California, San Diego
San Diego, California

Saad B. Chaudhary, MD, MBA
Center for Spine Health
The Cleveland Clinic
Cleveland, Ohio

Morgan N. Chen, MD
Orthopedic Associates of Long Island, LLP
East Setauket, New York

Kirk W. Dabney, MD
Associate Director of the Cerebral
  Palsy Program
Alfred I. duPont Hospital for Children
Wilmington, Delaware

John P. Dormans, MD
Chief of Orthopaedic Surgery
The Children's Hospital of Philadelphia
Philadelphia, Pennsylvania

Denis S. Drummond, MD
Professor of Orthopaedic Surgery
University of Pennsylvania School of
  Medicine
Attending Surgeon
Emeritus Chief of Orthopaedic Surgery
The Children's Hospital of Philadelphia
Philadelphia, Pennsylvania

Mark Dumonski, MD
Resident
Department of Orthopaedic Surgery
Rush University Medical Center
Chicago, Illinois

John B. Emans, MD
Professor of Orthopedic Surgery
Children's Hospital Boston
Harvard Medical School
Boston, Massachusetts

Reginald S. Fayssoux, MD
Department of Orthopaedic Surgery
The Emory Spine Center
Emory University School of Medicine
Atlanta, Georgia

Ira L. Fedder, PharmD, MD
Scoliosis and Spine Center of Maryland
Towson Orthopaedic Associates
Towson, Maryland

Richard G. Fessler, MD, PhD
Professor of Neurological Surgery
Department of Neurological Surgery
Northwestern University
Feinberg School of Medicine
Chicago, Illinois

Michael A. Finn, MD
Assistant Professor of Neurosurgery
University of Colorado School of Medicine
Aurora, Colorado

Todd B. Francis, MD, PhD
Spine Surgery Fellow
The Cleveland Clinic
Cleveland, Ohio

Steven R. Garfin, MD
Professor and Chairman of
  Orthopaedic Surgery
Chief of Spine Surgery
University of California, San Diego
San Diego, California

James T. Guille, MD
Division of Spinal Disorders
Brandywine Institute of Orthopaedics
Pottstown, Pennsylvania

James S. Harrop, MD
Associate Professor of Neurological and
  Orthopedic Surgery
Thomas Jefferson University
Philadelphia, Pennsylvania

Andrew C. Hecht, MD
Co-Chief, Spine Surgery
Assistant Professor of Orthopaedic and
  Neurosurgery
Mt. Sinai Medical Center and School of
  Medicine
New York, New York

Daniel J. Hedequist, MD
Associate Professor of Orthopedic Surgery
Children's Hospital Boston/Harvard
  Medical School
Boston, Massachusetts

John Heflin, MD
Resident
Department of Orthopaedic Surgery
Emory University School of Medicine
Atlanta, Georgia

John G. Heller, MD
Professor of Orthopaedic Surgery
Spine Fellowship Director
The Emory Spine Center
Emory University School of Medicine
Emory University Orthopaedics & Spine
  Hospital
Atlanta, Georgia

Harry N. Herkowitz, MD
Department of Orthopaedic Surgery
Beaumont Health System
Royal Oak, Michigan
Professor and Chairman
Orthopaedic Surgery
Oakland University William Beaumont
School of Medicine
Rochester, Michigan

William C. Horton III, MD
Adjunct Professor of Orthopedic Surgery
The Emory Spine Center
Emory University School of Medicine
Atlanta, Georgia

Victor Hsu, BA, MD
Attending Spine Surgeon
Department of Orthopaedic Surgery
Orthopaedic Specialty Center
Willow Grove, Pennsylvania

Claude Jarrett, MD
Resident
Department of Orthopaedic Surgery
Emory University School of Medicine
Atlanta, Georgia

S. Babak Kalantar, MD
Assistant Professor of Orthopaedics
Georgetown University Hospital
Washington, DC

Christopher G. Kalhorn, MD
Associate Professor of Neurosurgery
Georgetown University Hospital
Washington, DC

Norio Kawahara, MD, PhD
Clinical Professor of Orthopaedic Surgery
Kanazawa University School of Medicine
Ishikawa, Japan

Khaled M. Kebaish, MD, MSc, FRCS(C)
Associate Professor of Orthopaedic Surgery
The Johns Hopkins University
Johns Hopkins Outpatient Center
Baltimore, Maryland

Michael P. Kelly, MD
Assistant Professor of Orthopaedic Surgery
Washington University Orthopaedics
St. Louis, Missouri

Christopher K. Kepler, MD, MBA
Instructor of Orthopaedic Surgery
Thomas Jefferson University Hospitals
Philadelphia, Pennsylvania

James S. Kercher, MD
Resident
Department of Orthopaedic Surgery
Emory University
Atlanta, Georgia

Choll W. Kim, MD, PhD
Spine Institute of San Diego
Center for Minimally Invasive Spine
Surgery at Alvarado Hospital
Associate Clinical Professor
University of California San Diego
Executive Director
Society for Minimally Invasive Spine Surgery
San Diego, California

Youjeong Kim, MD
Orthopaedic Consultants of North Texas
Baylor University Medical Center
Dallas, Texas

Michael J. Lee, MD
Assistant Professor of Sports Medicine and
Orthopaedic Surgery
University of Washington Medical Center
Seattle, Washington

Yu-Po Lee, MD
Associate Clinical Professor of
Orthopaedic Surgery
Spine Surgery
University of California, San Diego
San Diego, California

Ronald A. Lehman, Jr., MD
Director
Pediatric and Adult Spine
Assistant Professor of Surgery, USUHS
Department of Orthopaedics and
Rehabilitation
Walter Reed Army Medical Center
Potomac, Maryland

Lawrence G. Lenke, MD
The Jerome J. Gilden Distinguished
Professor of Orthopaedic Surgery
Chief, Orthopaedic Spine Surgery
Codirector, Adult and Pediatric Spinal
Deformity Surgery
Professor of Neurological Surgery
Washington University School of Medicine
St. Louis, Missouri

Steven C. Ludwig, MD
Associate Professor of Orthopaedics
Chief of Spine Surgery, Department of
Orthopaedics
Codirector, University of Maryland Spine
Center
University of Maryland Medical Center
Baltimore, Maryland

Satyajit V. Marawar, MD
Fellow in Spine Surgery
Department of Orthopaedic Surgery
Medical College of Wisconsin
Milwaukee, Wisconsin

Christopher T. Martin, MD
Department of Orthopaedic Surgery
University of Iowa Hospitals and Clinics
Iowa City, Iowa

Paul C. McAfee, MD
Chief of Spine Surgery
St. Joseph's Hospital
Towson, Maryland

Richard E. McCarthy, MD
Professor of Orthopaedics
Chief of Spinal Deformities
Arkansas Children's Hospital
Little Rock, Arkansas

Kevin M. McGrail, MD, FACS
Professor and Chair of Neurosurgery
Georgetown University Hospital
Washington, DC

Keith W. Michael, MD
Spine Fellow
Emory University
Atlanta, Georgia

Gokce Mik, MD
Department of Orthopaedic Surgery
The Children's Hospital of Philadelphia
Philadelphia, Pennsylvania

Freeman Miller, MD
Al duPont Hospital for Children
Wilmington, Delaware

Hideki Murakami, MD
Lecturer of Orthopaedic Surgery
Department of Orthopaedic Surgery
Kanazawa University School of Medicine
Ishikawa, Japan

Daniel Park, MD
Resident
Department of Orthopaedic Surgery
Rush University Medical Center
Chicago, Illinois

Ankur D. Patel, MD
Department of Orthopaedic Surgery
University of California, San Diego
San Diego, California

Adam M. Pearson, MD
Department of Orthopaedic Surgery
Dartmouth Medical School
Dartmouth-Hitchcock Medical Center
Lebanon, New Hampshire

Victor M. Popov, MD
Department of Orthopaedic Surgery
Rothman Institute
Philadelphia, Pennsylvania

Sheeraz A. Qureshi, MD
Assistant Professor of Orthopaedic Surgery
Mount Sinai Hospital
Chief, Spinal Trauma
Elmhurst Hospital Center
New York, New York

Raj Rao, MD
Professor of Orthopaedic Surgery
Medical College of Wisconsin
Milwaukee, Wisconsin

Daniel Refai, MD
Assistant Professor of Orthopaedic and
Neurosurgery
Emory University School of Medicine
Atlanta, Georgia

Mitchell F. Reiter, MD
Assistant Professor of Orthopedic Surgery
The New Jersey Medical School/UMDNJ
Summit, New Jersey

John M. Rhee, MD
Assistant Professor of Orthopaedic Surgery
Emory University School of Medicine
Atlanta, Georgia

K. Daniel Riew, MD
Mildred B. Simon Distinguished Professor
of Orthopaedic Surgery
Professor of Neurological Surgery
Chief, Cervical Spine Surgery
Washington University Orthopedics
Director, Orthopedic-Rehab Institute for
Cervical Spine Surgery
St. Louis, Missouri

Gerald E. Rodts, Jr., MD
Professor of Neurosurgery
The Emory Spine Center
Emory University School of Medicine
Atlanta, Georgia

Samer Saiedy, MD
Department of Surgery
St. Joseph's Hospital
Towson, Maryland

Matthew N. Scott-Young, MBBS, FRACS, FAOrthA
Associate Professor of Health Science and Medicine
Bond University
Gold Coast, Australia

Gursukhman Sidhu, MD
Department of Orthopaedic Surgery
Thomas Jefferson University
The Rothman Institute
Philadelphia, Pennsylvania

Kern Singh, MD
Assistant Professor of Orthopaedic Surgery
Rush University Medical Center
Chicago, Illinois

Nicholas P. Slimack, MD
Department of Neurological Surgery
Northwestern University
Feinberg School of Medicine
Chicago, Illinois

Thomas Stanley, MD
Resident
Department of Orthopaedic Surgery
Rush University Medical Center
Chicago, Illinois

Selvon St. Clair, MD, PhD
Orthopaedic and Spine Surgeon
Orthopaedic Institute of Ohio
Lima, Ohio

Daniel J. Sucato, MD, MS
Associate Professor
University of Texas at Southwestern Medical Center
Staff Orthopaedic Surgeon
Texas Scottish Rite Hospital
Dallas, Texas

Katsuro Tomita, MD
Professor of Orthopaedic Surgery
Kanazawa University School of Medicine
Ishikawa, Japan

P. Justin Tortolani, BA, MD
Towson Orthopaedic Associates
Towson, Maryland

Alexander R. Vaccaro, MD
Department of Orthopaedic Surgery
Thomas Jefferson University
The Rothman Institute
Philadelphia, Pennsylvania

David H. Wei, MD
Department of Orthopaedic Surgery
Columbia University Medical Center
New York Presbyterian Hospital
New York, New York

Bradley K. Weiner, MD
Associate Professor of Orthopaedic Surgery
Chief of Spinal Surgery
The Methodist Hospital
Houston, Texas

Andrew P. White, MD
Instructor
Harvard Medical School
Department of Orthopaedic Surgery
Beth Israel Deaconess Medical Center
Boston, Massachusetts

Sam W. Wiesel, MD
Professor and Chair of Orthopaedic Surgery
Georgetown University Medical School
Washington, District of Columbia

Bart Wojewnik, MD
Resident
Department of Orthopaedic Surgery
Loyola University Health System
Maywood, Illinois

Adam L. Wollowick, MD
Assistant Professor of Surgery
Montefiore Medical Center
Bronx, New York

S. Tim Yoon, MD, PhD
Assistant Professor of Orthopaedic Surgery
Emory University
Atlanta, Georgia

Lukas P. Zebala, MD
Assistant Professor of Orthopedic Surgery
Department of Neurological Surgery
Washington University School of Medicine
St. Louis, Missouri

Aristidis Zibis, MD
Fellow in Spinal Surgery
Department of Orthopaedic Surgery
Penn State Hershey Medical School
Hershey, Pennsylvania

PREFACE

When a surgeon contemplates performing a procedure, there are three major questions to consider: Why is the surgery being done? When in the course of a disease process should it be performed? And, finally, what are the technical steps involved? The purpose of this text is to describe in a detailed, step-by-step manner the "how to do it" of the vast majority of orthopaedic procedures. The "why" and "when" are covered in outline form at the beginning of each procedure. However, it is assumed that the surgeon understands the basics of "why" and "when" and has made the definitive decision to undertake a specific case. This text is designed to review and make clear the detailed steps of the anticipated operation.

Operative Techniques in Spine Surgery differs from other books because it is mainly visual. Each procedure is described in a systematic way that makes liberal use of focused, original artwork. It is hoped that the surgeon will be able to visualize each significant step of a procedure as it unfolds during a case.

Each chapter has been edited by a specialist who has specific expertise and experience in the discipline. It has taken a tremendous amount of work for each editor to enlist talented authors for each procedure and then review the final work. It has been very stimulating to work with all of these wonderful and talented people, and I am honored to have taken part in this rewarding experience.

Finally, I would like to thank everyone who has contributed to the development of this book. Specifically, Grace Caputo at Dovetail Content Solutions and Dave Murphy and Eileen Wolfberg at Lippincott Williams & Wilkins, who have been very helpful and generous with their input. Special thanks, as well, goes to Bob Hurley at LWW, who has adeptly guided this textbook from original concept to publication.

SWW

RESIDENCY ADVISORY BOARD

The editors and the publisher would like to thank the resident reviewers who participated in the reviews of the manuscript and page proofs. Their detailed review and analysis was invaluable in helping to make certain this text meets the needs of residents today and in the future.

Chapter 1

Anterior Cervical Discectomy and Fusion With and Without Instrumentation

John M. Rhee, Claude Jarrett, and Sam Wiesel

DEFINITION

▪ Cervical spondylosis refers to degenerative conditions affecting the cervical spine, including disc degeneration, herniation, facet arthrosis, and osteophytic spur formation. Depending on the nature and location of the spondylotic changes, pathologic compression of neural structures in the cervical spine may occur.

▪ This chapter focuses on anterior cervical discectomy and fusion (ACDF) as a surgical treatment option for patients with cervical radiculopathy. Cervical myelopathy can also be treated with ACDF as long as the spinal cord compression occurs at the disc, rather than the retrovertebral, level.

▪ All techniques described in this chapter can apply to the decompression of the spinal cord in myelopathic patients as well as the nerve root in radiculopathic patients.

ANATOMY

▪ The anterior longitudinal ligament is a wide band of ligaments stretching along the anterior surface of the vertebral bodies. Its dense longitudinal fibers widen as they travel caudally and are intimately associated with the intervertebral discs as well as the vertebral endplates.

▪ The posterior longitudinal ligament (PLL) is a smooth and shiny group of dense ligaments that course along the posterior surface of the vertebral bodies within the spinal canal. The PLL tends to be thicker centrally and thins out laterally as it attaches to the uncinate regions. Bulging or ossification of the PLL (OPLL) can cause spinal cord compression.

▪ The intervertebral disc comprises the outer annulus fibrosus and the central gelatinous nucleus pulposus. Each disc is attached to the subchondral bone of the adjacent vertebral bodies. The outermost rim of the vertebral endplate is not attached to the disc, leaving a ring of exposed bone that may be more prone to forming arthrotic spurs.

▪ The uncovertebral joints are critical bony landmarks for anterior cervical decompression (**FIG 1**). Spurs commonly arise from these articulations and cause impingement of the exiting roots as they enter the foramen.

  ▪ Depending on the cervical level, the vertebral artery may be as close as 5 mm away from the medial aspect of the uncinate process.

▪ Each cervical spinal nerve is composed of dorsal and ventral roots. The ventral root lies dorsal to the uncovertebral joint, while the dorsal root is ventral to the superior articular facet.

  ▪ It is important to keep in mind when performing uncovertebral osteophyte resection that the nerve root leaves the spinal cord at roughly a 45-degree angle ventrolaterally in the axial plane. Thus, care must be taken to hug the

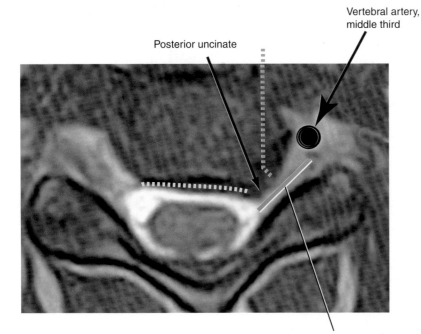

Posterior uncinate

Vertebral artery, middle third

Root exits ventrally at 45-degree angle

FIG 1 • Anterior foraminotomy anatomy: important anatomic relationships to consider when performing anterior cervical spine surgery. The exiting nerve root enters the foramen at a 45-degree ventrolateral angle. The posterior aspect of the uncinate joint marks the entry zone of the neuroforamen, and it is where osteophytes commonly arise to impinge the exiting root. Thus, the uncus should be decompressed when performing foraminotomy. It is critical to hug the posterior aspect of the uncinate during foraminotomy to avoid injuring the exiting root, which lies immediately dorsal. The vertebral artery is unlikely to be injured while working in the posterior disc space (eg, during decompression) because it is located at roughly the level of the middle third of the vertebra. The trajectory of discectomy should be bounded by the uncinates at all times, but it can widen posteriorly at the level of the nerve root to thoroughly decompress the root while avoiding vertebral artery injury (*dashed blue line*). The posterior longitudinal ligament (*dashed yellow line*) tends to be thicker and better defined centrally; it thins out laterally.

Table 1	Neurologic Examination of the Cervical Spine		
Root	**Sensory**	**Motor**	**Reflex**
C2	Sensation to posterior occiput		
C3	Sensation to neck		
C4	Sensation to upper shoulder, chest		
C5	Sensation along lateral arm	Motor to deltoid	Biceps reflex
C6	Sensation to lateral forearm and radial two digits	Motor to biceps, wrist extension, pronation	Brachioradialis reflex
C7	Sensation to middle finger	Motor to triceps and wrist flexion	Triceps reflex
C8	Sensation to medial forearm and ulnar two digits	Motor to finger flexors—grip	
T1	Sensation to medial arm	Motor to interossei	

posterior surface of the uncinate to avoid injury to the exiting root.[4]

PATHOGENESIS

▪ Neural impingement occurs in two main locations: within the spinal canal, affecting the spinal cord, the nerve root, or both; or within the foramen, where the exiting root can be affected.

▪ Depending on whether the involved structure is the spinal cord or the nerve root, patients can present with symptoms of myelopathy, radiculopathy, or both.

NATURAL HISTORY

▪ The natural history of cervical radiculopathy is generally favorable, with most patients having spontaneous resolution or considerable improvement of their symptoms over time.

▪ It is not common for radiculopathic patients to progress to myelopathy.[9,10]

HISTORY AND PHYSICAL FINDINGS

▪ Patients with radiculopathy typically present with radiating pain, paresthesia, or motor weakness (Table 1). However, the pattern of symptoms is not always dermatomal (**FIG 2**).

▪ On examination, patients with radiculopathy may have motor, sensory, or reflex changes along the affected nerve root distribution. However, the neurologic examination findings may be normal.

▪ Patients may express exacerbation of radicular pain with particular head positions (ie, head positions that narrow the size of the neural foramen, such as neck extension with rotation to the affected extremity).

  ▪ This can be elicited by performing the Spurling test. The Spurling sign is very helpful in differentiating cervical radiculopathy from extraspinal causes, such as cubital or carpal tunnel syndromes, as reproduction of symptoms should occur only with a cervical source of compression.

IMAGING AND OTHER DIAGNOSTIC STUDIES

▪ Plain radiographs, although of limited value in evaluating neural compression, remain a commonly acquired initial study and can be used to evaluate overall alignment, spinal instability, or bony pathology, including spur formation.

▪ MRI is the modality of choice for evaluating neural compression.

▪ CT-myelography provides outstanding resolution of bony and neural anatomy, but it is less appealing as it requires an invasive procedure. It is typically recommended for patients with contraindications for MRI (eg, prosthetic heart valve, pacemaker) or when MRI fails to provide sufficient detail.

▪ If a high-quality MRI is available but questions remain regarding bony anatomy for the purposes of surgical planning, a noncontrast CT scan provides complementary information (eg, differentiating OPLL from disc herniation) (**FIG 3**).

DIFFERENTIAL DIAGNOSIS

▪ Cervical radiculopathy
▪ Cervical myelopathy
▪ Brachial plexus injury
▪ Complex regional pain syndrome or reflex sympathetic dystrophy
▪ Thoracic outlet syndrome
▪ Inflammatory arthropathy
▪ Spinal cord tumor
▪ Angina

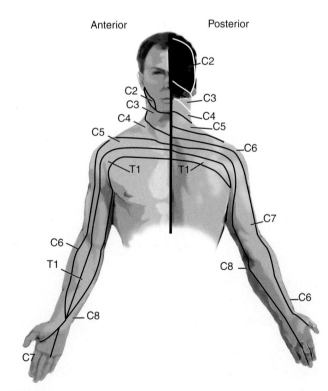

FIG 2 • Dermatomes of the cervical nerve roots. Symptoms do not always follow the textbook distribution of dermatomes. In particular, radiculopathies involving various nerve roots, such as C5, C6, or C7, can all produce periscapular pain, not uncommonly in the absence of radiating pain down the arm. If in doubt as to the offending level, a selective nerve root block can be performed for diagnostic purposes.

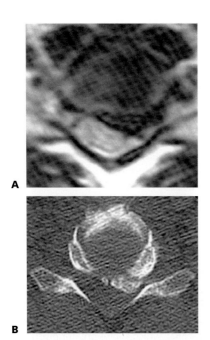

FIG 3 • MRI and CT scans may provide complementary information in delineating bony versus soft tissue masses. **A.** On the axial MRI, the compressive lesion appears to be a soft disc. **B.** A CT scan through the same level, however, demonstrates the pathology to be an ossified disc. Similarly, CT scans can help differentiate disc herniations from ossification of the posterior longitudinal ligament.

- Shoulder pathology
- Peripheral nerve compression (eg, carpal or cubital tunnel syndrome)
- Diabetic neuropathy
- Multiple sclerosis
- Syringomyelia
- Stroke
- Guillain-Barré syndrome
- Normal-pressure hydrocephalus
- Spinal cord tumor

NONOPERATIVE MANAGEMENT

- Nonoperative management should be considered as the initial mode of treatment for most patients with radiculopathy.
- Nonsurgical treatment typically includes physical therapy, traction, pain medication, cervical collars, and epidural injections.

SURGICAL MANAGEMENT

- Surgical intervention is indicated for radiculopathy in patients with persistent symptoms resistant to nonoperative care, progressive weakness, or instability.
- Common surgical approaches to radiculopathy include ACDF versus posterior laminoforaminotomy.[11]

Preoperative Planning

- The surgeon should evaluate imaging studies for anatomic variations, such as medial aberrancy of the vertebral artery.
- To perform a safe but complete and adequate neural decompression, high-quality illumination and magnification are essential.

- An operating microscope provides illumination and visualization superior to that of loupes and headlights, but either method can be used.
- Another advantage to the microscope is that the view obtained by the assistant is the same as that of the operating surgeon.
- If the surgeon chooses to use the microscope, given the smaller field of view, it is imperative to continuously adjust the viewing angle such that a line of sight parallel to the disc space is achieved (**FIG 4**). If this is not done, the surgeon may inadvertently stray away from the disc space, veer into one vertebral body or the other, and not proceed to the back of the disc space, where the decompression needs to occur.

Positioning

- The patient is positioned with a bump under the scapula and the occiput on a foam doughnut to prevent pressure necrosis.
- The amount of extension tolerated preoperatively without excessive pain or neurologic symptoms is recreated.

Approach

- A standard Smith-Robinson approach to the anterior cervical spine is used for most cases from C2 to T2.

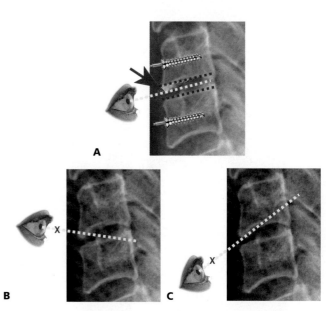

FIG 4 • Line of sight. When using the microscope, it must be angled properly to provide a parallel view of the disc space to facilitate decompression and endplate preparation. Endplate preparation should proceed in a parallel fashion (*dotted red lines*) (**A**) centered on the disc space to achieve a rectangular space for graft insertion. Parallel, wide preparation of the disc space also makes decompression easier to perform and ensures that the decompression is centered on the disc space (**C**). (**B,C**) If the line of sight is not maintained, one may err into the vertebral bodies above and below rather than progressing toward the area at the disc level that requires decompression. To achieve parallel surfaces, the inferior endplate of the cephalad vertebra typically requires greater preparation because it is concave. In contrast, the superior endplate of the caudal vertebra is flatter and requires less preparation. (**C**) Proper line of sight is facilitated by removing the anterior lip (*arrow, shaded yellow*), which allows for better visualization of, and access to, the posterior disc space.

ANTERIOR CERVICAL DISCECTOMY AND FUSION WITH INSTRUMENTATION

Initial Discectomy

- Once the disc is exposed, it is sharply incised with a no. 15 blade and removed with a combination of curettes and pituitary rongeurs.
- The disc and cartilaginous material should be removed until the PLL and both uncinate processes are visualized (**TECH FIG 1A**).
- An important maneuver to facilitate disc space visualization and neural decompression is to remove the anterior portion of the inferior endplate of the superior vertebral body (the anterior lip). Doing so provides a direct line of sight into the posterior disc space, which facilitates later foraminotomy and resection of the PLL, if necessary.
- This surface is almost always concave, with the anterior portion overhanging the disc space, thus preventing direct visualization of the posterior disc space.
- Removal can be done with either a Kerrison rongeur or a high-speed burr.
- Flattening this surface also facilitates optimal graft–endplate contact (**TECH FIG 1B,C**).
- Use of the burr to fashion the endplates, alternating with use of the curettes and pituitary rongeur to remove cartilage and disc material, is performed.

Use of Distraction: Pins, Tongs, and Spreaders

- Intervertebral body distraction pins can be placed to gently distract the disc space and improve visualization.
  - Generally, this is done after an initial superficial discectomy, which allows greater disc space mobilization with the pins.
- Because greater preparation of the inferior endplate of the superior vertebra is usually needed, the Caspar pin should be placed more cephalad in the cephalad vertebral body (**TECH FIG 2**).
- Overdistraction of the disc space is not desired. If the disc space is fused in an overdistracted position, postoperative neck pain may result. If there is a significant compressive lesion on the spinal cord, distraction should

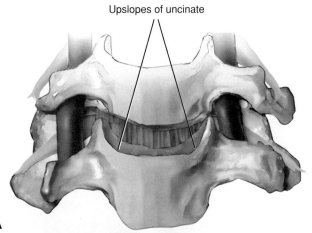

Upslopes of uncinate

A

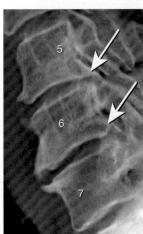

B

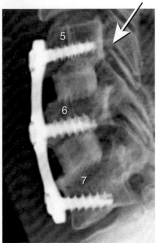

C

TECH FIG 1 • **A.** The discectomy should begin lateral (*red lines*) to the medial border of the uncinates. The upslope of the uncinate is clearly defined with curettes and Kerrison rongeurs until these borders are unquestionably identified. Having a wide discectomy allows for placement of larger grafts or supplemental grafts in the uncinate regions. **B,C.** Anterior cervical discectomy and fusion graft carpentry. Creating parallel disc spaces facilitates graft–host bone contact, securing an intimate fit, as well as allowing for wide decompression of spurs arising from the posterior disc space. Spurs are removed off the inferior vertebrae of C5 and C6 (*arrows*). More bone than usual was removed from the inferior portion of C6 because of the extensive spondylotic bar causing spinal cord compression along the floor of the canal in this patient.

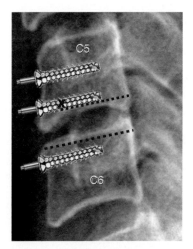

TECH FIG 2 • Caspar pin placement. Because greater preparation of the inferior endplate on the cephalad vertebra is necessary, the surgeon should place the upper Caspar pin (C5) further away from the endplate (eg, in the midbody of C5 or more cephalad), while being cognizant of not entering the adjacent disc space above. The Caspar pins are placed in the midline to avoid compromising later screw fixation during plating. To achieve parallel distraction, the pins should be placed parallel to the disc space. If the tips (ie, the leading ends) converge, relative kyphosis of the disc space occurs with placement of the Caspar pin spreader and distraction; if the tips diverge, relative segmental lordosis occurs with placement of the Caspar pin spreader and distraction.

be avoided until the compression has been relieved to prevent stretching or tenting of the cord over that lesion.
- An additional benefit of the Caspar pins is that they help to retract the soft tissues in a cephalad–caudal direction without the use of a secondary set of retractor blades.
- Alternatively, a small laminar spreader can be used in the contralateral disc space instead of Caspar pins to provide distraction.

Endplate Preparation

- The inferior endplate of the cephalad level is concave, whereas the superior endplate of the inferior level tends to be relatively flatter. Thus, to achieve intimate contact of bone graft with both endplates, a rectangular space is created by parallel decortication of the endplates.
  - This generally requires greater preparation of the inferior endplate of the cephalad level versus the superior endplate of the inferior level.
  - It is important not to remove too much bone off the inferior endplate of the cephalad level, however, as doing so limits the bone available in the vertebra to accommodate a plate and screws. This is particularly the case in smaller patients who have smaller vertebrae.
- A high-speed burr is helpful in decorticating the endplates.
- The creation of a parallel rectangular space within the disc space allows insertion of a graft appropriately sized to match the larger height present at the center of the disc space.
- Both endplates should be thoroughly denuded of cartilage and decorticated to reveal bleeding bony surfaces to enhance the chance of successful fusion.[5]
- Alternating use of the high-speed burr, curettes, and the pituitary rongeur will allow the surgeon to reach the posterior disc space and the PLL.
- During ACDF, we are more aggressive with endplate preparation than during corpectomy, because ACDF grafts tend to be more stable than corpectomy grafts.
  - If major endplate resection is performed during corpectomy, significant settling or pistoning of the graft may occur, which is less likely with ACDFs. Furthermore, in cases of extensive spondylosis, wide disc space preparation facilitates decompression along the floor of the canal in ACDF surgery.
  - When performing corpectomy, on the other hand, the additional room is not usually necessary because removing the vertebral body creates wide access for work at the disc level.

Anterior Foraminotomy

- The discectomy is performed to the level of the PLL, with complete removal of the posterior annulus. It is safer to leave the PLL intact during the initial foraminotomy or resection of posterior osteophytes when the burr is being used, because it acts as a protective layer to the neural elements. Once the bony removal is complete, the PLL can then be resected.[2]
- The medial half of the posterior uncinate is thinned under direct visualization with a high-speed burr to unroof the entry zone of the foramen (**TECH FIG 3**).
  - The microscope is angled appropriately to visualize the uncinate.

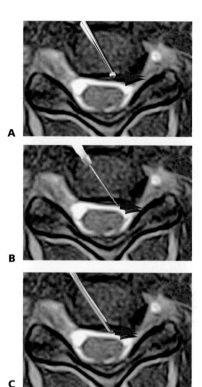

TECH FIG 3 • Anterior foraminotomy. **A.** The burr is used to thin down bone in the lateral aspect of the canal (*arrow*) until only a thin shell is left. The posterior longitudinal ligament (PLL) is left intact as a protective layer to the neural elements until burring is completed. **B.** A curette is used to outline the bony edges and ensure that they are thin enough for passage of a curette or Kerrison rongeur. The PLL does not necessarily need to be resected during foraminotomy if the pathology is due solely to uncinate bone spurs, although we routinely do so and do not consider the decompression complete until the lateral edge of the dura and the exiting root are clearly visualized and palpated to be free of compression. **C.** A 2-mm Kerrison is then used to remove bone spurs. It is critical to hug the posterior margin of the uncinate during this move to avoid injuring the root underneath, which exits the canal ventrolaterally at about a 45-degree angle.

- In general, it is easier to decompress the contralateral rather than the ipsilateral foramen, although decompression of both is certainly possible. Thus, in cases of unilateral radiculopathy, we prefer to approach the spine from the side opposite to the patient's symptoms.
- It is important not to force a large instrument into a severely narrowed foramen if it does not fit easily. Instead, the surgeon should use the burr to thin the uncus until the instrument can easily be passed into the foramen.
- Constant irrigation is performed to prevent thermal injury and to clear away bone debris.
- If visualization is adequate, continued thinning of the osteophyte can progress until only a thin shell of bone is left.
- A microcurette or 2-mm Kerrison is then used to resect the thinned osteophytes.

- Alternating between microcurettes or a Kerrison and the burr, the foramen can be gently and progressively carved out laterally.
    - The nerve root exits the spinal canal at roughly a 45-degree angle, ventrolaterally. Thus, it is imperative to avoid blindly placing a burr, curette, or Kerrison deep to the uncinate to avoid root injury. Instead, one should closely hug the uncinate while entering and decompressing the foramen (see Fig 1).
- Foraminotomy is complete when a micro nerve hook or curette can easily be passed into the foramen anterior to the exiting root without resistance.[6]

When and How to Resect the PLL

- With soft disc herniations, a defect in the PLL is often present through which the nuclear material extrudes (**TECH FIG 4A,B**).
- By delicately probing with a microcurette, the extruded fragment can be fished out from behind the PLL.
    - If necessary, the defect in the PLL should be enlarged with a 2-mm Kerrison until a satisfactory portal is available to remove the herniation and ensure that all loose disc fragments have been removed.
- It is debatable whether the PLL needs to be resected in every case. In general, we prefer to do so, especially in cases of disc extrusion, and do not consider the decompression complete until the dural sac or exiting nerve root (depending on which is compressed based on preoperative imaging) is inspected for the absence of any further compression.
    - If, however, the compressive lesion is an uncinate spur, with no evidence of subligamentous disc extrusion, satisfactory decompression can be achieved by removing the spurs without necessarily removing the PLL.
- If there is no rent in the PLL, one can be created by teasing a microcurette between the longitudinal fibers of the PLL until the curette is posterior to the PLL (**TECH FIG 4C,D**).
- Once the plane is identified between the PLL and dura, the fibers of the PLL can be resected with a curette or Kerrison rongeur.
- Placing tension on the PLL with gentle distraction will facilitate its removal.

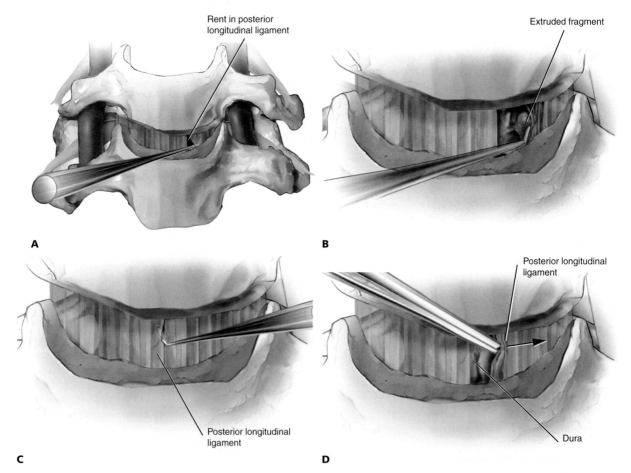

A

Rent in posterior longitudinal ligament

B

Extruded fragment

C

Posterior longitudinal ligament

D

Posterior longitudinal ligament

Dura

TECH FIG 4 A,B. • Removing herniated nucleus pulposus. **A.** With extruded herniations, a rent in the longitudinal fibers of the posterior longitudinal ligament (PLL) may be identified. A curette is then used to delineate the edges of the rent in the PLL. Once this is defined and the surgeon is certain of a plane between the PLL and underlying dura, a Kerrison is used to enlarge the edges of the rent. **B.** The rent has been enlarged to provide more room for finding the herniation. Curettes are then used to fish out the fragments and decompress the cord or root. **C,D.** Removing the PLL. **C.** If the PLL is intact, it can be removed by teasing in between the longitudinal fibers with a microcurette. Once a plane is established, a Kerrison can be used to remove the PLL. **D.** It is often easier to find this plane in the central portion of the PLL, where it is thicker, than laterally, where it is thinner and less defined.

- We generally find it easier to define a plane in the PLL centrally, where it tends to be thicker, than laterally, where it is thinner and the plane with the dura is less distinct. Often, there are multiple layers of PLL, and usually in chronic cases there is a membranous layer between the PLL and the dural sac that can be confused with dura itself. In general, if it does not look like dura, it probably is not.
- The portion of the PLL contralateral to the disc herniation or symptomatic foraminal stenosis does not routinely need to be removed.

Avoiding Vertebral Artery and Neural Injury

- Before surgery, the surgeon should always scrutinize the position of the vertebral arteries on the preoperative scans to rule out the presence of aberrancies in their course (**TECH FIG 5A,B,C**).
- Aberrations typically occur within the vertebral body. However, it is not uncommon for one vertebral artery to be closer to the uncinate on one side versus the other, which would mandate greater caution when approaching that side.[3]
- In the absence of vertebral artery aberrancy, laceration to the vertebral artery is most likely to occur from the surgeon's loss of orientation to the uncinates. The

uncinates define the safe zone for the vertebral artery and the effective zone for the decompression.
  - It is imperative to define and maintain orientation with both uncinates at all times during anterior cervical surgery.
- The vertebral artery is typically in the anterior two thirds of the disc space. When curetting disc material in this area, a vertebral artery laceration might occur if the curette strays lateral to the lateral border of the uncinate.
- If in doubt, a Penfield dissector can be used to identify the lateral border of the uncinate processes to avoid straying laterally and injuring the vertebral arteries, which are generally a few millimeters from the lateral edge of the uncinate (Tech Fig 5C).

Graft Sizing and Placement

- Ultimate graft height can be estimated preoperatively from the preoperative lateral film. In many cases, a graft height of 2 to 3 mm more than that measured on the preoperative lateral film will be the optimal choice.
- Ideally, the anteroposterior depth of the graft should be a few millimeters less than that of the disc space, such that the graft can be countersunk 2 mm without entering the spinal canal.
- The final height of the graft can be determined after endplate preparation with sizers that accompany commercial grafts (**TECH FIG 6**).
  - The trials should be lightly malleted into position under gentle Caspar pin distraction.
- A snug fit in the distracted position will ensure an excellent fit after removal of distraction pins.
- If the trial does not fit but the next smaller trial seems too loose, the surgeon should identify the area of impingement and lightly decorticate that area. Then, the trial is reinserted.

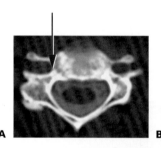 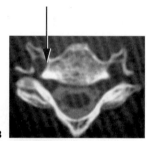

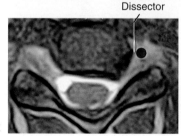

Dissector

TECH FIG 5 A,B. • Vertebral artery anomalies. **A.** The right transverse foramen (*arrow*) courses somewhat more medially than the one on the left. This is a subtle but potentially important anomaly to observe preoperatively. **B.** The anomaly occurs within the vertebral body rather than at the disc space level, where the right transverse foramen is now more normally positioned (*arrow*). **C.** Penfield lateral to the uncinate. In certain cases, especially if there is a deformity, the location of the lateral border of the uncinate (ie, the safe zone for the vertebral artery) may not be obvious after elevation of the longus colli. Placing a Penfield 4 dissector gently underneath the longus colli, retracting it laterally, and then hooking the dissector lateral to the uncinate will allow for safe orientation to the vertebral artery.

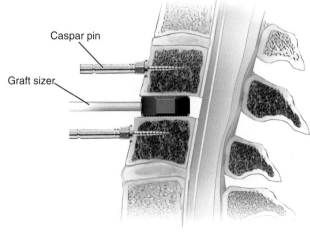

Caspar pin

Graft sizer

TECH FIG 6 • Commercially available sizers are used to determine optimal graft size. A trial that fits snugly under gentle Caspar distraction will suffice. If autograft is used, the appropriate trial is used as a template for cutting the autograft bone. The surgeon should try to place a graft that fills the space as much as possible without overdistracting, which can cause posterior neck pain, or entering the spinal canal.

- For multilevel ACDF, we prefer to decompress and graft each segment before proceeding to the next level.
- One way to enhance fusion rates is to place as much bone into the interspace as possible. A wide decompression also provides greater room for bone graft.
  - Space lateral to the structural bone graft in the uncinate regions can be packed with bone or bone graft substitutes. If the space is wide enough, two grafts can be placed side by side to fill the entire space.
- We generally prefer to use commercially prepared cortical allografts for ACDF, except in patients with poor healing potential. Alternatively, autograft iliac crest bone can be used.

Determining Plate Length

- Plating is optional for one-level ACDF with autograft. If allograft or multilevel surgery is performed, plating is recommended.
- Once the graft has been placed, the size of the plate is then determined.
- Optimal plate length is one that allows for the screws to be immediately adjacent to the endplates (**TECH FIG 7**).
  - This plate length allows for screws that angle away from the disc space, which in turn allows for screws that are longer than ones directed parallel to the disc space, yet are short enough to avoid entry into the supra- and infra-adjacent disc spaces.
  - This length also prevents impingement of the plate into the adjacent disc spaces.

Plating Techniques

- The plate should be contoured into lordosis to lie flush against the vertebral bodies.
  - It should also be centered coronally within the margins of the uncinate processes.
- Screws should also be angled medially to decrease the chance of lateral injury to nerve roots or vertebral arteries.
- The screw length can be estimated preoperatively by measuring the depth of the vertebral body on CT or MRI scans. The majority of levels will accommodate 14- to 16-mm screws.
- Dynamic plates can be used if desired (**TECH FIG 8**). They have the theoretical benefit of improving load sharing on the graft. There are several types of dynamic plates.
  - Variable screw systems allow for toggling within a fixed screw hole with settling of the construct. A potential downside is that the screw can loosen within bone as toggling occurs.
  - Slotted plates have holes that allow screws to translate longitudinally as the construct shortens. The screws are rigidly fixed to bone and do not toggle, but excessive translation may lead to adjacent-level plate impingement.
  - Telescoping plates use fixed screws in nonslotted holes, but the ends of the plate telescope with respect to each other as settling occurs. Postoperative adjacent-level plate impingement will not occur with this design if the plate is properly positioned at the time of surgery, as the distance from the end of the

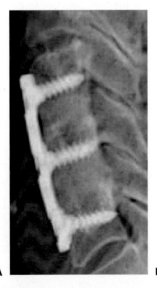
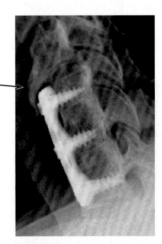

A   B

TECH FIG 7 • Proper plate sizing. **A.** The length of an optimally sized plate is such that the screw holes at the top and bottom of the construct are immediately adjacent to their respective endplates. In this example, even though this was done, the plate is still closer to the cephalad adjacent disc space than ideal because the vertebral bodies in this patient are relatively short. Nevertheless, adjacent-level disc degeneration did not occur in this patient at 2-year follow-up. Bicortical screw purchase is not routinely needed, but estimates of screw length can be obtained by measuring MRI or CT scans preoperatively. Screws should be angled away from the disc space to provide greater length and divergent fixation, which may better resist pullout. **B.** This patient also has short vertebrae. However, this plate was placed too close to the adjacent disc, resulting in adjacent-level ossification disease (*arrow*). The cephalad screws are not immediately adjacent to the endplate but rather inserted at roughly the midpoint of the vertebral body. Similarly, the caudal screws begin in the midportion of the vertebral body. The plate is too long distally and comes close to the subjacent disc as well. As demonstrated by these examples, proper plate sizing is especially important in patients with shorter vertebrae, where the adjacent discs are closer together.

Variable   Slotted   Telescoping

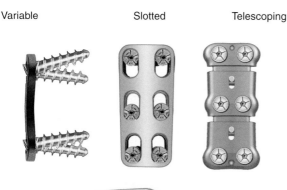

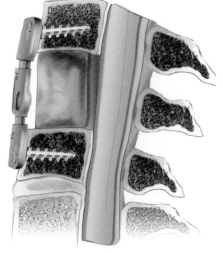

TECH FIG 8 • Dynamic plates generally fall into three categories: those with variable screws that fit into round holes that allow for toggling of the screws, those with slotted holes to allow for translation, and those in which the ends of the plate telescope or shorten. In contrast to the variable and slotted plates, with the telescoping plate design shown, the relationship between the ends of the plate and the adjacent disc spaces remains fixed as the plate dynamizes, because the plate shortens internally. Thus, progressive adjacent level disc impingement is less likely to occur with settling over time if it did not occur at the initial placement of the device.

plate to the endplate does not change with construct shortening. However, these plates tend to be somewhat thicker.

- If dynamic plates are used, the surgeon must perform the plating procedure to accommodate the anticipated settling without overlapping uninvolved adjacent discs.[8]

ANTERIOR CERVICAL DISCECTOMY AND FUSION WITHOUT INSTRUMENTATION

- ACDFs were traditionally performed without plating.
- Although plates may better preserve lordosis and achieve higher fusion rates in multilevel cases, avoiding plates may decrease operative time, decrease the amount of retraction on the soft tissue structures of the neck during surgery, and avoid plate-related complications such as screw backout or esophageal erosion.
- However, if one chooses not to use a plate, autograft should be used rather than allograft, and rigid postoperative immobilization in a cervical orthosis is mandatory.
- Up to three adjacent interbody cervical fusions can be safely performed without instrumentation.
  - The interspaces should be fused sequentially, meaning a decompression and fusion is completed at one interspace before the next is addressed.

Measuring the Space

- After appropriate decompression, the depth and height of the interspace are measured without distraction (**TECH FIG 9A,B**).

- A laminar spreader is then inserted to distract the interspace, and the height is again measured (**TECH FIG 9C,D**).
- Without distraction, the height is generally 6 mm; with distraction, it can be to up to 12 mm.
- This distraction is important in shaping the tricortical graft. The height of the graft should be greater than the resting height but less than the distracting height so that the inherent compression of the vertebral bodies will hold the graft firmly in place.

Inserting the Graft

- After the appropriate size of cortical graft is obtained, it is inserted with the laminar spreader distracted (**TECH FIG 10A,B**).
- The graft should have at least a 2-mm offset anteriorly, and the posterior edge of the graft should be 4 mm anterior to the dura and PLL.
- After the distraction is released (Tech Fig 10C,D), the graft should be tested for stability by trying to dislodge it using a smooth right-angle probe.
- Postoperatively, if the graft is stable, a simple soft collar should be used for 4 to 6 weeks.

TECHNIQUES

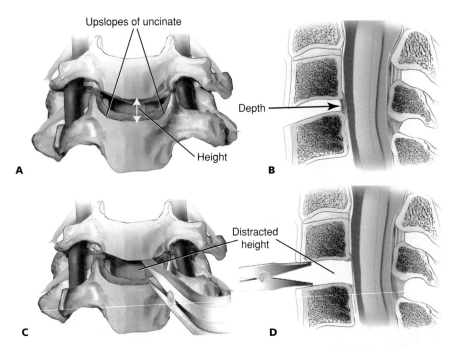

TECH FIG 9 • Measuring the interspace without (**A,B**) and with (**C,D**) distraction.

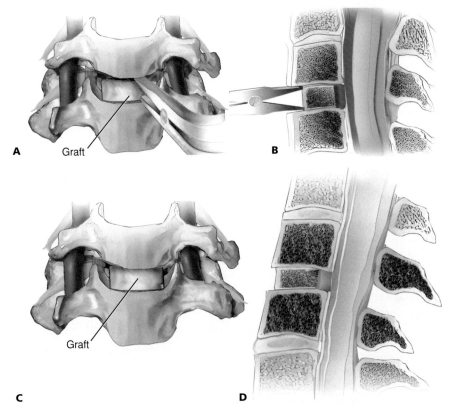

TECH FIG 10 • The cortical graft in place with (**A,B**) and without (**C,D**) distraction. Without distraction, the graft is compressed by the natural elasticity of the cervical spine. There is about 2 to 6 mm of free space between the posterior surface of the graft and the spinal cord.

PEARLS AND PITFALLS

Discectomy	▪ Removing the anterior portion of the inferior endplate allows for better visualization of the posterior disc space, particularly in narrow spondylotic discs, and facilitates subsequent decompression.
Endplate preparation	▪ The surgeon should create a rectangular space with parallel endplates. This will generally require greater preparation of the inferior endplate of the cephalad vertebrae. Excessive bone removal should be avoided to prevent excessive graft settling.
Foraminotomy	▪ The uncinate is the guide to the foramen. The surgeon should maintain orientation to it at all times. When entering the foramen to remove bone spurs, the curette or Kerrison should hug the posterior aspect of the uncinate to avoid the nerve root, which exits ventrally at a 45-degree angle. The uncinate should be thinned first with a burr so that a small instrument can be inserted into the foramen to complete the foraminotomy without injuring the underlying root.
Plate fixation	▪ The surgeon should choose the shortest plate that will fit, such that the screw holes are immediately adjacent to the endplates, to avoid adjacent-level plate or screw impingement.
Multiple fusions in ACDF without instrumentation	▪ In cases of multiple fusions, each decompression and fusion must be completed before the next interspace is addressed. If all the interspaces to be fused are decompressed before the first graft is inserted, it will lead to unbalanced grafts, with one bone plug being significantly wider than the others because of the inherent elasticity of the vertebral bodies.

POSTOPERATIVE CARE

▪ The utility of bracing after plated ACDF is debatable.
▪ We typically place the patient in a cervical collar for 6 weeks.
▪ A deep drain is placed in the retropharyngeal space to prevent hematoma formation. It is typically removed the morning after surgery unless its output is greater than 30 cc in the last 8 hours.
▪ The postoperative diet may be rapidly advanced as tolerated. Cold beverages and ice cream may help with dysphagia and reduce swelling in the immediate perioperative period.

OUTCOMES

▪ Over 90% of patients experience excellent relief of radicular symptoms with ACDF.
▪ Midline axial neck pain may improve if it is associated with radicular pain, but patients should be counseled that the primary goal of treatment is neural decompression and relief of radicular or myelopathic symptoms.
   ▪ Similarly, unilateral neck pain can be a manifestation of radiculopathy and also generally improves.
   ▪ However, isolated axial neck pain without radicular complaints does not predictably improve with surgery, and we recommend nonoperative treatment in such patients.

COMPLICATIONS

▪ Complications potentially associated with ACDF include dysphagia, dysphonia, pseudarthrosis, implant failure, neurologic injury, esophageal injury, airway compromise from swelling or hematoma, and vertebral artery injury.[1]
▪ Some degree of dysphagia is almost universal immediately after surgery. The majority of patients with dysphagia have only mild symptoms, with clinical improvement within 3 weeks. Long-term significant dysphagia is not common (about 4%).
▪ The superior laryngeal nerve innervates the cricothyroid muscle, which adjusts the tension on the vocal folds and also provides supraglottic sensation. Superior laryngeal nerve palsies therefore may lead to difficulty with singing high notes as well as aspiration.
▪ The recurrent laryngeal nerve innervates the muscles responsible for abducting the vocal folds. Recurrent laryngeal nerve palsy most commonly presents as hoarseness. Bilateral injuries can lead to airway obstruction and require tracheostomy.
▪ Even with modern surgical techniques, nonunions still occur. However, many cervical nonunions are asymptomatic and do not require further treatment. Symptomatic nonunions can be addressed with revision ACDF or posterior laminoforaminotomy and fusion.
▪ It is often argued that fusion accelerates adjacent-segment degeneration. Although biomechanical studies show increased disc pressures and mobility at discs adjacent to fusions, clinical series have not confirmed that adjacent-segment degeneration is truly accelerated by fusion versus simply being a manifestation of the patient's propensity toward spondylosis. In fact, the available evidence suggests that about 3% of patients will have symptomatic adjacent-segment disease regardless of whether the index operation was ACDF, ACD without fusion, or posterior foraminotomy without fusion.[7]

REFERENCES

1. Bazaz R, Lee MJ, Yoo JU. Incidence of dysphagia after anterior cervical spine surgery: a prospective study. Spine 2002;27:2453–2458.
2. Brigham CD, Tsahakis PJ. Anterior cervical foraminotomy and fusion: surgical technique and results. Spine 1995;20:766–770.
3. Curylo LJ, Mason HC, Bohlman HH, et al. Tortuous course of the vertebral artery and anterior cervical decompression: a cadaveric and clinical case study. Spine 2000;25:2860–2864.
4. Ebraheim NA, Lu J, Haman SP, et al. Anatomic basis of the anterior surgery on the cervical spine: relationships between uncus-artery-root complex and vertebral artery injury. Surg Radiol Anat 1998;20:389–392.
5. Emery SE, Bolesta MJ, Banks MA, et al. Robinson anterior cervical fusion: comparison of the standard and modified techniques. Spine 1994;19:660–663.
6. Henderson CM, Hennessy RG, Shuey HM Jr, et al. Posterior-lateral foraminotomy as an exclusive operative technique for cervical radiculopathy: a review of 846 consecutively operated cases. Neurosurgery 1983;13:504–512.
7. Hilibrand AS, Carlson GD, Palumbo MA, et al. Radiculopathy and myelopathy at segments adjacent to the site of a previous anterior cervical arthrodesis. J Bone Joint Surg Am 1999;81A:519–528.
8. Park JB, Cho YS, Riew KD. Development of adjacent-level ossification in patients with an anterior cervical plate. J Bone Joint Surg Am 2005;87A:558–563.
9. Radhakrishan K, Litchy WJ, O'Falon WM, et al. Epidemiology of cervical radiculopathy: a population-based study from Rochester, Minnesota, 1976 through 1990. Brain 1994;117:325–335.
10. Sampath P, Bendebba M, Davis JD, et al. Outcome in patients with cervical radiculopathy: prospective, multicenter study with independent clinical review. Spine 1999;24:591–597.
11. Smith GW, Robinson RA. The treatment of certain cervical spine disorders by anterior removal of the intervertebral disc and interbody fusion. J Bone Joint Surg Am 1958;40A:607–624.

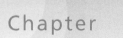

Chapter 2

Anterior Cervical Corpectomy and Fusion With Instrumentation

Claude Jarrett and John M. Rhee

DEFINITION

- Cervical myelopathy describes a constellation of signs and symptoms resulting from cervical spinal cord compression. Common symptoms include gait instability, clumsiness and loss of manual dexterity, and glovelike (rather than dermatomal) numbness of the hands.
- Because the presentation of myelopathy can be subtle, especially in its early manifestation, the diagnosis can be missed or wrongly attributed to "aging."
- Surgical decompression is the mainstay of treatment and can be accomplished anteriorly (ie, corpectomy, discectomy and fusion, or both) or posteriorly (ie, laminectomy and fusion or laminoplasty).
- Anterior corpectomy and fusion will be discussed in this chapter. Corpectomy is performed when retrovertebral compression of the spinal cord exists. If the compression is purely disc-based, corpectomy is not necessary, and an anterior cervical discectomy and fusion approach can be used instead.

PATHOGENESIS

- Spondylotic changes (eg, bone spurs, disc degeneration with annular bulging, disc herniations) are the most common causes of cervical cord compression.
- Ossification of the posterior longitudinal ligament (OPLL) is another not uncommon cause of cord compression. It may arise in discrete locations or be continuous (**FIG 1A,B**).[4]
- Kyphosis, whether primary or occurring after laminectomy, can also cause cord compression and myelopathy.
- Cervical myelopathy often arises in the setting of a congenitally narrowed cervical canal (**FIG 1C,D**). In these patients, the cord may have escaped compression during relative youth but not after the accumulation of a threshold amount of space-occupying spondylotic changes.
  - Although cervical spondylotic myelopathy tends to be a disorder seen in patients 50 years of age or older, depending on the degree of congenital stenosis and the magnitude of the accumulated spondylotic changes, it can be seen in patients who are much younger.

NATURAL HISTORY

- Patients with cervical myelopathy are generally thought to have a poor prognosis without surgical treatment, with a gradual stepwise progression of symptoms.[1]

HISTORY AND PHYSICAL FINDINGS

- Patients with cervical myelopathy present with a spectrum of upper and lower extremity complaints.
  - Upper extremity complaints include a generalized feeling of clumsiness of the arms and hands, "dropping things," inability to manipulate fine objects such as coins or buttons, trouble with handwriting, and diffuse (nondermatomal) numbness.
  - Lower extremity complaints include gait instability, a sense of imbalance when walking, and "bumping into walls" when walking. Family members may comment that the patient walks as if he or she is intoxicated.
- Patients with severe spinal cord compression may also complain of Lhermitte symptoms: electric shock-like sensations that radiate down the spine or into the extremities with certain offending positions of the neck (can occur with either flexion or extension).
- Many myelopathic patients deny any loss of motor strength. Similarly, bowel and bladder symptoms, if present, may arise in the later stages of disease. Despite advanced degrees of spondylosis, many myelopathic patients may have no neck pain.
- Symptomatic nerve root compression can coexist in patients with myelopathy and presents as a myeloradiculopathy.
- Physical examination should include:
  - Scapulohumeral reflex testing, which is positive with hyperactive elevation of the scapula or abduction of humerus
  - Jaw jerk reflex, which is positive with hyperactive jerking of the jaw. Because cervical cord compression alone will not cause this reflex to be positive, its presence suggests that the origin of upper motor neuron findings in a given patient may arise from the brain rather than the spinal cord.
  - Test for the Babinski sign, which is positive if the great toe extends while the remaining toes fan apart.
  - Test for the Hoffman sign, which is positive with flexion of the index finger and thumb.
  - Inverted radial reflex test, which is positive if one observes flexion of fingers rather than a reflex contraction of the brachioradialis. Positive result suggests cord and root compression at the C5–6 level.
  - Test for finger escape sign, which is positive if the little finger (also possibly the ring finger) cannot be held in this position without falling into abduction and flexion for more than 30 seconds. This is suggestive of cervical myelopathy.
  - Tandem gait test, which is positive if the patient demonstrates significant instability. A positive result confirms gait imbalance, but in no way specifies the source of the imbalance as being the cervical spinal cord.

IMAGING AND OTHER DIAGNOSTIC STUDIES

- A lateral radiographic view can be helpful in showing the amount of congenital cervical stenosis as well as sagittal alignment.
- Lateral views are consistent with congenital stenosis when the ratio of the diameter of the canal to the diameter of the vertebral body is less than 0.8.
- Particularly if OPLL is suspected, CT scans (with or without myelograms, depending on whether a high-quality MRI is available) are helpful in delineating bony versus soft tissue pathology.

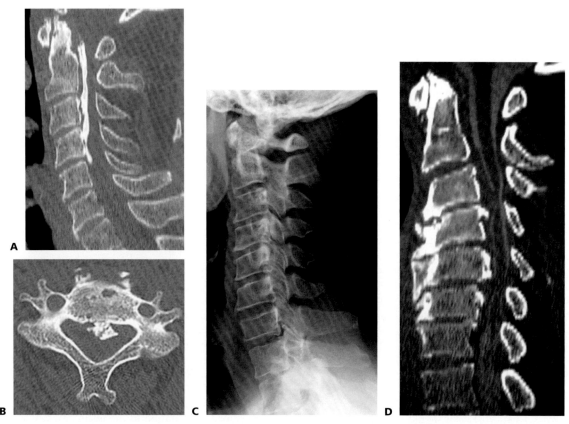

FIG 1 A,B. • Ossification of the posterior longitudinal ligament (OPLL). **A.** Continuous OPLL causing severe spinal canal stenosis from C1 to C4. **B.** Axial CT scan in a different patient demonstrating a central stalk of OPLL. **C,D.** Congenital canal. Congenital stenosis is defined as a ratio of the canal to the vertebral body of 0.8 or less, and it can be measured on lateral radiographs (**C**) or advanced imaging such as CT-myelography (**D**) (different patients). The CT-myelogram shows superimposed spondylotic changes that further narrow the canal dimensions and cause cord compression.

DIFFERENTIAL DIAGNOSIS

■ Of cervical myelopathy:
  ■ Amyotrophic lateral sclerosis
  ■ Myopathies
  ■ Peripheral neuropathy
  ■ Syringomyelia
  ■ Multiple sclerosis
  ■ Diabetic neuropathy
  ■ Brachial plexopathy

NONOPERATIVE MANAGEMENT

■ Surgery is the treatment of choice for symptomatic cervical myelopathy.

■ Nonoperative treatment of cervical myelopathy is reserved for patients who cannot tolerate surgery.

■ Controversy exists regarding the management of patients with asymptomatic spinal cord compression. In those with severe asymptomatic compression, consideration should be given to prophylactic surgery, particularly if cord signal changes are present, to prevent spinal cord injury with trauma (eg, central cord syndrome) (**FIG 2**).

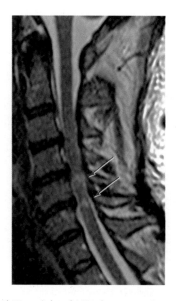

FIG 2 • Sagittal T2-weighted MRI demonstrating spinal cord signal changes.

SURGICAL MANAGEMENT

- The most common surgical options include anterior decompression and fusion (discectomy versus corpectomy, depending on the absence or presence of retrovertebral cord compression, respectively), laminoplasty, and laminectomy with fusion.
- In general, anterior surgery is preferred when cord compression arises from three or fewer disc segments, as the incidence of fusion and graft complications increases exponentially with greater number of segments fused. The presence of kyphosis or significant spondylotic neck pain also favors an anterior approach.
- Conversely, posterior approaches such as laminoplasty are favored when myelopathy arises from three or more motion segments and the cervical alignment is neutral or lordotic, particularly if the patient has minimal to no neck pain.
    - For posterior surgery to adequately decompress the cord, however, enough lordosis must be present to allow cord driftback after removal of the posterior tethers (lamina, flavum).
- Combined anterior and posterior surgery should be considered in cases of severe or postlaminectomy kyphosis.
- Multilevel corpectomy as a stand-alone operation is not recommended in patients with significant postlaminectomy kyphosis, as this creates a highly unstable construct that is prone to failure.

Preoperative Planning

- Preoperative CT and MRI scans should be scrutinized to analyze the course of the vertebral arteries and the width of the spinal canal requiring decompression.

- CT scans may provide additional information to MRI scans when it is unclear whether the compressive lesions are bony (OPLL, osteophytes) or soft disc material.

Positioning

- For anterior cervical corpectomy and fusion, patients are positioned as described in Chapter SP-1.
- However, greater caution is necessary in positioning the myelopathic versus radiculopathic patient. In particular, one must ensure that the patient is not excessively extended beyond the tolerance of the compressed cord. The amount of extension tolerated preoperatively should be assessed and not exceeded intraoperatively.
- Gardner-Wells tongs may be used for multilevel corpectomy but are not generally needed for one-level corpectomy.
- Weight, typically 30 to 40 lb, can be added to the tongs after decompression to allow for distraction during graft insertion. Significant distraction on the spine should be avoided until after the cord has been decompressed.

Approach

- The approach is similar to that for anterior cervical discectomy and fusion but generally needs to be more extensile to access multiple levels.
- The surgeon should ensure that wide exposure beyond the medial border of the uncinates is achieved, with appropriate elevation of the longus colli muscles bilaterally, to achieve a stable base for the self-retaining retractors as well as to provide orientation to the uncinates, which remain the critical landmarks for either corpectomy or discectomy surgery.

EVALUATING THE LIMITS FOR THE CORPECTOMY

- The corpectomy is performed after the initial discectomies above and below the vertebra to be resected. The discectomies are performed from uncinate to uncinate as detailed in Chapter SP-11.

- The width of the corpectomy required to decompress the cord should be based on preoperative imaging studies (TECH FIG 1).

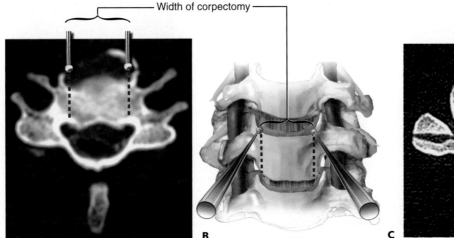
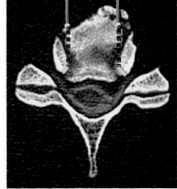

TECH FIG 1 • Limits of corpectomy. **A.** The width of the corpectomy is based on that necessary to decompress the spinal cord and can be estimated on preoperative imaging. **B.** In general, a corpectomy spanning from the medial border of one uncinate to the other will be sufficient at the vertebral body level. **C.** At the level of the disc space, a wider decompression may be necessary for satisfactory root decompression (*yellow lines*).

- Generally, sufficient decompression will occur if the width of the decompression spans from uncinate to uncinate.
- Wider decompressions beyond the medial border to the uncinates are typically performed at the disc level, where a combination of cord and root compression may occur, but are not necessary at the vertebral body level, where only the spinal cord is compressed.

- Staying within the uncinates will allow for thorough decompression while avoiding vertebral artery injury, unless a vertebral artery anomaly exists. Such anomalies are more likely to occur within the vertebral body rather than the disc spaces, and they should be recognized on preoperative imaging to avoid injury.

CERVICAL CORPECTOMY

- The edges of the corpectomy are longitudinally delineated with a high-speed burr from uncinate to uncinate to define the safe limits of the decompression.
- Next, a Leksell rongeur can be used to quickly remove large fragments of vertebral body bone (**TECH FIG 2**). This bone should be saved for grafting.
- Once the cancellous bone is removed grossly, fine decompression then proceeds with a high-speed burr.
- Under direct visualization, a high-speed burr is used to remove bone until a thin shell of posterior cortex remains.
- Microcurettes and Kerrisons are then used to flake off the remaining bone.
- Attention should be paid to maintaining the width of the corpectomy as it proceeds posteriorly toward the

canal, as the tendency is to cone the decompression narrowly as one proceeds posteriorly.
- Vertebral body bleeding often hinders visualization during bone removal.
  - The surgeon should take time to achieve hemostasis using bone wax (gently applied when the remaining vertebra is still thick) or powdered Gelfoam–thrombin (when the remnant vertebral body is very thin).
  - Significant dorsal pressure should be avoided during these maneuvers to avoid inadvertently plunging into the spinal canal.
- Epidural bleeding is best controlled with bipolar cautery as well as Gelfoam–thrombin.

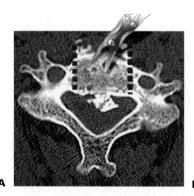 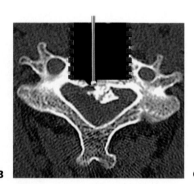 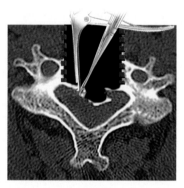

A   B   C

TECH FIG 2 • Steps in bone removal. **A.** Leksell rongeur is used to remove large pieces of vertebral body bone after delineating the lateral edges of the corpectomy longitudinally along the medial border of the uncinates with a high-speed burr. **B.** After removing the bulk of the vertebra, a burr is used to sequentially remove bone in layers until only a thin remnant of bone remains. **C.** Finally, curettes and Kerrison rongeurs are used to remove the remaining bone. Adequate thinning of all bone to be removed allows the passage of smaller instruments that do not exert pressure on the spinal cord.

REMOVING THE POSTERIOR LONGITUDINAL LIGAMENT

- If cord compression arises strictly from bony osteophytes or congenital narrowing of the spinal canal, the PLL does not necessarily need to be resected. In general, we favor removing the PLL to confirm adequate decompression.
- If, however, there is an extruded or sequestered herniated disc behind the vertebral body, or if OPLL is the cause of compression, the PLL should be resected.
- When resecting the PLL, a small curette is used to probe in between longitudinal fibers of the PLL until it can be passed dorsal to it. Once a plane is created, larger curettes or 2- or 3-mm Kerrisons can be used to complete the resection of the PLL (**TECH FIG 3**).

- If severe OPLL is present, the dura may be deficient or absent, and the surgeon should be prepared to perform a dural patch and possibly a subarachnoid lumbar drain.
  - The presence of severe OPLL may favor a posterior approach, all other factors being equal, to avoid complications related to dural deficiencies.
- In severe OPLL, instead of removing the entire OPLL, an alternative technique is to allow it to float anteriorly by releasing its tethers at nonossified portions, then allowing the ossified portion to float anteriorly along with the underlying adherent dura. However, one downside to this approach can be the potential for regrowth of the OPLL.[7]

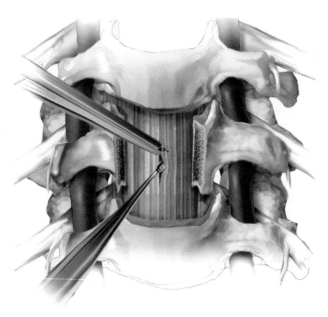

TECH FIG 3 • A curette is used to tease apart the longitudinal fibers and create a plane dorsal to the posterior longitudinal ligament (PLL). Once this plane is identified, a curette or pituitary rongeur is used to elevate the PLL while a small Kerrison removes it. The surgeon must be careful never to exert compression on the cord by passing large instruments.

GRAFTING OPTIONS

- Autograft, allograft, or cages can be used.
- Autograft options include structural iliac crest or autologous fibula. Both are excellent graft materials but can be associated with significant donor site morbidity. Because of its shape, iliac crest is generally suitable for one- or sometimes two-segment corpectomy reconstruction. Fibula is favored for two-segment or more corpectomy reconstruction.[6]
- Because of donor site morbidity issues, allograft fibula or cages filled with local autograft remain popular choices for corpectomy reconstruction.
- Local corpectomy bone can be used to provide the biologic stimulus for healing, allowing the allograft to serve both structural and osteoconductive roles. Local bone is packed in and around the allograft (**TECH FIG 4**).

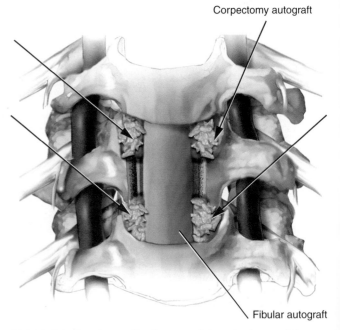

Corpectomy autograft

Fibular autograft

TECH FIG 4 • Local morselized autograft is packed around the strut graft and into the cleared-out uncinate regions. An additional benefit of wide discectomy is the ability to fuse the uncinate regions.

ENDPLATE PREPARATION

- The endplates above and below the corpectomy should be thoroughly decorticated and denuded of all cartilaginous material.
  - To prevent excessive subsidence, we prefer not to remove as much endplate when performing corpectomy reconstruction as is done when performing anterior cervical discectomy and fusion.

- Nevertheless, it is helpful to remove the anterior lip on the caudal surface of the cephalad vertebra to allow for better contact of the graft to the endplate. The anterior lip is flattened to be level with the central concavity of the endplate (**TECH FIG 5A**).
- The structural integrity of the endplate is maintained in the central third to allow a stable loading surface for the

graft. Preserving the curvature on the posterior third of the endplate protects the graft from kicking posteriorly into the canal.

- If the posterior lip needs to be removed to decompress the cord, it can be done along the floor of the canal with a Kerrison after the corpectomy is completed.

- Kickout is most likely to occur at the caudal end of the construct, where the compressive loads on the graft are translated into a shear force due to the relative lordosis of the caudal vertebra. To prevent kickout, the caudal endplate should be prepared parallel to the floor, such that the shear vector is minimized. The tradeoff is that doing so will result in a greater likelihood of subsidence (**TECH FIG 5B,C**).

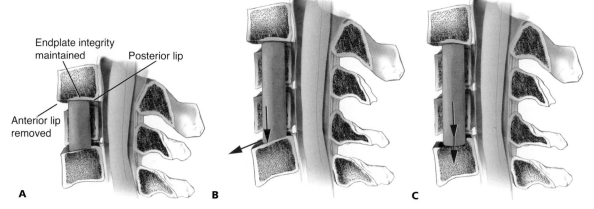

TECH FIG 5 • A. Carpentry of the inferior endplate of the cephalad level: preparing the inferior endplate of the cephalad segment (eg, the inferior endplate of C5 during a C6 corpectomy). Flattening the anterior lip and the anterior third of the endplate allows for proper insertion of a strut graft. They are flattened to be level with the central concavity of the endplate. The central third of the endplate is left as structurally sound as possible to resist excessive subsidence. The posterior third may be left intact to act as a barrier to posterior migration of the graft into the canal. The posterior lip, which is often a source of spondylotic compression, can be removed with a Kerrison after the corpectomy is completed to decompress the floor of the spinal canal. **B,C.** Carpentry of the superior endplate of the distal level. **B.** When performing corpectomy reconstructions in which the distal level is lordotic, if the superior endplate of that vertebra is not level with the ground, the graft is likely to kick out anteriorly as the compressive loads on the graft are converted into shear at the graft–endplate interface. **C.** The solution is to flatten the superior endplate of the caudal vertebra. The graft is now less likely to kick out, but the tradeoff is that it is more likely to piston.

GRAFT SIZING

- If a total corpectomy is performed, care is taken to find a graft that will fill most of the depth of the vertebral body but will still be small enough to stay well clear of the decompressed cord when recessed by 2 to 3 mm from the front of the vertebral body.

- A reasonable amount of distraction should be performed after the decompression. This can be done by the application of weights to cervical tongs or, in one- or some two-level situations, by Caspar pin distraction (the Caspar spreader is usually not long enough to span multilevel corpectomies).

- Care should be taken not to distract the spine until all compressive lesions on the cord have been removed, to avoid tenting the cord over the compressive lesions.

- In general, the amount of distraction should result in overall vertebral column length that is slightly longer than it was preoperatively. Excessive distraction is more likely to result in subsequent graft pistoning and subsidence, as the spine naturally recoils to its initial state once the patient is upright.

- The wooden end of a cotton applicator can be whittled away until it just fits into the corpectomy. This can be used as a template for cutting the graft to appropriate length (**TECH FIG 6**).

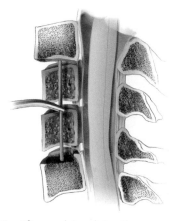

TECH FIG 6 • After applying distraction, a wooden applicator (Q-tip) serves as a useful device for measuring the length of the graft.

TECHNIQUES

GRAFT INSERTION

- The graft is gently tamped into the distracted corpectomy site (**TECH FIG 7**).
- Distraction is then released, and the stability of the graft is tested by gently pulling on the graft with a clamp.
- Because bony union is desired not only at the ends of the graft but also side to side between the shaft of the strut graft and the remaining vertebral bodies, intimate contact of graft to host is desirable in all regions. Any open spaces can be grafted with the local bone from the corpectomy.
- If autograft is scarce, it is best to save it for the ends of the allograft strut and fill the middle portion of the marrow cavity with a bone graft substitute.
- The uncinate regions at each disc level are a good surface for fusion and can be grafted with local bone. The residual disc spaces lateral to the medial border of the uncinates can be packed with local bone to facilitate fusion.

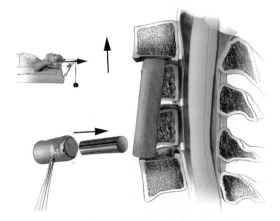

TECH FIG 7 • The graft is inserted under either tong traction or Caspar pin distraction. The superior end of the graft is inserted first, and then the inferior end is gently tamped into position.

ANTERIOR CERVICAL PLATING

- Plating is performed as noted during anterior cervical discectomy and fusion.
- Standalone plated multilevel corpectomies (three or more disc levels) have been reported to be associated with high failure rates. Consideration should be given in such cases to supplemental posterior fixation.[5]

PEARLS AND PITFALLS

Limits of corpectomy	■ The uncinates should be used as boundaries to prevent injury to the vertebral arteries while achieving wide enough cord decompression.
Carpentry of the caudal endplate of the cephalad vertebra	■ The endplates should be thoroughly decorticated but preserved in the area of contact with the graft to avoid excessive subsidence.
Carpentry of the cephalad endplate of the caudal vertebra	■ If the inferior end of the construct is at a lordotic segment, the endplate should be flattened such that the graft will sit parallel to the ground. Doing so will help avoid kickout.

POSTOPERATIVE CARE

■ If retraction time on the soft tissues of the neck has been more than 3 hours, a cuff-leak test should be considered before extubation to rule out the presence of edema that may lead to airway obstruction upon extubation.

■ This is performed by deflating the endotracheal tube while obstructing the lumen of the tube, and then determining if there is a leak around the deflated tube. If there is no leak, consideration should be given to keeping the patient intubated with the head elevated until a leak is detected. Steroids can also be given to decrease airway edema.

■ The head of the bed should be elevated above 45 degrees in all patients postoperatively to diminish edema.

■ Most patients are placed in a rigid cervical orthosis for 6 weeks.

■ If a drain is placed, it should be followed closely and removed once the output is below an acceptable limit (ie, 30 cc per shift), typically on postoperative day 1.

OUTCOMES

■ Although the primary goal of surgery in myelopathy is to prevent progression, most patients actually note neurologic improvement after successful corpectomy and fusion.[2]

COMPLICATIONS

■ Complications encountered during the anterior approach to the cervical spine are similar to those discussed in Chapter 11. The incidence of airway obstruction may be higher due to soft tissue edema from longer surgical retraction times.

■ Neurologic injury is rare (1% to 2%).

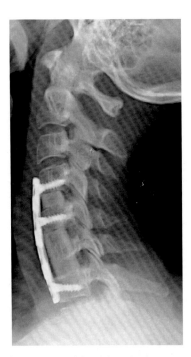

FIG 3 • Hybrid constructs. This patient had retrovertebral cord compression behind C6 and disc-based compression at C4–5. Rather than doing a two-level corpectomy of both C4 and C5, a discectomy–corpectomy construct allows for a shorter strut graft and intermediate points of screw fixation into C5.

■ Most complications associated with cervical corpectomies are related to graft and plate problems.[3]

■ Dislodgement and pistoning of the graft into the adjacent vertebral bodies with loss of lordosis are potential postoperative complications.[8]

   ■ The risk increases as the number of levels corpectomized and the length of the strut graft increases. The rate of graft dislodgement ranged from 7% to 50% despite plating in one early series of multilevel corpectomy.

   ■ To avoid such complications, hybrid corpectomy constructs can be used instead if the pattern of neural compression allows.

   ■ Hybrid constructs combine corpectomies at levels with retrovertebral compression along with discectomies at levels

demonstrating compression only at the level of the disc space (**FIG 3**).

   ■ For a three-disc–level problem, a single-level corpectomy can be combined with a single-level anterior cervical discectomy and fusion.

   ■ For a four-disc–level problem, two single-level corpectomies can be performed with an intervening intact vertebra, or a single-level corpectomy with two single-level anterior cervical discectomies and fusions.

■ Hybrid constructs avoid the negative biomechanical issues associated with long strut grafts and provide more points of segmental screw fixation, leading to constructs that are more stable and less likely to fail.

■ If a posterior approach can be used instead in the patient with multilevel myelopathy, we prefer to do so. Ideal candidates for posterior surgery such as laminoplasty are those with multilevel cervical myelopathy, preserved lordosis, and little to no spondylotic neck pain. In patients like these, fusion and its attendant complications can be avoided altogether with laminoplasty.

■ Exacerbation of axial neck pain can occur after laminoplasty in those who have significant complaints preoperatively, although it rarely becomes of significance in those who have little to no axial pain preoperatively. Also, adequate decompression may not occur after laminoplasty in those with kyphosis, as cord driftback away from anterior compressive lesions is unreliable in this setting.

REFERENCES

1. Clarke E, Robinson PK. Cervical myelopathy: a complication of cervical spondylosis. Brain 1956;79:483–510.
2. Ikenaga M, Shikata J, Tanaka C. Long-term results over 10 years of anterior corpectomy and fusion for multilevel cervical myelopathy. Spine 2006;31:1568–1574.
3. Riew KD, Sethi NS, Devney J, et al. Complications of buttress plate stabilization of cervical corpectomy. Spine 1999;24:2404–2410.
4. Tsuyama N. Ossification of the posterior longitudinal ligament of the spine. Clin Orthop Relat Res 1984;184:71–84.
5. Vaccaro AR, Falatyn SP, Scuderi GJ, et al. Early failure of long segment anterior cervical plate fixation. J Spinal Disord 1998;11:410–415.
6. Whitecloud TS, LaRocca H. Fibular strut graft in reconstructive surgery of the cervical spine. Spine 1976;1:33–43.
7. Yamaura I, Kurosa Y, Matuoka T, et al. Anterior floating method for cervical myelopathy caused by ossification of the posterior longitudinal ligament. Clin Orthop Relat Res 1999;359:27–34.
8. Yonenobu K, Hosono N, Iwasaki M, et al. Laminoplasty versus subtotal corpectomy: a comparative study of results in multisegmental cervical spondylotic myelopathy. Spine 1992;17:1281–1284.

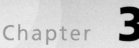

Chapter 3

Posterior Cervical Foraminotomy

Jacob M. Buchowski, Ronald A. Lehman, Jr., and K. Daniel Riew

DEFINITION

■ Cervical radiculopathy is a clinical diagnosis defined by the presence of motor or sensory changes or complaints in a specific dermatomal distribution.

ANATOMY

■ Cervical radiculopathy is largely due to mechanical compression of the exiting cervical nerve roots.
■ The intervertebral foramen is bounded by the following structures (**FIG 1**):
  ■ The disc and uncovertebral joint ventrally
  ■ The borders of the pedicles cranially and caudally
  ■ The superior articular facet of the caudal segment (eg, the superior articular facet of C6 at the C5-6 foramen) dorsally
■ In the subaxial cervical spine, the foramen averages 9 to 12 mm in height and 4 to 6 mm in width, and in a young person, the cervical nerve root occupies approximately one third of the available space in the foramen.
■ With increasing age, degenerative changes (osteophyte formation), disc protrusion, or cervical instability, this proportion may increase and signs of radiculopathy may develop.

PATHOGENESIS

■ Any process that causes impingement of the exiting cervical nerve roots can lead to cervical radiculopathy.
■ Potential etiologies of cervical radiculopathy include cervical spondylosis leading to foraminal stenosis due to uncinate or facet hypertrophy, disc herniation, instability, and anterolisthesis or retrolisthesis.

NATURAL HISTORY

■ The natural history of cervical radiculopathy is not well studied, but about half of the adult population will have neck and radicular symptoms at some point during their lifetime.
■ In patients treated nonoperatively, up to 66% will have persistent symptoms and up to 23% of patients with persistent neck or radicular pain will be unable to return to their original occupation.

PATIENT HISTORY AND PHYSICAL FINDINGS

■ When a patient presents with radiculopathy, a complete history and physical examination is of paramount importance.
■ Questions about the duration of the symptoms, location and nature of the pain, distribution of altered sensation and numbness (axial or radicular), presence of weakness, and any associated manifestations must be asked to understand the underlying pathology and target the offending level of cervical pathology.

■ Since radiculopathy can be associated with myelopathy, the presence or absence of balance difficulties, loss of bowel or bladder control, presence of constitutional symptoms, trauma, signs of dysdiadochokinesia, or change in neurologic status must be elucidated.
■ The physical examination should include motor and sensory evaluation (both gross and pinprick), reflex testing, upper and lower motor neuron signs, and cerebellar functional testing.

IMAGING AND OTHER DIAGNOSTIC STUDIES

■ Plain radiographs of the cervical spine, including anteroposterior (AP), lateral, odontoid, oblique, and lateral flexion/extension views, are used initially to evaluate for the presence of cervical pathology.
■ If symptoms have been present for at least 6 weeks, additional imaging is indicated and usually includes cervical spine MRI.
■ If MRI is contraindicated, a cervical CT myelogram may be beneficial.
■ A CT scan with coronal and sagittal reconstructions may be helpful in operative planning.

DIFFERENTIAL DIAGNOSIS

■ Cervical radiculopathy
■ Myelopathy
■ Myeloradiculopathy
■ Entrapment syndromes (eg, pronator syndrome, carpal tunnel syndrome, cubital tunnel syndrome)
■ Thoracic outlet syndrome

NONOPERATIVE MANAGEMENT

■ Although cervical radiculopathy is common, only a few patients require surgical intervention, and despite a heightened clinical acumen for the diagnosis and treatment of cervical spondylosis, the mainstay of treatment remains nonsurgical.
■ Nonsurgical modalities that are initiated first include physical therapy, nonsteroidal anti-inflammatory drugs, and activity modification.
■ If these methods fail, a selective nerve root injection at a designated level can be attempted with a high degree of safety and efficacy.
■ The purpose of the nerve root injection is twofold: to provide pain relief by decreasing inflammation through the use of a corticosteroid, and to serve as a diagnostic tool to localize the offending pathology.

SURGICAL MANAGEMENT

■ Posterior cervical foraminotomy is indicated for foraminal stenosis or a foraminal disc herniation resulting in a neurologic deficit such as a sensory deficit, motor weakness, and/or progressive symptoms that fail to respond to an appropriate course of nonsurgical treatment.

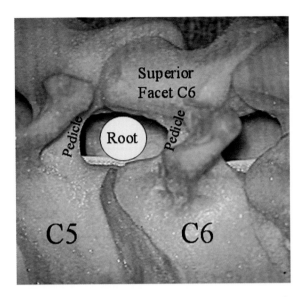

FIG 1 • Model showing the posterior element anatomy and boundaries of the foramen.

■ As with any surgical intervention, a thorough discussion with the patient and family about the desired outcomes and risks and benefits of the procedure must be undertaken before surgery.

Preoperative Planning

■ To perform an adequate foraminotomy, one must first understand the anatomy of the foramen.
■ The basic principle of the procedure is to unroof the foramen, which then allows the nerve root to displace dorsally away from the compressive pathology, which is anterior in most cases.
  ■ Less commonly, a portion of the superior facet may itself be a source of compression, which can then be directly removed by the posterior foraminotomy.
■ Since the superior articular facet of the caudal cervical segment forms the roof of the foramen, resection of the medial portion of the superior articular facet is necessary to adequately decompress the neuroforamen.
■ Similarly, since the pedicles form the cranial and caudal borders of the neuroforamen, adequate decompression requires resection of the superior articular facet to the lateral margin of the pedicles, as any overhang of the superior articular facet over the caudal pedicle can lead to persistent compression.
■ In contrast, because resection of more than 50% of the facet joint can lead to facet instability, resection of the superior facet lateral to the pedicle is unnecessary.

Positioning

■ Proper patient positioning is critical when performing posterior cervical foraminotomy to reduce blood loss and improve visualization of the operative field.
■ Although there are a variety of ways to position a patient, we routinely place the patient in bivector Gardner-Wells tong traction and position the patient prone on an open Jackson frame (OSI, Orthopaedic Systems, Inc., Union City, CA).
  ■ This table is quite versatile and allows for intraoperative alterations in patient positioning throughout the operation.
■ Typically, the table is tilted into reverse Trendelenburg to distribute blood into the abdomen and legs, thereby creating a

more physiologic state for the patient and providing better visualization in the operative field.
  ■ To facilitate this position, the head of the table is placed in the top rung and the foot of the bed is placed in the bottom rung.
■ The chest and abdomen are supported on bolsters that allow the abdomen to hang free, and the legs are supported in a sling with pillow support.
■ The shoulders are taped down on both sides to provide traction, thereby allowing better radiographic visualization of the lower cervical spine during intraoperative imaging.
■ Bivector traction is used with the aid of two separate ropes so the neck is maintained in proper alignment, depending on the procedure being performed (**FIG 2**).
■ One of the ropes is placed in-line and horizontal to the table through a pulley system, and the other is placed over a crossbar on the Jackson frame to facilitate placement of the head into extension.
■ It is imperative to maintain good coordination and communication with the anesthesia providers during change of positioning of the head, as the endotracheal tube may become dislodged if not secured properly.

Positioning

■ Foraminotomies are best accomplished with the neck in maximal flexion. This position unshingles the facets and exposes the underlying superior articular facet.

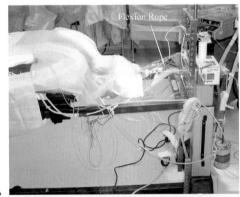

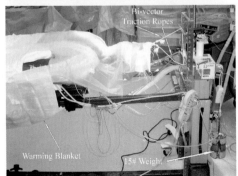

FIG 2 • Bivector traction technique using the open Jackson frame. Two separate ropes are used so the neck is maintained in proper alignment, depending on the procedure being performed: one of the ropes is placed in-line and horizontal to the table through a pulley system, and the other is placed over a cross-bar on the Jackson frame to facilitate placement of the head into extension. Although not necessary, a horseshoe may be used ventral to the face to catch the head if the tongs slip.

- If the neck is not adequately flexed during a foraminotomy, one must resect a large amount of the overhanging inferior articular facet to expose the underlying superior facet.
  - This may weaken the lateral mass and lead to a fracture, or more commonly it makes placement of the lateral mass

screw more difficult if a fusion is being performed in addition to a foraminotomy.

Approach

- A posterior cervical foraminotomy can be performed using open, endoscopic, or microscopically assisted approaches.

EXPOSURE

- For bilateral foraminotomies, typically a midline incision is used, whereas for a unilateral foraminotomy, an incision approximately 2 cm lateral to the midline can be made (**TECH FIG 1A–C**).
  - With either approach, the lamina, the junction between the lamina and the facet joint, and the facet

joint itself have to be exposed while preserving the facet capsule.
- After exposure, the intralaminar V is identified and the decompression is performed (**TECH FIG 1D,E**).

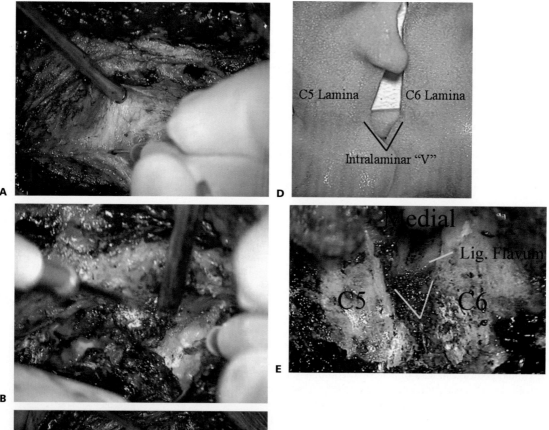

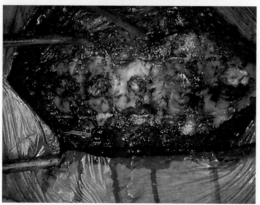

TECH FIG 1 • **A.** Dissection of the posterior cervical spine along the midline in the avascular plane. **B.** Continued dissection, showing midline splitting of the muscles. **C.** The posterior cervical spine after meticulous dissection of the posterior elements with lateral extension over the facet capsules. Bovie marks illustrate the lateral mass–laminar border. **D.** Model of the cervical spine showing the C5-6 interspace with the intralaminar V (*yellow lines*). This is the key anatomic landmark that must be recognized to perform an adequate foraminotomy. **E.** An intraoperative image showing the C5-6 interspace with the intralaminar V (*yellow lines*).

RESECTION OF INFERIOR ARTICULAR FACET

- A high-speed 2-mm acorn-shaped carbide-tip cutting burr is used to resect the overlying inferior articular facet and then the medial superior articular facet with the neck in neutral or flexed position (**TECH FIG 2**).
- Although the inferior articular facet does not cause impingement of the nerve root (the inferior articular facet lies dorsal to the superior articular facet), the overlying inferior articular facet must be resected to the lateral margin of the pedicles to expose the underlying superior articular facet.

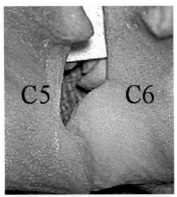

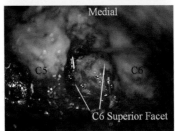

TECH FIG 2 • A. Model of the cervical spine showing the C5-6 interspace with resection of the inferior facet, which must be resected to the lateral margin of the pedicles to expose the underlying superior articular facet. To determine whether enough of the inferior facet has been resected, a small angled microcurette can be used to palpate the pedicle. **B.** An intraoperative image showing the C5-6 interspace with resection of the inferior facet. The probe illustrates the cranial extent of the C6 superior articular facet.

RESECTION OF SUPERIOR ARTICULAR FACET

- Once the inferior articular facet is resected, the superior articular facet underneath is resected out to the lateral border of the pedicles, completing the decompression (**TECH FIG 3**).
- During the decompression, copious irrigation (20-mL syringe with a 2-inch-long 18-gauge angiocath) must be used to prevent thermal damage to the surrounding tissues. It also aids in visualization.

- Typically we recommend the use of a burr over Kerrison rongeurs because inserting instruments (such as Kerrison rongeur, which may have a relatively thick footplate) into the already stenotic canal and foramen can cause neurologic damage. However, once most of the roof of the foramen has been removed, it is usually safe to use a 1-mm Kerrison rongeur to clean up any overhanging bone.

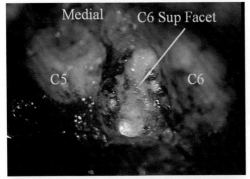

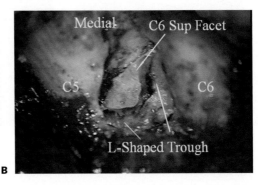

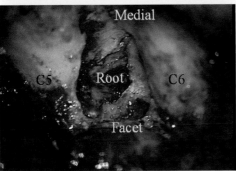

TECH FIG 3 • A. An intraoperative image showing that once the inferior articular facet is resected, the superior articular facet underneath can be identified. **B.** The superior articular facet is resected out to the lateral border of the pedicles; this is best performed using an L-shaped resection, as shown in the intraoperative image, to ensure there is no iatrogenic impingement on the nerve root, which can occur if a keyhole or a C-shaped resection of the superior articular facet is performed (see **E**). **C.** An intraoperative image showing the completed resection of the superior articular facet. The remaining small ledge of bone can be removed using a small angled microcurette or 1-mm Kerrison rongeur. *(continued)*

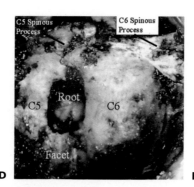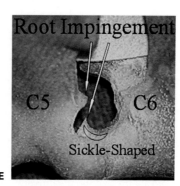

TECH FIG 3 • *(continued)* **D.** An intraoperative image showing the completed foraminotomy. **E.** Model of the cervical spine showing the C5-6 interspace showing C- or sickle-shaped decompression, which can lead to iatrogenic impingement on the nerve root.

DISCECTOMY

- If the patient has an intraforaminal disc herniation, then the nerve root must be manipulated to expose the herniated disc fragment that is ventral to the nerve root.
- If there is little room for the root to migrate cranially, the cranial 2 to 3 mm of the caudal pedicle may have to be burred down, and a microscopic right-angle probe can then be placed into this space and rotated ventrally to the root to sweep any herniated disc fragment out from under the root, and micro pituitary rongeurs can be used to remove the disc fragment.

CONFIRMATION OF ADEQUATE DECOMPRESSION

- After completing the decompression, a hemostatic agent such as FloSeal or Surgiflo is used to control any bleeding surfaces.
- Once the foraminotomy is completed, the lateral walls of the cranial and caudal pedicles should be readily palpable, and there should be no bone overhanging the medial and superior aspect of the caudal pedicle (**TECH FIG 4**).

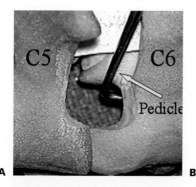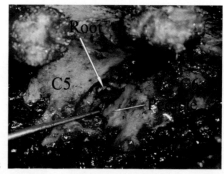

TECH FIG 4 • A. Model showing completion of the foraminotomy with complete decompression of the foramen. The microprobe shows the medial pedicle border. **B.** An intraoperative image showing palpation of the medial pedicle border after completion of the foraminotomy.

WOUND CLOSURE

- The posterior wound is closed in multiple layers.
- If meticulous midline exposure was performed, the preserved interspinous ligaments with the muscular attachments are used as the first layer of closure. The amount of muscle incorporated into the suture is minimized, since all such muscle will necrose.
- With a well-exposed spine, one can find a thin fascial layer enveloping the muscle that can be used to close the layers.
- The closure progresses from deep to superficial with the placement of deep, middle, and superficial drains.
- The multiple drains prevent isolated pockets of hematoma, which can act as a nidus for infection.

PEARLS AND PITFALLS

Positioning	▪ Bivector traction with the neck placed in flexion when the foraminotomy is being performed is crucial, as neck flexion unshingles the facets and exposes the underlying superior articular facet. ▪ Reverse Trendelenburg position helps to decrease blood loss. ▪ Good coordination and communication with the anesthesia providers during change of positioning of the head is critical.
Exposure	▪ Meticulous midline dissection through avascular raphe decreases blood loss and allows better closure. ▪ Care must be taken not to detach the semispinalis cervicis from the spinous process of C2 if a C2-3 foraminotomy is required. ▪ Care must be taken to remain superficial to the facet capsules during dissection to preserve them, as they provide some protection against postoperative kyphosis.
Decompression	▪ Adequate decompression requires resection of the superior articular facet (the roof of the foramen) to the lateral margin of the pedicles. ▪ About 50% (medial-lateral) of the overlying inferior articular facet must be resected to expose the underlying superior articular facet. ▪ Any overhang of the superior facet over the caudal pedicle can result in persistent nerve root compression.
Closure	▪ The posterior wound is closed in multiple layers to more closely reapproximate the normal anatomy.
Postoperative course	▪ Postoperatively, patients do not have any range-of-motion restrictions, nor are they required to wear a brace.

POSTOPERATIVE CARE

▪ Postoperative pain regimen includes patient-controlled analgesia and ketorolac (Toradol) for 36 to 48 hours in patients under age 65 who have normal renal function and no history of congestive heart failure.

▪ Patients typically remain in the hospital for 24 to 48 hours, depending on drain output. Patients are discharged on oral pain medication and are instructed to return to the clinic for routine follow-up at 6 weeks postoperatively.

▪ Although a soft collar is given for comfort, patients are encouraged to discontinue using the collar as soon as they can.

▪ There are no range-of-motion restrictions, and therapy with immediate motion can begin.

▪ Rapid return to normal activities and aerobic exercise is encouraged.

OUTCOMES

▪ Results of posterior cervical foraminotomy are encouraging, with good or excellent outcomes reported in about 90% to 95% of patients.

COMPLICATIONS

▪ Neurologic injury or worsening radiculopathy
▪ Infection
▪ Inadequate decompression or failure to relieve symptoms
▪ Instability and deformity secondary to overly aggressive decompression
▪ Air embolism if the procedure is done in a sitting position

REFERENCES

1. Albert TJ, Murrell SE. Surgical management of cervical radiculopathy. J Am Acad Orthop Surg 1999;7:368–376.
2. Aldrich F. Posterolateral microdiscectomy for cervical monoradiculopathy caused by posterolateral soft cervical disc sequestration. J Neurosurg 1990;72:370–377.
3. Brodsky A. Management of radiculopathy secondary to acute cervical disc degeneration and spondylosis by the posterior approach. In: The Cervical Spine. Philadelphia: Lippincott, 1983:395–402.
4. Emery SE. Cervical disc disease and cervical spondylosis. In: An HS, ed. Principles and Techniques in Spine Surgery, ed 1. Philadelphia: Williams & Wilkins, 1998:401–412.
5. Epstein JA. The surgical management of cervical spinal stenosis, spondylosis, and myeloradiculopathy by means of the posterior approach. Spine 1988;13:864–869.
6. Epstein NE. A review of laminoforaminotomy for the management of lateral and foraminal cervical disc herniations or spurs. Surg Neurol 2002;57:226–234.
7. Fager CA. Management of cervical disc lesions and spondylosis by posterior approaches. Clin Neurosurg 1977;24:488–507.
8. Fager CA. Posterior surgical tactics for the neurological syndromes of cervical disc and spondylotic lesions. Clin Neurosurg 1978;25:218–244.
9. Fager CA. Posterolateral approach to ruptured median and paramedian cervical disk. Surg Neurol 1983;20:443–452.
10. Grob D. Surgery in the degenerative cervical spine. Spine 1998;23:2674–2683.
11. Henderson CM, Hennessy RG, Shuey HM Jr, et al. Posterior-lateral foraminotomy as an exclusive operative technique for cervical radiculopathy: a review of 846 consecutively operated cases. Neurosurgery 1983;13:504–512.
12. Herkowitz H. Surgical management of cervical soft disc herniation: a comparison between the anterior and posterior approach. Spine 1990;15:1026–1030.
13. Levine MJ, Albert TJ, Smith MD. Cervical radiculopathy: diagnosis and nonoperative management. J Am Acad Orthop Surg 1996;4:305–316.
14. Ma DJ, Gilula LA, Riew KD. Complications of fluoroscopically guided extraforaminal cervical nerve blocks: an analysis of 1036 injections. J Bone Joint Surg Am 2005;87A:1025–1030.
15. Parker WD. Cervical laminoforaminotomy. J Neurosurg 2002;96(2 Suppl):254.
16. Williams RW. Microcervical foraminotomy: a surgical alternative for intractable radicular pain. Spine 1983;8:708–716.
17. Witzmann A, Hejazi N, Krasznai L. Posterior cervical foraminotomy: a follow-up study of 67 surgically treated patients with compressive radiculopathy. Neurosurg Rev 2000;23:213–217.
18. Woertgen C, Holzschuh M, Rothoerl RD, et al. Prognostic factors of posterior cervical disc surgery: a prospective, consecutive study of 54 patients. Neurosurgery 1997;40:724–729.
19. Zeidman SM, Ducker TB. Posterior cervical laminoforaminotomy for radiculopathy: review of 172 cases. Neurosurgery 1993;33:356–362.

Chapter 4

Cervical Laminoplasty: Open and French Door

S. Tim Yoon and James Kercher

DEFINITION

- Cervical laminoplasty is a surgical procedure designed to decompress the spinal cord from a posterior approach. The cervical laminae are reconstructed to create more available space for the spinal cord while at the same time preserving motion and normal alignment.
- Cervical myelopathy is pathologic spinal cord dysfunction due to spinal cord compression. Compression of neural elements results in a spectrum of cord dysfunction ranging from mild to quite severe. Cervical laminoplasty is most often used to treat cervical myelopathy associated with multilevel cervical stenosis.
- Multilevel cord compression is commonly due to cervical spondylotic stenosis. This is a degenerative process resulting in decreased space available for the spinal cord, with possible instability and loss of lordosis. Congenital stenosis of varying degrees is often associated with patients with symptomatic cervical spondylotic myelopathy.
  - Other conditions such as ossification of the posterior longitudinal ligament, trauma, infection, and neoplasm can result in stenosis that can be treated with laminoplasty.
- The key to treating this condition is to achieve multilevel decompression that alleviates circumferential compression and allows the spinal cord to drift away from ventral compressive lesions.

ANATOMY

- The cervical spine is composed of seven vertebrae normally arranged in an overall lordotic alignment. The occiput–C1 articulation is responsible for 50% of neck flexion and extension and the C1–C2 atlantoaxial articulation is responsible for 50% of total rotation. Lateral bending below the C2–C3 level is coupled with rotation due to the 45-degree inclination of the cervical facet joints.
- The subaxial vertebral segments of C3–C7 are similar to each other and distinct from C1 (atlas) and C2 (axis). The subaxial vertebrae articulate via zygapophyseal or facet joints posteriorly and laterally via the uncovertebral joints, or joints of Luschka.
- Intervertebral discs are located between vertebral bodies of C2–C7. The discs are composed of an inner nucleus pulposus and outer annular fibrosus.
- Anteriorly the spinal canal is bounded by the vertebral bodies, the intervertebral discs, and the posterior longitudinal ligaments; laterally and posteriorly by the vertebral arch; and posteriorly by the ligamentum flavum, which runs from the anterior surface of the superior lamina to the posterior surface of the inferior lamina (**FIG 1**).

PATHOGENESIS

- Cervical spondylotic myelopathy is the most common indication for cervical laminoplasty. It is the most common cause of myelopathy in patients older than 50 years. By age 40, most people will have radiographic evidence of degenerative changes.[3]
- The degenerative process typically begins in the intervertebral disc. The degenerated discs are more fibrotic as a result of proteoglycan loss within the nucleus pulposus. This is associated with lost water content from the nucleus pulposus and loss of normal shock-absorbing capacity.
- With disc degeneration, the disc height decreases and the annulus fibrosus bulges radially, resulting in ventral spinal canal narrowing. Collapse and loss of lordotic curvature can lead to a cascade of compensatory changes, including osteophyte formation around the uncovertebral joints, the facet joints, and the insertion of the annulus fibrosus. In the dorsal spinal canal, there is thickening or buckling of the ligamentum flavum, which causes a decrease in canal and foraminal dimensions.
- Protruded disc material, osteophytes, and thickened soft tissues within the canal or foramen result in extrinsic pressure on the nerve roots or spinal cord.
- Spondylotic changes and osteophyte compression may also impair the circulation within the cord, leading to cord ischemia and resultant myelopathy.

NATURAL HISTORY

- The true natural history of cervical spondylotic myelopathy is difficult to discern. This is due partly to the fact that most cases now are treated surgically and early studies of the disease took place several decades ago. At that time modern diagnostics were unavailable; therefore, confounding variables due to other neurologic conditions cloud the picture.
- What is known about the natural history is that the disease process progresses in a variable and unpredictable manner. Often there is stepwise deterioration of neurologic function, with periods of stable symptoms followed by decline.
- The clinical course may wax and wane over a period of years. Sensory symptoms may be transient, but motor symptoms tend to persist and progress. While surgical intervention may relieve symptoms and halt progression, some neurologic deficits are permanent and do not respond to surgical treatment.[4]

PATIENT HISTORY AND PHYSICAL FINDINGS

- The diagnosis of cervical myelopathy may be difficult to make due to the variability in clinical findings. Pain is frequently not a significant complaint in myelopathic patients unless associated with root compression or facet arthrosis. Patients may present with subtle findings or profound neurologic deficits.
- The diagnosis requires a high index of suspicion and careful evaluation of the patient's history, physical examination, and imaging studies.

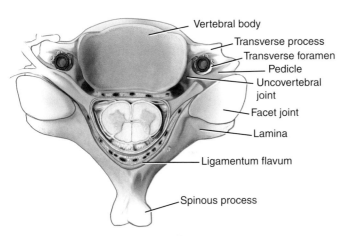

FIG 1 • Anatomy of cervical vertebrae.

■ Patients commonly present with insidious onset of gait disturbance, trouble with balance, and clumsiness in the hands and lower extremities. They may report burning pain in the upper extremities, difficulty in handwriting and fine motor control, diffuse numbness, and weakness of grasp. Advanced cases can present with flaccid weakness and bowel and bladder dysfunction.

■ The physical examination should begin with an assessment of gait, which may be wide-based, hesitant, stiff, or spastic. Patients may be unable to perform heel-toe walk or may have poor balance during toe raises. A careful neurologic examination should follow. Each dermatome should be tested.

■ Sensory findings may be variable. Pain, temperature, and vibratory and dermatomal sensation may all be decreased.

■ On the motor examination, depending on the level of cord compression as well as nerve root and peripheral nerve dysfunction, mixed upper and lower motor neuron findings may be present in the extremities. Patients may have weakness and atrophy as well as brisk reflexes.

■ The Lhermitte sign is said to be positive when extremes of neck flexion or extension result in paresthesias and weakness. This can be a sign of posterior column compression. Pathologic reflexes such as the scapulohumeral reflex (indicates compression above the C3 level), inverted radial reflex (indicates compression at the C5 to C6 levels), the Hoffman sign, clonus, the Babinski sign, and finger escape may be present.

IMAGING AND OTHER DIAGNOSTIC STUDIES

■ Plain AP and lateral radiographs are useful for initial evaluation of cervical spine sagittal alignment and the extent of spondylotic changes such as disc space narrowing, osteophytes, kyphosis, joint subluxation, and spinal canal stenosis (**FIG 2A**).

   ■ Flexion and extension views can provide information about possible spinal instability.

■ Magnetic resonance imaging (MRI) aids in determining accurate dimensions of the spinal cord and canal. MRI is also the technique of choice for visualization of soft tissues such as ligamentous hypertrophy, disc herniations, and changes within the cord parenchyma such as edema and myelomalacia (**FIG 2B**).

■ Computed tomography (CT) with and without contrast is superior to MRI for defining the bony anatomy and is the

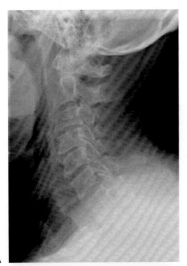 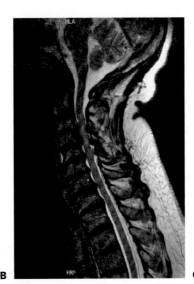 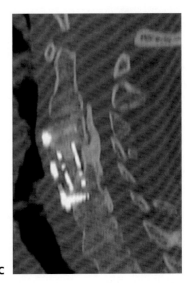
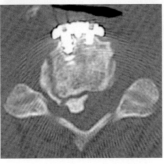

FIG 2 • **A.** Preoperative lateral cervical spine radiograph demonstrating spondylotic changes: diffuse disc height loss and osteophyte formation. **B.** Sagittal T2-weighted MRI showing multilevel cervical disc protrusions and circumferential stenosis at C3–4, C4–5, and C5–6, resulting in cord deformation. Cord signal changes can be seen at C3–4 and C4–5, indicative of cord damage. **C.** Sagittal CT reconstruction showing large ossified posterior longitudinal ligament extending from C2 to C6. There is evidence of failed anterior decompression by an outside facility. **D.** Axial CT image demonstrating vertebral canal compression from large ossified posterior longitudinal ligament.

study of choice for evaluating ossification of the posterior longitudinal ligament (**FIG 2C,D**).

DIFFERENTIAL DIAGNOSIS

- Cervical spondylosis
- Soft disc herniations
- Infectious discitis or epidural abscess
- Muscular dystrophy or dystonia
- Loss of normal sagittal alignment
- Neurogenic disorders (syringomyelia, multiple sclerosis, amyotrophic lateral sclerosis, cerebellar dysfunction)
- Instability of the cervical spine can cause myelopathic symptoms.
- Ossification of the posterior longitudinal ligament
- Peripheral neuropathy or nerve injury
- Drug intoxication
- Vascular disease
- Autoimmune disorders

SURGICAL MANAGEMENT

- Laminoplasty was specifically designed to prevent the kyphotic deformities seen with laminectomy alone and is associated with fewer complications than laminectomy and fusion.[1]
- Laminoplasty involves posterior decompression from C3 to C7, allowing for dorsal cord expansion and drift while preserving motion.
- Indications
  - Cervical spondylotic myelopathy involving three or more disc levels
  - Congenital stenosis of the spinal canal
  - Ossification of the posterior longitudinal ligament
  - Spinal cord tumors
- Contraindications
  - Kyphotic sagittal alignment of more than 10 to 14 degrees can lead to worsening of the kyphotic deformity and poor neurologic outcomes.
  - Significant segmental instability
- Relative contraindications
  - Ossification of the ligamentum flavum. This condition is associated with dural adhesions, which can make opening the posterior arch difficult.
  - Previous posterior cervical surgery such as foraminotomies. Scar formation can produce adhesions that can make opening the laminar arch difficult.
  - Primary axial neck pain in the setting of myelopathy. Laminoplasty preserves motion, and hence the procedure is not designed to address pain generation from facet arthrosis and disc degeneration. Fusion procedures provide greater benefit to patients with significant complaints of axial neck pain.

Preoperative Planning

- The patient's history, clinical examination, and imaging studies should be thoroughly reviewed and documented before the case.
- Evaluation of the patient's active range of motion in flexion and extension assists with head positioning. Passive flexion and extension outside of this range (eg, during positioning) can be dangerous in the setting of cord impingement.
- The presence of preoperative axial neck pain may be an indication for an alternative procedure, as listed above.
- Careful examination of CT scans to determine the bony

anatomy of the dorsal cortices can be helpful. Special attention should be given to the lamina-to-lateral-mass junction.
- If concomitant fusion is planned, the midline splitting laminoplasty ("French door") approach may be considered, but a unilateral open door technique can also be used with fusion and lateral mass instrumentation.

Positioning

- Intubation is preformed with caution to protect the cervical spine. This includes advanced notification to anesthesia personnel of spinal cord compression in severe cases. Care should be taken not to extend the neck more than the patient's comfortable range of motion before sedation. The use of fiberoptic assistance should be considered in high-risk cases.
- Application of a Mayfield head holder reduces risks to soft tissues and provides a stable platform for the head during the procedure (**FIG 3A**).
- The patient is placed prone onto chest bolsters. The abdomen should be as free as possible to reduce venous bleeding and prevent ventilatory difficulty. Arms are tucked in at the patient's side (**FIG 3B**).
- The head is positioned to allow for slight cervical flexion to tension skin on the posterior neck folds and decrease shingling (or overlap) of lamina. Intraoperative repositioning of the flexion–extension of the head is possible if necessary with the Mayfield tongs.
- The bed is then placed in reverse Trendelenburg to decrease venous bleeding and allow for horizontal positioning of the cervical spine.
- Spinal cord monitoring is routinely performed in myelopathic patients. This helps to monitor neurologic problems related to positioning as well as with the laminoplasty procedure itself.
- The surgical field should be prepared from the nuchal line to roughly T4 to allow for possible wound extension.

Approach

- A posterior midline incision is made over the spinous processes from C2 to T1. This can be extended to the occiput or further down the thoracic spine as necessary.

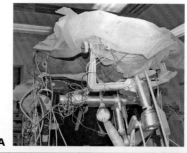
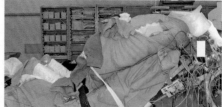

FIG 3 • **A.** The patient's head is placed in a Mayfield head holder. **B.** The patient is placed prone onto chest bolsters with arms tucked in at the sides. The head is placed in slight flexion. Spinal cord monitoring equipment is also seen.

INCISION AND DISSECTION

- A posterior midline approach to the spinous processes is made, using a longitudinal incision from C2 to T1.
- Electrocautery is used to divide the subcutaneous fat in the midline to reach the tips of the spinous processes.
- Once the tips of the spinous processes have been found, a subperiosteal dissection is performed to expose the C3–C7 lamina. Careful attention should be taken to stay in the midline avascular plane to reduce bleeding.
  - The dissection should extend laterally to fully expose the junction of the lateral mass and the lamina.
  - Exposure should not extend beyond the midportion of the lateral masses.
- The extensor muscle attachment to the C2 spinous process is carefully preserved. The inferior C2 laminar margin is usually broad and should be exposed to aid in visualization of the C2–3 junction.
- The spinous processes can be amputated at their base. Spinous processes are useful for bone graft (either for strutting open the lamina or for local bone graft for the hinge side).
  - Removing the spinous processes significantly improves exposure and reduces asymmetric posterior displacement of paraspinal musculature (TECH FIG 1A).
- The interlaminar ligamentum flavum between C2–3 and C7–T1 is removed. First, a rongeur is used to create a small opening in the interlaminar ligament flavum. Then a combination of curette and Kerrison rongeur is used to divide the rest of the interlaminar ligamentum flavum (TECH FIG 1B).

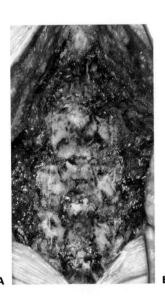 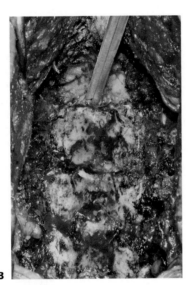

TECH FIG 1 • A. Lamina exposure after subperiosteal dissection and spinous process removal. The dissection should extend laterally to expose the junction of the lateral mass and lamina. Attempts should be made to minimize disruption of the facet capsule. This will decrease long-term postoperative neck pain. Planned lines for opening and hinge trough creation have been marked using electrocautery and marking pen. **B.** A Kerrison rongeur is used to divide the interlaminar ligamentum flavum.

TROUGH PREPARATION

Open-Side Trough

- A 3.0- or 4.0-mm round or oval low-aggression high-speed burr is used to form the trough.
- The trough location is at the junction of the lamina and lateral mass.
- For the opening side, bony layers should be removed in sequence: the outer cortex, next the cancellous middle layer, followed by the ventral cortex (TECH FIG 2A).
- Troughs should be made no deeper than 4 mm. Once at that depth, the burr should be directed medially to avoid the facets. Switching to a 3.0-mm burr can be beneficial after the initial work with the 4.0-mm burr to aid in more precise burring.
- As the bone is thinned, the surgeon should use a delicate instrument such as a microcurette or Penfield elevator to palpate and identify any bone bridges still attaching the lamina to the lateral masses. Completion of the bone separation can be performed with a microcurette, a 1.0-mm Kerrison rongeur, or a diamond burr (TECH FIG 2B).
- Care should be used at this time to avoid the epidural veins, which create significant bleeding. Bipolar electrocautery can be used to control bleeding epidural veins.

French Door (Midline Splitting)

- The French door technique involves creation of a midline opening trough and two hinge troughs.
- The midline of the posterior arch can be split by a variety of methods. One method is to remove the spinous process as described above and use a 4.0-mm low-aggression burr to create a complete midline trough. The burr is carefully manipulated to remove the dorsal midline bone down to the ventral bone (TECH FIG 3).
- Completion of the opening is then performed as described earlier and shown in Techniques Figure 2B.

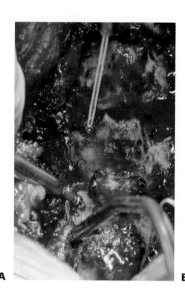 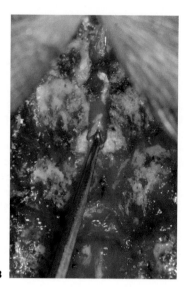

TECH FIG 2 • A. Creation of the opening trough requires sequential removal of bony layers. Figure demonstrates burring with irrigation and suction. **B.** After the initial burring, completion of the bone separation on the opening side can be performed using a microcurette, a 1.0-mm Kerrison rongeur, or a diamond burr. Figure demonstrates the careful removal of the opening trough ventral cortex with the use of a microcurette during a midline splitting French door laminoplasty.

Hinge-Side Trough

- The hinge side is prepared opposite the opening side at the same anatomic junction of lamina and lateral mass.
- The hinge trough is prepared in a similar manner; however, it entails removal of only the dorsal cortex and cancellous layers. The ventral cortex can be thinned to open the hinge, but the surgeon should preserve as much as possible to preserve a mechanically sound hinge (**TECH FIG 4**).

- Stiffness of the hinge should be tested periodically during preparation. This is the rationale for performing the hinge after the open side has been completed. The goal is to create a pliable yet firm hinge that yields to moderate opening force without breaking the hinge inner cortex.
- Hinge troughs used for the French door technique are prepared in the same anatomic location as troughs created for the open door technique. Similar to the open door technique, ventral cortex should be preserved to create stable hinges.

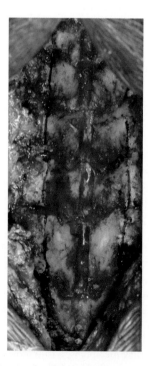

TECH FIG 3 • The French door technique uses a midline opening trough. Here the midline trough has been created. Planned lines for the hinge troughs are shown on either side.

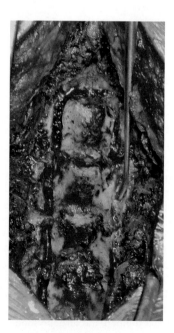

TECH FIG 4 • Opening and hinge troughs for the open door technique. Preserved ventral cortex for the hinge trough is seen at the tip of the Penfield dissector.

OPENING THE LAMINOPLASTY

- Proceeding from caudal to cranial, a nerve hook or curved curette is used to elevate the lamina on the opening side. Division of the residual ligamentum flavum and epidural veins proceeds from C3 to C7. A Kerrison rongeur can be used to divide ligamentous attachments, and bipolar forceps are used for cauterization of epidural veins.
- The laminae are then opened sequentially. This can be done with the assistance of a curved microcurette to raise the opening side and gently bend open each lamina hinge. Care should be taken to identify and lyse any epidural adhesions (**TECH FIG 5A**).
- Starting from C3 and proceeding to C7 allows for blood to flow away from the working area and reduces the overhang of the inferior edge of the superior lamina due to lamina shingling.
- Completion of opening laminae is carried out carefully with small curettes (**TECH FIG 5B**).

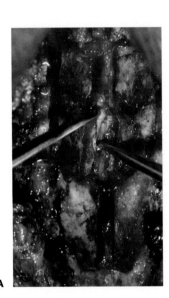 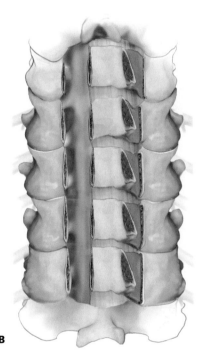

TECH FIG 5 • A. Completing the opening for the French door technique. With the assistance of a curved microcurette, the lamina is gently bent back upon its hinge. Care should be taken to identify and lyse epidural adhesions. **B.** Completion of open door laminoplasty.

A   **B**

POSTERIOR ARCH RECONSTRUCTION

- The laminoplasty door is held open using a variety of techniques.
- Plate reconstruction has become popular because of the immediate mechanical security that plates provide (**TECH FIG 6A,B**). However, eventual mechanical stability relies on hinge-side bony healing to permanently hold the posterior arch open.
- Bone struts can also be used; this was the most frequently used method for many decades. Autogenous spinous process grafts fashioned from the spinous processes of C6 and C7 can be used, as well as rib allograft or machined cortical grafts (**TECH FIG 6C**).
  - Reconstruction with bone has the advantage of allowing for full bony reconstruction of the lamina arch, as the bone struts usually fully incorporate with time. Furthermore, placing bone is easier and faster to place than plate and screws, but bone provides less initial mechanical stability to the arch and may (rarely) dislodge before healing of the hinge.
- Hybrid reconstruction with alternating plate and bone graft can also be used (**TECH FIG 6D**).
- With the French door technique, midline plates can be applied. Other structures have been used, including autograft, allograft, or hydroxyapatite (**TECH FIG 6E**).
- Alternatively, the lamina can be held open with sutures that go from the lamina to the lateral mass or facet capsules. Suture anchors have also been used.

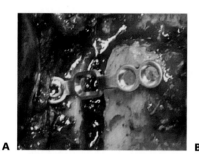

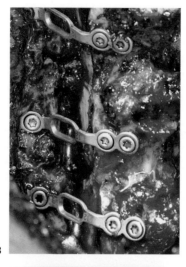

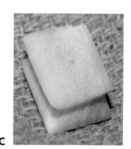

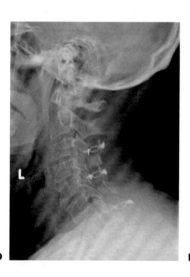

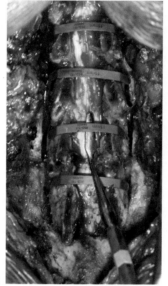

TECH FIG 6 A,B. • Open door plates. **A.** First, the lateral mass screw is placed with a 6-mm screw. **B.** Then the lamina is opened and held in place by subsequent 4-mm screws placed in the lamina. **C.** Machined cortical allograft. Grooves allow for better stability when interpositioned between lamina and lateral mass. **D.** Postoperative lateral radiograph after laminoplasty performed with alternating plate and graft technique. **E.** French door posterior arch reconstruction using midline plates. Adequate space must be maintained between the plate and cord to allow for expansion.

WOUND CLOSURE

- A deep drain is placed, followed by a layered fascial and subcutaneous closure.
- Skin is closed using a subcuticular stitch.

PEARLS AND PITFALLS

Physical examination	▪ The Hoffman reflex can indicate spinal cord compression but can be positive in normal individuals.
Patient position	▪ Slight cervical flexion facilitates exposure and closure by eliminating redundant posterior skin folds and decreases overlap of lamina (laminar shingling) for improved identification of adjacent levels.
Opening side	▪ If foraminotomies are planned, then the opening side should be made over the ipsilateral side of compression. If asymmetric compression is present, it may be beneficial to open the more affected side. ▪ While creating the opening hinge, a color change in the cortex can be appreciated. As the deep (ventral) cortex is thinned, yellow areas (which correspond to ligamentum flavum) and blue areas (which correspond to veins or dura) can be seen through the bone. Care should be taken at this point as the ventral bone is now very thin.

Hinge-side trough	▪ The surgeon should avoid removing excessive bone on the hinge side, thus creating a floppy hinge. ▪ The surgeon should always recheck to make sure that the opening side is complete if there is any difficulty elevating the hinge side. ▪ If the hinge is completely incompetent, then it can be reconstructed with a special plate that fixates on the hinge side (lamina-to-lateral-mass plate).
Epidural vein ligation	▪ The epidural veins should be ligated as far dorsal as possible. This decreases bleeding by avoiding the ventral longitudinal veins.

POSTOPERATIVE CARE

▪ Typically a soft cervical collar is worn for comfort.
▪ Most patients can begin immediate active range of motion.
▪ Drain output is monitored and drains are typically removed by 48 hours after surgery.
▪ The patient is weaned from the cervical collar over 2 to 4 weeks.

OUTCOMES

▪ Cervical laminoplasty is a valuable treatment option for myelopathic patients with multilevel stenosis. It provides cord decompression while preserving motion.
▪ With proper patient selection, neurologic outcomes are excellent, with few complications. In a meta-analysis of results on neurologic improvement, 80% of postoperative patients were reported to have excellent outcomes.[2]
▪ When compared with laminectomy with fusion, outcomes regarding neurologic improvement were similar. However, laminectomy with fusion had more frequent complications, such as progression of myelopathy, nonunion, instrumentation failure, development of a significant kyphotic alignment, persistent bone graft harvest site pain, subjacent degeneration requiring reoperation, and deep infection.[1]

COMPLICATIONS

▪ Segmental nerve root palsy: This is most commonly a motor deficit affecting the C5 root that occurs a day or two after surgery. It usually resolves to a large degree with time.
▪ Axial neck pain has been reported. However, the pain is typically mild and often described as stiffness.
▪ Loss of cervical motion: Up to 50% loss of range of motion has been reported with some laminoplasty techniques.
▪ Dural tears are infrequent. They can be handled with either direct repair or with fibrin glue with the addition of a lumbar diverting cerebrospinal fluid drain.
▪ The infection rate is very low. Good hemostasis and irrigation is recommended.

REFERENCES

1. Heller JG, Edwards CC II, Murakami H, et al. Laminoplasty versus laminectomy and fusion for multilevel cervical myelopathy: an independent matched cohort analysis. Spine 2001;26:1330–1336.
2. Sani S, Ratliff JK, Cooper PR. A critical review of cervical laminoplasty. Neurosurg Q 2004;14:5–16.
3. Teresi LM, Lufkin RB, Reicher MA, et al. Asymptomatic degenerative disk disease and spondylosis of the cervical spine: MR imaging. Radiology 1987;164:83–88.
4. Yoon TS. Cervical myelopathy. Semin Spine Surg 2004;16:4.

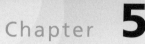
Posterior Cervical Fusion With Instrumentation

Raj Rao and Satyajit V. Marawar

SURGICAL MANAGEMENT

- Operative intervention in the posterior subaxial cervical spine is frequently carried out for decompression or stabilization.
  - Fusion and instrumentation of the posterior cervical spine may be required for unstable fractures or after extensive decompressive procedures.
  - Instrumentation reduces the need for postoperative immobilization and orthosis wear, augments fusion success, and allows better maintenance of sagittal alignment of the cervical spine.

Interspinous Wiring

- Interspinous wiring can be an alternative to lateral mass or pedicle screw fixation in stabilization of the posterior cervical spine.
  - Although it resists flexion reasonably well, it is generally not as strong in resisting extension, axial load, rotation, and lateral bending.
- The most commonly used implants are 18- or 20-gauge stainless steel wire or 1- to 1.2-mm titanium braided cable.
  - Alternatives include braided stainless steel or polyethylene cable. Multistrand braided steel, titanium, or polyethylene cables show superior fatigue resistance, greater flexibility, and improved stability on flexion–extension testing compared to a single-filament stainless steel wire.[31,34]
- In modern spine surgery, wiring techniques are generally limited to cases in which biomechanically superior techniques such as lateral mass fixation cannot be used, a somewhat less invasive midline-only exposure is desired, or the additional rigidity of lateral mass fixation is not necessary (eg, for posterior repair of relatively stable pseudarthroses, or to provide a tension band effect as an adjunct to anterior instrumentation).
- Techniques of wiring include simple interspinous wiring (eg, Rogers), Bohlman triple wiring (can be used also for occipitocervical fixation), and oblique wiring.
  - As a result of the direction of its stabilizing forces, oblique wiring may counter rotational instability better than simple interspinous wiring.

Lateral Mass Screw Fixation

- The lateral mass of the subaxial cervical vertebra is a quadrangular column of bone formed by the complex of the superior and inferior articular processes and the intervening bone.
- Lateral mass screws are the implants most commonly used at present for posterior fixation of the subaxial cervical spine.
- They are versatile in that they can be used when the posterior elements are deficient (eg, from trauma, tumors, or surgical resection for decompression).
- Lateral mass screw and rod–plate fixation provides superior flexion and torsional stiffness compared to posterior wiring.[9,32]
  - The improved strength of fixation allows instrumentation to be limited to the levels of fusion. When wiring techniques are used, the construct occasionally needs to be extended proximally or distally to obtain additional points of fixation.
- A lower incidence of postoperative kyphosis can be achieved with lateral mass screws versus wiring techniques.[13]
- Lateral mass screws have a low incidence of complications and are much easier to insert than cervical pedicle screws.
- The Magerl technique of lateral mass screw fixation has been shown to have superior pullout strength and higher load to failure when compared to screws inserted with the Roy-Camille technique.[26]
  - This may be related to the longer screw length generally obtained with the Magerl technique (18 mm with Magerl technique versus 14 mm with the Roy-Camille technique).[6,16]
- Pullout strength is significantly greater with a bicortical screw than with a unicortical purchase.
  - Because bicortical purchase engenders potential risk to nerve roots and the vertebral artery, however, unicortical purchase is used in most cases.

Pedicle Screw Fixation of the Cervical Spine

- Pedicle screw fixation allows superior, simultaneous stabilization of all three columns of the cervical spine.
- The risk of neurovascular injury from penetration of the small cervical pedicle restricts the widespread use of this technique.
- Pedicle screws are most commonly used at C2 and C7, where the pedicles are largest in the cervical spine.
  - They are often used at the cephalad or caudal ends of long instrumented constructs.
- At C7, most patients do not have a vertebral artery in the foramen transversarium, making pedicle screw fixation feasible.
  - At C2, the vertebral artery is generally lateral to the insertion site and trajectory of the pedicle, making pedicle screw fixation feasible.
  - From C3 to C6, the proximity of the vertebral artery and the small diameter of the pedicles make pedicle screw fixation challenging and not feasible for routine use.
  - Whenever pedicle screw fixation in the cervical spine is contemplated, careful scrutiny of preoperative CT and MRI scans is essential.
- The cervical pedicle is generally taller than it is wide, with the mean height of all cervical pedicles around 7 mm (range 6 to 11 mm).[27]
  - The width of the pedicle is the critical determinant for feasibility of pedicle screw placement.
  - Pedicle outer diameters less than 4 mm may preclude pedicle screw insertion.[12]
  - Multiple morphologic studies have found that the mean cervical pedicle outer width varies from 4 to 7 mm, with significant variation in width at different levels (Table 1).[12,24,27]

Table 1	Cervical Pedicle Outer Width

Pedicle	Width (mm)
C2	6.9 ± 1.6
C3	5.3 ± 0.8
C4	5.4 ± 0.8
C5	5.7 ± 0.8
C6	5.9 ± 0.9
C7	6.7 ± 1.0

(Adapted from Callahan RA, et al. Cervical facet fusion for control of instability following laminectomy. J Bone Joint Surg Am 1977;59A:991–1002.)

- The pedicles of C2 and C7 are generally large enough to accommodate either 3.5- or 4-mm screws.
- The length of the pedicles from C3 to C6 ranges from 12 to 18 mm.[12] Screw lengths are generally slightly longer to obtain purchase within the vertebral body.
- The axial angle of the pedicle (medial angle to the sagittal plane) is the least at C2 (25 to 30 degrees)[10] and increases to a mean of 44 degrees (25 to 55 degrees) at C3. From C3 to C7 it gradually reduces to a mean of 37 degrees (33 to 55 degrees).[24]

POSTERIOR CERVICAL FUSION

- Although it is tempting to focus on instrumentation techniques, performing a meticulous fusion technique is just as important, if not more so, to the success of surgery.
- In virtually all cases, posterior fusion is supplemented by some form of instrumentation.
- To maximize the surface area for fusion, all posterior bony surfaces that do not need to be resected for the decompression should be left intact for fusion.
  - The main priority, however, should always be to first achieve adequate neural decompression.
- After exposure, all soft tissues, including the interspinous ligaments and muscles, facet joint capsules, and paraspinal soft tissue, are meticulously resected so that the cortical surfaces lie exposed.
- Facet joint cartilage is removed with a curette or 3-mm burr within the facet joint.
- The posterior cortical surfaces of the laminae and spinous processes are decorticated with a 3-mm burr to expose bleeding subcortical bone (**TECH FIG 1**).
- Bone graft obtained from the iliac crest is morselized into small cancellous and corticocancellous chips and onlaid over the bleeding bone.
- Cancellous chips of bone are directly inserted into the facet joint.
- Bone placed between the spinous processes has the additional benefit of being readily visualized on postoperative lateral radiographs obtained to radiographically assess the presence of fusion.

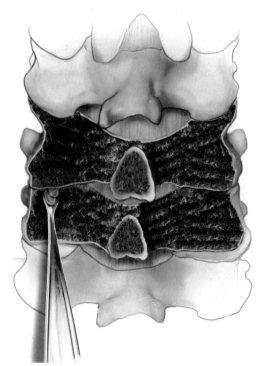

TECH FIG 1 • Decortication of the laminae and facet joints at the levels selected for fusion. Onlay iliac crest bone graft is placed over the decorticated areas.

INTERSPINOUS WIRING

Simple Interspinous Wiring

- The spinous processes and laminae at the level to be instrumented should be confirmed to be intact and instrumentable on preoperative imaging studies.
  - Closed or operative reduction of spinal fracture-dislocations should be carried out before instrumentation if possible.
  - In some cases of flexion–distraction injury, sequential tightening of the wires can be done to reduce the spine.

- Two- to 3-mm drill holes are made through the cortex at the junction of the spinous process and laminae bilaterally, at the levels to be included in the fusion.
- Attention should be paid to the ventral location of the dural sac, and the drill should be directed coronally to minimize the risk of inadvertent spinal cord injury (**TECH FIG 2A**).
- The drill holes should be positioned at the proximal aspect of the cephalad spinous process and the distal aspect of the caudal spinous process to provide the widest margin of safety against the wire cutting through the spinous process.

TECHNIQUES

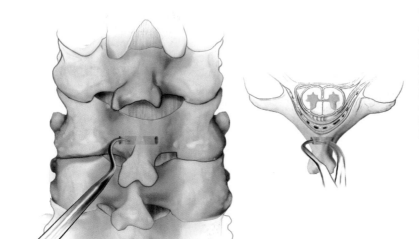

TECH FIG 2 • Simple interspinous wiring. **A.** Safe position of the drill hole for passage of spinous process wire is dorsal to the spinal laminar line. **B.** The wire or cable selected is passed through and around the base of the cranial and caudal spinous processes at the levels selected for fusion, so that both ends of the wire are on the same side of the spine. **C.** Ends of wire are twisted together after releasing any cervical traction.

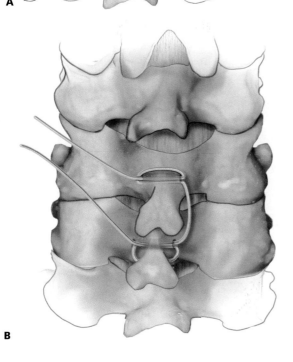

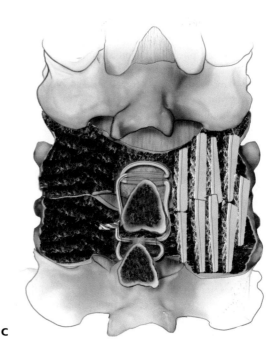

- The tips of a towel clip or a tenaculum clamp are placed in the cortical holes on either side of the base of the spinous process.
  - A gentle side-to-side rocking movement is used to create a continuous tract in the cancellous bone at the base of the spinous process.
- The wire or cable selected for use is passed through and around the base of the cranial spinous process (**TECH FIG 2B**).
  - One end of this wire is similarly passed through and around the base of the caudal spinous process so that both the ends of the wire end up on the same side of the spine.
- A plate of corticocancellous bone graft is harvested from the iliac crest and divided into halves.

- The graft should be long enough to extend from the superior edge of the cephalad lamina to the inferior edge of the caudal lamina within the fusion levels.
  - The cancellous surface of this bone is placed on the decorticated laminae on either side of the spinous process.
  - The free ends of the wire are then tightened over the graft (**TECH FIG 2C**).
- Additional cancellous bone graft is placed over the decorticated laminae and spinous processes and within the facet joint at the fusion levels.

Triple Wire Technique

- The wire or cable selected is passed through and around the spinous processes at the cephalad and caudal ends of the fusion levels, as with routine interspinous wiring.

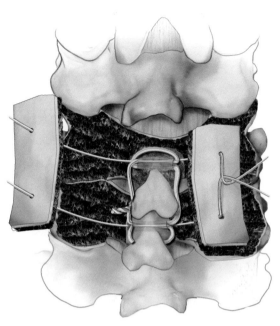

span the fusion construct and wide enough to cover the decorticated laminae within the fusion levels.

- Two- to 3-mm drill holes are created in the proximal and distal portions of the harvested bone grafts.
  - Two additional 22-gauge wires are passed through the holes in the proximal and distal spinous processes.
  - These wires are then passed on either side through the holes made in the bone graft.
  - The wires are tightened over the grafts on both sides to hold the bone graft rigidly against the decorticated lamina and spinous process (TECH FIG 3).

Oblique Wiring

- A periosteal elevator is carefully inserted into the facet joint to slightly distract and clearly identify the plane of the facet joint.
- A 2-mm drill bit is used to make a channel in the sagittal plane through the midportion of the inferior articular process, exiting through the articular surface into the joint.
  - The periosteal elevator within the joint confirms penetration by the drill and prevents overpenetration by the drill (TECH FIG 4A).
- A 20-gauge wire or cable is passed through this drill hole and is guided distally through and out of the facet joint using a periosteal elevator in a "shoehorn" fashion.
  - One end of the wire is then passed either around or through a hole in the intact spinous process of the vertebra one or two levels caudal to the level of injury.
  - This procedure is done bilaterally, and the free ends of the ipsilateral wires are twisted together to the appropriate tension (TECH FIG 4B). The absence of

TECH FIG 3 • Triple wiring technique. After simple interspinous wiring, additional wires are passed through the cranial and caudal spinous processes at the levels selected for fusion. These wires are used to firmly hold corticocancellous plates of bone graft against the decorticated laminae at the fusion levels.

- A pair of corticocancellous plates of bone graft including the full thickness of the cancellous bone of the iliac crest but excluding the inner cortical table is harvested from the posterior iliac crest.
  - The length of the bone block should be adequate to

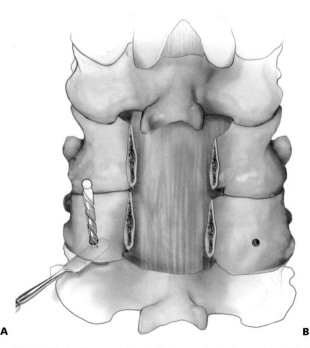 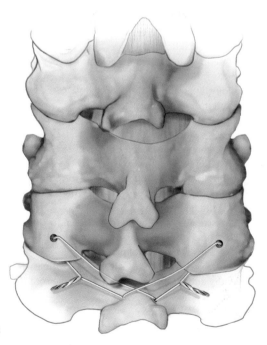

A   B

TECH FIG 4 • Facet wiring techniques. **A.** A channel is drilled in the sagittal plane through the midportion of the inferior articular process, exiting through the articular surface into the joint. A periosteal elevator held within the joint space prevents overpenetration by the drill and can be used to guide the wire out through the joint space. **B.** Facet wires may be obliquely looped around the spinous process when the lamina is deficient at a level.

laminae or spinous processes is often a reason to consider oblique wiring over interspinous wiring.

■ Supplemental midline interspinous or triple wiring is frequently added when the bony anatomy permits.

Multilevel Buttress Facet Wiring

■ Posterior stabilization after multilevel laminectomy can also be obtained by posterolateral facet fusion with multilevel facet wiring.[8]

■ Oblique facet wires are passed bilaterally through the inferior articular processes at all facet joints included in the fusion.

■ Two wires are passed through a hole in the spinous process of the most caudal vertebra.

■ Rib grafts, iliac crest strut grafts, or metal rods have all been used with the multilevel facet wires (**TECH FIG 5**).[8,14]

■ The graft or rod is placed over the decorticated lateral masses and in between the free ends of the wires, and the wires are twisted together at each level to the appropriate tension.

Postoperative Immobilization

■ Rigid external bracing is recommended in all posterior cervical wiring procedures until solid bony fusion is obtained. Six to 12 weeks of halo vest or rigid cervicothoracic bracing should be used after interspinous or oblique wiring, depending on the stability of the construct and the number of levels included in the fusion.

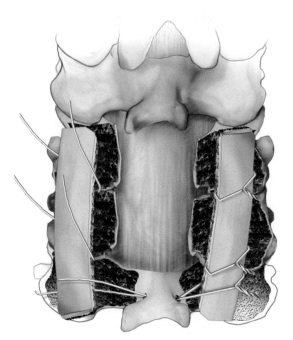

TECH FIG 5 • Facet wires may be tightened over rib grafts bilaterally in cases of multilevel laminectomy.

■ Radiographs should show a continuous fusion mass and absence of mobility in flexion and extension before immobilization is discontinued.

LATERAL MASS SCREW FIXATION

■ The quadrilateral posterior surface of the lateral mass is clearly exposed.

■ A ridge between the lamina and lateral mass identifies the medial border.

■ The lateral edge of the lateral mass can be easily palpated.

■ The joint lines above and below delineate the superior and inferior borders.

■ The center of the quadrilateral posterior surface of the lateral mass is identified.

■ Several techniques have been described for lateral mass screw insertion.

■ Roy-Camille et al[30] proposed an entry point for the lateral mass screw at the center of the posterior surface of the lateral mass.

■ The screw is directed perpendicular to the posterior surface of the lateral mass, angled laterally 10 degrees to the sagittal plane.

■ This trajectory aims to exit lateral to the vertebral artery and inferior to the exiting nerve root (**TECH FIG 6A–C**).

■ Magerl et al[25] proposed an entry point 1 mm medial to the center of the posterior surface of the lateral mass.

■ The screw is directed parallel to the plane of the facet joint with 25 degrees of lateral angulation in the axial plane.

■ Magerl et al recommended inserting a needle into the facet joint to determine the plane of the joint.

■ We use lateral-plane fluoroscopy to determine the direction of the screw in the sagittal plane, aiming to keep the screw parallel to and between the articular surfaces of the lateral mass.

■ This trajectory aims to exit lateral to the vertebral artery and superior to the exiting nerve root (**TECH FIG 6D,E**).

■ A modification of the Magerl et al technique by An et al[5] uses a similar starting point but recommends angling the screw 30 degrees laterally in the axial plane and 15 degrees cranially in the sagittal plane.

■ This trajectory again aims to exit lateral to the vertebral artery and superior to the exiting nerve root at the junction of the transverse process and the lateral mass.

■ Lining up the screw heads for subsequent fixation to the rod is easier if the most proximal and distal screws are inserted initially, followed by the screws in between.

■ Most current instrumentation systems use a rod to connect the screws after they have been precisely positioned and inserted into the lateral mass.

■ Polyaxial screw heads compensate for minor variations in insertion or anatomy.

■ The rods can be contoured in multiple planes and allow for application of compressive, distractive, and rotatory forces for correction of deformity.

■ A rod–screw construct can easily be extended to the occipital and thoracic region.

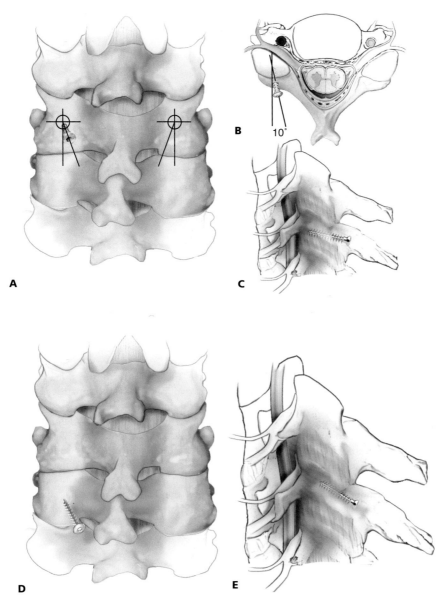

TECH FIG 6 • Lateral mass screw insertion techniques. **A–C.** In the Roy-Camille method, the entry point is at the center of the posterior surface of the lateral mass, with the screw directed perpendicular to the posterior surface of the lateral mass and angled laterally 10 degrees to the sagittal plane. **D,E.** In the Magerl technique, the entry point is 1 mm medial to the center of the posterior surface of the lateral mass, and the screw is directed parallel to the plane of the facet joint and angled laterally 25 degrees to the sagittal plane.

- Bicortical screws should be considered in certain cases:
  - Patients with rheumatoid arthritis or metastatic bone tumors in whom bone quality may be suboptimal.

- Longer fixation constructs extending to the occipital or thoracic regions, to reduce the chances of implant pullout.

PEDICLE SCREW FIXATION OF THE CERVICAL SPINE

Insertion of Pedicle Screws from C3 to C7

- Preoperative radiographs and CT images should be reviewed to assess pedicle dimensions and orientation and to confirm the feasibility of obtaining intraoperative radiographs; this is especially important in patients with short, stocky necks.

- Inserting pedicle screws before decompression allows better identification of morphologic landmarks and reduces the risk of inadvertent injury to an exposed spinal cord during the insertion process.
- The most commonly used technique relies on identification of topographic landmarks combined with fluoroscopy.[1]
- The entry point to the pedicle is 1 to 2 mm inferior to the caudal edge of the inferior articular process and 2 to

- 3 mm lateral to the midline or 2 to 3 mm medial to the lateral edge of the lateral mass.
  - Occasionally, degenerative changes at the joint may obscure true landmarks.
- The dorsal cortex of the lateral mass is penetrated using a high-speed burr.
  - The cancellous bone of the pedicle in many cases can be visualized in this pilot hole.
- A blunt, fine pedicle probe is advanced through this cancellous bone to find the medially angled pedicle (**TECH FIG 7A**).
- Fluoroscopy is used to guide the trajectory in the sagittal plane.
  - In general, the screws should be parallel to the superior endplate of the vertebral body from C5 to C7 and angled slightly rostral to the endplate from C2 to C4.
- Some authors recommend that a keyhole laminoforaminotomy be performed after locating the entry point.[4]
  - The superior and medial walls of the pedicle are directly palpated through this foraminotomy with a right-angled nerve hook to direct the trajectory of the pedicle probe (**TECH FIG 7B**).
- The pilot hole is tapped before inserting the screw.
  - Size 3.5- or 4-mm screws are generally used, based on preoperative imaging of pedicle dimensions.
  - Small pedicle diameters may require a 2.7-mm screw.[19]
- The length of the screw ranges from 18 to 26 mm, depending on the length of the pedicle as determined on preoperative CT scans.
  - The screw should be inserted to a depth no longer than two thirds of the anteroposterior width of the vertebral body, as confirmed on the lateral fluoroscopy image.
  - Since the C7 pedicle is longer, a screw up to 30 mm can usually be inserted at this level.
- Computer-assisted image guidance systems have been used for pedicle screw insertion in the cervical spine.
  - Preoperative CT data are used by the computer-assisted system to prepare a three-dimensional model of the vertebra.
  - After registration of surface landmarks during surgery, a registered probe or drill bit can be used to locate the entry point and guide a fine drill bit through the pedicle into the vertebral body.

C2 Pedicle Screw Insertion

- The entry point for the C2 pedicle is located on the superior medial quadrant of the posterior aspect of the lateral mass of C2, 3 mm lateral to the medial edge of the isthmus, and in line with or slightly distal to the superior margin of the C2 lamina.
  - The cortex is penetrated with a 3-mm burr.
  - The underlying cancellous bone is probed with a fine curette or pedicle probe to locate the pedicle channel.
  - The entry point and trajectory for subsequent drilling are confirmed by palpating the medial and superior margins of the C2 pedicle with a Penfield probe, and with fluoroscopy to determine sagittal angulation.
  - The drill is generally angled 15 to 25 degrees medially and 20 to 30 degrees cranially.
  - The integrity of the drilled hole is verified with a blunt probe and tapped, and a 3.5- to 4.0-mm screw is inserted.
- Twenty- to 22-mm screw lengths are generally used. C2 pedicle screws longer than 24 mm are likely to penetrate the anterior surface of the vertebral body and may provide superior fixation in some situations.[28]
- Using a polyaxial screw head allows easier compensation for the difference in medial angulation between the C2 and other subaxial pedicles when connecting to a rod.

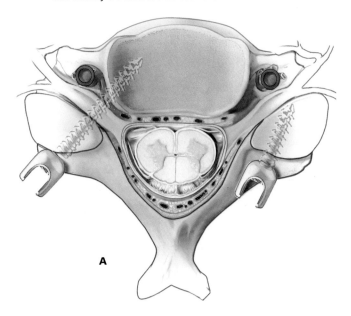

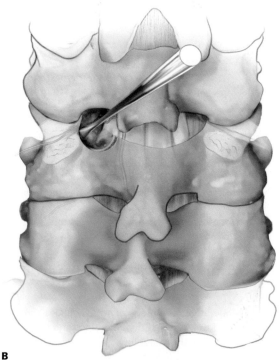

TECH FIG 7 • A. Comparative trajectories of cervical pedicle screw and lateral mass screw in the axial plane. **B.** Palpation of the superior and medial pedicle walls through the laminoforaminotomy window helps determine the trajectory of the pedicle probe.

PEARLS AND PITFALLS

Posterior cervical fusion	▪ The surgeon should ensure meticulous decortication of the laminae and spinous processes within the fusion levels. ▪ Facet joint cartilage should be resected at fused levels.
Posterior cervical instrumentation	▪ We prefer to insert lateral mass or pedicle screws before neural decompression. This allows better identification of morphologic landmarks and offers a degree of protection against inadvertent injury to the spinal cord.
Posterior wiring techniques	▪ Drill holes should be positioned at the proximal aspect of the cephalad spinous process and the distal aspect of the caudad spinous process to allow greater purchase of the wires in bone. ▪ Wires should be positioned dorsal to the spinolaminar line.
Lateral mass fixation	▪ Preoperative templating allows selection of appropriate screw length to minimize the risk of spinal nerve injury. ▪ Linking the screws to the rod is easier if the most proximal and distal screws are inserted initially, followed by the screws in between.
Pedicle screw fixation	▪ Pedicle screw dimensions and orientation should be identified on preoperative imaging studies. ▪ Osteophytes can distort bony margins and should be resected to allow identification of morphologic landmarks for screw insertion. ▪ A burr is used to expose cancellous bone at the pedicle screw insertion point. A blunt, fine pedicle probe is advanced through this cancellous bone to find the medially angled pedicle. ▪ The screw should be inserted to a depth no greater than two thirds of the anteroposterior width of the vertebral body.

OUTCOMES

Posterior Wiring Techniques

▪ Long-term successful fusion rates of 94% to 96% have been reported with interspinous wiring techniques when used for trauma, degenerative conditions, and tumors of the cervical spine.[22,29]

▪ Weiland and McAfee[33] reported a fusion rate of 100% when a triple-wire technique was used for subaxial posterior cervical fusion in 60 patients.

  ▪ Two of the 60 patients required halo vest immobilization, while the rest fused with a two-poster orthosis.

▪ Cahill et al[7] reported stable fusion and acceptable alignment in all 18 patients with facet dislocations treated using bilateral oblique wiring.

  ▪ Fusion generally occurred within 3 to 4 months. No patients developed neurologic deterioration after wiring.

▪ Callahan et al[8] reported solid fusion in 50 of 52 cases with multilevel facet fusion done after, using iliac crests or rib graft for fixation along with facet wires.

  ▪ Two patients who failed to achieve solid fusion were followed up with regular assessments and did not require any further management.

▪ Fusion rates with interspinous wiring have been found to be comparable to those obtained from lateral mass plating.[23]

Lateral Mass Screw Fixation

▪ Ebraheim et al[11] retrospectively reviewed the radiographic and clinical outcomes in 36 patients treated with lateral mass plate–screw fixation for traumatic instability, post-laminectomy instability, or metastatic disease. Fusion occurred at an average of 3 months in all patients. One patient demonstrated postoperative neurologic deterioration, but this resolved with subsequent decompression.

▪ Fehlings et al[13] reported successful arthrodesis in 39 (93%) of 42 patients treated with lateral mass plate–screw fixation for

cervical instability at a mean follow-up of 46 months. Revision of posterior plating was required in two patients for a screw pullout. Another patient required supplementary anterior plating for progressive postoperative kyphosis.

Cervical Pedicle Screws

▪ Screw loosening or pullout has not been an issue with cervical pedicle screw use.

  ▪ Abumi et al[3] used pedicle screw–rod fixation after correction of cervical kyphosis in 30 patients and reported excellent correction and no adverse mechanical or neurovascular sequelae related to the pedicle screws.

COMPLICATIONS

Wiring

▪ The most common complication reported with interspinous wiring is loss of reduction and recurrence of the deformity.

  ▪ Loss of reduction is more common when posterior wiring is done across a level with fractured posterior elements by bypassing that level.[22]

▪ Osteoporosis or excessive tensioning of the wires may result in intraoperative or postoperative fracture of a spinous process.

▪ Wire breakage can occur with use of a single-strand wire.

  ▪ Use of multistrand cable reduces the risk of wire breakage.[18,34]

▪ Inadvertent passage of spinous process wire through the spinal canal can lead to spinal cord injury.

  ▪ Appropriate placement of drill holes at the spinolaminar line and avoiding a ventrally placed tract between the holes on either side should avoid this complication.

Lateral Mass Screw Fixation

▪ In a cadaveric comparison of different screw placement techniques, Xu et al[35] found that violation of either the dorsal or ventral nerve root was least likely using the modification of the Magerl technique described by An et al.[5]

- Clinical studies with lateral mass screw insertion have reported a 6% incidence of nerve root injury[17] and a 6% incidence of screw malposition.[15]
  - Three percent of the patients required screw removal for radiculopathy.[15]
- Screw loosening is reported to occur with a incidence ranging from 2% to 6%.[13,15,17]
- In addition to direct contact of the nerve root by the screw, radiculopathy can also occur from foraminal stenosis as the lateral mass gets pulled up to the rod during final tightening of the construct.
  - Precise screw length and placement and appropriate contouring of the rod should minimize the incidence of this problem.
- Vertebral artery injuries have not been reported after lateral mass plating.

Cervical Pedicle Screws

- The medial pedicle wall is the thickest, making medial perforation and spinal cord injury less likely.
  - The lateral pedicular wall is thin, increasing the risk of lateral perforation during pedicular screw insertion.
  - There is little to no space between the superior border of the pedicle and the superior nerve root, while there is a mean gap of 1.4 to 1.6 mm between the inferior border of the pedicle and the inferior nerve root.[36]
  - Thus, cortical perforations of the pedicle walls by the pedicular screws are more likely to damage the vertebral artery or superior nerve roots.
- Abumi et al[2] reported a 6.7% (45/669 pedicle screws) incidence of cortical perforation by the screw in 180 consecutive patients.
  - Three of the 180 patients developed screw-associated neurovascular complications, with two patients developing radiculopathy that resolved with nonoperative management.
  - One patient developed vertebral artery injury without neurologic sequelae.
- Kast et al[20] reported lateral cortical perforation with more than 25% narrowing of the vertebral artery foramen in 4 of 94 pedicular screws implanted in 26 patients.
  - No vascular or neurologic sequelae occurred with these breaches.
  - Three screws encroached on the intervertebral foramen; one of these screws was revised for a sensory radiculopathy.
- Kotani et al[21] reported reduced pedicle perforation when an image-guided system was used, while other authors[24] have not shown significant improvement in safety or accuracy with these systems.

REFERENCES

1. Abumi K, Kaneda K, Shono Y, et al. One-stage posterior decompression and reconstruction of the cervical spine by using pedicle screw fixation systems. J Neurosurg 1999;90:19–26.
2. Abumi K, Shono Y, Ito M, et al. Complications of pedicle screw fixation in reconstructive surgery of the cervical spine. Spine 2000;25:962–969.
3. Abumi K, Shono Y, Taneichi H, et al. Correction of cervical kyphosis using pedicle screw fixation systems. Spine 1999;24:2389–2396.
4. Albert TJ, Klein GR, Joffe D, et al. Use of cervicothoracic junction pedicle screws for reconstruction of complex cervical spine pathology. Spine 1998;23:1596–1599.
5. An HS, Gordin R, Renner K. Anatomic considerations for plate-screw fixation of the cervical spine. Spine 1991;16:S548–S551.
6. Barrey C, Mertens P, Jund J, et al. Quantitative anatomic evaluation of cervical lateral mass fixation with a comparison of the Roy-Camille and the Magerl screw techniques. Spine 2005;30:E140–147.
7. Cahill DW, Bellegarrigue R, Ducker TB. Bilateral facet to spinous process fusion: a new technique for posterior spinal fusion after trauma. Neurosurgery 1983;13:1–4.
8. Callahan RA, Johnson RM, Margolis RN, et al. Cervical facet fusion for control of instability following laminectomy. J Bone Joint Surg Am 1977;59A:991–1002.
9. Coe JD, Warden KE, Sutterlin CE III, et al. Biomechanical evaluation of cervical spinal stabilization methods in a human cadaveric model. Spine 1989;14:1122–1131.
10. Ebraheim N, Rollins JR Jr, Xu R, et al. Anatomic consideration of C2 pedicle screw placement. Spine 1996;21:691–695.
11. Ebraheim NA, Rupp RE, Savolaine ER, et al. Posterior plating of the cervical spine. J Spinal Disord 1995;8:111–115.
12. Ebraheim NA, Xu R, Knight T, et al. Morphometric evaluation of lower cervical pedicle and its projection. Spine 1997;22:1–6.
13. Fehlings MG, Cooper PR, Errico TJ. Posterior plates in the management of cervical instability: long-term results in 44 patients. J Neurosurg 1994;81:341–349.
14. Garfin SR, Moore MR, Marshall LF. A modified technique for cervical facet fusions. Clin Orthop Relat Res 1988;230:149–153.
15. Graham AW, Swank ML, Kinard RE, et al. Posterior cervical arthrodesis and stabilization with a lateral mass plate: clinical and computed tomographic evaluation of lateral mass screw placement and associated complications. Spine 1996;21:323–329.
16. Heller JG, Carlson GD, Abitbol JJ, et al. Anatomic comparison of the Roy-Camille and Magerl techniques for screw placement in the lower cervical spine. Spine 1991;16:S552–S557.
17. Heller JG, Silcox DH III, Sutterlin CE III. Complications of posterior cervical plating. Spine 1995;20:2442–2448.
18. Huhn SL, Wolf AL, Ecklund J. Posterior spinal osteosynthesis for cervical fracture/dislocation using a flexible multistrand cable system: technical note. Neurosurgery 1991;29:943–946.
19. Jones EL, Heller JG, Silcox DH, et al. Cervical pedicle screws versus lateral mass screws. Anatomic feasibility and biomechanical comparison. Spine 1997;22:977–982.
20. Kast E, Mohr K, Richter HP, et al. Complications of transpedicular screw fixation in the cervical spine. Eur Spine J 2006;15:327–334.
21. Kotani Y, Abumi K, Ito M, et al. Improved accuracy of computer-assisted cervical pedicle screw insertion. J Neurosurg 2003;99:257–263.
22. Lovely TJ, Carl A. Posterior cervical spine fusion with tension-band wiring. J Neurosurg 1995;83:631–635.
23. Lowry DW, Lovely TJ, Rastogi P. Comparison of tension band wiring and lateral mass plating for subaxial posterior cervical fusion. Surg Neurol 1998;50:323–331.
24. Ludwig SC, Kramer DL, Balderston RA, et al. Placement of pedicle screws in the human cadaveric cervical spine: comparative accuracy of three techniques. Spine 2000;25:1655–1667.
25. Magerl F, Seeman PS, Grob D. Stable dorsal fusion of cervical spine (C2-T1) using hook plates. In: The Cervical Spine. New York: Springer Verlag; 1987.
26. Montesano PX, Juach EC, Anderson PA, et al. Biomechanics of cervical spine internal fixation. Spine 1991;16:S10–S16.
27. Panjabi MM, Duranceau J, Goel V, et al. Cervical human vertebrae: quantitative three-dimensional anatomy of the middle and lower regions. Spine 1991;16:861–869.
28. Resnick DK, Lapsiwala S, Trost GR. Anatomic suitability of the C1-C2 complex for pedicle screw fixation. Spine 2002;27:1494–1498.
29. Rogers WA. Fractures and dislocations of the cervical spine: an end result study. J Bone Joint Surg Am 1957;39A:311–376.
30. Roy-Camille R, Sallient G, Mazel C. Internal fixation of the unstable cervical spine by posterior osteosynthesis with plates and screws. In: The Cervical Spine, ed 2. Philadelphia: JB Lippincott; 1989.
31. Scuderi GJ, Greenberg SS, Cohen DS, et al. A biomechanical evaluation of magnetic resonance imaging-compatible wire in cervical spine fixation. Spine 1993;18:1991–1994.

32. Ulrich C, Worsdorfer O, Claes L, et al. Comparative study of the stability of anterior and posterior cervical spine fixation procedures. Arch Orthop Trauma Surg 1987;106:226–231.

33. Weiland DJ, McAfee PC. Posterior cervical fusion with triple-wire strut graft technique: one hundred consecutive patients. J Spinal Disord 1991;4:15–21.

34. Weis JC, Cunningham BW, Kanayama M, et al. In vitro biomechanical comparison of multistrand cables with conventional cervical stabilization. Spine 1996;21:2108–2114.

35. Xu R, Haman SP, Ebraheim NA, et al. The anatomic relation of lateral mass screws to the spinal nerves: a comparison of the Magerl, Anderson, and An techniques. Spine 1999;24:2057–2061.

36. Xu R, Kang A, Ebraheim NA, Yeasting RA. Anatomic relation between the cervical pedicle and the adjacent neural structures. Spine 1999;24:451–454.

Chapter 6

Occipitocervical and C1–2 Fusion with Instrumentation

S. Babak Kalantar, Youjeong Kim, Maneesh Bawa, John Rhee, and John G. Heller

DEFINITION

The term *occipitocervical* and *atlantoaxial instability* encompasses a number of varied conditions that compromise the normal function of the O–C1 and C1–2 joints, resulting in either pain, spinal cord dysfunction, or the threat thereof.

▪ Instability can result from trauma, including fractures of the articular masses and occipital condyles, rupture of the transverse ligament, odontoid fracture, or Jefferson fracture. Nontraumatic causes include inflammatory arthropathy (most commonly rheumatoid arthritis), osteoarthritis, congenital anomalies, rotatory subluxation, tumor, and infection.

▪ Several methods have been described for stabilizing the atlantoaxial complex, as well as the occipitocervical junction including wiring techniques, transarticular screw fixation, plate and screw fixation, and screw and rod fixation.

▪ We describe our technique for occipitocervical plating; transarticular screw fixation; articular mass screw and rod construct to achieve atlantoaxial arthrodesis with C2 pars, pedicle, and translaminar screw fixation; and C1–2 wiring techniques.

ANATOMY

▪ The base of the skull is comprised of the external occipital protuberance, the occipital condyles (which articulate with the C1 lateral masses), and foramen magnum. Landmarks noted on posterior dissection are the posterior edge of the foramen magnum, the superior nuchal line, the inferior nuchal line, and the external protuberance (**FIG 1**).

▪ The nuchal lines serve as attachments to the paired neck muscles. The trapezius attaches to the superior line and the rectus capitis attaches to the inferior line

▪ The nuchal ligament attaches to the external protuberance.

▪ The thickness of the bone in the suboccipital region varies depending on location. In the midline, the internal occipital crest has a mean thickness of 8.3 mm at the level of the inferior nuchal line, increasing to a mean of 13.8 mm at the external occipital protuberance. The lateral bone is thinner, ranging from a mean of 3.7 mm at the level of the inferior nuchal line and increasing to a mean of 8.3 mm at the level of the superior nuchal line.[1]

▪ The first cervical vertebra, or the atlas (C1), is unlike any other in that it lacks a vertebral body and spinous process. It consists of an anterior and posterior arch connected by two articular masses, forming a ring that pivots about the odontoid process of C2 (**FIG 2A**).

▪ On each side of the cranial surface of the C1 posterior arch there is a groove for the vertebral artery, the first cervical nerve, and their associated venous complex (**FIG 2B**). In a small subset of the population, this groove is covered by an arch of bone, the ponticulus posticus. The resulting foramen is identified as the *arcuate foramen*.[2]

▪ The articular masses of C1 give rise to the superior and inferior articular facets, which are broad and articulate with the occipital condyles superiorly and the axis inferiorly. A synovial joint also is located between the posterior aspect of C1 and the odontoid process of the axis.

▪ The axis (C2) has thicker laminae and a larger bifid spinous process than the subaxial cervical vertebra. It is characterized further by an odontoid process that projects upward from the vertebral body. Lateral to the odontoid process, or dens, are the sloping superior articular surfaces, which articulate with the inferior articular facets of C1, forming the atlantoaxial

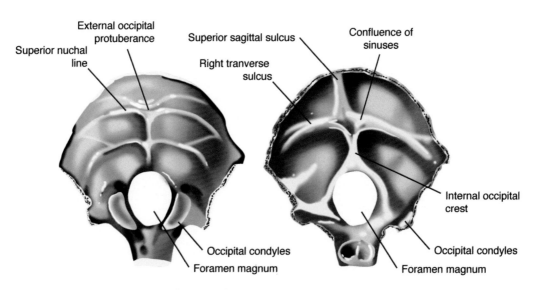

FIG 1 • Anatomic landmarks and features of the occiput.

joint. The C2 pedicle can be identified in a zone between the lamina and vertebral body, projecting superomedially (**FIG 2C,D**).

- O–C1 articulation: The kidney-shaped lateral masses of the atlas articulate cranially with the kidney-shaped occipital condyles. The joint allows for 15 to 20 degrees flexion and extension with 5 to 10 degrees of lateral bending.[3] Stability depends on the joint ligaments, the tectorial membrane, and the longitudinal bands of the cruciate ligaments.
- C1–2 articulation: The C1–2 complex is composed of three articulations—two laterally comprised of the inferior C1 and superior C2 articular facets, and one anteriorly between the dens and the posterior aspect of the anterior C1 arch.

  - The C1–2 articulation allows for 47 degrees of rotation to either side, which is approximately 50% of the lateral

rotation of the entire cervical spine.[4] Panjabi and associates[5] showed that in the healthy spine, C1–2 flexion is 11.5 degrees, extension is 10.9 degrees, lateral bending 6.7 degrees, and axial rotation to each side 38.9 degrees.

- The vertebral artery, which is the first branch of the subclavian artery medial to the anterior scalene muscle, ascends behind the common carotid artery. It then ascends through the foramina transversaria from C6 to C1. After traversing through the foramina transversaria at C1, the artery takes a sharp turn medially and posteriorly to course behind the C1 articular mass along the groove in the posterior arch of C1. It then passes through the posterior atlanto-occipital membrane before ascending through the foramen magnum as it merges with its counterpart to form the basilar artery (**FIG 2E,F**).

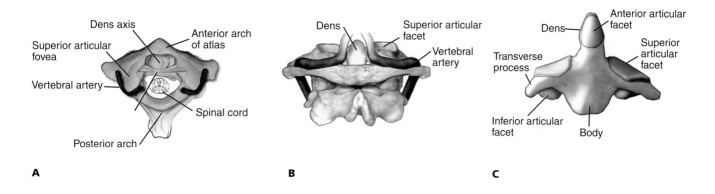

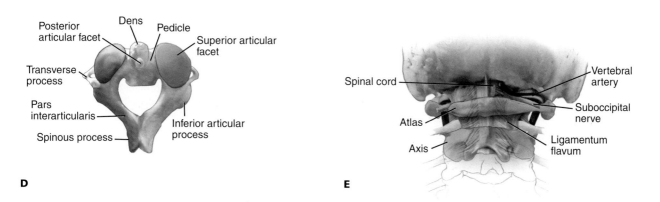

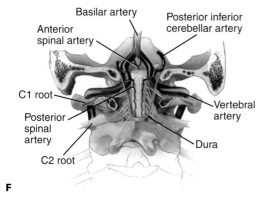

FIG 2 • **A.** The atlas consists of an anterior and posterior arch connected by two articular masses. **B.** Anteroposterior view of first and second cervical vertebrae. Anterior (**C**) and posterior (**D**) views of the axis, demonstrating the odontoid process projecting upward from the vertebral body. The pedicle connects the lamina and the vertebral body, projecting superomedially. The pars interarticularis lies between the superior and inferior articular processes. **E.** The vertebral artery ascends through the foramina transversaria from C6 to C3. It takes a turn laterally through C2 underneath the pars interarticularis. Once it traverses the transverse foramen at C1, it turns medially and lies on the superior surface of the C1 ring. **F.** After passing medially on the superior surface of the C1 ring, the vertebral artery passes through the foramen magnum and merges with its counterpart to form the basilar artery.

■ The C1 nerve root, or the suboccipital nerve, exits cranial to the posterior arch of C1 and innervates muscles of the suboccipital triangle. The C2 nerve root, or greater occipital nerve, exits between the posterior arches of C1 and C2, posterior to the superior C1–2 articulation. It does not exit through a true foramen like the remaining subaxial cervical nerve roots. It traverses inferior to the obliquus capitis inferiorly to ascend through the semispinalis capitis to lie superficial to the rectus capitis. Injury to the greater occipital nerve can lead to dysesthesia of the posterior scalp and can be troublesome to patients.

PATHOGENESIS

■ Stability of the O–C1 articulation relies on the ligamentous support and anatomic contour of the occipital condyles on the lateral masses of C1. Occipital condyle fractures may be stable or represent the bony component of an occipitocervical dissociation (OCD). OCD involves disruption of the ligamentous constraints resulting in an injury with high mortality rate.[6]

■ Stability of the C1–2 articulation relies heavily on its ligamentous restraints, including the transverse, alar, and apical ligaments, and the facet capsules. Trauma may disrupt these ligamentous restraints. Also, with the advanced degeneration found in arthritic conditions, these ligamentous structures may become incompetent.

■ Up to 3 mm of anterior translation of C1 on C2, as measured by the anterior atlantodental interval (AADI) on a lateral cervical radiograph, is normal. An atlantodental interval of 3.5 to 5 mm in an adult indicates potential damage to the transverse ligament, whereas an interval greater than 5 mm indicates probable injury to the transverse ligament and accessory ligaments (**FIG 3A**).

■ In cases of trauma, an atlantodental interval greater than 3.5 mm probably is an indication for further evaluation and most likely requires C1–2 arthrodesis.

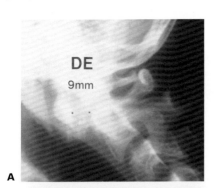

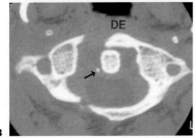

FIG 3 • A. An anterior atlantodental interval greater than 5 mm indicates likely injury to the transverse ligament and, in the setting of trauma, necessitates operative stabilization. **B.** An avulsion (*arrow*) of the transverse ligament from the ring of C1 indicates instability and may require arthrodesis of C1–2.

■ In patients with inflammatory arthropathy, including rheumatoid arthritis, a canal diameter identified as posterior atlantodental interval (PADI) smaller than 14 mm is associated with a worse outcome and is an indication for decompression and fusion.[7] The exact anterior atlantodental interval measurement is not as relevant in these patients as with trauma patients.

■ Fractures that involve the osseous structures of C1 and C2 also may result in atlantoaxial instability and require arthrodesis (**FIG 3B**).

NATURAL HISTORY

■ In the event of trauma to the occipital condyles, careful evaluation with CT and possibly MRI is indicated to rule out associated OCD. In the setting of an OCD, patient mortality can be high and operative management is recommended. Any translation or distraction at that level is an indication for intervention. Traction is contraindicated. Immediate immobilization followed by occipitocervical fusion is indicated.

■ In the event of C1–2 trauma, the potential need for surgery arises in the setting of ligamentous instability, fractures, or a combination of the two. Atlantoaxial instability due to rupture of the transverse ligament represents a threat to the cervical spinal cord with a low likelihood of successful healing. Thus, C1–2 fusion is indicated.

■ Transverse ligament disruption in association with a Jefferson fracture may represent an exception to this rule, in that successful nonoperative fracture treatment (halo vest) can lead to a "stable" C1–2 segment on flexion–extension radiographs.

■ Fractures of the odontoid process may represent a primary indication for C1–2 fusion if nonoperative means (eg, halo vest immobilization) cannot obtain or maintain an appropriate reduction, or if a patient elects surgery to avoid the use of a halo. Displaced odontoid fractures have an increased likelihood of resulting in either non- or malunion in the cases of type II and III fractures, respectively (**FIG 4A**).

■ Primary atlantoaxial osteoarthritis is quite painful and responds poorly to nonoperative means. C1–2 fusion affords a high likelihood of symptom relief (**FIG 4B**).

■ Cervical myelopathy due to either rheumatoid pannus or pseudopannus formation, as seen in older individuals with extensive subaxial spondylosis and spontaneous fusion, is unlikely to improve without fusion of the C1–2 segment (**FIG 4C**).

■ C1–2 instability due to rheumatoid arthritis may be neither symptomatic nor a neurologic threat. Thus, in this case, an ADI exceeding 3.5 mm is not, by itself, an indication for surgery. A PADI of less than 14 mm or the presence of myelopathy is a poor prognostic sign and indicates the need for surgery. Painful C1–2 rheumatoid involvement in the face of adequate medical therapy also indicates the need for surgery.

■ Basilar invagination or cranial setting of the occipitocervical junction due to rheumatoid arthritis can result in cervicomedullary cord compression. Especially in the presence of myelopathic symptoms, occipitocervical fusion with or without decompression is indicated.

■ Progressive C1–2 subluxation, especially with cranial settling, also has an unfavorable natural history. C1–2 fusion in this instance will obviate the need for a future occipitocervical fusion, which has a less favorable influence on the overall condition of the cervical spine (**FIG 4D,E**).

■ The natural history of asymptomatic C1–2 instability associated with miscellaneous conditions such as os odontoideum

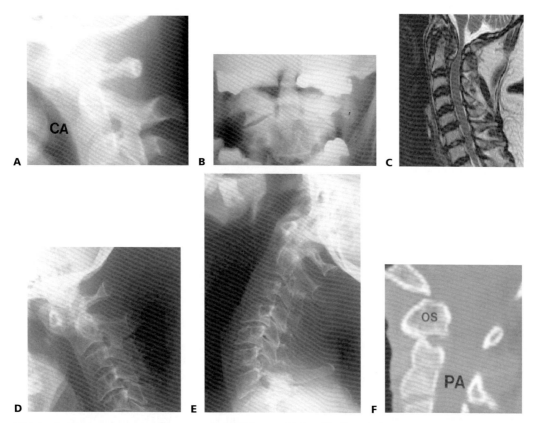

FIG 4 • **A.** Displaced odontoid fractures (type II) have a higher likelihood of a nonunion and may require a primary C1–2 fusion. **B.** Joint space narrowing is a sign of C1–2 osteoarthritis and responds poorly to nonoperative management. **C.** Pseudopannus formation behind the dens in patients with rheumatoid arthritis can lead to cervical stenosis and myelopathy. It rarely improves without surgery, but will dissolve after C1–2 fusion. Flexion (**D**) and extension (**E**) lateral radiographs demonstrate C1–2 instability in a patient with rheumatoid arthritis. **F.** Os odontoideum is another condition associated with instability in which part of the dens is not attached to the axis body.

(**FIG 4F**) and Down syndrome is less clear. When such patients have symptoms, myelopathic signs, or an insufficient PADI, the potential benefits of a C1–2 fusion probably outweigh the risks of the natural history. The patient's age, lifestyle, and activity level also must be considered in determining the need for surgery.

HISTORY AND PHYSICAL FINDINGS

- A complete history and physical examination, including a thorough neurologic examination, should be performed when evaluating a patient with occipitocervical and/or C1–2 pathology. The complaints offered will vary with the presentation (eg, trauma, inflammatory arthritis, developmental, congenital).
- Patients with a traumatic injury may complain of isolated pain but also may present with neurologic deficits. A low threshold of suspicion should be maintained for patients with blunt trauma to the head or face or with known noncontiguous fractures of the spine.
- Some patients with rheumatoid arthritis may complain only of axial neck pain, whereas others may present with deteriorating gait and bilateral hand numbness or clumsiness without significant neck pain.
- Patients with primary atlantoaxial arthritis will complain of severe neck and head pain, most often unilateral, with varying degrees of refusal to rotate their head, especially ipsilaterally toward the pain. Locking or crepitation of the affected joint may be both audible and palpable.

- Physical examination should include the following:
  - Active self-limited rotation of the head, especially toward the side of the pain. Normal rotation is up to 50 degrees of rotation to either side. C1–2 pathology often causes pain that limits rotation.
  - Palpation of the suboccipital area near the interval between the posterior arches of C1 and C2 may elicit pain. When asked, the patient often can point to the source of their pain.
  - Response to traction versus compression combined with passive C1–2 rotation. The patient is examined supine with his or her head resting comfortably on a pillow. Passive lateral head rotation is measured with slight manual traction. In cases of C1–2 arthritis, this maneuver should provide more motion and less pain than similar motion with an axial load. With slight manual traction, head rotation is increased, whereas an axial load may cause pain and result in decreased rotation.
- In the setting of potential traumatic instability, however, these examination maneuvers are not applicable. The cervical spine must be immobilized until the radiographic and CT findings are known.

IMAGING AND OTHER DIAGNOSTIC STUDIES

▪ In the setting of blunt trauma, plain radiographs of the cervical spine, specifically the upper cervical spine, have been shown to be inadequate. McCulloch et al.[8] reported that plain radiographs have a sensitivity of 52%, a specificity of 98%, a positive predictive value (PPV) of 81%, and a negative predictive value (NPV) of 93%, whereas helical CT had a sensitivity and specificity of 98%, PPV of 81%, and NPV of 93%. They concluded that although helical CT has limited ability to detect pure ligamentous injury, it is superior to plain radiographs when evaluating patients with high-energy trauma for cervical spine fractures.

▪ MRI scan is the most effective diagnostic tool for identification of ligamentous and other soft-tissue injury.[9]

▪ Patient-controlled flexion-extension plane radiographs may be beneficial in certain situations. However, studies have shown that even extensive damage to the intervertebral structures may inconsistently result in abnormal findings using this tool.[10] In addition, patient effort may play a role in the ability to obtain reliable results.[11]

▪ CT with sagittal and coronal reconstruction is done routinely for diagnostic purposes as well as for preoperative planning.

▪ Fractures of either C1 or C2 indicate a significant likelihood of additional cervical spine fractures. As many as 50% of C1 fractures may be associated with other fractures.

▪ A vertebral artery angiogram is recommended when there is any question of acute injury or history of injury to the vertebral arteries. A unilateral vertebral artery injury rarely is symptomatic because of sufficient collateral flow through the contralateral vertebral artery as well as the circle of Willis. A patient with a vertebral artery injury who presents with neurologic deficits due to a concomitant spinal cord injury may be especially difficult to diagnose clinically.

▪ We recommend imaging with either an angiogram or an MRA in all patients presenting with a significant flexion–distraction injury, fracture that extends into the transverse foramen, or facet dislocation (**FIG 5**).

▪ The method of treatment of vertebral artery injuries associated with cervical trauma remains controversial, especially with asymptomatic injuries. When discovered, symptomatic vertebral artery injuries may be treated with anticoagulation to prevent thromboembolic complications. If a surgical procedure is necessary, anticoagulation is stopped before and restarted after surgery.[12]

DIFFERENTIAL DIAGNOSIS

▪ Rheumatoid arthritis: instability, pannus accumulation, cranial settling
▪ Degenerative osteoarthritis
▪ Trauma: occipital condyle fracture, occipitocervical disassociation, articular mass fracture, odontoid fracture, Jefferson fracture, transverse ligament rupture
▪ Tumor
▪ Infection
▪ Atlantoaxial rotatory subluxation: recurring subluxation, irreducible and fixed subluxation
▪ Miscellaneous: Down syndrome, os odontoideum

NONOPERATIVE MANAGEMENT

▪ Stable occipital fractures can be treated with rigid cervical collar immobilization. Stable injuries are typically those that involve the occipital condyle without injury to the tectorial membrane or alar ligaments. Unstable injuries are those that involve occipital avulsion fractures or extensive comminution signaling ligamentous injury. These injuries need halo vest immobilization versus occiput to C2 instrumentation and fusion.

▪ In most instances, a hard collar is not adequate for immobilizing an unstable C1–2 articulation, but one may be considered in an elderly patient who is not a surgical candidate and otherwise cannot tolerate a halo or Minerva vest (Variteks, Istanbul, Turkey).[13]

▪ For certain fractures, use of a halo vest may be appropriate, and the patient is treated in the orthosis for 3 months. It is a time-tested "nonoperative" option with well-defined success/failure rates.

▪ Some patients may require a halo for postoperative immobilization, depending on the fixation quality, the anticipated level of patient compliance with a hard collar, and other unusual circumstances.

SURGICAL MANAGEMENT

▪ Occipitocervical fusion with plate and rod fixation is widely used and is described below.

▪ Several different techniques have been described for successful posterior C1–2 fixation and fusion.

▪ Before Jeanneret and Magerl[14] described the transarticular screw technique, posterior fixation was accomplished with Gallie's sublaminar wiring and grafting[15] or by the Brooks wiring method.[16]

▪ Some of the newer methods include the C1 articular mass and C2 pedicle screw and rod construct described by Goel and Laheri,[17] the use of C1 articular mass and C2 pars screw, and the use of C2 translaminar screw combined with C1 articular mass screw and rod construct.[18]

▪ Biomechanically, the Magerl technique of transarticular fixation provides the best stability compared with traditional wiring methods, but it may be technically more demanding than either the Brooks or Gallie method of fixation as well as C1 lateral mass and C2 screw fixation.

▪ Malreduction of C1–2, anomalous position or size of the vertebral arteries, and collapse of the lateral masses of C2 are

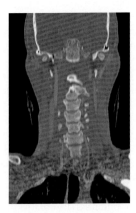

FIG 5 • Coronal reconstruction of a CT angiogram demonstrating occlusion of flow through the left vertebral artery (right side of the image) in a patient with a C4–5 facet fracture-subluxation.

relative contraindications to the use of the transarticular screw method because of the risk for inadvertent penetration of the vertebral artery.

▪ Because of the restrictions on screw trajectory through the C2 pedicle and C1–2 joint without endangering the vertebral artery, up to 20% of patients cannot have safe placement of bilateral screws using the Magerl technique.[19] Using C1 and C2 independently placed screws, more patients can receive rigid fixation in the setting of anatomic variations.

▪ The C2 pars and C2 pedicle are distinct structures. Placement of screws into either the pars or pedicle puts the vertebral artery at risk.

▪ C2 translaminar screws involve placement of polyaxial screws into the laminae of C2 in a bilateral, crossing fashion. This screw technique does not put the vertebral artery at risk and does not require fluoroscopic guidance. It does, however, require intact posterior elements at C2.[20]

PREOPERATIVE PLANNING

▪ All imaging studies should be reviewed with regard to osseous anatomy as well as the course of the vertebral artery. Preoperative CT scanning with reconstructed images in the sagittal plane or in the plane of planned screw trajectory is necessary to view the pertinent anatomy and to avoid injury to the vertebral artery. This should be in addition to standard radiographs to assess overall alignment and MRI to assess neurologic compression.

POSITIONING

▪ The patient under general anesthesia with an orally placed endotracheal tube is placed in the prone position.

▪ The head is rigidly held in place using Mayfield tongs or previously placed halo. The shoulders and arms are tucked at the patient's side. The torso is placed on vertical rolls or gel pads that allow for the abdomen to be free lowering the intraabdominal pressure.

▪ The table is adjusted into a reverse Trendelenburg orientation, with the knees bent and well-padded (**FIG 6**).

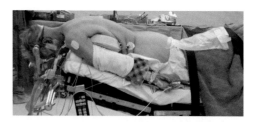

FIG 6 • The patient is positioned prone with the head flexed and posteriorly translated to allow the instruments to achieve the correct C1–2 trajectory. It is important to confirm reduction of an unstable C1–2 joint radiographically before proceeding further.

The shoulders can be depressed with wide tape if necessary to obtain a true lateral view of the C1–2 complex.

▪ After the patient is positioned, the proper alignment and anatomic reduction of an unstable C1–2 joint should be confirmed radiographically before proceeding further. Reduction is preferable to avoid vertebral artery injury, neurologic injury, and inadequate bony purchase of the screw. However, mild anterior displacement of C1 on C2 is well tolerated and may facilitate fixing the C1 lateral mass, as long as the PADI remains large enough to accommodate the spinal cord. It is important to confirm that the head is in neutral rotation, to avoid an iatrogenic torticollis. Visualization of overlapping of the mandibular rami and the C2–3 facets can aid in confirmation of a true lateral image.

▪ C1–2 reduction in most trauma conditions can be achieved with longitudinal traction in the awake patient. After successful reduction, a halo vest may be applied to facilitate prone positioning of the patient under anesthesia.

▪ The patient's hair should be shaved to above the occipital protuberance especially if occipitocervical fusion is planned.

▪ The occiput, posterior neck, and posterior iliac crest should be prepped and draped in standard fashion.

EXPOSURE

▪ A midline posterior skin and subcutaneous incision is made from the occiput to as far distal as necessary. For C1–2 fusion, the deep subperiosteal dissection is confined from the upper edge of C1 to the inferior margin of the C2 laminae (**TECH FIG 1**). For occipitocervical fusion, the external occipital protuberance should be exposed with full-thickness lateral and subperiosteal dissection of the muscular attachments of the trapezius and semispinalis capitis.

▪ When performing Magerl screw fixation, a longer skin incision permits the correct trajectory of the drill guides, which often are tunneled through the posterior cervical extensor muscles.

  ▪ A shorter skin incision could be used, with the drills, guides, and other instruments passed through percutaneous stab wounds, but we have found the cosmetic results less desirable.

▪ Muscular infiltration with local anesthetic and epinephrine will reduce bleeding.

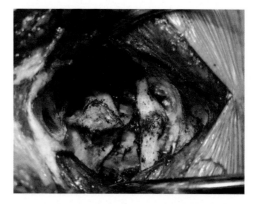

TECH FIG 1 • The posterior arch of C1 down to the inferior margin of the lamina of C2 is exposed with meticulous subperiosteal dissection.

TECHNIQUES

- Care should be taken to identify and dissect within the nuchal ligament. This will allow for a relatively avascular dissection to the spinous processes.
- The extensor musculature should carefully be dissected off of the C2 spinous process. The C2 spinous process should be preserved in a C1–2 fusion to allow for suturing of the extensor musculature back to bone through drill holes.
- The posterior tubercle of the atlas is palpated and musculature attached to the arch is detached with care on both sides. This is done to about 1.5 cm from midline

bilaterally to avoid damage to the vertebral artery located in the sulcus of the posterior arch.

- Dissection lateral to C1 and C2 should be limited to the zygapophyseal joint and not between as there can be significant bleeding from the venous plexus located at that level.
- A small-angled curette can be used to detach the soft tissues from the edges of the lamina of C2 and posterior arch of C1 for sublaminar suturing versus wiring at the end of the procedure.

OCCIPITOCERVICAL FUSION

- Posterior dissection is done by exposing to 2 cm above the occipital protuberance and 2 to 3 cm lateral to midline and down to the foramen magnum.
- Locate and palpate suboccipital midline keel and paramedian cranium. This will be the location of plate fixation.
- Midline screws offer the best bone purchase. Bicortical screws have 50% greater pullout strength than either unicortical screws or wires.[21]
- Size the appropriate occipital plate. Plate size should depend on the rod connection to suboccipital screws. Attempt should be made to minimize medial-lateral rod bending to meet the C1 or C2 screws by appropriately sizing the plate.
- Cranial thickness can be measured on preoperative CT; however, typical thickness for midline keel is 8 to 16 mm (thickest at the EOP, and progressively thinner proceeding caudally from the EOP) and 6 mm for paramedian screws.
- With the plate held in position, pilot holes are drilled using a handheld power drill with drill guides. Drill guides set to 6 to 8 mm are used for the central keel initially and can be increased up to 14 to 16 mm for maximal purchase at the external occipital protuberance. Smaller screws are placed distal to the EOP as determined by patient anatomy.
- Bicortical screws can be placed with care to maximize bone purchase. Occasionally, CSF or slow venous bleeding can emanate from screw holes. If this occurs, this is typically controlled with placement of the screw.
- C1, C2, and other subaxial screws are placed as described below and connected to the occipital plate with a rod and set screw construct.

- Decortication to bleeding bone of the arch of C1, posterior occiput, C2, and other fusion levels is completed using a high-speed burr. Bone grafting is performed using local bone and autologous iliac crest or rib, depending on the anatomic circumstances. Corticocancellous harvested graft can be secured between suboccipital bone and arch of C1 or C2 by performing a modified Gallie technique and heavy suture (**TECH FIG 2**).

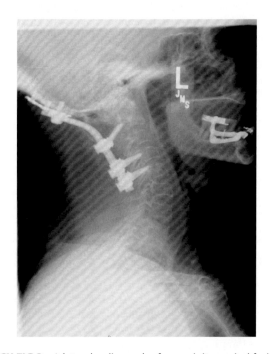

TECH FIG 2 • A lateral radiograph of an occipitocervical fusion.

MAGERL METHOD OF C1–2 TRANSARTICULAR SCREW FIXATION[14]

- Sagittal and axial CT images are scrutinized preoperatively. The isthmus of the C2 pars must measure at least 4.5 mm in height and width to accommodate a transarticular screw.[22] An abnormally large or malpositioned vertebral artery might lead to increased risk of harm to this important structure.
- C1–2 reduction and the ability to obtain a true lateral view of C1–2 with a fluoroscope are confirmed.

- A midline incision is made from the occiput far enough caudally to allow a steep enough angulation of the drill and other instruments.
- Posterior C1 and C2 exposure is carried out laterally to visualize the superior and medial surfaces of the C2 pars. Care also should be taken to avoid disturbing the C2–3 facet capsule.

- The starting point for the transarticular screw is at the posterior cortex of the C2 inferior articular process 2 mm cephalad and 2 to 3 mm lateral to the medial border of the C2–3 facet joint.
- The starting point is confirmed with a direct lateral C-arm image and marked with a 2-mm burr to provide a secure starting point for the tip of the drill bit. Caudal–cranial angulation is determined via lateral C-arm fluoroscopic guidance. The sagittal plane orientation is confirmed visually with reference to the superior and medial surfaces of the C2 pars. A Penfield 4 dissector can be placed on the dorsal surface of the C2 pars to serve as a guide on the lateral fluoroscopy view.
- The K-wire is directed superiorly along the C2 pars while aiming toward the anterior arch of C1 as seen on the lateral fluoroscopic images, with slight medial angulation

of 0 to 10 degrees (**TECH FIG 3A,B**). Advance the drill or wire slowly with frequent fluoroscopic visualization.
- We recommend leaving the drill bit or K-wire in place on the initial side to transfix the C1–2 joint, then proceeding to the opposite side. The screw on the second side is inserted before returning to the initial side to remove the drill bit, then tap and insert the second screw. This avoids any problems with loss of reduction (**TECH FIG 3C–F**).
- Bone grafting is performed with autologous iliac crest. After careful decortication of the posterior arches, a modified Gallie technique is employed using either heavy suture or braided titanium cable to secure the graft in place (as described under Gallie Method of Sublaminar Wiring and Grafting).
- The extensors at C2 are repaired with drill holes placed through the spinous process.

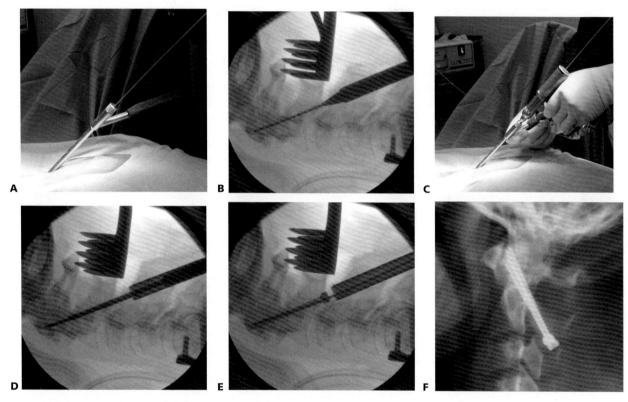

TECH FIG 3 • **A,B.** The guidewire is placed superiorly through the pars, aiming toward the anterior arch of C1 on lateral fluoroscopic images. With the first guidewire in place, a second guidewire is placed on the other side. The K-wire is overdrilled with a drill bit (**C,D**) and tapped, and the screw is placed on the second side (**E**) before the same is done on the first side. **F.** Postoperative radiograph of transarticular screw fixation in a patient who sustained a C1–2 fracture-dislocation.

HARMS/GOEL METHOD OF C1 ARTICULAR MASS FIXATION[17]

- The ponticulus posticus is a common anomaly that can easily be mistaken for a broad posterior arch of the atlas, and the lateral radiograph must be reviewed to check for the presence of an arcuate foramen to avoid injuring the vertebral artery.[23]
- The starting point for the C1 screw is in the middle of the junction of the C1 posterior arch and the midpoint of the posterior inferior part of the C1 lateral mass. The entry point is marked with a 2-mm high-speed burr (**TECH FIG 4**).

- The C2 nerve root is retracted in a caudal direction for proper screw placement. If divided, the patient may experience troubling neuralgia and numbness postoperatively.
- The initial drill hole is made in a straight or slightly convergent trajectory in the sagittal plane and parallel to the plane of the C1 posterior arch in the coronal plane, with the tip of the drill aimed toward the anterior arch of C1 (**TECH FIG 5A**).

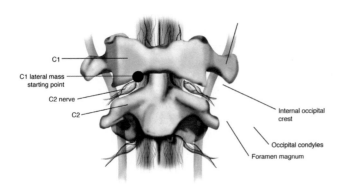

TECH FIG 4 • C1 lateral mass starting point.

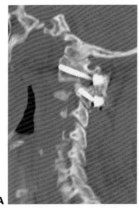 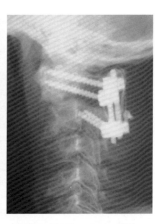

TECH FIG 5 • Postoperative CT scan (**A**) and lateral radiograph (**B**) of a patient with a displaced, kyphotic, chronic C2 fracture who underwent C1–2 posterior fusion using C1 articular mass screws and C2 pars screws.

- The hole is tapped and measured, and a 3.5-mm polyaxial screw of appropriate length is placed allowing the polyaxial portion of the screw to lie above the arch of C1. An 8-mm unthreaded portion of the C1 screw will also stay above the lateral mass to avoid any irritation to the greater occipital nerve.
- Care should be taken when dissecting around the C1–2 articulation to avoid excessive bleeding from the epidural venous plexus in this area. Hemostasis can be achieved using bipolar electrocautery, powdered Gelfoam with thrombin, and cotton pledgets.
- The center of the lateral mass of C1 is the ideal exit point of the C1 lateral mass screw, and the proximity of the

internal carotid artery (ICA) places it in danger when placing a bicortical screw. The ICA can vary in location from side to side and may be within 1 mm of the ideal exit point of a bicortical transarticular screw or a C1 lateral mass screw.[24]
- Medial angulation of the screw in the lateral mass of C1 may increase the margin of safety for the ICA, but care should be taken to avoid penetrating the occipitocervical joint by aiming caudally.

C2 PEDICLE/PARS SCREW PLACEMENT

- The starting point of the C2 pedicle is in the midline of the C2–3 facet joint, 3 to 5 mm cranial to the C2–3 articulation. The trajectory is 25 degrees of medial convergence and is aimed 25 degrees cephalad, while keeping in mind that individual anatomy will vary (**TECH FIG 6A**).
- The starting point of the C2 pars screw is 2 mm superior and lateral to the inferior C2–3 articulation. It is placed in a craniocaudal trajectory similar to the transarticular screw but does not need to be aimed as much cephalad. It is aimed 20 to 25 degrees medial (**TECH FIG 6B**).
- A no. 4 Penfield dissector is used to feel the medial border of the C2 pars interarticularis, and the superior and medial aspects of the isthmus are palpated during the drilling process.

- The drilled hole is then palpated with a blunt ball-tipped probe. The hole is tapped, and a 3.5-mm or 4.0-mm polyaxial screw is inserted.
- C2 pars screw length is typically 16 to 22 mm, depending on the anatomy of the vertebral artery and thickness of the pars. Preoperative CT will aid in estimating length.
- The polyaxial screw heads are connected with two rods. If necessary, a reduction of the C1–2 articulation is performed before fixation with the rods.
- The posterior elements of C1 and C2 are decorticated, and a corticocancellous H-graft is secured using a modified Gallie technique (**TECH FIG 5B**).
- The extensors at C2 are repaired using drill holes through the spinous process.

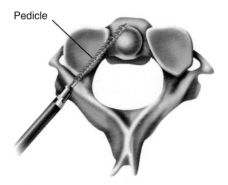 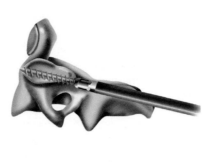

A **C2 Pedicle Screw**

TECH FIG 6 • Screw trajectory and correct identification of the pedicle (**A**) and pars (**B**) of the C2 or axis.

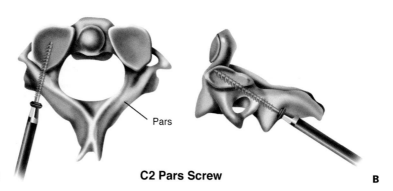

TECH FIG 6 • *(continued)*   **C2 Pars Screw**   **B**

C2 TRANSLAMINAR SCREW PLACEMENT[25]

- A high-speed burr with a 2-mm tip is used to open a small cortical hole at the junction of the C2 spinous process and lamina starting on the right side. This is done in the cranial half of the C2 lamina.
- A hand drill is used to drill the contralateral or left lamina with the drill aligned along the angle of that lamina. This is done to a depth of 25 to 30 mm. Care must be taken to allow the trajectory to be slightly less than the downslope of the lamina so that any cortical breakthrough would occur dorsally and not ventrally toward the spinal canal.
- A small ball probe is used to evaluate the drilled hole for any cortical breaches.
- Typically a 4.0 × 30 mm screw is placed with the head of the screw at the junction of the spinous process and lamina on the right. A smaller diameter screw may be

needed depending on the height of the lamina in order to accommodate two screws.
- Using the high-speed burr, a small cortical hole is made at the junction of the spinous process and lamina on the left in the caudal half of the lamina. Using a similar technique as described above, a 4.0 × 30 mm screw is placed in the right lamina with the screw head at the junction of the spinous process and lamina on the left (**TECH FIG 7A–C**).
- C1 lateral mass screws and/or subaxial screws are placed as described.
- The posterior elements of C1 and C2 are decorticated, and a corticocancellous H-graft is secured using a modified Gallie technique (**TECH FIG 5B**).
- If possible, the extensors at C2 are repaired using drill holes through the spinous process.

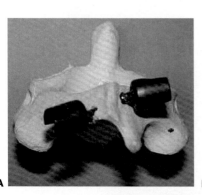
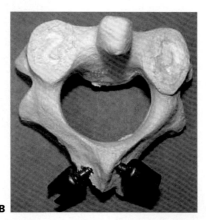
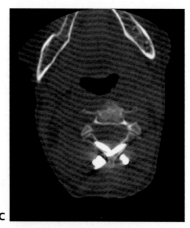

A   **B**   **C**

TECH FIG 7 • Saw bones model demonstrating coronal (**A**) and axial (**B**) appearance of the translaminar screw technique. Axial CT image of translaminar fixation (**C**).

BROOKS METHOD OF WIRE FIXATION

- Brooks wiring is the most reliable of the traditional wire fixation methods. It does not provide as much stability as other screw options, however, and so must be used in conjunction with significant postoperative immobilization, often a halo vest, for optimal likelihood of fusion.[16] It also requires passing sublaminar wires at C2, which can be technically demanding.

- Midline posterior subperiosteal exposure of C1 and C2 laminae is carried out with careful attention to dissect from midline laterally at C1 to prevent injury to the vertebral artery. The occipital nerves emerge through the interlaminar space between C1 and C2.
- The ligamentum flavum between C1 and the occiput and also between C1 and C2 is sharply divided. A Woodson

instrument is used to confirm that there are no dural adhesions in the sublaminar space.

- Although Brooks originally described the use of two doubled 20-gauge stainless steel wires passed under each side of the arch of C1 followed by C2 with the aid of a no. 2 Mersilene suture in a cephalad-to-caudal direction, we routinely use pairs of braided titanium cables rather than stainless steel wire.
- After the cables are passed with a loop at the end, two full-thickness rectangular bone grafts measuring approximately 1.25 × 3.5 cm are taken from the iliac crest. The sides of each graft are beveled to fit in the interval between the C1 and C2 laminae and placed on each side.
- The bone grafts are then held in place by securing the cables (**TECH FIG 8**).

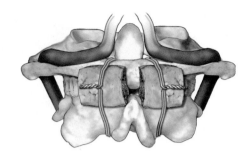

TECH FIG 8 • Brooks wiring technique.

GALLIE METHOD OF SUBLAMINAR WIRING AND GRAFTING

- The Gallie method is less stable than the Brooks method and is relatively contraindicated in the presence of any posterior C1–2 instability.[15] Biomechanically, this method provides minimal stabilization in rotation with only comparable stabilization in anteroposterior motion in response to motion.[26] It also requires significant postoperative immobilization.
- Dissection similar to that of the Brooks method is performed.
- A sublaminar wire or braided titanium cable is passed under the arch of C1 and looped around the spinous process of C2. We use a suture for this technique when the Gallie graft is employed in conjunction with Magerl transarticular fixation because the Gallie configuration is relied on for maintenance of graft position, not for mechanical stability (**TECH FIG 9**).
- A corticocancellous bone graft from the iliac crest (**TECH FIG 10A**) is taken and placed with the cancellous side facing down on the posterior elements after the cortical bone has been burred to reveal a nice bleeding cancellous bed (**TECH FIG 10B**). The small grooves are placed on the superior and inferior edges of the graft to hold the cables in place.
- The cable is tightened, and the graft is secured (**TECH FIG 10C**).

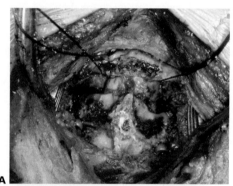

A

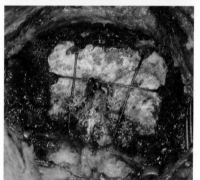

B

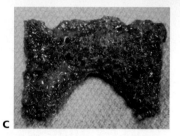

C

TECH FIG 10 • **A.** The posterior arches of C1 and C2 are decorticated. **B.** A corticocancellous graft is taken from the iliac crest. This is fashioned into an H shape, and the cancellous side is placed facing down on the decorticated posterior elements of C1–2. **C.** A modified Gallie technique is used to secure the graft in place.

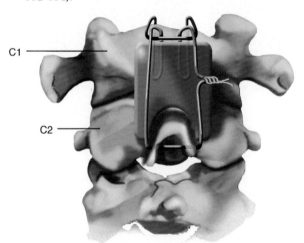

C1

C2

TECH FIG 9 • Gallie wiring technique.

PEARLS AND PITFALLS

Bone grafting	■ A Gallie H-graft is fashioned from the iliac crest and contoured to fit over the posterior arches of C1 and C2, with its cancellous surface applied directly opposing the decorticated surfaces of C1 and C2.
Frameless stereotactic navigation	■ This method registers only one vertebra, and the relation of C1 and C2 obtained on the CT scan may differ from that resulting after positioning on the operating table, resulting in aberrant screw placement and possible injury to the vertebral artery, whereas intraoperative fluoroscopy yields real-time information. Caution should be used in interpreting the information presented on the "virtual" images during surgery.
Injury to the vertebral artery	■ Careful preoperative planning will guide selection of the appropriate procedure to reduce the risk of injury. In the event of injury to a vertebral artery during a Magerl procedure, a short screw may be placed to contain the bleeding. If this occurs while drilling or tapping the first side, it is unwise to attempt a C1–2 screw on the contralateral side. An alternative fixation technique which does not place the contralateral artery at risk should be employed, such as a Brooks or Gallie procedure.
Venous bleeding in the C1 lateral mass	■ Gentle tamponade of the venous sinuses, along with application of hemostatic agents, is recommended. Once the surgical instruments are removed along with the pressure from the retractors, the bleeding is usually controlled with ease. Avoid indiscriminate use of cautery.
Supplemental wire/cable fixation	■ Supplemental wiring in conjunction with screw fixation methods at C1 and C2 provides no significant mechanical advantage. However, a suture configuration of a similar nature will hold the graft surfaces in proper apposition to the decorticated host bone, possibly improving the fusion rates.
C1–2 facet fusion	■ Originally described as a component of the Magerl procedure, direct exposure, decortication, and grafting of the posterior aspect of the C1–2 facets is not routinely necessary. It may be indicated for revision procedures, patients with incompetent posterior C1 arches, certain fracture patterns, or for high-risk hosts.

POSTOPERATIVE CARE

■ Whereas patients undergoing the Brooks or Gallie procedure obtain a maximal fusion rate with postoperative halo vest immobilization, the modern screw fixation methods yield fusion rates in excess of 90% with only cervical collars worn for 6 to 12 weeks.

■ The type of collar used and duration of wear should be in accordance with surgeon judgment about host bone, security of fixation, anticipated patient compliance, and so forth.

OUTCOMES

■ Jeanneret and Magerl[14] achieved solid fusion in 13 patients stabilized with the transarticular screw technique.

■ McGuire and Harkey[27] showed solid fusion in 8 patients using a transfacet screw technique.

■ Fielding and associates[28] achieved fusion in 45 of 46 patients with fractures using the Gallie technique.

■ Brooks and Jenkins[16] used a C1–2 sublaminar wiring technique to achieve fusion in 14 of 15 patients.

■ Harms[29] reported fusion in all 37 patients with C1 lateral mass and C2 pedicle mini-polyaxial screw and rod construct.

COMPLICATIONS

■ Vertebral artery and internal carotid artery injuries
■ Infection
■ Malpositioned screw
■ Nonunion
■ C2 neuralgia
■ C1–2 hyperextension with Brooks or Gallie procedure if the C1 and C2 arches are compressed together

REFERENCES

1. Roberts DA, Doherty BJ, Heggeness MH. Quantitative anatomy of the occiput and the biomechanics of occipital screw fixation. Spine (Phila Pa 1976) 1998;23(10):1100–1107; discussion 1107–1108.
2. Stubbs D. The arcuate foramen. Variability in distribution related to race and sex. Spine 1992;17(12):1502–1504.
3. Wang JC, Mummaneni PV, Haid RW Jr. Fixation options in the occipitocervical junction. In: Mummaneni PV, Lenke LG, Haid RW Jr, eds. Spinal Deformity: A Guide to Surgical Planning and Management. St Louis, MO: Quality Medical Publishing; 2008: 223–2400.
4. White A, Panjabi M. The clinical biomechanics of the occipitoatlantoaxial complex. Orthop Clin North Am 1978;9(4):867–878.
5. Panjabi M, Dvorak J, Duranceau J, et al. Three-dimensional movements of the upper cervical spine. Spine 1988;13(7):726–730.
6. Ben-Galim PJ, Sibai TA, Hipp JA, et al. Internal decapitation: survival after head to neck dissociation injuries. Spine (Phila Pa 1976) 2008;33(16):1744–1749.
7. Boden SD, Dodge LD, Bohlman HH, et al. Rheumatoid arthritis of the cervical spine: a long-term analysis with predictors of paralysis and recovery. J Bone Joint Surg Am 1993;75A:1282–1297.
8. McCulloch PT, France J, Jones DL, et al. Helical computed tomography alone compared with plain radiographs with adjunct computed tomography to evaluate the cervical spine after high-energy trauma. J Bone Joint Surg Am 2005;87(11):2388–2394.
9. Muchow RD, Resnick DK, Abdel MP, et al. Magnetic resonance imaging (MRI) in the clearance of the cervical spine in blunt trauma: a meta-analysis. J Trauma 2008;64(1):179–189.
10. Brown T, Reitman CA, Nguyen L, et al. Intervertebral motion after incremental damage to the posterior structures of the cervical spine. Spine 2005;30(17):E503–E508.
11. Hwang H, Hipp JA, Ben-Galim P, et al. Threshold cervical range-of-motion necessary to detect abnormal intervertebral motion in cervical spine radiographs. Spine. 2008;33(8):E261–E267.
12. Cothren CC, Moore EE, Ray CE Jr, et al. Cervical spine fracture patterns mandating screening to rule out blunt cerebrovascular injury. Surgery 2007;141(1):76–82.

13. Chaudhary A, Drew B, Orr RD, et al. Management of Type II odontoid fractures in the geriatric population: outcome of treatment in a rigid cervical orthosis. J Spinal Disord Tech 2010;23(5):317–320.

14. Jeanneret B, Magerl F. Primary posterior fusion of C1/2 in odontoid fractures: indications, techniques, and results of transarticular screw fixation. J Spinal Disord 1992;5(4):464–475.

15. Gallie W. Fractures and dislocations of the cervical spine. Am J Surg 1939;46:495–499.

16. Brooks AL, Jenkins EW. Atlanto-axial arthrodesis by the wedge compression method. J Bone Joint Surg Am 1978;60(3):279–284.

17. Goel A, Laheri V. Plate and screw fixation for atlanto-axial subluxation. Acta Neurochir (Wien)1994;129(1–2):47–53.

18. Gorek J, Acaroglu E, Berven S, et al. Constructs incorporating intralaminar C2 screws provide rigid stability for atlantoaxial fixation. Spine 2005;30(13):1513–1518.

19. Madawi AA, Casey AT, Solanki GA, et al. Radiological and anatomic evaluation of the atlantoaxial transarticular screw fixation technique. J Neurosurg 1997;86(6):961–968.

20. Wright NM. Posterior C2 fixation using bilateral, crossing C2 laminar screws: case series and technical note. J Spinal Disord Tech 2004;17(2):158–162.

21. Haher TR, Yeung AW, Caruso SA, et al. Occipital screw pullout strength: a biomechanical investigation of occipital morphology. Spine 1999;24(1):5–9.

22. Mandel IM, Kambach BJ, Petersilge CA, et al. Morphologic considerations of C2 isthmus dimensions for the placement of transarticular screws. Spine 2000;25(12):1542–1547.

23. Young JP, Young PH, Ackermann MJ, et al. The ponticulus posticus: implications for screw insertion into the first cervical lateral mass. J Bone Joint Surg Am 2005;87(11):2495–2498.

24. Currier BL, Todd LT, Maus TP, et al. Anatomic relationship of the internal carotid artery to the c1 vertebra: a case report of the cervical reconstruction for chordoma and pilot study to assess the risk of screw fixation of the atlas. Spine 2003;28(22):E461–E467.

25. Menendez JA, Wright NM. Techniques of posterior C1-C2 stabilization. Neurosurgery 2007;60(1 suppl 1):S103–S111.

26. Grob D, Crisco JJ III, Panjabi MM, et al. Biomechanical evaluation of four different posterior atlantoaxial fixation techniques. Spine 1992;17(5):480–490.

27. McGuire RA, Harkey HL. Modification of technique and results of atlantoaxial transfacet stabilization. Orthopaedics. 1995;18(10):1029–1032.

28. Fielding JW, Hawkins RJ, Ratsan SA. Spine fusion for atlanto-axial instability. J Bone Joint Surg Am 1976;58(3):400–407.

29. Harms J, Melcher RP. Posterior C1–2 fusion with polyaxial screw and rod fixation. Spine 2001;26(22):2467–2471.

Chapter 7

Cervical Disc Replacement

Michael Finn and Paul Anderson

INDICATIONS

- Single level symptomatic degenerative disease of the cervical spine including disc degeneration/herniation and osteophyte formation causing radiculopathy or myelopathy.
- Symptoms remittent to conservative care for >6 weeks or progressive neurologic deficit.
- Indicated for the treatment of levels from C2–3 to C6–7.
- Controversial in multilevel disease, adjacent level disease.

Expanded Indications (Off Label Use or Worldwide)

- Multilevel disease
- Adjacent to prior fusion or concurrent fusion (ie, hybrid construct)

CONTRAINDICATIONS

- Significant sagittal plane deformity (angulation >20 degrees)
- Instability (>3.5 mm of motion in flexion/extension or spondylolisthesis)
- Severe disc space collapse with limited range of motion (<2 degrees of motion)
- Significant facet arthrosis
- Ossification of the posterior longitudinal ligament (OPLL)
- History of fractures, infections, and tumors
- Osteoporosis
- Multilevel cervical spondylotic myelopathy

ANATOMY

- Familiarity with the anterior cervical anatomy is a necessity, particularly in regard to muscular, fascial, vascular, visceral, nervous, and bony structures (**FIG 1**)
  - Approach level can be estimated by overlying anatomy:
    - C3: hyoid bone
    - C4–5: thyroid cartilage
    - C6: cricoid cartilage, carotid tubercle
  - Muscular anatomy. The only muscle transected in the approach is the platysma, which lies superficially, just under the subcutaneous fat layer. The sternocleidomas-

toid extends from the mastoid inferomedially to the sternomanubrial articulation and provides a lateral border for the exposure. The omohyoid traverses the approach to the anterior cervical spine at approximately the C6 level and may be retracted or divided. The longus colli muscles lie on the anterolateral surface of the cervical spine and are more widely spaced caudally than cephalad. The position of the longus colli muscles is helpful in identifying the midline of the vertebral bodies.

- Fascial planes
  - Superficial cervical fascia lies just deep to the dermis and surrounds the platysma.
  - Deep cervical fascia
    - Superficial layer (AKA investing layer) forms a collar around the neck and contains the sternocleidomastoid, among other structures, and blends with the lateral aspect of the carotid sheath.
    - Middle layer is the muscular part that surrounds the strap muscles and great vessels whereas the visceral part (AKA pretracheal fascia) encloses the anteromedial structures of the neck (aerodigestive tract and thyroid gland). It blends laterally with the carotid sheath.
    - Deep layer is the prevertebral part closely surrounding the vertebral column and prevertebral muscles. The alar part lies between the prevertebral and pretracheal fascia and defines the posterior border of the retropharyngeal space.
- Vascular structures. The anterior and external jugular veins take variable courses superficial to the sternocleidomastoid and deep to the platysma. The carotid artery and internal jugular vein are contained in the carotid sheath and help define the lateral margin of the deep exposure. The vertebral arteries enter the transverse foramen at the C6 level in most (~90%) of the cases. The vertebral artery usually lies 1.5 mm laterally to the uncovertebral joints in the middle cervical spine, although this is somewhat variable. The course the vertebral artery takes is more medial, closer to the uncinate processes more rostrally.[1]
- Neural structures. The recurrent laryngeal nerve ascends from the thoracic cavity in the tracheoesophageal groove to innervate the intrinsic muscles of larynx, with the exception of the cricothyroid. The right recurrent laryngeal nerve arises anterior to the subclavian artery and takes a more anterior course in the neck than does the left nerve, which arises more distally near the arch of the aorta. Superiorly, the superficial laryngeal nerve crosses lateral to medial at the level of the hyoid to pierce the thyrohyoid membrane, at the level of the C3–4 interspace, and provides innervation to the cricothyroid muscle as well as sensory innervation to the posterior phaynx.[2,3] The spinal radicular nerve exits the spinal canal through the neural foramen at approximately a 45-degree angle to the cord in the axial plane.

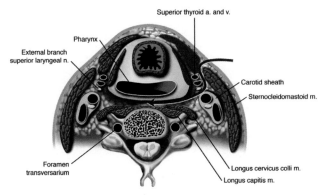

Superior thyroid a. and v.

Pharynx

External branch superior laryngeal n.

Carotid sheath

Sternocleidomastoid m.

Foramen transversarium

Longus cervicus colli m.

Longus capitis m.

FIG 1 • Cross-sectional view of the cervical spine with avenue of Smith-Robinson approach drawn.

- Bony and ligamentous structures. The anterior longitudinal ligament (ALL) overlies the anterior aspect of the vertebral column and is closely adherent to the intervertebral disc and endplate. The intervertebral disc lies deep to the ALL and is composed of a tough outer annulus fibrosis surrounding a soft gelatinous core, the nucleus pulposus. The annular fibers are attached to the subchondral bone of the adjacent vertebral bodies. The posterior longitudinal ligament (PLL) extends down the posterior aspect of the vertebral column. At each intervertebral space the PLL widens and becomes more fan-shaped. The uncovertebral joints, or uncinate joints, form from projections on the posterior lateral corner of the vertebral bodies and are often hypertrophied causing foraminal stenosis. Identifying the midline, which is essential in cervical arthroplasty, is aided by examination of the location of the left and right uncinate processes.

PATHOGENESIS

- Symptoms are usually the result of arthritic degeneration and can affect any mobile component of the spine
  - Facet joint: neck pain (not treated with arthroplasty)
  - Uncovertebral joints: foraminal stenosis causing radiculopathy
  - Disc space
    - Osteophytic degeneration can cause central stenosis and myelopathy or radiculopathy
  - Herniated disc fragments can be associated with significant inflammatory response and profound acute symptoms of radiculopathy or myelopathy.[4] Most common levels are C5–6 and C6–7.
- Risk factors for degeneration[5,6]
  - Genetic predisposition
  - Age
  - Tobacco use
  - Activity/occupation (heavy manual labor, exposure to vibrational stresses)
  - Obesity (body mass index >30)

NATURAL HISTORY

- The natural history of cervical radiculopathy is most often benign, with ~70% of patients having spontaneous improvement.[7–9]
  - Symptoms can recur or take on a intermittent course
  - Between 6% and 35% of patients require surgical intervention

- The natural history of myelopathy is less well known and most often has a course of episodic or steady decline while improving with conservative treatment in only a minority of patients.[10]
- Cases of mild myelopathy or asymptomatic stenosis may have a favorable prognosis but do require close follow-up.

HISTORY AND PHYSICAL FINDINGS

- Radiculopathy
  - Patients often present with dermatomal pain, sensory changes (numbness, paresthesias), and weakness (Table 1)
  - May have dull ache in neck, shoulder, and scapula
  - Cervicogenic headache is seen in over 80% of cases[11]
  - Often worse with extension, lateral rotation, and bending toward symptomatic side or when straining, sneezing, or coughing
  - Neurologic examination may be normal or reveal segmental weakness (myotomal), sensory impairment (dermatomal), and reflex deficit
- Myelopathy
  - More than 50% of patients may present without significant painful complaints[12]
  - Often presents as insidious decline of upper and lower extremity motor function
    - Clumsiness of hands
    - Gait instability
    - Sensory dysfunction
  - Physical exam can reveal
    - Weakness, often greatest in hands
    - Muscle wasting, often greatest in hands
    - Spasticity
    - Hyperreflexia with pathologic reflexes (Hoffman's sign, Babinski sign, and clonus)

IMAGING AND OTHER DIAGNOSTIC STUDIES

- Plain radiographs may demonstrate degenerative or age-related changes such as disc space narrowing, subchondral sclerosis, or osteophyte formation. Foraminal stenosis maybe visualized on oblique views. The overall alignment of neck and evidence of instability are assessed and are important determinants of treatment.
- CT more clearly delineates bony changes and may demonstrate bony foraminal compression. CT may be useful in evaluating for suspected OPLL when considering arthroplasty. CT myelography is useful in evaluating for the presence of neural

Table 1	Cervical Radicular Function		
Root	**Motor Function**	**Sensory Distribution**	**Reflex**
C3	Diaphragm	Upper neck	
C4	Diaphragm	Neck, upper shoulder, and chest	
C5	Shoulder abduction (deltoid) > elbow flexion (biceps) > external rotation of arm (supraspinatus/infraspinatus; diaphragm)	Shoulder, lateral arm to anterior forearm	Biceps, brachioradialis
C6	Wrist extension > elbow flexion > forearm supination	Anterior arm and forearm to thumb and index finger	Biceps, brachioradialis
C7	Elbow extension, wrist flexors > finger extensors	Lateral arm, dorsal forearm to middle three fingers	Triceps
C8	Intrinsics, thumb extension, wrist ulnar deviation	Back of arm to little and index fingers	Pronator

compression in patients who are unable to undergo MRI and in those who have been previously instrumented. Significant facet joint degeneration is a contraindication to disc replacement and is best assessed on CT. It has been recommended that a CT be included in the preoperative workup for cervical arthroplasty.[13]

▪ MRI is the imaging modality of choice for the evaluation of cervical radiculopathy or myelopathy and is sensitive in detecting disc herniations, osteophytes, spinal cord signal abnormalities, and central and foraminal stenosis.

▪ Other modalities including electrodiagnostic studies (EMGs) and selective injections may be used to clarify a diagnosis in difficult cases.

DIFFERENTIAL DIAGNOSIS

▪ Cervical radiculopathy
▪ Cervical myelopathy
▪ Tumor (cranial or spinal)
▪ Stroke
▪ Motor neuron disease
▪ Multiple sclerosis
▪ Syringomyelia
▪ Brachial plexopathy
  ▪ Parsonage-Turner syndrome
  ▪ Thoracic outlet syndrome
  ▪ Radiation plexopathy
▪ Peripheral nerve entrapment
▪ Musculoskeletal
  ▪ Shoulder disease (eg, rotator cuff)
  ▪ Myofascial pain syndrome
  ▪ Infection
  ▪ Tumor
  ▪ Tendinitis
  ▪ Inflammatory arthropathy
▪ Cardiac ischemia
▪ Chest pathology
▪ Reflex sympathetic dystrophy

NONOPERATIVE MANAGEMENT

▪ Nonoperative treatment should be attempted in most patients with radiculopathy
  ▪ Physical therapy or placement of a cervical collar have both been shown to be efficacious in acute (<1 month duration) symptoms and nonefficacious in cases of longstanding (>3 months) radiculopathy.[9,14,15]
  ▪ Medications
    ▪ Anti-inflammatory medications
    ▪ "Nerve medications": gabapentin, pregabalin, antidepressants
    ▪ Opioids, limited role
  ▪ Injections: Epidural steroid injection and selective nerve root block can be therapeutic and predictive of surgical outcome.[16,17] Long-term results indicate <20% responsiveness (unpublished data).
▪ Cervical myelopathy can be treated conservatively with a collar in patients unable or unwilling to undergo surgical decompression[18,19] or in mild cases.

SURGICAL MANAGEMENT

▪ Surgical intervention is indicated in cases of radiculopathy resistant to conservative care and in cases of progressive weakness.
▪ Surgical intervention is indicated for cervical myelopathy in the presence of a compressive spinal cord lesion.

▪ Cervical arthroplasty indications and contraindications are listed above.

Preoperative Planning

▪ Images should be thoroughly examined for anomalous anatomy, such as an aberrant vertebral artery course, and for other possible causes of the patient's symptoms. The depth and height of the disc space can be measured to estimate the size of the potential implant. Preoperative measurements should always be confirmed intraoperatively as endplate preparation will alter dimensions.

Positioning

▪ The patient is positioned supine with a small bump under the shoulders and the head in a doughnut in slight extension. A towel roll can also be placed behind the neck to offer support against rebound when placing the device. A radiolucent table is used to allow for anteroposterior and lateral fluoroscopy. The patient should not be placed in hyperextension but placed in a neutral position similar to that on the preoperative standing radiograph.

▪ The shoulders may need to be retracted inferiorly with tape to allow visualization of more caudal levels in large patients. If proper intraoperative imaging cannot be obtained then fusion should be performed. Overly aggressive retraction should be avoided to reduce risk of brachial plexus injury.

Approach

▪ A standard Smith-Robinson approach is used to access the anterior cervical spine.

▪ Upon initial exposure, the level of interest is confirmed radiographically and the midline of immediately adjacent cephalad and caudad levels are marked with Bovie electrocautery prior to elevation of the longus muscles (**FIG 2**). Using a marking

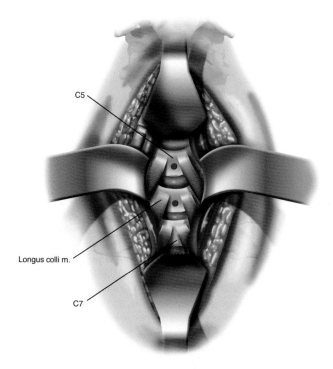

C5

Longus colli m.

C7

FIG 2 • Illustration showing exposure of the anterior cervical spine. The longus colli are used to identify the midline, which is then marked with Bovie electrocautery and a marking pen.

pen over the cauterized bone can help more clearly delineate and preserve midline markings.

■ After the midline is clearly marked, the medial border of the longus colli muscle is incised with the Bovie electrocautery and a longus flap is elevated. The longus should be elevated over

approximately one-half the height of the adjacent vertebral body with care taken to preserve the annular attachments of the adjacent level. A self-retaining retractor is placed underneath the flap.

■ It is essential to place the device exactly in the midline so its identification is essential for the rest of the procedure.

DISCECTOMY

■ The disc space is incised with a no. 15 blade scalpel and a partial discectomy is performed with pituitary rongeurs.
  ■ A 3–0 curette is then used to separate the attachment of the annular fibers to vertebral endplate at the lateral margins of the disc space.
    ■ The separation with the curette proceeds from lateral to medial and superficial to deep, allowing for the lateral aspect of the disc to be removed en bloc.
    ■ This technique allows for rapid identification and exposure of the uncovertebral joints, and thus the lateral margins of the exposure. The location of the uncinate process can be used to confirm midline location previously marked.
  ■ The disc is removed posteriorly to the PLL.

Use of Distraction: Pins, Tongs, Spreaders

■ Distraction posts may be placed before or after the discectomy, although placing posts after the discectomy allows better definition of the vertebral endplates and an improved understanding of their trajectory.
■ Although we place distraction posts in a mildly divergent trajectory when performing fusion, to reestablish cervical lordosis, we place them parallel to the endplates of the treated level in arthroplasty so as not to introduce hyperlordosis and to ensure the best orientation of the

implant. The ProDisc system has unique distraction posts which should be placed parallel to the adjacent endplate as outlined below.
■ The posts should be placed approximately two-thirds of length of the vertebral body away from the interspace, allowing for a sufficient working corridor at the level of interest.
■ Distraction about the endplate should be employed only to aid in visualization for neural decompression. Over distraction during implant sizing and placement may lead the placement of an oversized implant, which will have suboptimal mobility.

Endplate Preparation

■ The cartilaginous endplates are removed with care taken to preserve the integrity of the bony endplate as this structure will prevent subsidence. The cartilaginous endplates can be removed with curettes or the high-speed drill.
■ The inferior endplate of the superior level is usually concave in the sagittal plane, with an inferiorly protruding lip at the anteroinferior aspect, whereas the superior endplate of the inferior level slightly concave in the coronal plane. Milling the endplate flush is not necessary and may predispose the implant to settling, as the strong bony endplate will be violated.

FORAMINOTOMY AND OSTEOPHYTECTOMY

■ An aggressive foraminotomy is needed with arthroplasty as motion will be preserved and incomplete decompression will result in recurrent radicular symptoms. Furthermore, foraminal expansion by means of distraction is not utilized in arthroplasty as an oversized implant will result in reduced motion due to increased ligamentous tension.
■ The PLL is left intact for the initial foraminotomy to protect the underlying neural elements.
■ The high-speed burr is used to perform the majority of the foraminotomy. We use the burr with a horizontal back and forth motion to remove posteriorly protruding osteophytes from the uncinate processes. The burr can also be used in circular motion at the foraminal opening to enlarge the foramen. The burr should be operated under continuous motion and with frequent irrigation to prevent thermal injury to the underlying nerve root.
  ■ Final osteophytectomy can be accomplished with a small upgoing curette used in a rotational motion.

The cutting edge of the curette can be angled in to bone for safe removal with minimal intrusion into the foraminal space.
■ A small (2-mm) Kerrison rongeur can also be used to expand the foraminotomy. Care should be taken to angle the butt of the instrument directly against the thecal sac to minimize chances of injuring the underlying exiting nerve.
  ■ Small instruments should be used when enlarging to foraminal opening to avoid traumatic damage to the exiting nerve.
■ Adequate foraminal decompression is confirmed by placing a nerve hook out the neural foramen without resistance.
■ The high-speed burr can also be used to remove posteriorly protruding osteophytes. The burr should be angled to attack the junction of the osteophyte and normal vertebral body, to reduce the chances of drilling out the endplate, and more efficiently disconnect and remove the osteophyte. Final osteophytectomy can be

accomplished with an upward angle curette used in a twisting motion.

- Resection of posterior osteophytes can be confirmed by placing a nerve hook or upgoing curette posterior to the vertebral bodies and taking a fluoroscopic image. The

instrument should lie flush with the posterior aspect of the vertebral body (**TECH FIG 1**).

- Anterior osteophytes should also be removed, either with a rongeurs or a high-speed burr, to ensure flush fitment of devices with anterior flanges (eg, Prestige ST).

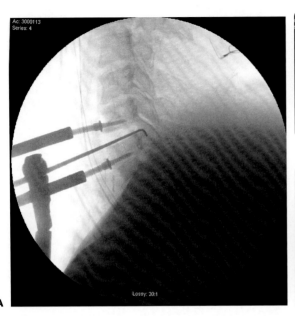 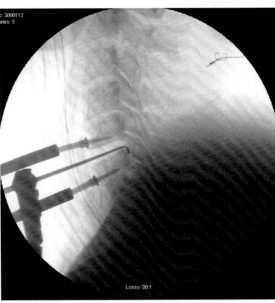

A   **B**

TECH FIG 1 • A. Fluoroscopic image demonstrating residual posterior osteophyte underlying nerve hook. **B.** Image after osteophyte has been removed, showing flush apposition of the nerve hook to the posterior vertebral body.

PLL RESECTION

- The question of whether to resect the PLL in all cases of cervical arthroplasty is controversial. You should check with the manufacturer regarding this question.
- PLL resection results in increased segmental motion without instability, which may aid the goal of arthroplasty.[20,21] PLL resection may further aid in the adequate posterior positioning of the implant, especially in cases of significant degeneration, and may aid in restoration of a physiologic instantaneous axis of rotation.
- PLL resection should be performed in all cases of posterior disc extrusion in which a fragment may be situated dorsal to the ligament.
- The first step in resecting the PLL is the creation (or identification) of a rent in the ligament allowing access to the epidural space. A rent may be present in cases of

posteriorly herniated fragments, whereas one can otherwise be created with an upgoing curette. The curette can be used in a rotational cephalocaudad fashion to slip between the fibers of the PLL and enter the epidural space.

- Once the rent is identified or created, it can be expanded with an upgoing curette. A small (2-mm) Kerrison can then be used to resect the ligament. Using the Kerrison at the intersection of the ligament and vertebral body ensures efficient resection. Care must be taken to minimize dorsal pressure on fragment herniated behind the PLL with the butt end of the Kerrison rongeurs. Care is also taken when resecting the ligament laterally to avoid grasping the exiting nerve root with the Kerrison rongeur.

IMPLANT SIZING AND SELECTION

Prestige ST (TECH FIG 2)

- The size of the implant can be estimated preoperatively by measuring endplate depth and height on the preoperative MRI or CT. As large a footprint as possible should be chosen. The disc space after endplate preparation is used to determine device height. In general, smaller

heights are better and more stable than large ones. If between sizes, select the one with less height.

- After decompression is complete, a trial spacer is used to confirm implant size. The spacer should slide smoothly into the disc space without distraction applied. If distraction is needed to place the trial, a smaller trial should be

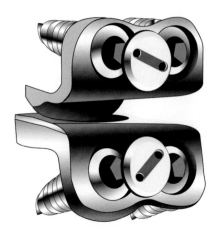

TECH FIG 2 • The Prestige ST implant.

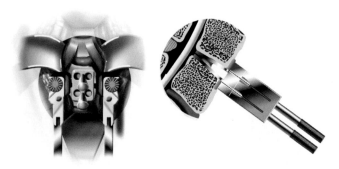

TECH FIG 4 • Anterior (**A**) and lateral (**B**) views of the implant inserted into the disc space, mounted on the inserter with incorporated drill guide.

placed or the endplates should be further milled. Care is taken to ensure midline placement of the trial, as marked previously. Final position is confirmed with biplanar fluoroscopy with anteroposterior (AP) views used to confirm midline position.

- Anterior osteophytes are removed with rongeurs or the high-speed burr to ensure that the implant sits flush with anterior vertebral body. The Profile Trial, which is angled to slide into the prepared disc space, is then used to confirm adequate anterior osteophyte resection and flush fitment of the implant (**TECH FIG 3**).

- Following preparation, the appropriate size implant is loaded into the loading block and inserted into the disc space. The implant is directional, with a slight cranial inclination, and should slide easily into the disc space although gentle tamping with a mallet is sometimes needed.

- Prospective screw tracts are then created using the drill placed through a guide in line with the holes in the insertion device. The 13-mm drill guide is typically used (**TECH FIG 4**).

- The drill guide is removed and the screws are then partially placed through the inserter. All four screws are then sequentially tightened and the inserter is removed. Locking screws are then placed over the screw heads to prevent backout.

- Final position of the implant is confirmed with AP and lateral fluoroscopy. Motion can be confirm by manipulating the patient's head through the drapes.

ProDisc-C (TECH FIG 5)

- The size of the implant can be estimated on preoperative imaging studies.

- Upon initial exposure, the midline is marked using the fluoroscopy. A lasting mark is made by using the Bovie to burn down to bone and then using a marking pen over this mark.

- The distraction screws are then placed in the distal one-third of the adjacent vertebral bodies. An initial perforation of the anterior cortex is created and then the screws are placed parallel to the adjacent endplates. The screws are placed under fluoroscopic guidance as deeply as possible. It is important to place the screws distally enough to allow for the implant keels to be placed between them (**TECH FIG 6**). The retainer is then placed over the screws and a partial discectomy is performed. The vertebral distractor is then placed in the disc space and the distraction is applied across the operated level. The distraction is maintained in a parallel fashion with the retainer and the distractor is removed.

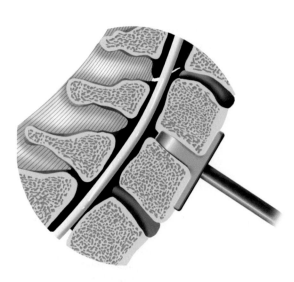

TECH FIG 3 • The Profile Trial spacer is used to confirm adequate milling of anterior osteophytes.

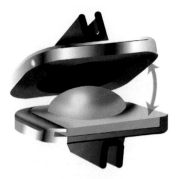

TECH FIG 5 • The Prodisc-C implant.

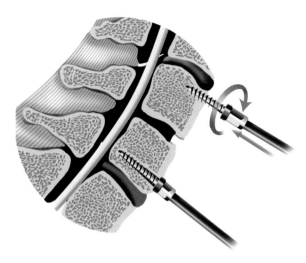

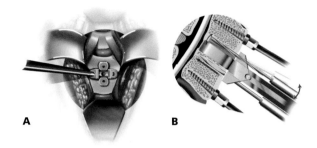

TECH FIG 8 • Anterior (**A**) and lateral (**B**) depictions of the milling guide placed over the trial. The guide sets the limits of bone removal to accommodate the implant keel.

TECH FIG 6 • The distraction posts are placed parallel to the adjacent endplates.

- The discectomy and decompression are completed. Trial implants are then placed into the disc space. The implant with the largest possible footprint is chosen. The trial should be inserted flush with the posterior aspect of the vertebral body in the midline. Distraction should be released and the trial handle is removed to leave the trial in the disc space. Care is taken not to overdistract the interspace, which may compromise implant motion. A 5-mm implant is most commonly selected. AP and lateral fluoroscopy images are then taken to confirm adequate position (**TECH FIG 7**).
- The milling guide is next placed over the shaft of the trial implant and secured with a locking nut. A retention pin is placed through the superior hole of the guide.

A power drill is used to create the inferior hole under fluoroscopic guidance. The drill is sunk to the level of the stop and then rotated to the limits of the stop in a cephalad and caudad angulation. The drill is removed, a retention pin is placed in its spot, and the process is repeated at the cephalad level (**TECH FIG 8**).

- The box chisel is next placed over the shaft of the trial and advanced into the vertebral bodies with a mallet under fluoroscopic visualization. Prior to impaction, it is confirmed that the trial stop is seated securely against the anterior face of the vertebral bodies. The box cutting chisel is next used over the implant. Prior to removal of the box cutting chisel, a small amount of distraction is reintroduced around the operated level through the distraction pins.
- Excess bone is removed from the keel tracts with the keel cut cleaner. Symmetric depth of the superior and inferior keel cuts is also confirmed—the posterior edge of both keels should be identical when measured from the posterior vertebral body wall. A position gauge can be used to confirm adequacy of the final bone work to accept the implant.
- The implant is prepared in the implant inserter with the appropriately sized spacer and keels with care taken to maintain the superior and inferior directionality of the keels. The implant is then advanced into the prepared disc space under fluoroscopic control. The inserter, retainer, and retainer screws are then removed and final position is confirmed with AP and lateral fluoroscopy (**TECH FIG 9**).

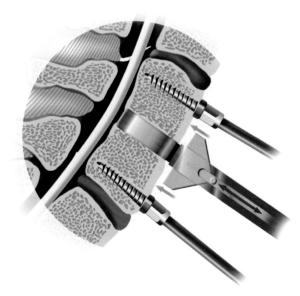

TECH FIG 7 • The trial is placed to be flush with the posterior vertebral body line. The stops can be adjusted for optimal depth positioning.

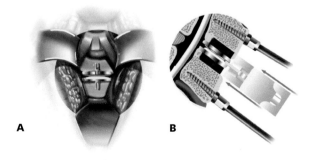

TECH FIG 9 • **A.** The implant is tamped into the defect under fluoroscopic guidance with care taken to ensure that is fully seated posteriorly. **B.** Anterior view of the final implant.

POSTOPERATIVE CARE

- Postoperatively, bracing is not used.
- A drain may be placed depending on surgeon preference.
- Most patients are admitted for a single hospital day, although some surgeons perform single level arthroplasties as an outpatient.
- Diet is advanced as tolerated. Dysphagia, when experienced, is usually transient and may mandate a slower advance of diet.
- Nonsteroidal anti-inflammatory drugs (NSAIDs) may be given postoperatively and may have a role in decreasing the incidence of heterotopic ossification.[22]
- Activity is restricted with no heavy lifting or high impact activity for 6 weeks. After 6 weeks, patients are encouraged so slowly resume their activity to preoperative levels.

OUTCOMES

- Recent reports from randomized trials of all three devices described demonstrate significant improvements or trends toward significant improvements in Neck Disability Index (NDI), arm pain, neck pain, SF-36, and reduced need for further surgery when compared with fusion at 4 and 5 years.[23–25]
- Maintenance of or small improvements in segmental motion have been demonstrated immediately postoperatively and at long-term follow-up.
- The impact of cervical arthroplasty on the incidence of adjacent segment disease is controversial and, as yet, indeterminate.[26,27]

COMPLICATIONS

- Complications can be grouped as approach and device related.
  - Approach-related complications:
    - Dysphagia: Frequent complication and often self-limited. The incidence and severity of dysphagia may be lower after arthroplasty compared with fusion, potentially as a result of the lower profile of the constructs or the decreased need for esophageal retraction.[28]
    - Nerve palsies: recurrent laryngeal nerve, superior laryngeal nerve
    - Nerve root injury
    - Spinal cord injury
    - Cerebrospinal fluid leak
    - Hematoma
      - Prevertebral
      - Epidural
    - Esophageal injury
  - Device-related
    - Device failure: Loosening or migration is rare but has been reported more frequently in the perioperative period in devices not secured with screw fixation.[29]
    - Arthrosis of the facet at the operated level and heterotopic ossification have been reported to occur in up to 20% and 50% of patients, respectively, but neither have been shown to have a correlation with clinical outcome.[30,31]
      - The incidence of same level facet arthrosis may be influenced by suboptimal positioning of the implant.
      - The incidence of heterotopic ossification may be reduced by thoroughly irrigating the wound to eliminate bone dust, coagulating exposed bone with electrocautery, and administering NSAIDs in the perioperative period.
    - Segmental kyphosis is likely attributable to improper endplate preparation and device insertion.[32] Arthroplasties are not likely to correct preoperative segmental kyphosis and should be avoided in such cases.
    - Subsidence: Risk increased with osteoporosis and minimized by placing as large an endplate footprint as possible.
    - Continued neurologic deficit can be caused by the maintenance of motion in the setting of inadequate decompression.
      - Persistent radiculopathy may be treatable with a posterior foraminotomy.
      - Persistent myelopathy or pain may require fusion.
    - Sagittal split fracture of the vertebral body is rare and may be predisposed by osteoporosis and the use of a keeled device.[33]

REFERENCES

1. Pait TG, Killefer JA, Arnautovic KA. Surgical anatomy of the anterior cervical spine: the disc space, vertebral artery, and associated bony structures. Neurosurgery 1996;39(4):769–776.
2. Melamed H, Harris MB, Awasthi D. Anatomic considerations of superior laryngeal nerve during anterior cervical spine procedures. Spine (Phila Pa 1976) 2002;27(4):E83–E86.
3. Sant'Ambrogio G, Sant'Ambrogio FB. Role of laryngeal afferents in cough. Pulm Pharmacol 1996;9(5–6):309–314.
4. Olmarker K, Blomquist J, Stromberg J, et al. Inflammatogenic properties of nucleus pulposus. Spine (Phila Pa 1976) 1995;20(6):665–669.
5. Shiri R, Karppinen J, Leino-Arjas P, et al. Cardiovascular and lifestyle risk factors in lumbar radicular pain or clinically defined sciatica: a systematic review. Eur Spine J 2007;16(12):2043–2054.
6. Hassett G, Hart DJ, Manek NJ, et al. Risk factors for progression of lumbar spine disc degeneration: the Chingford Study. Arthritis Rheum 2003;48(11):3112–3117.
7. Radhakrishnan K, Litchy WJ, O'Fallon WM, et al. Epidemiology of cervical radiculopathy. A population-based study from Rochester, Minnesota, 1976 through 1990. Brain 1994;117(pt 2):325–335.
8. Heckmann JG, Lang CJ, Zobelein I, et al. Herniated cervical intervertebral discs with radiculopathy: an outcome study of conservatively or surgically treated patients. J Spinal Disord 1999;12(5):396–401.
9. Kuijper B, Tans JT, Beelen A, et al. Cervical collar or physiotherapy versus wait and see policy for recent onset cervical radiculopathy: randomised trial. BMJ 2009;339:b3883.
10. Lees F, Turner JW. Natural history and prognosis of cervical spondylosis. BMJ 1963;2(5373):1607–1610.
11. Riina J, Anderson PA, Holly LT, et al. The effect of an anterior cervical operation for cervical radiculopathy or myelopathy on associated headaches. J Bone Joint Surg Am 200;91(8):1919–1923.
12. Crandall PH, Batzdorf U. Cervical spondylotic myelopathy. J Neurosurg 1966;25(1):57–66.
13. Lehman RA Jr., Helgeson MD, Keeler KA, et al. Comparison of magnetic resonance imaging and computed tomography in predicting facet arthrosis in the cervical spine. Spine (Phila Pa 1976) 2009;34(1):65–68.
14. Persson LC, Carlsson CA, Carlsson JY. Long-lasting cervical radicular pain managed with surgery, physiotherapy, or a cervical collar. A prospective, randomized study. Spine (Phila Pa 1976) 1997;22(7):751–758.
15. Pain in the neck and arm: a multicentre trial of the effects of physiotherapy, arranged by the British Association of Physical Medicine. BMJ 1966;1(5482):253–258.
16. Stav A, Ovadia L, Sternberg A, et al. Cervical epidural steroid injection for cervicobrachialgia. Acta Anaesthesiol Scand 1993;37(6):562–566.
17. Sasso RC, Macadaeq K, Nordmann D, et al. Selective nerve root injections can predict surgical outcome for lumbar and cervical radiculopathy: comparison to magnetic resonance imaging. J Spinal Disord Tech 2005;18(6):471–478.

18. Kadanka Z, Mares M, Bednarik J, et al. Approaches to spondylotic cervical myelopathy: conservative versus surgical results in a 3-year follow-up study. Spine (Phila Pa 1976) 2002;27(20):2205–2210; discussion 2210–2211.
19. Kadanka Z, Mares M, Bednarik J, et al. Predictive factors for spondylotic cervical myelopathy treated conservatively or surgically. Eur J Neurol 2005;12(1):55–63.
20. Roberto RF, McDonald T, Curtiss S, et al. Kinematics of progressive circumferential ligament resection (decompression) in conjunction with cervical disc arthroplasty in a spondylotic spine model. Spine (Phila Pa 1976) 2010;35(18):1676–1683.
21. McAfee PC, Cunningham B, Dmitrieve A, et al. Cervical disc replacement-porous coated motion prosthesis: a comparative biomechanical analysis showing the key role of the posterior longitudinal ligament. Spine (Phila Pa 1976) 2003;28(20):S176–S185.
22. Mehren C, Suchomel P, Grochulla F, et al. Heterotopic ossification in total cervical artificial disc replacement. Spine (Phila Pa 1976) 2006; 31(24):2802–2806.
23. Fessler RG, Sasso R, Papadopoulos S, et al. Cervical disc replacement: four-year follow-up results from the United States prospective randomized Bryan clinical trial. Neurosurgery 2009;65(2):407–408.
24. Burkus JR, Haid RW, Traynelis VC, et al. Long-term clinical and radiographic outcomes of the PRESTIGE-ST cervical disc replacement: results from a prospective randomized controlled clinical trial. J Neurosurg Spine 2010;13(3):308–318.
25. Murrey, D. Janssen ME, Delamarter RB, et al. 5-year results of the prospective, randomized, multi-center FDA investigational device exeomption ProDisc-C TDR clinical trial, in CSRS2009.
26. Jawahar A, Cavanaugh DA, Kerr EJ III, et al. Total disc arthroplasty does not affect the incidence of adjacent segment degeneration in cervical spine: results of 93 patients in three prospective randomized clinical trials. Spine J 2010;10(12):1043–1048.
27. Botelho RV, Moraes OJ, Fernandes GA, et al. A systematic review of randomized trials on the effect of cervical disc arthroplasty on reducing adjacent-level degeneration. Neurosurg Focus 2010; 28(6):E5.
28. McAfee PC, Cappuccino A, Cunningham BW, et al. Lower incidence of dysphagia with cervical arthroplasty compared with ACDF in a prospective randomized clinical trial. J Spinal Disord Tech 2010; 23(1):1–8.
29. Goffin J, Van Calenbergh F, van Loon J, et al. Intermediate follow-up after treatment of degenerative disc disease with the Bryan Cervical Disc Prosthesis: single-level and bi-level. Spine (Phila Pa 1976) 2003;28(24):2673–2678.
30. Ryu KS, Park CK, Jun SC, et al. Radiological changes of the operated and adjacent segments following cervical arthroplasty after a minimum 24-month follow-up: comparison between the Bryan and Prodisc-C devices. J Neurosurg Spine 2010;13(3):299–307.
31. Yi S, Kim KN, Yang MS, et al. Difference in occurrence of heterotopic ossification according to prosthesis type in the cervical artificial disc replacement. Spine (Phila Pa 1976) 2010;35(16):1556–15561.
32. Pickett GE, Sekhon LH, Sears WR, et al. Complications with cervical arthroplasty. J Neurosurg Spine 2006;4(2):98–105.
33. Datta JC, Janssen ME, Beckman R, et al. Sagittal split fractures in multilevel cervical arthroplasty using a keeled prosthesis. J Spinal Disord Tech 2007;20(1):89–92.

Chapter 8

Cervical Osteotomies for Kyphosis

Michael P. Kelly, Adam L. Wollowick, and K. Daniel Riew

DEFINITION

▪ The precise definition of cervical kyphosis is not clearly described. Normal alignment from C2 to C7 in the sagittal plane is approximately 20 degrees of lordosis.

ANATOMY

▪ With normal alignment, the load bearing axis of the cervical spine lies in the posterior third of the vertebral bodies.
▪ The foramen transversarium of C7 generally contains only veins; however, vertebral artery anomalies do exist and careful examination of the preoperative MRI is necessary.[1]
▪ As the C7 foramen transversarium is usually "empty," this level is the most amenable to a pedicle subtraction osteotomy.

PATHOGENESIS

▪ There are many etiologies of cervical kyphosis, including degenerative disease, trauma (acute and chronic onset), tumor, infection, inflammatory arthropathies, and iatrogenic causes.
  ▪ Ankylosing spondylitis is the most common inflammatory cause.
    ▪ Caused by contraction and ossification of the ligaments of the spine.
    ▪ Associated with the HLA-B27 haplotype in 80–90% of patients.
  ▪ Iatrogenic causes include postlaminectomy kyphosis, pseudarthrosis, and postradiation syndromes.

NATURAL HISTORY

▪ As there are many etiologies of cervical kyphosis, the natural history is quite variable.
  ▪ In patients with fixed deformities, such as ankylosing spondylitis, the deformity may progress due to stress fracture or an unrecognized fracture, often indicated by an acute increase in the magnitude of the deformity or the level of pain.
  ▪ As the axis of loading moves anterior to the vertebral body, the tendency is for progression of the deformity.
  ▪ With more deformity, the spinal cord may become draped over the vertebral bodies, and the patient may become myelopathic, quadriparetic, or quadriplegic.

PATIENT HISTORY AND PHYSICAL FINDINGS

▪ The chief complaint of the patient should be elicited. The patient may present with swallowing and/or breathing difficulties. Forward gaze is often affected. Patients may also note low back pain, as they hyperextend the lumbar spine to maintain a horizontal gaze.
  ▪ The patient should be asked to stand with hips and knees extended, allowing for an accurate assessment of the deformity and sagittal balance.

▪ Any sudden change in deformity or pain should be considered a fracture, until proven otherwise.
▪ An accurate history of previous cervical procedures is needed, as this is essential for preoperative planning.
▪ The patient should be asked to lay supine to assess the rigidity of the deformity.
▪ The gait should be observed for evidence of myelopathy. Other affected joints should be assessed to determine the need for treatment prior to addressing the cervical deformity.
▪ The exam should include a full neurologic exam, to check for evidence of myelopathy or spinal cord dysfunction.
▪ All patients should undergo a full medical evaluation, as respiratory and gastrointestinal dysfunction are not uncommon in this population. In severe cases of respiratory compromise, a preoperative tracheostomy may be advisable.

IMAGING AND OTHER DIAGNOSTIC STUDIES

▪ Radiographic evaluation should begin with anteroposterior (AP), lateral, and flexion/extension radiographs of the cervical spine (**FIG 1A–C**).
  ▪ This allows for assessment of both the degree and flexibility of the deformity.
▪ Standing AP and lateral radiographs of the entire spine, with the hips and knees in maximal extension, are obtained to assess global coronal and sagittal balance. We also obtain standing AP and lateral photographs, to post in the operating room, to aid in planning correction (**FIG 2A,B**).
▪ A CT scan with 1-mm cuts and sagittal, coronal, and three dimensional reconstructions are obtained. This allows for assessment of the fusion mass and helps provide landmark guidance for instrumentation (**FIG 3**).
  ▪ If one is deciding between Smith-Petersen osteotomies (SPO) and a pedicle subtraction osteotomy (PSO), then careful evaluation of the disc spaces is necessary. If there is a circumferential fusion, then a PSO is required.
▪ An MRI is obtained to visualize the neural elements. If the patient cannot tolerate a closed MRI (sometimes precluded by the deformity), then an open MRI or CT myelogram may be obtained.

DIFFERENTIAL DIAGNOSIS

▪ Degenerative disease
▪ Inflammatory arthropathy
  ▪ Ankylosing spondylitis
  ▪ Rheumatoid arthritis
▪ Posttraumatic kyphosis
  ▪ Acute
  ▪ Chronic
▪ Infection

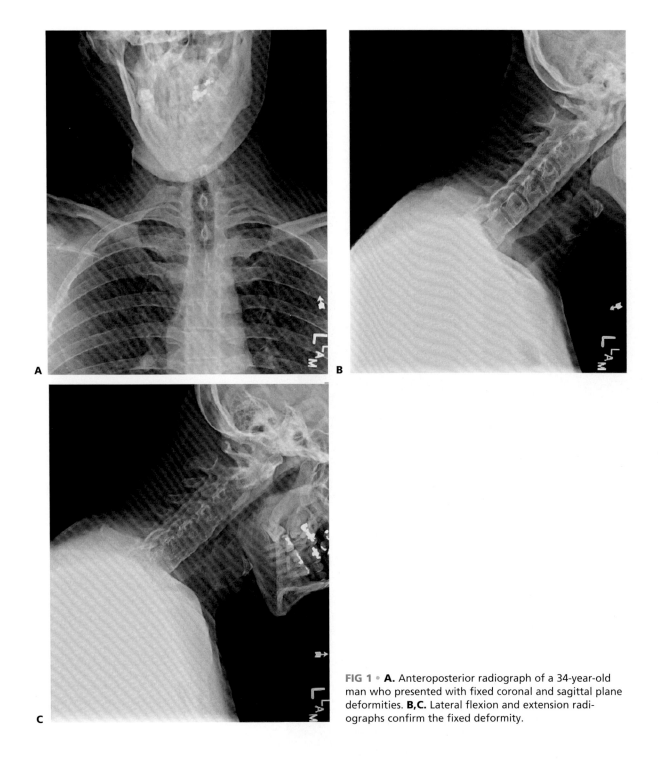

FIG 1 • A. Anteroposterior radiograph of a 34-year-old man who presented with fixed coronal and sagittal plane deformities. **B,C.** Lateral flexion and extension radiographs confirm the fixed deformity.

■ Tumor
  ■ Includes intradural pathologies
■ Iatrogenic
  ■ Postlaminectomy
  ■ Pseudarthrosis
  ■ Postradiation

NONOPERATIVE MANAGEMENT

■ Nonoperative management of symptomatic cervical kyphosis is limited, as the patient has minimal compensatory mechanisms to maintain horizontal gaze.

■ Pain may be controlled with anti-inflammatory and narcotic medications.

■ Bracing of flexible deformities is not ideal, as any improvement in symptoms will only occur when the brace is worn. Bracing of fixed deformities is not possible. Chronic brace use runs the risk of pressure ulcer formation.

SURGICAL MANAGEMENT

■ Surgical management is necessary when the patient is suffering from respiratory compromise, has difficulty eating, or has significant difficulty maintaining horizontal gaze.

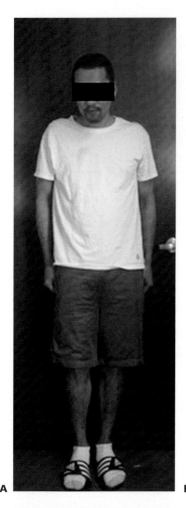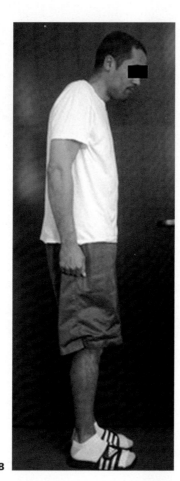

FIG 2 • Standing (**A**) anteroposterior and (**B**) lateral photographs of the patient in FIG 1, showing mild coronal plane deformity in addition to the sagittal plane deformity.

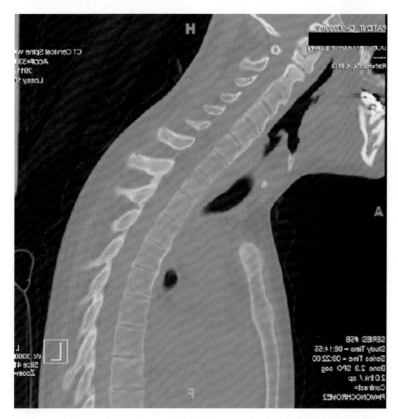

FIG 3 • Midsagittal CT scan image of the patient in FIG 1, showing fusion from C2 to the thoracic spine.

■ In many cases, correction of cervical kyphosis is an elective procedure that is performed when the patient can no longer tolerate the symptoms, most of which are not life threatening.

Preoperative Planning

■ All joints should be evaluated prior to a cervical osteotomy because hip and knee flexion contractures may require intervention prior to addressing the cervical spine.

■ Patients may present with concomitant thoracolumbar (TL) kyphosis, and a corrective osteotomy of the TL spine may be necessary. In this case, the TL procedure should be performed first, as horizontal gaze may correct with the TL osteotomy.[2] If the cervical osteotomy is performed first, a subsequent TL osteotomy may leave the patient in a position with the head fixed in too much extension.

■ The chin-brow angle should be measured.
  ■ We also measure the angle of deformity with a midsagittal CT scan image. This allows for more accurate planning in severe deformities.
  ■ The goal of correction should be to create a chin-brow angle of approximately 10 degrees.
    ■ With the head in slight flexion, the patient is able to see both their feet and straight ahead.
    ■ We aim to align the posterior vertebral line of C2 with the anterior vertebral line of C7.
    ■ Although aesthetically pleasing to the layman, a neutral chin-brow angle is not well-tolerated by the patient, as they cannot see directly in front of their body.[2]
  ■ For smaller deformities, with only a posterior fusion, we may perform single or multiple SPOs. For larger deformities (>30 degrees) or circumferential fusion, we will perform a PSO.

Positioning

■ Gardner-Wells tongs are used to secure the head, and 15 lb of traction is applied.
  ■ Bi-vector traction is applied through the frame. One vector pulls axially and is used to position the head until the osteotomy closure. At the time of closure, an extension moment is applied by switching the weight to the second rope which facilitates closure and holds the head in the appropriate position until the head is fixed in place (**FIG 4A,B**).

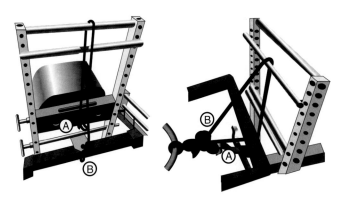

FIG 4 • Bi-vector traction is achieved through two traction ropes. *Rope A* pulls longitudinally. *Rope B* is placed over the "H-bar" and pulls with an extension moment.

■ We position the patient prone on a Jackson frame with a chest bolster, anterior iliac crest pads, and a leg sling. In the case of severe deformity, the chest bolster may be built up with pillows to allow appropriate positioning of the surgical field.
  ■ Although historically performed in a seated position, we prefer the prone position, as upper cervical implant placement is easier.[3]

■ The arms are wrapped with blankets at the patient's side and the elbows and wrists padded.

■ Gentle traction is applied to the shoulders with tape.

■ The patient is placed in a maximal reverse Trendelenburg position. This brings the operative site into the surgeon's field of view and allows for pooling of blood in the lower extremities.

Approach

■ A standard midline approach is used. We minimize blood loss by staying within the midline raphe down to the spinous processes.

■ The lateral masses are exposed in their entirety, but not more laterally in an effort to minimize bleeding.

SMITH-PETERSEN OSTEOTOMY

Placement of Instrumentation

■ Lateral mass screws are placed at C6, and above, to achieve six to eight points of proximal fixation. If the patient is fused from C2 down, then we will place C2 pedicle screws or lamina screws as the anatomy allows. In patients who are autofused to the skull, if the fixation from the axis distally is not adequate, we extend the instrumentation to the skull.

■ Place pedicle screws at C7 and distally, again to achieve six to eight points of distal fixation.

■ Place the implants in line to minimize the contouring needed to seat the rods.

Osteotomy

■ Most commonly performed at the C7/T1 level.

■ Begin with a laminectomy of C7, performed with a high speed burr. We undercut the laminae of C6 and T1 to prevent cord compression during extension of the osteotomy.
  ■ The ligamentum flavum is excised with Kerrison rongeurs or curettes. If ossified, it is removed with a high-speed burr.
  ■ The C7 lamina is preserved for use as local bone graft.

■ The inferior articular facet of C7 and superior articular facet of T1 are removed. A chevron shaped cut, as opposed to a straight transverse cut, is made to maintain stability of the osteotomy after closure.

- Ensure that the C8 nerve root is fully decompressed to minimize the chance of postoperative radiculopathy. This may require partial removal of the C7 pedicle.

Osteotomy Closure

- At this point, the surgeon takes a firm hold of the Gardner-Wells tongs and the traction weight is shifted to the extension rope. The surgeon extends the neck and the osteotomy is closed.
- The rods are placed in the screw heads and fixed in place.
- Intraoperative radiographs are obtained to check implant position and to check the correction of the deformity.
- The wound is closed as described later.

PEDICAL SUBTRACTION OSTEOTOMY

Placement of Instrumentation

- Similar to the Smith-Petersen osteotomy. At C2, pedicle screws are placed if the anatomy allows. Laminar screws may also be used, although rod placement may require cross connectors. A combination of laminar screws and pedicle screws may be used as well. We may extend to skull if the occipitocervical joint is already fused.
- From C3 to C5, lateral mass screws are placed. Attention is paid to place the screws inline with one another, as this facilitates placement of the final rod.
- Lateral mass screws are placed at C6, if T1 is not instrumented.
- Pedicle screws are placed from T1 to T3 or T4, with T1 omitted if C6 is instrumented. The instrumentation is placed distally to T3 or T4, to ensure six to eight points of distal fixation (**TECH FIG 1**).

C7 Laminectomy

- A laminectomy of C7 is performed using a high-speed burr. The lamina is removed in one piece and reserved for use as local bone graft (**TECH FIG 2**).
- The laminae of C6 and T1 are undercut to provide additional room for the neural elements following closure of the osteotomy.
- The ligamentum flavum is excised with Kerrison rongeurs and/or curettes. If ossified, a burr is used.
- The lateral masses of C7 are removed in piece meal fashion, with a Leksell rongeur and a high-speed burr. A chevron shaped cut is made so that there is rotational stability after closing the osteotomy (**TECH FIG 3**).
- The inferior facets of C6 and superior facets of T1 are excised. The inferior borders of the C6 pedicles and superior

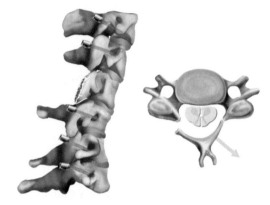

TECH FIG 2 • The laminectomy is performed en bloc and the bone is saved for use as bone graft.

borders of the T1 pedicles must be visualized. This allows adequate room for the C7 and C8 nerve roots following osteotomy closure.

Decancellation

- Cotton patties and Penfield retractors are place around the C7 pedicle to protect the C7 and C8 nerve roots. Resection of the C7 pedicle begins by passing the high-speed burr down the pedicle.
  - Care must be taken to preserve the walls of the pedicle.
- The pedicle walls are then removed, piecemeal, with pituitary rongeurs and reverse angle curettes (**TECH FIG 4**).
  - The pedicle walls must be removed entirely, to prevent nerve root impingement following closure of the osteotomy.

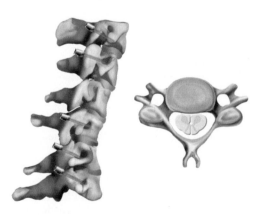

TECH FIG 1 • Instrumentation has been placed.

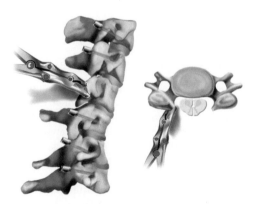

TECH FIG 3 • The lateral masses are removed with the Leksell rongeur, and the superior facets of T1 and inferior facets of C6 are removed.

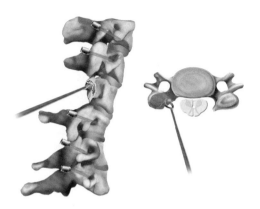

TECH FIG 4 • Resection of the pedicle walls begins with a curette.

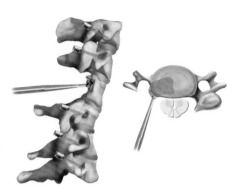

TECH FIG 5 • A void is created within the vertebral body with a small bone tamp.

- A void is created in the posterosuperior portion of the vertebral body, with reverse angle curettes or small bone tamps (**TECH FIG 5**).
- Decancellation is completed with curettes and pituitary rongeurs, with the cancellous bone removed and preserved for local graft or pushed anteriorly within the vertebral body (**TECH FIG 6**).
- The same procedure is performed at the contralateral pedicle. Decancellation should continue until the pedicles freely communicate with each other.
  - An "egg shell" of C7 should now remain.
- With a Woodson elevator or angled dural elevator, the posterior wall of the vertebral body is impacted, completing the osteotomy of C7. This should not require much force. If it does, then more decancellation of the body is necessary (**TECH FIG 7**).

Osteotomy Closure

- Pre-bent rods, or articulating rods (our preference), are placed in the distal screw heads (**TECH FIG 8**).
- The surgeon now grabs a hold of the Gardner-Wells tongs and the weight is switched to the extension moment rope. The neck is gently extended by the surgeon to the desired position (**TECH FIG 9**).
  - If enough bone has been removed from C7, this action should take little force.

- The rods are fixed in place.
- The C7 and C8 nerve roots are checked to ensure that there is no impingement.
- The electrophysiologist checks the neuromonitoring signals to ensure there have been no changes during closure of the osteotomy.
  - If there are changes, we relax the closure and perform a rehearsed Stagnara wake-up test.
- Radiographs are checked to assess implant position, deformity correction, and the integrity of the anterior column.
  - In some cases, the anterior column may book open. This usually happens when corrections greater than 40 degrees are attempted. In these cases, we will sometimes turn the patient supine and place a plate across the opening, with an allograft placed within the deficient area. We also do this in osteoporotic patients with poor fixation. If we instrumented to the skull and the screws have excellent purchase, this is not necessary.

Bone Grafting

- The laminae, spinous processes, and lateral masses/transverse processes of C6 and T1 are decorticated with a high-speed burr.
  - Irrigation is used to minimize thermal necrosis.

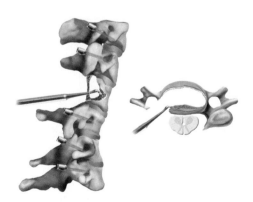

TECH FIG 6 • The void has been expanded so that the pedicles communicate freely with each other.

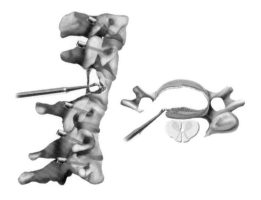

TECH FIG 7 • A Woodson elevator is used to impact the posterior aspect of the vertebral body, completing the osteotomy. This is performed on both sides of the body.

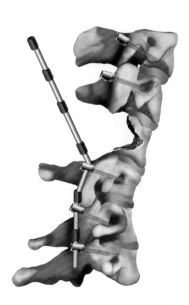

TECH FIG 8 • An articulating or contoured rod is then placed.

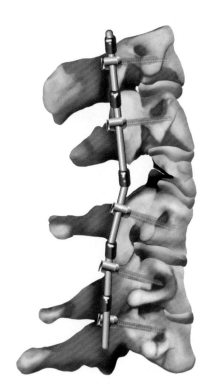

TECH FIG 9 • The head is extended, and the osteotomy site closed.

- The C7 lamina, which had been preserved, is split in the sagittal plane. The two pieces are then placed along the decorticated spinous processes of C6 and T1 and then cabled into place.
- The remainder of the local bone graft is packed around the closed osteotomy site.

Wound Closure

- Meticulous attention is paid to wound closure to minimize dead space and to ensure a good cosmetic appearance.
  - We close the paraspinals in multiple layers, minimizing the amount of muscle within each suture bite.
  - Prior to closure of the fascial layer, a thrombin-soaked Gelfoam sheet is placed in the wound.

- Prior to closure, 500 mg of vancomycin powder is sprinkled in the wound.
- Redundant skin is inevitable, but, with an accurate closure, the wound will smooth as it heals.
  - In the case of excessive redundancy, we will excise ellipses of full thickness skin from the proximal and distal aspects of the wound.
- Drains are placed deep and superficial to the fascia.
  - These drains are removed when over 8 hours output is less than 30 mL, usually on postoperative day 1.
- Hemostasis is verified after the closure of each layer.
  - Pressure is applied for 30 seconds after the closure of each layer.

PEARLS AND PITFALLS

Preoperative planning	▪ The preoperative physical examination should evaluate other joints that may be affected by the disease process and require intervention before the cervical spine. ▪ Thoracolumbar kyphosis, if severe enough to warrant surgery, should be corrected before the cervical spine. ▪ Careful examination of the vertebral artery using pre-operative imaging will minimize the risk of injury **(FIG 5)**. ▪ A detailed pulmonary history and exam is necessary, as some extreme cases may require a preoperative tracheostomy. ▪ The goal of correction should be to 10 to 20 degrees of flexion, allowing the patient to see directly in front of their body. ▪ Use Gardner-Wells tongs and bivector traction to help with intraoperative positioning of the head. ▪ Position the patient prone, in maximal reverse Trendelenburg. This brings the operative site into the field of view and minimizes blood loss through pooling in the lower extremities.
Implant placement	▪ Lamina screws may be placed at C2, if the anatomy is not amenable to pars screws. Lamina screws may also be placed as an adjunct to pars screws in cases of poor bone stock. ▪ Place the implants in a straight line, so that contouring of the rods is minimized.

Osteotomy	■ Remove the C7 lamina in one piece and reserve for use as local bone graft. ■ The inferior articular facet of C6 and superior articular facet of T1 must be removed entirely, to reduce the risk of C7 or C8 nerve root impingement. ■ Protect the nerve roots with cotton patties and Penfield retractors. ■ Impaction of the posterior wall should proceed with minimal force. If significant force is required, then remove more bone from the body itself.
Wound closure	■ Close the wound in many layers, with meticulous attention to tissue apposition. ■ Achieve hemostasis with compression and pharmacologic means (thrombin, Gelfoam, etc.) after closure of each layer. ■ Place drains deep and superficial to the fascia. This will minimize dead space. ■ In cases of extreme tissue redundancy, ellipses may be excised from the proximal and distal aspects of the wound. ■ A plastic surgery consultation may be appropriate in the most extreme cases (redundant skin, previous surgery, etc.).
Postoperative care	■ Immobilize the patient in a hard collar for 6 to 12 weeks. ■ Mobilize the patient on postoperative day 1.

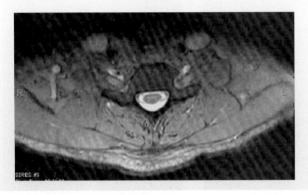

FIG 5 • Axial T2-weighted MRI of the patient in FIG 1, showing intraforaminal vertebral artery at C7. For this reason, multiple Smith-Petersen osteotomies were performed.

POSTOPERATIVE CARE

■ Most patients can be extubated without difficulty immediately following the procedure.
■ All patients are immobilized in a hard collar for 6–12 weeks.
■ All patients are out of bed and walking on postoperative day 1.
■ Patients are, generally, discharged to home on postoperative day 1 or 2.

OUTCOMES

■ With proper planning, horizontal gaze is reliably restored.[3–8] (**FIG 6B–D**)
■ Belanger et al. reported improved neck pain scores in 88% (21/24) of ankylosing spondylitis patients.[4]
    ■ Subjective dysphagia was improved in 95% (18/19).
■ Subjective satisfaction scores are often good to excellent.[3,8]

COMPLICATIONS

■ Neurologic injury, including paralysis, has been reported with extension osteotomies, with an overall rate of approximately 23%.[9]
    ■ The most commonly affected nerve root is C8, with transient palsies more common than permanent injury.[8]
■ In cases of osteoporosis and osteopenia, implant failure and pseudarthrosis are concerns.
    ■ Pseudarthrosis rates with modern implants have been reported from 0% to 13%.[4,6–8]
■ The vertebral artery is at risk; however, performing the osteotomy at C7 and careful planning may minimize the risk. Make sure that there is no anomalous vertebral artery in the foramen transversarium of C7.

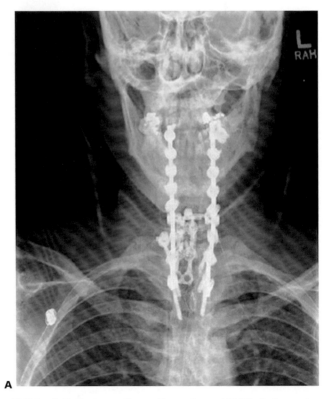

FIG 6 • **A,B.** Postoperative radiographs and (**C,D**) photographs of the patient in FIG 1. He underwent anterior osteotomies at C6–7 and C7–T1 with Smith-Petersen osteotomies at C6–7 and C7–T1 and instrumentation from C2–T3.

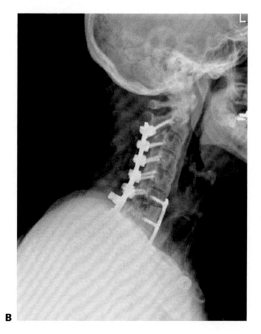

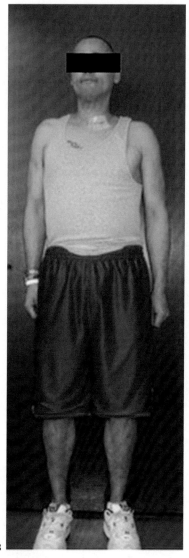

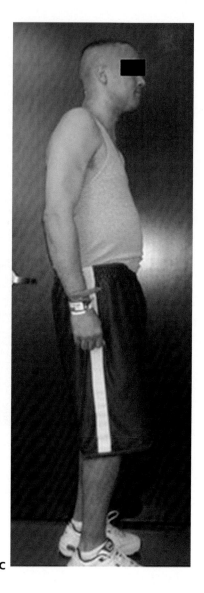

FIG 6 • *(continued)* **B**   **C**

- As with any posterior procedure, wound infection and wound dehiscence are potential risks. A plastic surgery consultation is appropriate for the most extreme wounds.

REFERENCES

1. Hong JT, Park DK, Lee MJ, et al. Anatomical variations of the vertebral artery segment in the lower cervical spine: analysis by three-dimensional computed tomography angiography. Spine (Phila Pa 1976) 2008;33(22):2422–2426.
2. Suk KS, Kim KT, Lee SH, et al. Significance of chin-brow vertical angle in correction of kyphotic deformity of ankylosing spondylitis patients. Spine (Phila Pa 1976) 2003;28(17):2001–2005.
3. Simmons ED, DiStefano RJ, Zheng Y, et al. Thirty-six years experience of cervical extension osteotomy in ankylosing spondylitis: techniques and outcomes. Spine (Phila Pa 1976) 2006;31(26):3006–3012.
4. Belanger TA, Milam RA, Roh JS, et al. Cervicothoracic extension osteotomy for chin-on-chest deformity in ankylosing spondylitis. J Bone Joint Surg Am 2005;87(8):1732–1738.
5. El Saghir H, Boehm H. Surgical options in the treatment of the spinal disorders in ankylosing spondylitis. Clin Exp Rheumatol 2002;20(Suppl. 28):S101–S105.
6. Langeloo DD, Journee HL, Pavlov PW, et al. Cervical osteotomy in ankylosing spondylitis: evaluation of new developments. Eur Spine J 2006;15(4):493–500.
7. McMaster MJ. Osteotomy of the cervical spine in ankylosing spondylitis. J Bone Joint Surg Br 1997;79(2):197–203.
8. Tokala DP, Lam KS, Freeman BJ, et al. C7 decancellisation closing wedge osteotomy for the correction of fixed cervico-thoracic kyphosis. Eur Spine J 2007;16(9):1471–1478.
9. Etame AB, Than KD, Wang AC, et al. Surgical management of symptomatic cervical or cervicothoracic kyphosis due to ankylosing spondylitis. Spine (Phila Pa 1976) 2008;33(16):E559–E564.

Chapter 9

Reduction Techniques for Cervical Fractures and Dislocations

Adam M. Pearson, Gursukhman Sidhu, and Alexander R. Vaccaro

INTRODUCTION

- Cervical spine fractures occur in approximately 5% of trauma patients being evaluated at level I trauma centers.
- Dislocations and displaced fractures require reduction and frequently surgical stabilization.
- This chapter focuses on the cervical fractures that often require reduction and the closed and open techniques used to manage them.

GENERAL PRINCIPLES OF CLOSED REDUCTION

Traction

- Application of longitudinal traction assists in the reduction of cervical spine fractures through ligamentotaxis and the ability to apply rotational moments to the cervical spine.
- Traction can be performed urgently in the emergency room.
- Successful reduction requires an understanding of the biomechanics of both injury and reduction.
- Traction is contraindicated in extension distraction injuries and type IIA Hangman's fractures (see later section).
- Placement of a towel roll between the scapulae can help to raise the head off the bed and allow for better control of the flexion or extension moment.
- Low weight (10 lb) should initially be placed in order to ensure there is no craniocervical instability or unsuspected distraction.
- Weight is generally added in 10-lb increments with lateral radiographs obtained every 10 to 15 minutes after adding weight in order to allow for the viscoelastic tissues to creep and for the muscles to fatigue. Serial neurologic exams should also be performed and documented with each addition of weight.
- If not successful, open reduction in the operating room is generally indicated.

Gardner-Wells Tongs

- Available in stainless steel and titanium. Stainless steel tongs offer the advantage of being able to safely use more weight, whereas titanium tongs are MRI compatible yet are limited in the amount of weight they can safely support (no more than 50 lb).[1]
- Imaging of the skull (plain films or CT scan) should be obtained prior to pin placement to ensure there are no skull fractures.
- Pin placement is extremely important. The pins should generally be placed 1 cm above the pinna, in line with the external auditory meatus and below the equator of the skull (**FIG 1**). Placement more anteriorly results in an extension moment, whereas placement more posterior results in a flexion moment (sometimes desirable for facet dislocations).
- The pin sites should be prepped with Betadine. Since these pins are temporary, the hair does not need to be shaved.

Lidocaine is injected subcutaneously and subperiosteally at the planned pin sites.

- Pins should be tightened until the indicator protrudes at least 1 mm, which corresponds to 30 lb of compression at the pin site. Undertightened pins can disengage and cause scalp lacerations. Do not overtighten pins as penetration of the inner table of the skull can occur.
- Gardner-Wells tongs are temporary devices used for reduction. Use of halo ring traction should be considered if a halo is to be used for definitive management, although the amount of weight that can be applied to a halo ring is also less than what can be added to stainless steel Gardner-Wells tongs. We generally prefer to perform a reduction using Gardner-Wells tongs and then convert to a halo if surgery is going to be delayed and the patient needs to be stabilized in the interim.

Halo Vest Application

- Most halo vest systems are now MRI compatible.
- Proper application of the ring is essential to prevent nerve injury, skin problems, and provide a method of immobilization with long-term durability.
- At least two providers familiar with halo application are required.
- The first step is to size the vest and the ring using the manufacturer's instructions. The vest should extend down to the level of the xiphoid and be snug but allow access to the skin. The ring should fit as close to the skull as is possible without contacting the skin at any point.
- The patient can be logrolled to place the posterior portion of the vest.
- One person then holds the halo ring in place, ensuring that it does not contact the ears or the head, is symmetrically and appropriately aligned, and is below the equator of the skull.
- Another person then plans the pin placement (**FIG 1**). The two anterior pins are generally placed 1 cm cranial to the lateral third of the orbital rim to avoid the supraorbital and supratrochlear nerves. The pins can be placed into the eyebrow in patients concerned about scar cosmesis. The posterior pins are generally placed 1 cm above the helix of the ear posterior to the external auditory meatus and below the equator of the skull.
- If the halo is going to remain in place for an extended period, the posterior pin sites should be shaved prior to starting the procedure. The pin sites should be prepped with Betadine, and lidocaine should be injected subcutaneously and subperiosteally.
- While one person holds the ring in place (various devices like suction cups and blunt pins can be used to assist with this), the other person screws the pins in until they all just contact the skin. Opposing pins should then be tightened simultaneously, going back and forth between the two pairs. The pins

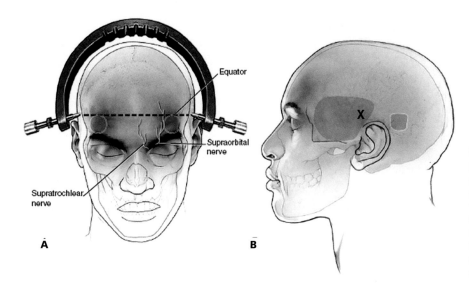

FIG 1 • Gardner-Wells tongs are to be placed with pins approximately 1 cm above the pinna inline with the external auditory meatus, below the equator of the skull. Anterior halo pins are placed over the lateral third of the eyebrow in order to avoid the supraorbital and supra-trochlear nerves, while posterior pin sites are posterior to the pinna, below the equator of the skull.

should be tightened to 8 inch-pounds using either a torque-limiting breakaway applicator or a torque wrench.

■ The halo ring can then be attached to traction using the appropriate metal bail or to the uprights of the halo vest. The head should be positioned appropriately, and radiographs should be obtained to determine if the alignment is appropriate.

■ Pins should be retightened to 8 inch-pounds in 24 to 48 hours.

■ Loose pins can be retightened once and should then be replaced through another hole if they loosen again.

■ Meticulous pin site care is required, although pin site infection can still occur. If infection is present but the pin is still tight, it can be treated with local care and oral antibiotics. If the pin loosens in the presence of infection, it should be replaced.

Bivector Traction

■ Bivector traction allows for simultaneous control of longitudinal traction and a flexion moment using a specially designed traction apparatus on a RotoRest bed (**FIG 2**).

■ The patient is positioned on a RotoRest bed with the head pad removed and shoulder roll in place to allow for freedom of motion of the head in the sagittal plane.

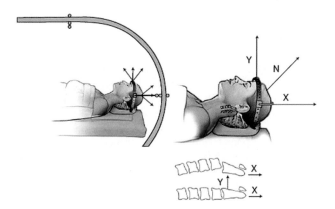

FIG 2 • Bivector traction with Gardner-Wells tongs. Two cables are used in order to adjust anterior and superior traction individually in order to affect a reduction.

■ Longitudinal traction is applied to the ring using an S-clip and anterior traction is applied via a cord attached to both of the pins. The two forces should initially be at 90 degrees to each other and can then be fine-tuned as needed.

■ Application of weight to the anterior pulley allows flexion to be "dialed-in" without having to change the position of the longitudinal traction, which can be difficult when heavy weight has been applied.

■ Bivector traction is indicated for most cervical spine reductions as it allows for more precise control of the traction vector than a single vector traction setup.

ODONTOID FRACTURES

Definition

■ Fracture through the odontoid process that can be located from the tip of the dens to its base.

■ Odontoid fractures are very common, accounting for 10% to 20% of all cervical fractures.[2]

Anatomy

■ Two ossification centers fuse in utero, separating the dens ossification center from the primary ossification center of the C2 vertebral body.[3] These two ossification centers are separated by the dentocentral synchondrosis, which fuses by age 7. Another secondary ossification center, the ossiculum terminale, forms at the tip of the dens around age 9 and fuses by age 13.

■ There is a rich vascular supply around the dens originating from the vertebral arteries and ascending pharyngeal artery. Although it was thought that type II dens fractures were predisposed to nonunion due to the presence of a watershed area at the base of the dens, this has been shown to be untrue.[4]

■ The transverse atlantal ligament runs posterior to dens and connects to the posterior aspect of the anterior C1 ring bilaterally, preventing anterior translation of C1 on C2. The alar ligaments run from the tip of the dens to the skull base and restrict axial rotation. The weak apical ligament connects the tip of the dens to the occiput (**FIG 3**).

■ The C2 nerve root exits posterior to the C1–2 joint in contrast to nerve roots below this level, which exit anterior to the facet joints. This puts the C2 nerve root at risk during posterior C1–2 fusions.

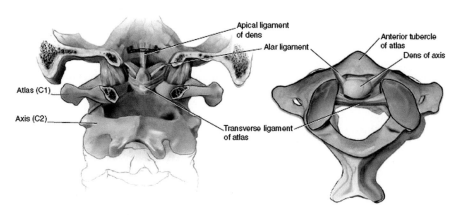

FIG 3 • Ligamentous anatomy of the upper cervical spine.

- Fifty percent of axial rotation of the cervical spine occurs at C1–2.
- A fracture of the dens results in atlantoaxial instability.

Classification

- Anderson and D'Alonzo (**FIG 4**)[5]
- Type I fractures are avulsions of the apical portion of dens and generally represents a stable fracture with a high union rate.[6] Occipital cervical dissociation should be suspected and ruled out.
- Type II fractures involve the base of the odontoid and do not extend into the C2 body. These are generally considered unstable and are associated with a nonunion rate of at least 32% with nonoperative treatment.[7]
- Type III fractures extend into the vertebral body of C2. These are relatively stable fractures that have a union rate of 85% to 90% with nonoperative treatment.[6]

Patient Presentation

- Studies of traffic fatalities suggest that high energy dens fractures could be associated with a mortality rate of up to 40%.[8] The mortality rate in low energy trauma is much lower.
- The vast majority of patients who survive the initial injury present neurologically intact, although a wide variety of neurologic deficits associated with odontoid fractures have been described.[5]
- Delayed presentation is common, and patients frequently present with neck pain and may have varying degrees of myelopathy. Respiratory depression and death have been reported.[9]

Imaging

- Plain films including an open mouth view of the odontoid should be obtained. However, nondisplaced dens fractures are frequently missed on plain films.[10]

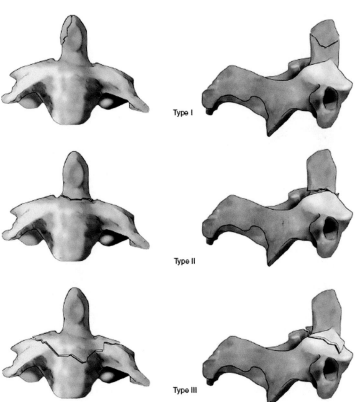

Type I

Type II

Type III

FIG 4 • Anderson and D'Alonzo classification of odontoid fractures. Type I involves the apex, type II the base of the dens, and type III enters the body of C2.

■ CT scan with thin cuts and sagittal and coronal reformations is the study of choice to detect and characterize odontoid fractures.

■ MRI is indicated in patients with neurologic deficit and can be useful to assess the ligaments of the upper cervical spine.

Closed Reduction and Treatment

■ Gardner-Wells tongs are applied and bivector traction is used to reduce displaced odontoid fractures.[11] If definitive treatment in a halo vest is planned, reduction can be performed with a halo ring. Although single vector traction can be used for the reduction of odontoid fractures, bivector traction allows for more precise control of the traction vector.

■ In posterior displaced fractures, there is a risk of respiratory compromise during the reduction maneuver that typically requires flexion of the neck. This is most likely due to compression of the airways by the retropharyngeal hematoma, although others have suggested it is due to the

displaced odontoid compressing the respiratory pathways that run in the anterolateral portion of the upper spinal cord.[12,13] As such, nasotracheal intubation of these patients prior to reduction is recommended.

■ A relatively low amount of weight is generally required (20–30 lb), and serial plain X-rays or fluoroscopy should be used with bivector traction to fine tune the reduction.

■ Type I and III fractures rarely need reduction and can be managed with a halo vest or cervical collar. It has been recommended that type II fractures, particularly in elderly patients who cannot tolerate a halo vest, should be treated surgically.[14]

Surgical Treatment

■ Indicated for elderly patients with type II fractures and for failure to hold reduction or nonunion in younger patients.

■ Options include odontoid screw, transarticular C1–2 fusion, and Harms posterior C1–2 fusion (**FIG 5**). Posterior C1–2

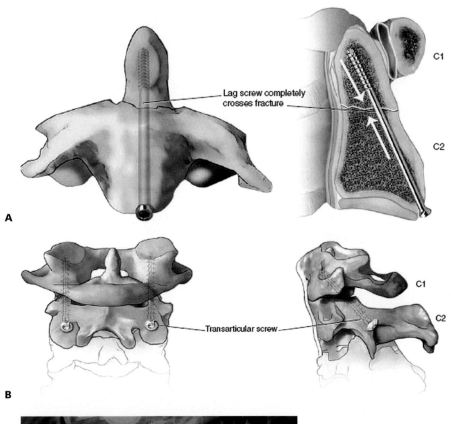

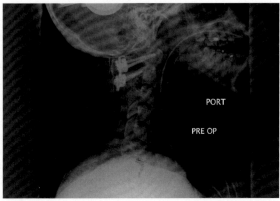

FIG 5 • Fixation techniques for odontoid fractures. **A.** Anterior lag screw. **B.** Transarticular fusion. **C.** Harms fusion.

wiring is an older technique that also had acceptable results, although a lower fusion rate than transarticular fixation.[15] Anterior screw fixation allows for some preservation of C1–2 rotation, although it is associated with a higher rate of technical problems and nonunions compared to posterior C1–2 fusion.[16]

Outcomes

■ In type II fractures, union rates are approximately 51% with collar treatment, 65% with halo vest orthosis, 82% with odontoid screw fixation, and 93% with posterior C1–2 fusion.[17]
■ In type III fractures, collar immobilization results in a union rate of approximately 92% compared to 95% with halo vest orthosis.[17]

Complications

■ In patients over 70 years old, inpatient mortality can be as high as 35%.[18]
■ In patients over 65 years old treated with a halo vest orthosis, mortality can be as high as 42%, primarily due to pneumonia and cardiac arrest.[19]
■ Operative treatment of dens fractures in the elderly is also associated with high mortality rates of 40% with anterior screw fixation and 22% for posterior C1–2 fusion.[18,20]
■ Anterior screw fixation can result in nonunion and screw cut out, particularly in elderly, osteoporotic bone.[21]
■ Posterior screw placement at C1 and C2 can result in vascular injury to the vertebral or internal carotid arteries.[22]

PEARLS AND PITFALLS

Bivector traction	■ Can be extremely helpful in the reduction of displaced odontoid fractures
Posterior-displaced fractures	■ Should be intubated prior to closed reduction
Elderly patients with a halo vest	■ Treatment is associated with high morbidity and mortality in elderly patients, so operative treatment is often favored ■ We prefer a posterior Harms C1–2 fusion in these patients

TRAUMATIC SPONDYLOLISTHESIS OF THE AXIS ("HANGMAN'S FRACTURE")

Definition

■ Fracture through the C2 pars interarticularis. A similar lesion is seen in judicial hangings, although the mechanisms and outcomes are obviously quite different.

Anatomy

■ C2 is a unique vertebra in that it serves as the transition from the upper cervical spine to the lower cervical spine.
■ The superior articular processes are anterolateral to the spinal canal, biconcave, articulate with the inferior articular processes of C1, and allow for rotation around the dens. The inferior articular processes are posterolateral to the spinal canal and articulate with the superior articular processes of C3. The pars connects the superior and inferior articular processes of C2 and is an area of frequent injury due to its relative weakness (**FIG 6**).
■ The vertebral artery runs through the C2 foramen on the lateral aspect of the C1–2 joint.
■ The spinal canal is quite capacious at C2, explaining the low rate of neurologic injuries with fractures at this level.

Pathogenesis and Classification

■ The most commonly used classification is Levine and Edward's modification of Effendi's classification system (**FIG 7**).[23]
■ Type I fractures are nondisplaced (<3 mm) and nonangulated vertical fractures just posterior to the vertebral body that

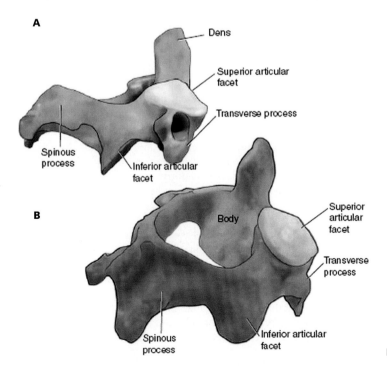

A

Dens

Superior articular facet

Transverse process

Spinous process

Inferior articular facet

B

Body

Superior articular facet

Transverse process

Spinous process

Inferior articular facet

FIG 6 • C2 bony anatomy.

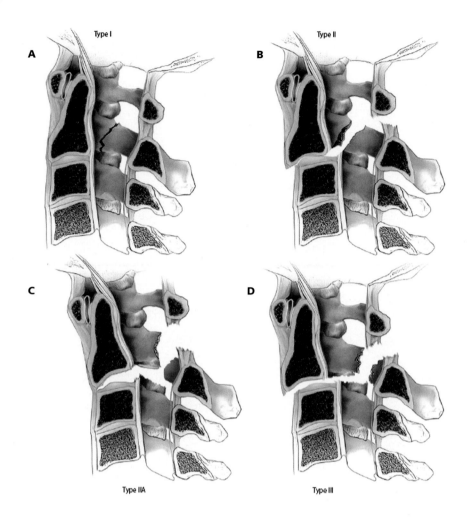

FIG 7 • Levine and Edward's classification of traumatic spondylolisthesis of the axis (Hangman's fracture). Type I fractures are minimally displaced (<3 mm). Type II fractures are displaced (>3 mm), angulated fractures. Type IIA fractures are angulated but minimally translated, usually with an intact anterior longitudinal ligament. Type III fractures have an accompanying bilateral facet dislocation.

are parallel and symmetric to each other. These typically result from hyperextension and axial loading. The discal and ligamentous structures are generally intact, and these represent stable fractures.

■ Type IA, or atypical, fractures are nondisplaced (<3 mm) and nonangulated vertical fractures that are asymmetric (ie, the fracture lines are located at slightly different locations in the neural arch and are not parallel). These typically result from hyperextension and lateral bending. These generally represent stable fractures. Starr and Eismont also described two displaced "atypical" Hangman's fractures that were associated with neurologic deficit due to the spinal cord becoming impaled on the posterior fragment at the fracture site.[24]

■ Type II fractures are displaced (>3 mm), angulated fractures that tend to be vertically oriented just posterior to the vertebral body. The pars fractures occur with initial hyperextension, which is then followed by flexion which disrupts the disc, elevates the anterior longitudinal ligament off of C3, and often fractures the anterosuperior corner of C3.

■ Type IIA fractures are angulated (often >15 degrees), minimally translated fractures that are oriented obliquely, running from anteroinferior to posterosuperior through the pars. The mechanism of injury is distraction-flexion, resulting in the pars failing in tension. The disc fails from posterior to anterior, and the ALL is usually intact. It is important to recognize this variant because traction will exacerbate the deformity rather than reduce it.

■ Type III fractures are typically type I fractures through the pars combined with a bilateral C2–3 facet dislocation. The mechanism leading to type III fractures is unclear, but it has been hypothesized that a distraction-flexion injury resulting in facet dislocation occurs initially, followed by an extension force that fractures the pars. Due to the discontinuity between the vertebral body and the dislocated facets, closed reduction generally fails, and this injury requires operative treatment.

Patient History and Physical Findings

■ The most common mechanism of injury is motor vehicle accident.

■ Neurologic injury is uncommon due to the large diameter of the spinal canal at this level, occurring in only 6.5% of patients in one series.[25] The majority of patients with neurologic injuries have type III fractures, although neurologic injury can also be seen in atypical type IA fractures due to asymmetric canal narrowing.

■ Concomitant fractures elsewhere in the spine are common, so the remainder of the spine needs to be assessed with physical exam and imaging.

Imaging

■ Cross-table lateral radiographs generally demonstrate the fracture lines through the pars and the traumatic spondylolisthesis if present. The exception is the type IA fracture, in which the fracture lines are in different planes and are not always seen on the X-ray.

■ Type II fractures can reduce when the patient is supine, so upright X-rays should be obtained in patients with type I fractures. Some authors have even suggested physician supervised flexion-extension radiographs in neurologically intact patients with apparent type I fractures to ensure that it does not actually represent a type II fracture.[26]

■ CT scan of the cervical spine should be obtained to better characterize the fracture and rule out other cervical spine fractures. Imaging of the thoracic and lumbar spine should also be obtained to rule out noncontiguous fractures, as multiple spine fractures are present in up to 30% of patients with traumatic spondylolisthesis of the axis.[27]

■ MRI is indicated in patients with neurologic deficits or type III fractures, which must be evaluated for a disc herniation in association with the facet dislocation.

Nonoperative Management

■ Type I and type IA fractures can be treated with a cervical collar for 3 months. Upright X-rays are obtained to make sure the fractures is not actually a type II fracture.

■ Type II fractures often are reduced by closed reduction. Because the mechanism causing displacement of these fractures is flexion and compression, reduction requires extension and traction.

■ This is generally best performed using halo ring traction as it allows for conversion to a halo vest orthosis.

■ To obtain reduction, a towel roll is generally placed at approximately C6 to extend the spine, and traction is applied. Reduction is generally obtained with 25 to 40 lb.

■ Following reduction, a halo vest orthosis is applied, and upright X-rays are obtained to ensure that reduction can be maintained with the halo vest.

■ In patients with more than 5 mm of anterior translation or 11 degrees of angulation, reduction is difficult to maintain in the halo vest.[28] These patients can be treated with prolonged skeletal traction (up to 6 weeks) followed by halo vest immobilization after the fracture becomes stable or with surgery. Many physicians forgo prolonged traction due to patient discomfort and cost and will accept fracture displacement while immobilized in a halo orthosis.

■ Type IIA fractures result from flexion-distraction, so traction is ABSOLUTELY CONTRAINDICATED and will increase the deformity. These fractures are characterized by angulation without translation and oblique fracture lines.

■ Type IIA fractures should be reduced with gentle hyperextension and axial compression. An acceptable reduction is less than 10 degrees of angulation. Prior to reduction, a halo ring should be placed and then attached to the halo vest with the neck in mild extension and compression in order to maintain the reduction. The halo vest is generally maintained for 3 months. Failure to obtain or maintain an acceptable reduction is an indication for surgery.

■ Type III fractures cannot be managed with closed treatment.

■ For Type II and type IIA fractures in which an acceptable reduction cannot be maintained with a halo vest, surgery is indicated.

■ Open reduction and osteosynthesis with placement of C2 pedicle screws across the fracture site is the surgical treatment of choice (**TECH FIG1**).

■ This is done with a posterior approach using Mayfield tongs or halo ring attached to the operating table to hold the head in a reduced position. The posterior elements of C2 are completely exposed, and the isthmus of C2 is palpated to help guide screw placement. Care is taken to protect the C2 nerve root. Lag screws are then placed across the fracture site using fluoroscopy guidance, if desired.

■ A C2–3 anterior cervical decompression and fusion (ACDF) is another option for fractures that lose reduction or go onto nonunion.

■ Type III fractures require open reduction and fixation of the facet dislocation and subsequent positioning of the head in an extended position if needed to reduce the spondylolisthesis.

■ The head is positioned in Mayfield tongs, and the posterior elements of C2 and C3 are completely exposed. Towel clips or tenaculums are then used to reduce the dislocated facets, and any remaining spondylolisthesis is reduced by positioning the head in extension.

■ Following reduction, C2 pedicle screws are placed across the fracture site using a lag technique to promote osteosynthesis of the pars fractures. Lateral mass screws are then placed at C3 and connected to the C2 pedicle screws using rods. The remaining cartilage in the C2–3 facet joint is removed using a burr and bone graft applied in order to obtain a C2–3 fusion (**TECH FIG 2**). Alternatively, the pars fracture may be treated nonoperatively with halo immobilization.

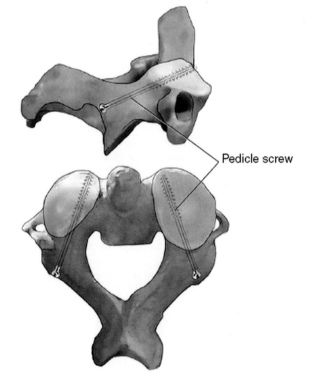

Pedicle screw

C2 pedicle screws for osteosynthesis

TECH FIG 1 • C2 osteosynthesis using pedicle screws placed across the pars fractures in traumatic spondylolisthesis of the axis (Hangman's fracture).

TECHNIQUES

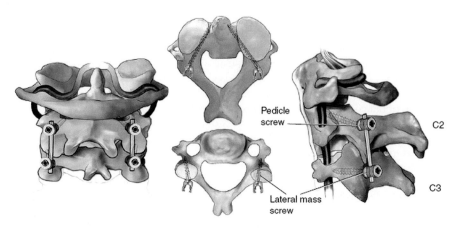

Pedicle screw

C2

C3

Lateral mass screw

C2-3 fusion with C2 pedicle screws and C3 lateral mass screws

TECH FIG 2 • C2–3 posterior fusion for type III traumatic spondylolisthesis of the axis (Hangman's fracture) using C2 pedicle screws across the pars fractures and lateral mass fixation at C3 following open reduction of the facet dislocation.

PEARLS AND PITFALLS

Type I and IA fractures	▪ Stable and should not be overtreated ▪ A collar is sufficient
Type IIA fracture	▪ Must be identified and traction is ABSOLUTELY CONTRAINDICATED in these patients as it will increase the deformity ▪ These patients should undergo closed reduction with gentle extension and axial compression
Type III fracture	▪ The only absolute indication for surgery

Outcomes

▪ The union rate for type I and IA fractures approaches 100%.[26]

▪ Some patients can develop C2–3 facet arthritis due to cartilage damage that occurs with hyperextension at the time of injury.

▪ Patients with type II fractures usually develop anterior ankylosis at C2–3 due to the injury to the disc and elevation of the ALL. If this fails to occur, nonunion can occur, although the rate of this is unknown.

▪ Patients with type III fractures typically have worse outcomes if they suffered a neurologic injury. No long-term outcome data on this group are available, likely due to the very low incidence of this injury.

Complications

▪ Nonunion is rare and can be treated with C2 pedicle screw osteosynthesis or a C2–3 ACDF.

▪ Injury to the spinal cord or vertebral artery can occur with improper C2 pedicle screw placement. Characterization of the course of the vertebral artery is necessary prior to performing this procedure.

SUBAXIAL FACET DISLOCATIONS

Definition

▪ Facet dislocations occur when the inferior articular process (IAP) of the cranial vertebra dislocates anterior to the superior articular process (SAP) of the caudal vertebra.

▪ This occurs with a distraction-flexion mechanism.

▪ Distraction-flexion injuries can present as subluxations with gapping of the facet joint, "perched" facets with the IAP resting on the SAP or "jumped" facets where the IAP has dislocated anterior to the SAP.

▪ These injuries can be unilateral or bilateral.

Anatomy

▪ The cervical spine can be viewed as having an anterior column (ALL, vertebral body, disc, PLL) and a posterior column (pedicle, lateral masses, facet joints, facet capsules, ligamentum flavum, inter- and supraspinous ligaments) that provide stability.

▪ The facet joints in the subaxial cervical spine are oriented in the coronal plane and inclined approximately 45 degrees to the horizontal (**FIG 8**). This orientation allows for axial rotation, lateral bending, and flexion-extension, with coupled lateral bending and axial rotation.

▪ The cervical nerve roots exit directly laterally and exit above the pedicle of the vertebra for which they are named (ie, C7 nerve root exits above the C7 pedicle), posterior to the vertebral artery.

▪ The vertebral artery runs through the foramina transversarium from C2 through C6 but generally not through the foramen at C7. It is located anterior to the medial aspect of the lateral masses.

Pathogenesis and Classification

▪ A popular classification for subaxial cervical spine injuries was published by Allen et al. in 1982.[29]

▪ Facet dislocations are classified in the distractive flexion (DF) phylogeny (**FIG 9**).

▪ The SLIC (Subaxial Cervical Spine Injury Classification) system would classify this injury as a translational cervical injury with facet dislocation, with disruption of the discoligamentous complex with or without a neurologic deficit.

▪ The majority of facet dislocations are due to shallow diving injuries or motor vehicle accidents in which the head is axially loaded anterior to the midsagittal plane, resulting in flexion and posterior distraction.

▪ A biomechanical model demonstrated that the posterior ligamentous structures fail first, allowing for flexion and

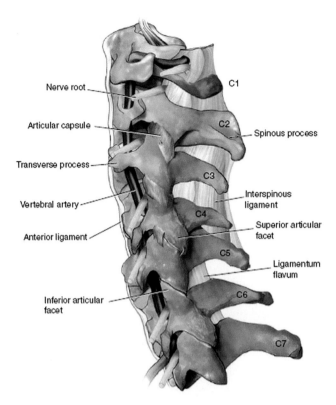

FIG 8 • Osteoligamentous anatomy of the cervical spine.

Nerve root

Articular capsule

Transverse process

Vertebral artery

Anterior ligament

Inferior articular facet

C1

C2

Spinous process

C3

C4

Interspinous ligament

Superior articular facet

C5

Ligamentum flavum

C6

C7

separation of the facet joints. As anterior column soft tissue structures fail, including the PLL and posterior anulus, anterior translation and facet dislocation can then occur.[30]

■ In Allen's DF phylogeny, DF stage 1 (DF-1) injuries include facet subluxation without dislocation, DF-2 injuries are unilateral facet dislocations with approximately 25% anterior translation of the cranial vertebra on the caudal vertebra, DF-3 injuries are bilateral facet dislocations with approximately 50% anterior translation, and DF-4 injuries represent 100% anterior translation (ie, the "floating vertebra").

Patient History, Physical Findings, and Initial Management

■ There is a high rate of spinal cord injury (SCI) associated with facet dislocations, at least 25% with unilateral dislocations and over 50% with bilateral dislocations.[31]

■ Patients should undergo full trauma resuscitation with immobilization of the cervical spine in the field.

■ The use of methylprednisolone in SCI patients is controversial. The NASCIS 2 and 3 trials concluded that SCI patients presenting within 8 hours of injury should receive methylprednisolone (30 mg/kg bolus followed by 5.4 mg/kg/hr infusion for 24 hours if presentation is within 3 hours of injury and for 48 hours if presentation is between 3 to 8 hours after injury).[32,33] However, these recommendations are based on minimal neurologic improvements found only in subgroup analyses, and many centers have abandoned the use of steroids in SCI.[34]

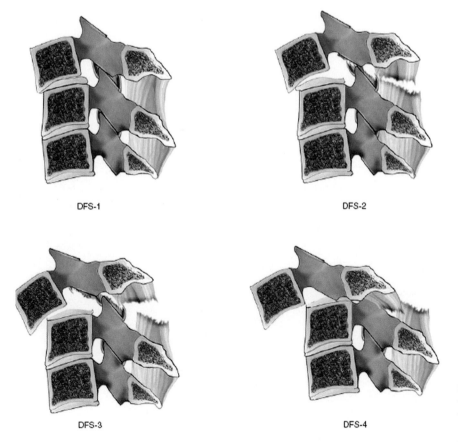

DFS-1

DFS-2

DFS-3

DFS-4

Distractive flexion phylogeny

FIG 9 • Allen and Ferguson's distraction flexion (DF) phylogeny. DF-1 injuries involve subluxation of the facet joints. DF-2 is a unilateral dislocation. DF-3 is a bilateral dislocation. DF-4 is 100% anterior translation of the vertebra.

■ An attempt should be made to maintain mean arterial pressure above 85 mm Hg for the first 5 to 7 days following SCI in order to maintain perfusion of the injured cord.[35]

Imaging

■ Standard radiographic evaluation of a suspected cervical spine injury includes anteroposterior (AP), lateral, and open mouth views. In order to be sufficient, both the occipitocervical and the cervicothoracic junctions should be visualized.

■ Most trauma centers now obtain CT scans of the cervical spine in all trauma patients since they are much more sensitive in diagnosing subtle cervical spine fractures and fractures at the occipitocervical and cervicothoracic junctions.[36]

■ MRI is indicated in all patients with facet dislocations to assess the status of the spinal cord, ligamentous structures, and the intervertebral disc. The timing of MRI relative to reduction is controversial. Many physicians experienced in the management of cervical dislocations advocate an immediate closed skeletal reduction in the absence of MRI only in an awake, alert, oriented, and cooperative patient in order to closely follow the patients neurologic status during the process of reduction .[37,38]

■ There is almost absolute consensus that patients with a complete SCI should also undergo immediate closed reduction prior to MRI because the potential downside neurologically is small compared to the potential benefit of immediate neurologic decompression. Obtunded patients should undergo MRI prior to closed reduction since they are unable to cooperate with serial neurologic examinations.

■ All patients need an MRI prior to surgical treatment to assess the need for an anterior discectomy.

■ Imaging of the entire spine should be performed due to the high rate of noncontiguous injuries (10% to 15%).[39]

Nonoperative Management

■ All patients with facet dislocations need to undergo reduction in order to decrease the pressure on the spinal cord as soon as possible. The timing of MRI relative to closed reduction is discussed above.

■ Most facet dislocations occur in the lower cervical spine, and large amounts of weight can be required (up to 140 lb) to obtain a closed reduction. As such, stainless steel Gardner-Wells tongs should be used.

■ An initial flexion moment should be applied along with axial traction in order to unlock the facet joints. This may be accomplished with bivector traction, although positioning the tongs posterior to the external auditory meatus will also produce a flexion moment.

■ Once the facets are "perched," the physician can then gently extend the patient's neck in order to obtain a reduction. This is done by using the treating physician's thumbs to control the traction pins while the other fingers are used to provide an anterior counterforce to the posterior aspect of the lower cervical spine. A towel roll between the scapulae and removal of the foam pad beneath the patient's head on the RotoRest bed can allow for unencumbered extension (**FIG 10**).

■ During the reduction maneuver, an assistant can decrease the amount of traction. If reduction is successful (it is oftentimes accompanied by a palpable clunk), the patient can be left with 10 lb of traction in extension to control the head and maintain reduction.

■ Reduction should be confirmed radiographically, and the patient's neurologic status should be documented. A decline in neurologic function with reduction suggests possible cord compression by herniated disc material.

■ An MRI should be obtained prior to going to the operating room in order to assess for the possibility of a herniated disc impinging on the cord. If present in a neurologically intact or incomplete patient, an anterior discectomy is indicated.

■ If operative treatment is delayed, application of a halo vest orthosis should be considered to maintain the reduction.

■ For unilateral facet dislocations, a reduction maneuver is often required.[40] Following the application of traction, the

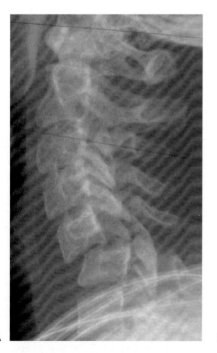 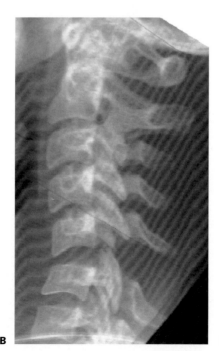 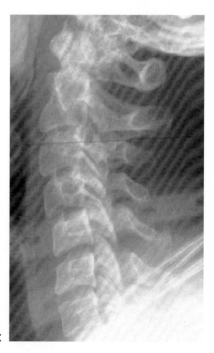

A   B   C

FIG 10 • Reduction of C5–6 bilateral facet dislocation. **A.** Injury film showing dislocated facets. **B.** Axial traction with slight flexion has been applied, and the facets are perched. **C.** Extension was applied at this point, resulting in reduction.

physician must axially rotate the head away from the side of the dislocation while flexion is applied in order to unlock the facet. Once imaging suggests the facet is perched, a reduction maneuver can be performed in which the neck is extended and axially rotated toward the side of the dislocation.

Operative Treatment

▪ Facet dislocations represent unstable injuries, and surgical intervention should be strongly considered. A variety of situations can be encountered that necessitate different approaches to treatment (**FIG 11**).

▪ If the dislocation is irreducible, the patient should be taken to the operating room for an open reduction and stabilization. An MRI should be obtained prior to going to the operating room in order to assess for a disc herniation and the need for an anterior discectomy prior to reduction.

▪ For anesthesia, awake fiberoptic intubation avoids excessive cervical extension and allows for a neurologic exam after intubation. Neurophysiologic baselines are recorded after the administration of general anesthesia as well as after prone positioning and shoulder taping. We generally obtain prepositioning baselines in all patients, and it is required in neurologically intact patients or those with incomplete spinal cord injuries.

▪ Neurophysiologic spinal cord monitoring during open reduction is extremely helpful. If a change in neurologic status is detected, the reduction maneuver can readily be reversed, potentially avoiding permanent neurologic injury.

▪ Multimodality monitoring is preferred, including motor-evoked potentials, somatosensory-evoked potentials, and spontaneous EMG recordings.

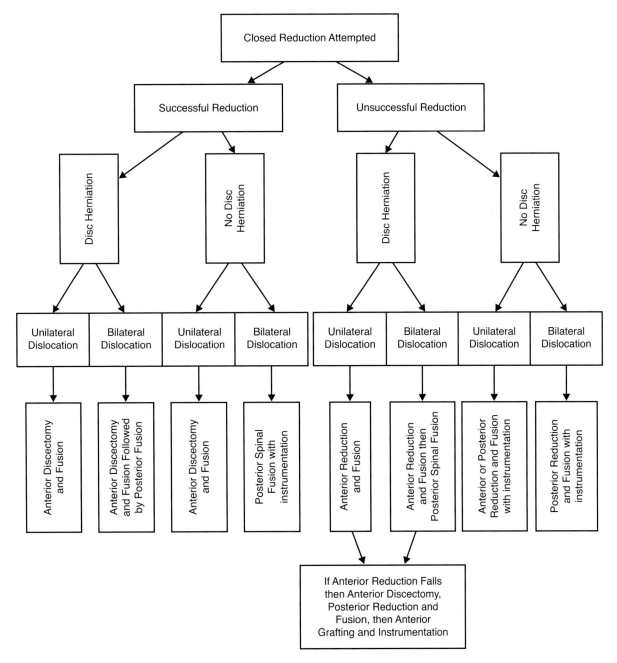

FIG 11 • Algorithm for treatment of facet dislocations.

POSTERIOR OPEN REDUCTION

- If the dislocation is irreducible with closed methods and there is no significant disc herniation, a posterior open reduction is favored because it allows direct access to the dislocated facet joints (**TECH FIGS 3 AND 4**).
- For prone positioning, the patient can remain in their halo ring or Mayfield tongs can be applied. The patient can then be rotated into the prone position on a Stryker frame or Jackson table. Traction can be applied during the rotation maneuver in order to increase stability.
- After prone positioning and establishment of neurophysiology baseline recordings, a standard subperiosteal dissection of the posterior cervical spine is performed.
- Care should be taken to avoid violating the facet capsules and interspinous ligaments of levels not involved in the intended fusion.
- The dislocated level can often be detected by a step-off between the spinous processes and the presence of hematoma and posterior ligamentous injury.
- Once the dislocation is identified clinically and/or radiographically, the lateral masses are exposed completely.
- The dislocation can be reduced by grasping the involved cephalad and caudal spinous process with a tenaculum or towel clip at the spinolaminar junction.
- The neurophysiologist should be warned of the possibility of an acute signal change. If any significant neurophysiologic changes are detected, the procedure should be halted.
- Axial caudal traction is applied to the caudal tenaculum. A gentle distraction and kyphotic moment is applied to the cephalad tenaculum to disengage the dislocated IAP.

- A rotational force may also be required for unilateral facet dislocations. The maneuver is applied until the IAP(s) of the cephalad vertebra is freed from the SAP(s) of the caudal vertebra.
- After disengaging the IAP(s), reduction can be obtained by applying cranial traction to the cranial vertebra until the IAP(s) clear the SAP. Caudal traction is then performed to reduce the IAP(s) posterior to the SAP(s).
- If this maneuver fails to achieve reduction, a Penfield or nerve hook along with the traction maneuvers can be used to lever the dislocated IAP over the SAP. Care must be taken to avoid fracturing the articular processes.
- The cranial edge of the SAP can also be trimmed using the burr in order to eliminate a barrier to reduction, although the surgeon should avoid overresection of the SAP as this decreases stability.
- Following reduction, lateral mass or pedicle screws are then placed in the standard fashion at the level of the dislocation. A one level fusion can be performed if there is no soft tissue injury at the adjacent levels and the lateral masses are intact and allow for good screw purchase. If these criteria are not met, additional levels must be included in the fusion.
- Many surgeons use local bone and bone graft extender for the fusion, although autograft harvested from the iliac crest is widely used.
- To achieve anatomic alignment, compression can be applied across the lateral mass screws.

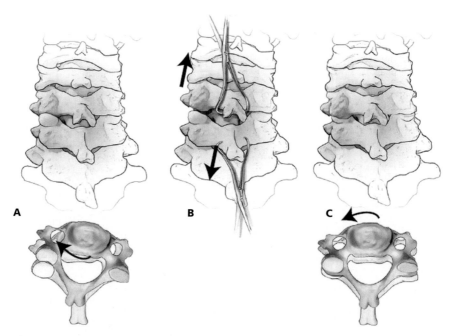

TECH FIG 3 • Posterior open reduction technique for unilateral facet dislocation. Tenaculums can be used to apply rotational and flexion moments to unlock the facet, followed by axial traction and reduction.

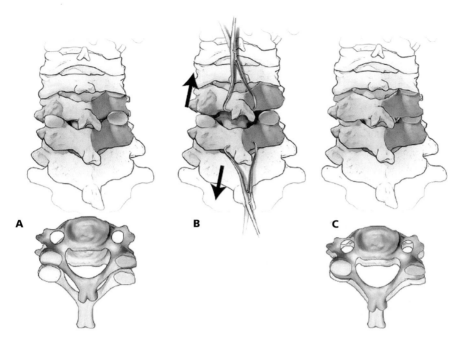

TECH FIG 4 • Posterior open reduction technique for bilateral facet dislocation. Tenaculums can be used to unlock the facet joints with axial traction and slight flexion followed by extension to affect the reduction.

ANTERIOR OPEN REDUCTION

- Although posterior open reduction is generally preferred for unreducible facet dislocations, if a disc herniation is present, an initial anterior approach is required. If the dislocation can be reduced through an anterior approach following discectomy, a posterior procedure may be avoided.
- The patient is positioned supine with a shoulder roll and the head supported in slight extension on a gel roll.
- Plain X-ray or fluoroscopy is essential to monitor the reduction maneuver.
- A standard ACDF approach is used.
- Once adequate exposure had been obtained, a discectomy is performed along with resection of the posterior longitudinal ligament. A complete, aggressive discectomy prior to reduction is of paramount importance to reduce the risk of neurological injury.
- Vertebral body pins (Caspar or equivalent devices) are placed into the vertebral bodies, diverging from each other approximately 10 to 20 degrees in order to produce a bending moment.
- Gently manipulating the pins into parallel orientation in the distraction device creates a flexion moment to unlock the facets. Subsequent distraction often results in perching of the facets.
- The cranial vertebral body is then translated dorsally with leverage through an interbody distractor or Cobb in order to obtain reduction. This can be done with simple manual manipulation of the distraction pins or by placing a Cobb under the inferior endplate of the dislocated vertebra and applying a gentle superoposterior force

once the facets are perched. Clearly, care must be taken to avoid overly aggressive reduction maneuvers or plunging into the spinal canal with the Cobb.
- In the case of a unilateral dislocation, the distraction pins should be applied with a divergent angle in the axial plane to accentuate the rotational deformity as traction is applied in order to unlock the facets. For example, if the right C5–6 facet joint is dislocated, the C5 pin would be placed rotated toward the right (in the opposite direction that the C5 vertebra is rotated) such that a rotational moment will be applied that will help to unlock the dislocation after traction is applied. Once the facet is perched, manual pressure or a Cobb can be used to affect reduction.
- Following radiographic confirmation of reduction, an interbody structural bone graft and anterior plate are placed. In general, we prefer to use allograft in the traumatic setting to prevent creating a wound at the iliac crest harvest site that could be at higher risk of infection in the trauma population. Autograft could be considered in patients at high risk of nonunion (ie, smokers). We use traditional fixed plates rather than dynamic plates when treating trauma patients since we are usually fixing a single level, and there is no evidence that dynamic plates improve fusion rates in single level cases. In addition, if an anterior-only construct is performed, a dynamic plate could allow for collapse into kyphosis due to injury to the posterior ligamentous complex that accompanies these injuries.

TECHNIQUES

DETERMINING THE TYPE OF STABILIZATION FOLLOWING REDUCTION

- If a successful closed reduction is performed, the surgeon must determine what approach to use for stabilization (ie, anterior, posterior, or circumferential).
- Posterior fixation has been shown to be biomechanically superior to ACDF[41]; however, clinical results of ACDF have been shown to be equivalent to posterior fusion even for bilateral facet dislocations.[42] Posterior surgery is generally associated with more surgical morbidity and postoperative pain due to the stripping of the paraspinal muscles off the posterior elements.
- Circumferential fusion is certainly the strongest construct and is preferred for bilateral facet dislocations by some authors. Additionally, it can avoid the need for multiple

level fusion, which is sometimes necessary if a posterior-only approach is used.

- If an anterior approach is necessary to remove herniated disc material, an ACDF is probably sufficient. Posterior fixation can also be added to improve the strength of the construct.
- If a posterior approach is needed to obtain reduction, posterior fixation alone is typically sufficient. An ACDF can also be performed to strengthen the construct.
- In cases where closed reduction is successful and there is no disc herniation, the approach is left to the surgeon's discretion.

PEARLS AND PITFALLS

Closed reduction	■ Should be performed urgently, and prereduction MRI is not necessary in awake, alert, alert, cooperative patients who can comply with a neurologic exam
Closed reduction of lower cervical spine facet dislocations	■ Can sometimes require high amounts of weight (up to 140 lb), but efforts should be made to obtain a rapid closed reduction in order to decrease pressure on the cord and simplify surgical treatment
Preoperative MRI	■ Always required to determine if a disc herniation is present
Open reduction	■ Much easier to perform via a posterior approach, although reduction with an anterior approach is technically feasible and often performed

Outcomes

■ The neurologic status of the patient is the main determinant of outcome.

■ Union rates following operative stabilization of facet dislocations are over 90%.[42]

Complications

■ Neurologic deterioration during closed reduction or surgery is a feared complication. This risk can be minimized with frequent neurologic examinations in an awake, alert, cooperative patient during closed reduction and neurologic monitoring during surgery.

■ Vertebral artery injury has been reported in up to 11% of patients with cervical spine injuries.[43] However, the majority are asymptomatic and treatment is controversial. For patients who are symptomatic, anticoagulation is an option, but the risks and benefits of anticoagulation in the presence of a spine injury must be weighed.

■ Cervical SCI patients are at risk for many complications including deep venous thrombosis, decubitus ulcers, contractures, osteoporosis, and respiratory failure (particularly with higher SCI). Coordination of care with a SCI rehab team is essential to avoid these and other complications.

REFERENCES

1. Blumberg KD, Catalano JB, Cotler JM, et al . The pullout strength of titanium alloy MRI-compatible and stainless steel MRI-incompatible Gardner-Wells tongs. Spine 1993;18(13):1895–1896.
2. Greene KA, Dickman CA, Marciano FF, et al. Acute axis fractures. Analysis of management and outcome in 340 consecutive cases. Spine 1997;22(16):1843–1852.
3. Ogden JA. Radiology of postnatal skeletal development. XII. The second cervical vertebra. Skeletal Radiol 1984;12(3):169–177.
4. Haffajee MR. A contribution by the ascending pharyngeal artery to the arterial supply of the odontoid process of the axis vertebra. Clin Anat 1997;10(1):14–18.
5. Anderson LD, D'Alonzo RT. Fractures of the odontoid process of the axis. J Bone Joint Surg Am 1974;56(8):1663–1674.
6. Julien TD, Frankel B, Traynelis VC, et al. Evidence-based analysis of odontoid fracture management. Neurosurg Focus 2000;8(6):e1.
7. Clark CR, White AA III. Fractures of the dens. A multicenter study. J Bone Joint Surg Am 1985;67(9):1340–1348.
8. Bucholz RW, Burkhead WZ, Graham W, et al. Occult cervical spine injuries in fatal traffic accidents. J Trauma 1979;19(10):768–771.
9. Fairholm D, Lee ST, Lui TN. Fractured odontoid: the management of delayed neurological symptoms. Neurosurgery 1996;38(1):38–43.
10. Blacksin MF, Lee HJ. Frequency and significance of fractures of the upper cervical spine detected by CT in patients with severe neck trauma. AJR Am J Roentgenol 1995;165:1201–1204.
11. Rushton SA, Vaccaro AR, Levine MJ, et al. Bivector traction for unstable cervical spine fractures: a description of its application and preliminary results. J Spinal Disord 1997;10(5):436–440.
12. Przybylski GJ, Harrop JS, Vaccaro AR. Closed management of displaced Type II odontoid fractures: more frequent respiratory compromise with posteriorly displaced fractures. Neurosurg Focus 2000; 8(6):e5.
13. Clarke A, Hutton MJ, Chan D. Respiratory failure due to a displaced fracture of the odontoid. J Bone Joint Surg Br 2010;92(7):1023–1024.
14. Lennarson PJ, Mostafavi H, Traynelis VC, et al. Management of type II dens fractures: a case-control study. Spine 2000;25(10):1234–1237.
15. Dickman CA, Sonntag VK. Posterior C1–C2 transarticular screw fixation for atlantoaxial arthrodesis. Neurosurgery 1998;43(2):275–280; discussion 80–81.
16. White AP, Hashimoto R, Norvell DC, et al. Morbidity and mortality related to odontoid fracture surgery in the elderly population. Spine 2010;35(suppl 9):S146–S157.

17. Hsu WK, Anderson PA. Odontoid fractures: update on management. J Am Acad Orthop Surg 2010;18(7):383–394.
18. Müller EJ, Wick M, Russe O, et al. Management of odontoid fractures in the elderly. Eur Spine J 1999;8(5):360–365.
19. Tashjian RZ, Majercik S, Biffl WL, et al. Halo-vest immobilization increases early morbidity and mortality in elderly odontoid fractures. J Trauma 2006;60(1):199–203.
20. Frangen TM, Zilkens C, Muhr G, et al. Odontoid fractures in the elderly: dorsal C1/C2 fusion is superior to halo-vest immobilization. J Trauma 2007;63(1):83–89.
21. Andersson S, Rodrigues M, Olerud C. Odontoid fractures: high complication rate associated with anterior screw fixation in the elderly. Eur Spine J 2000;9(1):56–59.
22. Inamasu J, Guiot BH. Vascular injury and complication in neurosurgical spine surgery. Acta Neurochir (Wien) 2006;148(4):375–387.
23. Levine AM, Edwards CC. The management of traumatic spondylolisthesis of the axis. J Bone Joint Surg Am 1985;67(2):217–226.
24. Starr JK, Eismont FJ. Atypical hangman's fractures. Spine 1993;18(14):1954–1957.
25. Francis WR, Fielding JW, Hawkins RJ, et al. Traumatic spondylolisthesis of the axis. J Bone Joint Surg Br 1981;63-B(3):313–318.
26. Levine AM, Dacre A. Traumatic spondylolisthesis of the axis. In: Clark CR, ed. The Cervical Spine 4th ed. Philadelphia, PA: Lippincott Williams & Wilkins; 2005:629–650.
27. Gleizes V, Jacquot FP, Signoret F, et al. Combined injuries in the upper cervical spine: clinical and epidemiological data over a 14-year period. Eur Spine J 2000;9(5):386–392.
28. Vaccaro AR, Madigan L, Bauerle WB, et al. Early halo immobilization of displaced traumatic spondylolisthesis of the axis. Spine 2002;27(20):2229–2233.
29. Allen BL Jr, Ferguson RL, Lehmann TR, et al. A mechanistic classification of closed, indirect fractures and dislocations of the lower cervical spine. Spine (Phila Pa 1976) 1982;7(1):1–27.
30. Panjabi MM, Simpson AK, Ivancic PC, et al. Cervical facet joint kinematics during bilateral facet dislocation. Eur Spine J 2007;16(10):1680–1688.
31. Vives MJ, Garfin SR. Flexion injuries. In: Clark CR, ed. The Cervical Spine 4th ed. Philadelphia, PA: Lippincott Williams & Wilkins; 2005.
32. Bracken MB, Shepard MJ, Collins WF, et al. A randomized, controlled trial of methylprednisolone or naloxone in the treatment of acute spinal-cord injury. Results of the Second National Acute Spinal Cord Injury Study. N Engl J Med 1990;322(20):1405–1411.
33. Bracken MB, Shepard MJ, Holford TR, et al. Administration of methylprednisolone for 24 or 48 hours or tirilazad mesylate for 48 hours in the treatment of acute spinal cord injury. Results of the Third National Acute Spinal Cord Injury Randomized Controlled Trial. National Acute Spinal Cord Injury Study. JAMA 1997;277(20):1597–1604.
34. Kwon BK, Vaccaro AR, Grauer JN, et al. Subaxial cervical spine trauma. J Am Acad Orthop Surg 2006;14(2):78–89.
35. Blood pressure management after acute spinal cord injury. Neurosurgery 2002;50(3 suppl):S58–S62.
36. LeBlang SD, Nunez DB Jr. Helical CT of cervical spine and soft tissue injuries of the neck. Radiol Clin North Am 1999;37(3):515–532, v–vi.
37. Eismont FJ, Arena MJ, Green BA. Extrusion of an intervertebral disc associated with traumatic subluxation or dislocation of cervical facets. Case report. J Bone Joint Surg Am 1991;73(10):1555–1560.
38. Vaccaro AR, Falatyn SP, Flanders AE, et al. Magnetic resonance evaluation of the intervertebral disc, spinal ligaments, and spinal cord before and after closed traction reduction of cervical spine dislocations. Spine 1999;24(12):1210–1217.
39. Vaccaro AR, An HS, Lin S, et al. Noncontiguous injuries of the spine. J Spinal Disord 1992;5(3):320–329.
40. Cotler HB, Miller LS, DeLucia FA, et al. Closed reduction of cervical spine dislocations. Clin Orthop Relat Res 1987;(214):185–199.
41. Ulrich C, Woersdoerfer O, Kalff R, et al. Biomechanics of fixation systems to the cervical spine. Spine 1991;16(3 suppl):S4–S9.
42. Razack N, Green BA, Levi AD. The management of traumatic cervical bilateral facet fracture-dislocations with unicortical anterior plates. J Spinal Disord 2000;13(5):374–381.
43. Management of vertebral artery injuries after nonpenetrating cervical trauma. Neurosurgery 2002;50(3 suppl):S173–S178.

Chapter 10

Minimally Invasive Posterior Cervical Laminoforaminotomy

Nicholas P. Slimack and Richard G. Fessler

DEFINITION

- Cervical radiculopathy is a neurologic condition characterized by dysfunction of a cervical spinal nerve, the roots of the nerve, or both.
- It usually presents with unilateral pain that radiates from the neck to the arm and/or the hand.
- There can be a combination of sensory loss, loss of motor function, and reflex changes in the affected nerve root distribution.
- This chapter focuses on minimally invasive posterior cervical laminoforaminotomy as a surgical treatment option for patients with cervical radiculopathy.

ANATOMY

- The external occipital protuberance (EOP) can be palpated in the midline of the skull. The superior nuchal line is the thickened ridge that extends laterally from the EOP (**FIG 1A**).
- Beneath the skin and subcutaneous fat of the posterior cervical spine is located the superficial fascia (**FIG 1B**).
- Deep to the superficial fascia, structures are anatomically compartmentalized by an organized deep fascia and several interfascial planes (**FIG 2**).
- There are three principle deep fascial layers: a superficial, middle, and deep layer.
  - One layer is attached to the external occipital protuberance, the superior nuchal line, the ligamentum nuchae, and the spinous processes of the cervical vertebrae.
  - It divides to surround the trapezius.
  - The deep layer of the deep cervical fascia is attached to the ligamentum nuchae in the midline.
- The most superficial muscle on the posterior aspect of the neck is the trapezius which arises from the external occipital protuberance and the medial part of the superior nuchal line of the occipital bone, the spinous processes of C7–T1 through T12, the supraspinal ligament, and the ligamentum nuchae (**FIG 3**).
- The next muscle is the splenius capitis and arises from the ligamentum nuchae and spinous processes of C7 through T3 and inserts on the lateral portion of the superior nuchal line (**FIG 1**).
- The erector spinae lie deep in the cervical region and include the iliocostalis cervicis, longissimus cervicis, the splenius cervicis, and the splenius capitis.
- The deep layer of the deep cervical musculature includes the semispinalis cervicis and the semispinalis capitis (**FIG 1**).
- The spinous process projects posteriorly from the junction of the laminae.
- The lateral mass forms at the junction of the lamina and pedicle and gives rise to the superior and inferior articular processes or facets (**FIG 4**).
- The superior facet at each level faces upward and posteriorly; the inferior facet faces downward and anteriorly.
- A superior facet articulates with the corresponding inferior facet of the vertebral body cephalad to form the osseous elements of the zygapophyseal joints.

- A vertebral notch is located on the superior and inferior aspect of each pedicle, such that adjacent notches contribute to the intervertebral foramen, through which the spinal nerve exits the spinal canal.
- The foramen is bound superiorly and inferiorly by the pedicle, posteriorly by the facets, and anteriorly by the intervertebral discs, uncovertebral joints, and vertebral bodies (**FIG 5**).
- The vertical diameter of the foramen is approximately 9 mm, the horizontal diameter is 4 mm, and the length ranges from 4 to 6 mm.
- Foramina exit at an angle of 45 degrees from the midsagittal plane.
- The spinal cord is cylindrical and slightly flattened in the anteroposterior (AP) direction, and thus usually has a larger transverse than AP diameter.
- The spinal cord enlarges from C3 to C6, where it usually attains a maximal transverse diameter of 13 to 14 mm (**FIG 6**).
- In the lower cervical spine, the anterior and posterior root entry zones are located approximately one disc level higher than the corresponding intervertebral foramen through which will pass the nerve root formed from its rootlets.
- The rootlets pass obliquely laterally and caudally within the canal, entering the root sleeve where the sensory and motor roots are separated by the interradicular septum, a lateral extension of the dura mater.
- Each dorsal root presents an oval enlargement, the spinal ganglion, as it approaches or enters the intervertebral foramen.
- Just distal to this ganglion, the dorsal and ventral roots combine to form a spinal nerve.
- The cervical nerve root occupies one-third of the foraminal space in a normal spine, usually the inferior aspect, with the superior aspect being filled with fat and associated veins.
- The ventral (motor) roots emerge from the dura mater more caudally than the dorsal (sensory) roots, and the ventral roots course along the caudal border of the dorsal roots within intervertebral foramina.
- Thus, compression of the ventral roots, dorsal roots, or both depends on the anatomic structures around the nerve roots, such as a prolapsed disc (ventral root compression) or osteophytes from the facet joint (dorsal root compression).
- The most likely site of compression of the radicular nerve is at the entrance zone of the intervertebral foramen because the medial entrance zone of the foramen is smaller in diameter than the lateral exit zone, whereas the nerve roots are widest at their takeoff from the central thecal sac and become more narrow laterally.
- Nerves C2 to C7 exit above the correspondingly numbered vertebrae.
- The C8 nerve root exits the intervertebral foramen formed between C7 and T1.
- The dorsal root ganglion is usually located between the vertebral artery and the superior articular process.

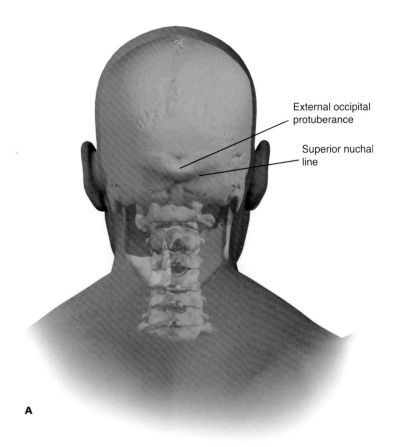

External occipital
protuberance

Superior nuchal
line

A

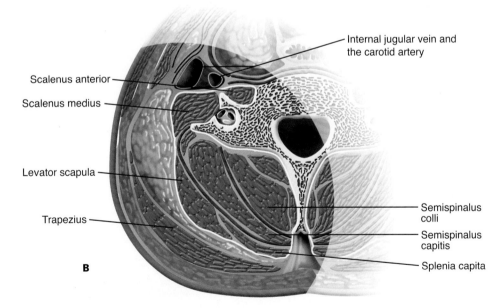

Internal jugular vein and
the carotid artery

Scalenus anterior

Scalenus medius

Levator scapula

Trapezius

Semispinalus
colli

Semispinalus
capitis

Splenia capita

B

FIG 1 • **A.** Superficial anatomical landmarks of the posterior cervical spine. **B.** Cross-sectional
anatomy of posterior cervical spine: superficial fascial layer (*blue*) and the muscles underneath.

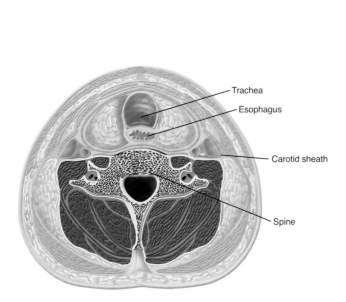

FIG 2 • Cross-sectional anatomy of posterior cervical spine: deep fascial layer (*blue*) and the muscles underneath.

Trachea
Esophagus
Carotid sheath
Spine

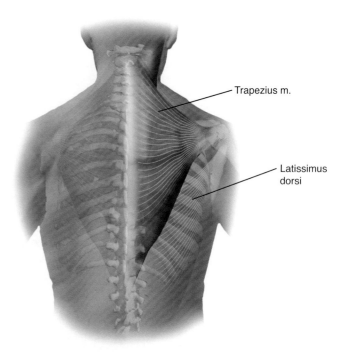

FIG 3 • Trapezius muscle anatomy and its insertion points.

Trapezius m.
Latissimus dorsi

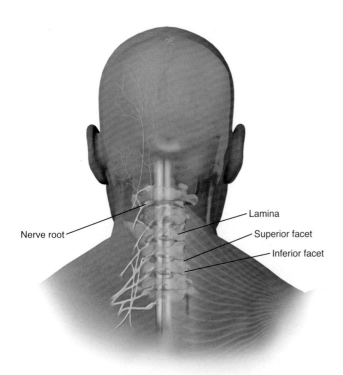

FIG 4 • Bone anatomy of the posterior cervical spine demonstrating the relationships of the superior and inferior facets, the lamina, and the exiting nerve roots.

Nerve root
Lamina
Superior facet
Inferior facet

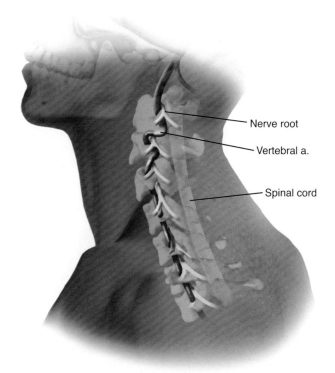

FIG 5 • Lateral view of cervical spine depicting exiting nerve roots and vertebral artery within the region of the neural foramen.

Nerve root
Vertebral a.
Spinal cord

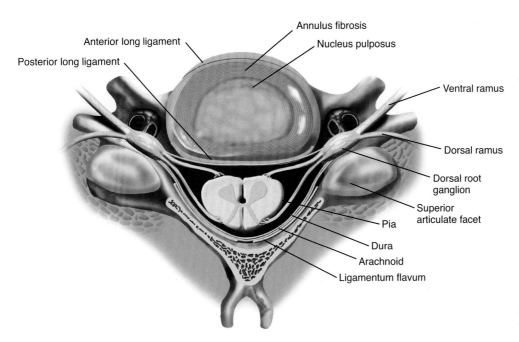

FIG 6 • Cross-sectional anatomy of the cervical spine.

■ In the sagittal plane, cervical nerve roots C3 through C8 in the intervertebral foramina lie midway between the posterior midpoints of the lateral masses situated an average of 5.5 mm above or below each lateral mass point.

■ Thus, cervical nerve roots enter their intervertebral foramina and leave the spinal canal at the level of the disc and above the pedicle of the same numbered level, except for C8, which exits above the T1 pedicle.

■ The vertebral artery enters the transverse foramen of C6 and ascends through the transverse foramen to the level of the atlas.

■ In this region, it lies just in front of (ventral) to the ventral rami of cervical nerves C6 to C2 and is surrounded by a venous plexus and sympathetic nerve fibers.

■ The transverse interforaminal distance and thus the transverse distance between vertebral arteries at the same cervical level increases slightly from C3 to C6.

PATHOGENESIS

■ The most common cause of cervical radiculopathy is foraminal compression of the spinal nerve.

■ Contributing factors include disc herniations and bulges, decreased disc height, degenerative changes of the uncovertebral joints anteriorly, and the zygapophyseal joints posteriorly (**FIGS 7–10**).

■ Other rare causes include tumor and spinal infections (**FIGS 11 AND 12**).

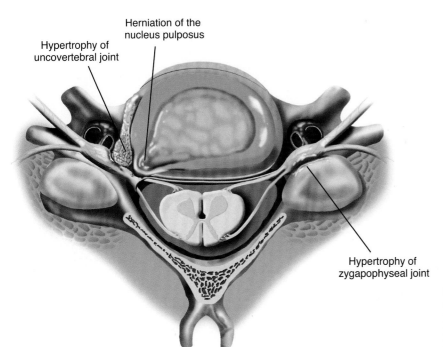

FIG 7 • Cross-sectional anatomy of the cervical spine depicting several pathologic states: hypertrophy of the uncovertebral joints, hypertrophy of zygapophyseal joints, and herniation of the nucleus pulposus.

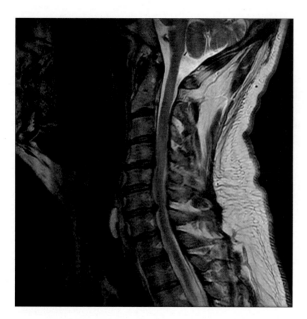

FIG 8 • Sagittal T2-weighted image of a patient with a right C7 radiculopathy due to a C6–7 lateral disc herniation.

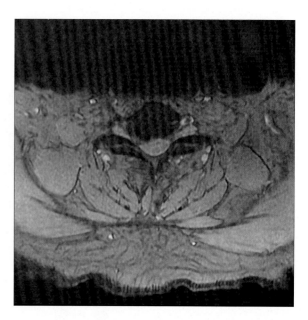

FIG 10 • Axial T2-weighted image of the same patient with a right C7 radiculopathy due to a C6–7 lateral disc herniation.

▪ Normal disc itself does not contain nociceptive nerve fibers and is insensitive to pain.

▪ When the nucleus pulposus ruptures through the annulus fibrosus, there is little or no localized pain until nociceptive fibers of the sinuvertebral nerves in the lateral posterior ligament and the dura of the nerve root sleeves are stimulated.

▪ This stimulation generates localized back and neck pain.

▪ In cases of cervical spondylosis, vertebral bodies subside and lose height, the ligamentum flavum and facet joint capsule tend to fold, which further decreases foraminal dimensions.

▪ Some have postulated that nerve root compression by itself does not always lead to pain and note that the dorsal-root ganglion must also be compressed.[1]

  ▪ Mechanical distortion of the nerve root leads to a cascade of events in the microenvironment of the nerve.

▪ Hypoxia of the nerve root and dorsal ganglion can aggravate the effect of compression.

▪ Evidence indicates that inflammatory mediators—including matrix metalloproteinases, prostaglandin E, interleukin-6, substance P, and nitric oxide—are released by herniated cervical intervertebral discs.

  ▪ These observations underlie the reason that anti-inflammatory agents often suffice to treat the radicular pain.

NATURAL HISTORY

▪ Cervical radiculopathy occurs annually in 85 out of 100,000 people.

▪ It is estimated that 75% to 90% of patients with acute cervical radiculopathy due to disc herniation will improve without surgery.

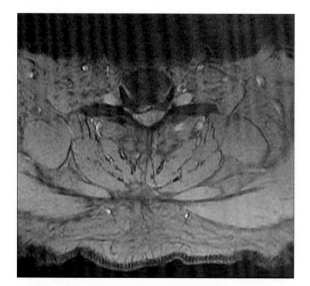

FIG 9 • Axial T2-weighted image of the same patient with a right C7 radiculopathy due to a C6–7 lateral disc herniation.

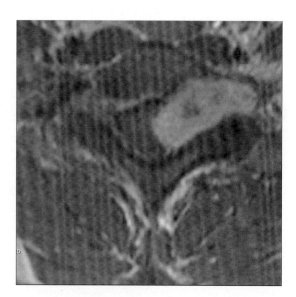

FIG 11 • Axial T1-weighted MRI with contrast showing a left C5–6 nerve sheath tumor.

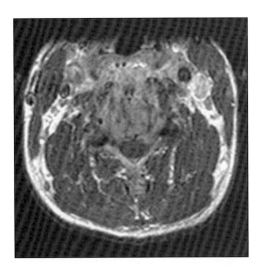

FIG 12 • Axial T1-weighted MRI with contrast showing a disc space infection with left foraminal epidural abscess.

■ In a 1994 population-based study from Rochester, MN, 26% of patients with cervical radiculopathy underwent surgery within 3 months of the diagnosis (typically for the combination of radicular pain, sensory loss, and muscle weakness), whereas the remainder were treated medically.

  ■ Recurrence, defined as the reappearance of symptoms of radiculopathy after a symptom-free interval of at least 6 months, occurred in 32% of patients during a median follow-up of 4.9 years. At the last follow-up, 90% of the nonoperated patients had normal findings or were only mildly incapacitated owing to cervical radiculopathy.

PATIENT HISTORY AND PHYSICAL FINDINGS

■ Patients with cervical radiculopathy exhibit the hallmark symptoms of unilateral neck and/or arm pain, sensory disturbances, and possibly motor deficits (Table 1).
■ Central to the patient's history are descriptors that include location, onset, duration, severity, associated symptoms, and triggers.
■ Pain is most prominent in acute cervical radiculopathy and it may be described as sharp, electric, achy, or burning.
■ It can be located in the neck, shoulder, arm, or chest, depending on the nerve root involved.
■ Classically, an acute radiculopathy presents with pain radiating in a myotomal distribution.
■ Sensory symptoms, predominantly paresthesias and numbness, are more common than motor loss and diminished reflexes.

■ The clinician should keep in mind that the sensory symptoms frequently do not follow classic dermatomal patterns as there is normal anatomic variation from individual to individual (**FIG 13**).
■ For patients with acute cervical radiculopathy, arm pain is present in nearly 100%, sensory deficits in 85%, neck pain in 79%, reflex deficits in 71%, motor deficits in 68%, scapular pain in 52%, anterior chest pain in 17%, headaches in 9%, anterior chest and arm pain in 5%, and left-sided chest and arm pain in 1%.
■ Radicular pain is often accentuated by maneuvers that stretch the involved nerve root, such as coughing, sneezing, Valsalva, and certain cervical movements and positions.
■ The Spurling test is performed by maximally extending and rotating the neck toward the involved side (**FIG 14**).
■ When positive, this test is particularly useful in differentiating cervical radiculopathy from other etiologies of upper extremity pain, such as peripheral nerve entrapment disorders, because the maneuver stresses only the structures within the cervical spine.
■ It is important to note that the physical examination can be normal.
■ The presence of "red flags" in the patient's history (including fever, chills, unexplained weight loss, unremitting night pain, previous cancer, immunosuppression, or intravenous drug use) should alert clinicians to the possibility of more serious disease, such as tumor or infection.

IMAGING AND OTHER DIAGNOSTIC STUDIES

Plain Films

■ Plain films offer the advantage of showing the spinal column in a weight-bearing state.
■ Degenerative changes on plain radiographs become more prevalent as individuals age.
  ■ However, it has been shown that degenerative changes are present in both symptomatic and asymptomatic individuals.
■ They are inexpensive, readily available, and provide information regarding sagittal balance, congenital abnormalities, fractures, deformity, and instability.
■ Flexion-extension lateral cervical spine radiographs can reveal instability that may be the cause of intermittent or positional symptoms.

Myelography

■ Changes in the contrast-filled spinal canal can serve as indirect measure of neural compression.
■ The major disadvantage of plain myelography is its invasive nature.
■ Accuracy rates for cervical myelography in the diagnosis of clinical nerve root compression ranges between 67% and 92% when compared with intraoperative findings.

| TABLE 1 | Distribution of Cervical Disc Herniations and Anatomic Correlates |

Level	Percentage of Cervical Discs	Compressed Root	Muscles Affected	Sensory Region	Reflex
C4–5	2%–5%	C5	Deltoid	Shoulder	Deltoid and pectoralis
C5–6	15%–20%	C6	Forearm flexion	Upper arm, thumb, radial forearm	Biceps and brachioradialis
C6–7	65%–70%	C7	Triceps and forearm extenders	2nd and 3rd fingers	Triceps
C7–T1	10%	C8	Hand intrinsics	4th and 5th fingers	Finger jerk

Methods for Examining the Cervical Spine for Nerve Root Syndromes

Examination	Technique	Illustration	Grading	Significance
Deltoid	Patient abducts arm against examiner's resistance; sensation tested in deltoid region and along lateral arm		Muscle strength graded 0–5	Deficits reveal abnormal function of C5 nerve root
Biceps, wrist extension	Patient flexes elbow and extends wrist against examiner's resistance; sensation lateral forearm and radial two digits		Muscle strength graded 0–5	Deficits reveal abnormal function of C6 nerve root
Triceps and wrist flexion	Patient extends elbow and flexes wrist; sensation to middle finger		Muscle strength graded 0–5	Deficits reveal abnormal function of C7 nerve root

(continued)

Methods for Examining the Cervical Spine for Nerve Root Syndromes

Examination	Technique	Illustration	Grading	Significance
Handgrip	Sensation to medial forearm and ulnar two digits; motor to finger flexors—grip		Muscle strength graded 0–5	Deficits reveal abnormal function of C8 nerve root
Finger abduction	Sensation to medial arm; motor to interossei		Muscle strength graded 0–5	Deficits reveal abnormal function of T1 nerve root

■ Myelography is associated with few false-positive results, a 15% false-negative rate, and an overall accuracy rate of 85% in a study of 53 patients who had surgical confirmation of the cervical spine pathology.

Computed Tomography

■ CT allows for the direct visualization of pathology causing compression of neural structures.
■ CT also has a high spatial resolution and is especially helpful in visualizing the foraminal region.
■ Another important advantage of CT is that it can distinguish neural compression caused by soft tissue from compression related to bony structures, such as facet hypertrophy.
■ The main disadvantage of CT is the partial volume averaging effect and streak artifacts.
  ■ These can cause distortion of images, particularly at the lower cervical levels, or in individuals with wide shoulders.
■ The reported accuracy of CT of the cervical spine ranges from 72% to 91%.

■ By combining myelography with CT scan, the diagnostic accuracy approaches 96%.

Magnetic Resonance Imaging

■ MRI can detect neural structures directly and noninvasively.
■ The accurate assessment of disc herniations and spinal stenosis is due to the intrinsic contrast and good spatial resolution.
■ MRI correctly predicts 88% of the lesions as opposed to 81% for CT myelography, 57% for plain myelography, and 50% for CT.
■ Disc herniations are commonly observed with MRI scans of asymptomatic individuals.
■ They may be observed in 10% of asymptomatic people younger than 40 years of age and 5% of those older than 40 years of age.
■ Degenerative disc disease may be observed in 25% of asymptomatic people less than 40 years of age and 60% of those older than 40.

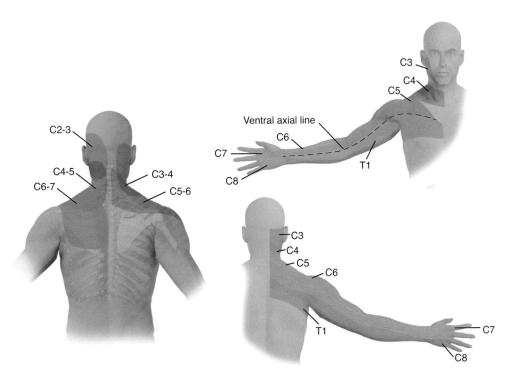

FIG 13 • Cervical dermatomes and sites of sensory symptoms.

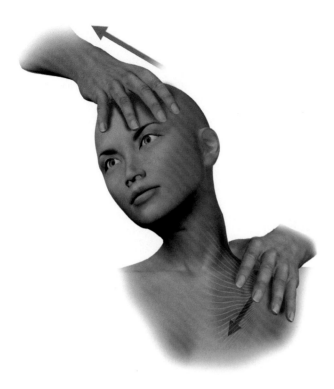

FIG 14 • Spurling maneuver.

■ Therefore, the imaging findings should be carefully correlated with the neurologic examination.

Electrodiagnostic Studies

■ Electrophysiologically, identify physiological abnormalities of the nerve root and rule out other neurologic causes of the patient's symptoms.

■ However, in patients with well-defined radiculopathy and good imaging correlation, the pain and added expense of electrodiagnostic studies are usually not justified.

■ The electrodiagnostic study has two parts: the nerve conduction velocities (NCV) and the needle electrode examination (EMG).

■ NCV are performed to exclude peripheral nerve pathology.

■ The EMG is performed by analyzing multiple muscles within the same myotome and in adjacent myotomes.

■ The presence of fibrillation potentials and positive sharp waves at rest is indicative of denervation, but these changes may not occur until 3 weeks after the onset of neural injury.

■ They are noted in the paraspinal musculature before they become apparent in the appendicular muscles.

■ EMG may be normal in the presence of mild radiculopathy or a predominantly sensory radiculopathy and are less likely to be positive in patients with no demonstrable weakness.

■ Nerve conduction studies and EMG have been shown to be useful in diagnosing nerve root dysfunction and distinguishing cervical radiculopathy from other lesions that are unclear on physical examination.

■ They have also been found to correlate well with findings on myelography and surgery.

DIFFERENTIAL DIAGNOSIS

■ Carpal tunnel syndrome
■ Cubital tunnel syndrome

■ Anterior interosseous syndrome
■ Posterior interosseous syndrome
■ Suprascapular nerve entrapment
■ Infection (discitis, osteomyelitis, epidural abscess)
■ Primary bone neoplasm
■ Nerve sheath tumor
■ Metastatic disease (epidural and/or bony element)
■ Inflammatory arthropathy
■ Cervical facet syndrome
■ Peripheral brachial plexus nerve tumor
■ Acute brachial neuritis (Parsonage–Turner syndrome)
■ Cervical sprain/strain injuries
■ Disorders of rotator cuff and shoulder
■ Thoracic outlet syndrome
■ Herpes zoster
■ Pancoast's tumor
■ Sympathetically mediated syndromes
■ Myocardial infarction/angina

NONOPERATIVE MANAGEMENT

■ Activity modification
  ■ Patients should be educated regarding the cause of their pain and basic activity modifications that may improve it.
  ■ Simple activity modifications to keep the head and neck in a midline and unflexed position may minimize stress on the cervical spine and thereby relieve pain and reduce root compression.
  ■ The effectiveness of these measures, however, is unproved.[2] Cervical orthoses (or collars) sometimes are recommended for this same purpose but should be used for less than 1 to 2 weeks, given the counterproductive effects of prolonged immobilization.
  ■ Lifting objects greater than 5 to 10 lbs is generally advised to be avoided during an acute stage of cervical radiculopathy.
■ Physical therapy
  ■ Core strengthening of neck musculature
  ■ Arm and hand exercises
  ■ Cervical traction
■ Medications
  ■ Nonsteroidal anti-inflammatory drugs (NSAIDs) and acetaminophen generally are the medications recommended most frequently early in the course of radiculopathy.
  ■ These agents are believed to reduce the inflammatory response that may underlie the pain in these conditions. NSAIDs have the potential for renal and gastric toxicity.
  ■ This is important to remember in high-risk patients (eg, the elderly or those treated with anticoagulants).
    ■ Coadministration of gastric protective agents, such as proton pump inhibitors, may be needed.
  ■ Steroids often are used in the acute period of radiculopathy as a pulse treatment.
  ■ Many regimens are described but generally an initial oral dose (approximately 1 mg/kg of ideal body weight daily) is followed by a tapered reduction over 2 to 3 weeks.
    ■ Steroids are associated with side effects, such as impaired glycemic control, worsening hypertension, and gastritis, but short-term use generally results in few long-term complications.
■ Epidural injections
  ■ Few randomized clinical trials are available and those available generally do not provide assessment with validated outcome measures.

- Multiple studies suggest that these injections may be beneficial, with decreased pain reported in up to 60% of patients.
  - These procedures may have significant complications, although the current use of fluoroscopic guidance may minimize the risk.

SURGICAL MANAGEMENT

- The primary indication for a posterior cervical foraminotomy is cervical radiculopathy that can be correlated to radiographic findings of a lateral herniated cervical disc or cervical foraminal stenosis.
- Open posterior cervical foraminotomy was historically the treatment for foraminal stenosis.
- Advances in the anterior approach to cervical disease made the anterior cervical discectomy and fusion (ACDF) the preferred method for spine surgeons.
- Anterior cervical approach allowed for decreased muscle injury, decreased postoperative pain, and decreased length of stay as compared to the classic open posterior foraminotomy.[3–5]
- Many studies have shown that posterior cervical foraminotomy is still a highly effective treatment option.[4, 6–8]
- Posterior cervical laminoforaminotomy has been shown to provide symptomatic relief in 92% to 97% of these patients.[4]
- Other indications for cervical foraminotomy include multilevel foraminal narrowing without central stenosis, persistent radicular symptoms after anterior cervical discectomy and fusion, and patients with relative contraindications for anterior cervical surgery (infection, prior radiation, multiple anterior surgeries).
- However, there are several major drawbacks to the posterior open procedure. These included the need for extensive subperiosteal stripping of the paraspinal musculature. This approach-related morbidity leads to significant postoperative pains and muscle spasms. This pain and dysfunction can be debilitating in 18% to 60% of patients.[2,9,10]
- Compared with an ACDF, there remain several key advantages to the posterior approach, including the direct visualization of the lateral cervical spinal cord and exiting cervical nerve root. The nerve root can be followed out into the neuroforamen and the source of compression can be directly visualized and addressed.
- The other significant advantage of the posterior approach is the preservation of motion segments in the cervical spine. This is especially important in young patients and athletes. In the elderly population, by avoiding a fusion, the risk of accelerated degenerative changes at the levels above and below the pathologic segment can be avoided as well.[9,11]
- The posterior cervical microendoscopic foraminotomy (CMEF) is a minimally invasive approach that was developed to exploit the advantages of a posterior cervical decompression while minimizing the approach-related morbidity.
- The major contraindication for CMEF is the presence of a large central herniated disc causing symptoms of radiculopathy.
- Utilizing a posterior approach, the cervical cord cannot be retracted to adequately address a central pathology.
- Other contraindications include cervical instability or a kyphotic cervical deformity.

Preoperative Planning

- A complete history and physical examination identifies patients with probable cervical pathology.

- Acute onset of symptoms, report of pain or paresthesias in a dermatomal distribution, and weakness are good historical clues that nerve root compression may exist.
- If this is corroborated on examination by findings of weakness, decreased sensation, presence of the Spurling sign, or diminished reflexes in a specific nerve root distribution, there is high clinical suspicion of root compression.
- It is paramount to exclude the presence of myelopathy (hyperreflexia, ataxia, presence of upper motor signs), which would suggest spinal stenosis and not root pathology.
- Plain cervical spine radiographs with flexion and extension views are essential for beginning the evaluation process.
- Oblique views are sometimes helpful in correlating foraminal stenosis with clinical symptoms.
- These studies reveal areas of foraminal stenosis, significant osteophytes, and the presence of spinal instability.
- A cervical spine MRI is next used to look for any disc herniations or foraminal stenosis and to exclude the presence of central stenosis.
- In patients with previous cervical surgery in whom hardware was implanted or in patients whose clinical history and examination findings do not correlate with MRI findings, a CT myelogram of the cervical spine is warranted.
- MRI is notorious for inadequately showing the degree of compression from osteophytes—these can be clearly seen on CT myelograms.
- We employ the METRx system (Medtronic Sofamor-Danek; Memphis, TN) of endoscopic retractors, camera, and instruments for our MEF procedures (**FIG 15**).

Positioning

- The patient is placed under general endotracheal anesthesia in the standard fashion. Throughout the procedure, somatosensory evoked potentials and myotomal EMG monitoring are used to monitor the spinal cord. An arterial line and a precordial Doppler may be used as well.
- The patient's head is secured in the three-point Mayfield head clamp.
- The patient is positioned in a semi-sitting position with the head slightly flexed. This position significantly reduces the blood loss and allows for better visualization of the affected stenosis and disc pathology. All extremities are carefully padded and the neck is once again examined to ensure adequate venous drainage (**FIG 16**).
- The organization of the operating room is as follows: The anesthesiologist is located to the left of the operating table; the scrub table, fluoroscopic monitor, and video cart are on the right side (**FIG 17**).
- The fluoroscopy unit is brought in from the right side as well.
- The C-arm is brought either over or under the patient's head, according to the surgeon's preference.
- Suction canisters and a Bovie unit are generally located at the patient's feet.
- The Midas drill is placed on a sterile Mayo stand on the left side behind the patient.
- We use a standard blue sterile drape, similar to the one used for routine hip surgery, to create our surgical field (**FIG 18**).
- A single dose of antibiotics (either cefazolin or vancomycin) is routinely given before skin incision.
- Intravenous steroids are not routinely administered.
- A Foley catheter is generally not needed.
- A C-arm fluoroscopic image is taken to identify the correct operative level.

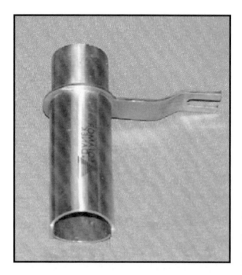
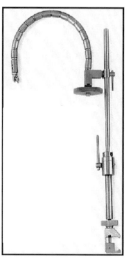
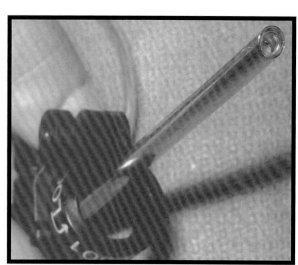

FIG 15 • The METRx system (Medtronic Sofamor-Danek; Memphis, TN) of endoscopic retractors, camera, and instruments for our microendoscopic foraminotomy procedures.

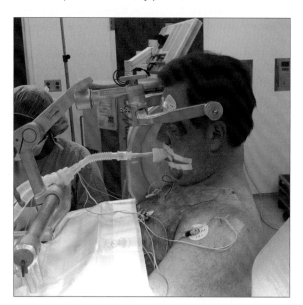

FIG 16 • Intraoperative picture of the patient in the Mayfield three-point fixation device and the sitting position.

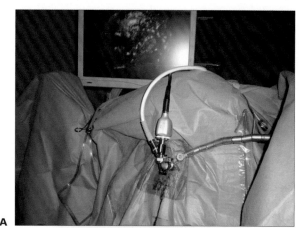

A

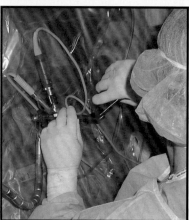

B

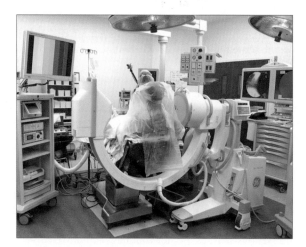

FIG 17 • Intraoperative picture of the operating room setup.

FIG 18 • **A.** Intraoperative picture showing the operative field with the sterile drape over the C-arm and the surgeon's operating screen in view. **B.** Example of this operative arrangement with a close-up view of the endoscopic apparatus in place as it would appear during the procedure.

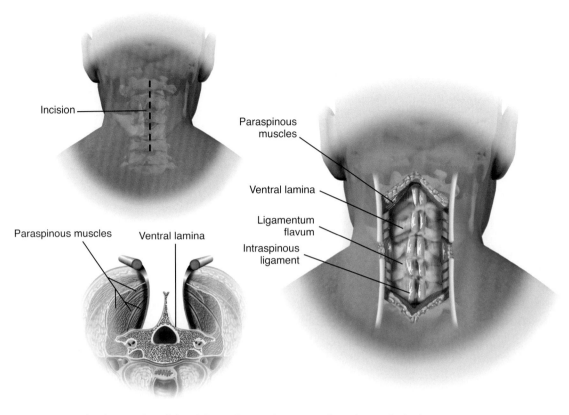

FIG 19 • Sample picture of traditional "open" posterior approach to the cervical spine.

Approach

- Traditionally, the posterior cervical laminoforaminotomy is performed via a midline incision in the region of interest. This approach, typically referred to as an "open" technique, requires an incision long enough such that the exposure can be carried laterally to the facet complex. The paraspinal muscles are then stripped from the spinous process, which requires violation of their ligamentous attachments to the midline. The muscular attachments are also stripped from their position on the bony elements of the facet capsule, spinous process, and lamina. To achieve this amount of muscular retraction, it is necessary to mobilize muscles above and below the targeted region (**FIG 19**).

SURGICAL TECHNIQUE FOR MINIMALLY INVASIVE CERVICAL LAMINOFORAMINOTOMY

- An 18-mm longitudinal incision is made 1.5 cm off the midline at the appropriate level.
- The muscle is spread and the fascia is incised under direct vision to the length of the incision.
- After the fascia is opened, a Metz scissors is used to carefully dissect down to the facet.
- The smallest dilator is introduced slowly in a perpendicular trajectory with no medial angulation.
- Fluoroscopy is used to visualize the dilator docking onto the inferomedial edge of the rostral lateral mass of the appropriate level (**TECH FIG 1**). The tubular muscle dilators are placed in a sequential fashion to the width of the retractor and endoscopic system that is used (**TECH FIGS 2 AND 3**).
- A 25-degree angled endoscope is then affixed to the retractor system.
- Radiography reveals a tubular rectractor docked at the C6–7 interspace (**TECH FIGS 4 AND 5**).
- Monopolar cautery and pituitary rongeurs are used to identify the lateral mass and lamina.

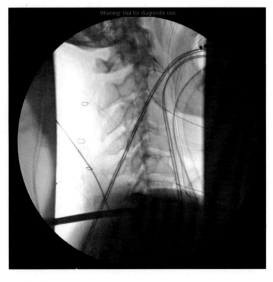

TECH FIG 1 • First dilator in position at C6–7.

TECHNIQUES

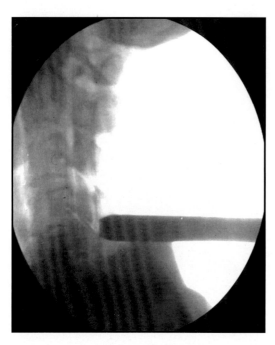

TECH FIG 2 • Intraoperative X-ray of final tube docked on facet complex.

- It is best to begin this dissection laterally where the bone is clearly felt. The dissection can then be continued medially to expose the laminofacet junction, with attention paid to not slip into the interlaminar space at this point.

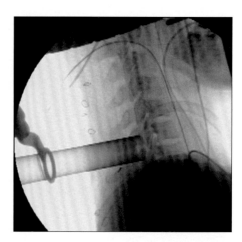

TECH FIG 4 • Intraoperative X-ray of tube secured at the C6–7 level.

- The possibility exists that there is a large interlaminar space medially and care must be used to remain over bony landmarks during this dissection.
- For a CMEF/D procedure, it is important to visualize the medial one-third of the rostral and caudal lateral mass and lateral one-third of the rostral and caudal lamina of interest (**TECH FIG 6**).
- A small-angled curette is used to detach the ligamentum flavum from the undersurface of the inferior edge of the rostral lamina (**TECH FIG 7**).

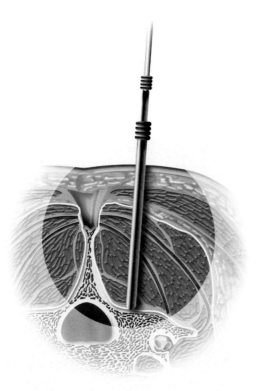

TECH FIG 3 • Drawing of final tube docked on facet complex.

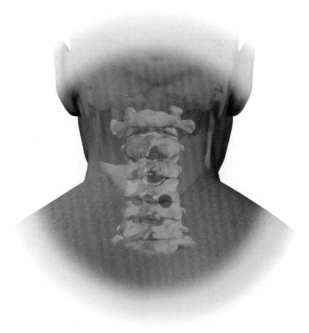

TECH FIG 5 • Schematic drawing of the area on the facet used to dock the dilators and working channel.

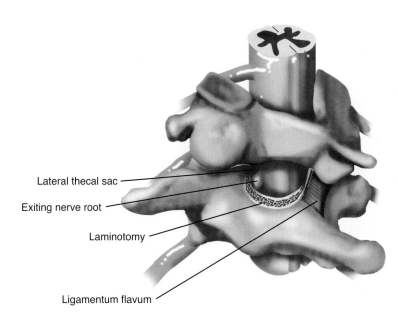

Lateral thecal sac

Exiting nerve root

Laminotomy

Ligamentum flavum

TECH FIG 6 • Illustration of the area of desired bone resection with the exiting nerve root and lateral thecal sac in view.

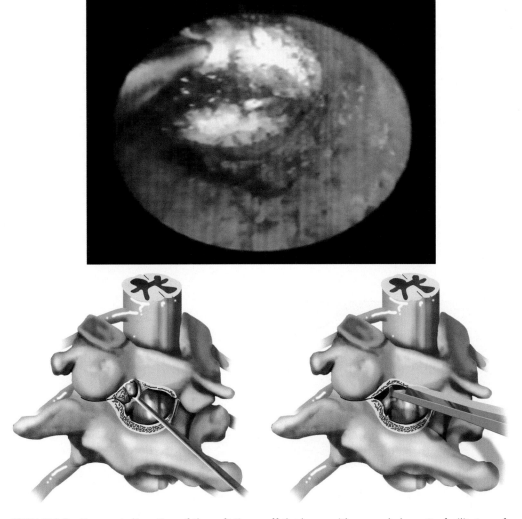

TECH FIG 7 • Frequent dissection of the soft tissue off the bone with an angled curette facilitates safe use of the Kerrison rongeur.

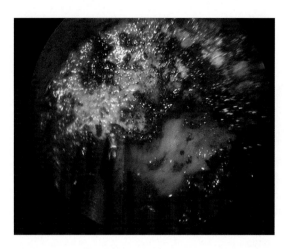

TECH FIG 8 • Kerrison punch with joint synovium in view.

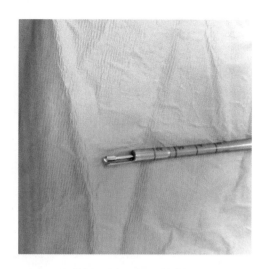

TECH FIG 10 • Drill bit with safety shield.

- Proper placement of the curettes can be confirmed under fluoroscopy to double check that it is indeed under the lamina of the correct level. Good dissection of the underlying flavum and dura from the bone defines the relevant anatomy and helps to prevent incidental dural tears.
- Bleeding from epidural veins and the edge of the flavum is controlled via a long-tipped endoscopic bipolar cautery. For bleeding underneath the edge of the lamina, angled bipolar forceps with a 45-degree angle are often useful.
- A 1- or 2-mm Kerrison rongeur is then used to create a small laminotomy to visualize the lateral border of the cervical dura and the proximal exiting cervical nerve root.
- The Kerrison is used to begin the medial facetectomy over the exit of the cervical root (**TECH FIG 8**).
- Periosteal and bone bleeding is addressed with bone wax and cautery.
- Often, the lamina can be oriented in quite a vertical fashion making it difficult to bite it with a Kerrison punch.
- In such instances, it is best to use a drill to simultaneously thin and flatten the lamina down.

- Frequent dissection of the soft tissue off the bone with an angled curette facilitates safe use of the Kerrison rongeur.
- The drill with a fine cutting bit is often useful to finish the medial facetectomy and guarantee an adequate foraminal decompression (**TECH FIG 9**).
- We prefer a drill bit with a safety shield on one side to prevent inadvertent injury to the thecal sac (**TECH FIG 10**).
- After the bony decompression of the dorsal cervical foramen is complete, bipolar coagulation is used to dissect the venous plexus that surround the nerve root.
- The nerve root can then be mobilized in a superior or inferior direction to visualize and palpate the ventral foramen and to identify the osteophytes or cervical disc fragments.
- To increase exposure to this ventral space without over distraction of the nerve root, the superomedial quadrant of the caudal pedicle can be drilled.
- Disc fragments can be teased out with the use of a nerve hook and micropituitary (**TECH FIG 11**). Osteophyte fragments can be manipulated and fractured through

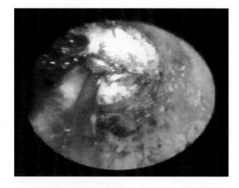

TECH FIG 9 • A drill with a long endoscopic bit (eg, AM-8 bit with Midas Rex, or TAC bit with MEDNext drill) can be used to further thin the medial facet and lateral mass.

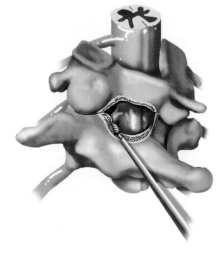

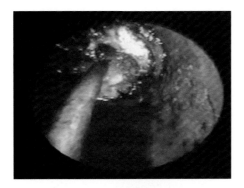

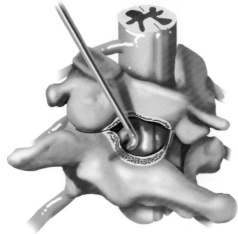

TECH FIG 11 • The adequacy of the decompression should be confirmed by palpating the root along its course with a small nerve hook.

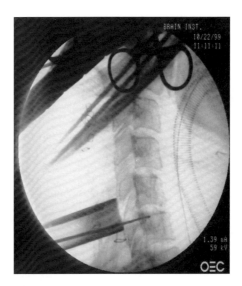

TECH FIG 13 • Intraoperative X-ray demonstrating that the foraminotomy is probed with a blunt nerve hook for tactile feedback on the completeness of decompression.

- the use of angled curettes or tamped down with down-angled curettes.
- The foramen should be inspected one final time to assure no ventral or dorsal compression of the exiting nerve root (TECH FIGS 12, 13, AND 14).
- After hemostasis is achieved and the wound is irrigated with antibiotic irrigation, the tubular retractor is removed and the wound is closed in layers and Dermabond (Ethicon, Somerville, NJ) is applied over the incision.

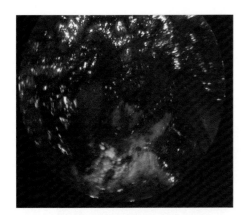

TECH FIG 12 • Intraoperative photograph showing that the foraminotomy is probed with a blunt nerve hook for tactile feedback on the completeness of decompression.

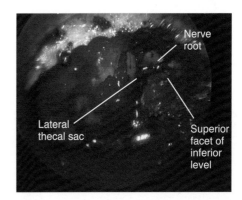

TECH FIG 14 • Intraoperative photograph at completion of the laminoforaminotomy. The lateral edge of the thecal sac can be seen, as well as the exiting nerve root.

PEARLS AND PITFALLS

Positioning	■ Care should be directed to ensuring that the cervical spine and neck musculature are not kinked or held in an unfavorable position. The neck, chin, and chest must be allowed to remain loose and free of compression. Precordial Doppler monitoring can be used to detect air emboli within the atrium.
Localization	■ The incision should be 1.5 cm from the midline to ensure that the surgical exposure is not too medial. The incision length and the tubular retractor width should be the same to ensure adequate stability of the final tube.

Incision and tube dilation	▪ A mini-open approach is used to avoid the need for K-wire insertion, and potential spinal cord injury, in the cervical spine. The first dilator is docked directly on the bony lamina. As sequential dilators are placed, care is taken to not apply too much pressure, which could result in an inadvertent plunge through the interlaminar space.
Surgical approach	▪ After the initial induction of anesthesia, we have refrained from the use of neuromuscular paralytics to allow for improved feedback from the nerve root during the operation. It is best to begin this dissection laterally where the bone is clearly felt. The dissection can then be continued medially to expose the laminofacet junction with attention paid to not slip into the interlaminar space at this point.
Bone exposure	▪ Good dissection of the underlying flavum and dura from the bone defines the relevant anatomy and helps to prevent incidental dural tears. For bleeding underneath the edge of the lamina, angled bipolar forceps with a 45-degree angle are often useful.
Foraminotomy	▪ Often, the lamina can be oriented in quite a vertical fashion making it difficult to bite it with a Kerrison punch. In such instances, it is best to use a drill to simultaneously thin and flatten the lamina down. Frequent dissection of the soft tissue off the bone with an angled curette facilitates safe use of the Kerrison rongeur. The adequacy of the decompression should be confirmed by palpating the root along its course with a small nerve hook.

POSTOPERATIVE CARE

▪ Most of our patients can be safely discharged home the same day of surgery.

▪ Patients are counseled to expect neck/muscle and incisional pain for the first week or two after surgery.

▪ They are given prescriptions for a narcotic pain medication and a muscle relaxant; we typically prescribe hydrocodone/acetaminophen and baclofen.

▪ Patients are also placed on a bowel regimen consisting of daily stool softeners to avoid constipation from the narcotic medication.

▪ They are encouraged to walk as tolerated and discouraged from lifting more than 10 lbs.

▪ Most patients can return to light work duties by 4 weeks.

▪ All patients begin a short course of physical therapy 4 to 6 weeks after surgery to improve neck strength and mobility.

▪ Most patients return to work, are able to drive, and have discontinued narcotic pain medication by 6 to 8 weeks following surgery.

OUTCOMES

▪ Good to excellent outcomes are reported in up to 96% of patients following laminoforaminotomy performed for radiculopathy.[11]

▪ Poor prognostic factors include long-term preoperative complaints and long-standing preoperative neurologic deficits.[12]

▪ Additionally, patients appear to exhibit continued good long-term outcomes in which 86% of patients were still doing well 15 years later (**FIG 20**).[12]

COMPLICATIONS

▪ Potential complications following either a minimally invasive cervical decompression include injury to the cervical

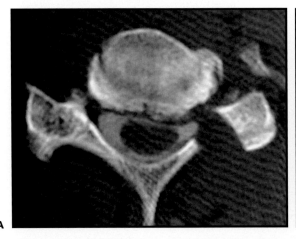
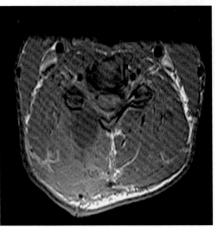

FIG 20 • **A.** Postoperative CT scan demonstrating the typical foraminotomy defect that is obtained after microendoscopic foraminotomy with good preservation of the lateral mass integrity. **B.** Postoperative MRI.

spinal cord or nerves, cerebrospinal fluid leak, and infections.

▪ The treatment of an unintended durotomy include direct repair of a visible tear, or placement of muscle, fat, or Gelfoam (Pfizer, New York, NY) over the tear and the application of a dural sealant such as DuraSeal (Confluent Surgical, Waltham, MA).

▪ The limited volume of dead space created with the minimally invasive approach has led to a decreased incidence of postoperative pseudomeningocele.

▪ The potential exists for injury to the cervical cord or the cervical nerve root. By careful dilation technique through the direct visual incision of the cervical fascia and placement of the first dilator tube directly perpendicular to the spine without any medial angulation, the risk of direct injury to the spinal cord can be minimized.

▪ To minimize injury to the cervical nerve root, adequate bony decompression must be achieved prior to manipulation of the nerve root.

▪ Venous bleeding from the plexus surrounding the cervical nerve root must be carefully monitored and controlled with bipolar coagulation and Gelfoam (Pfizer, New York, NY) packing. The use of the semi-sitting position helps decrease the amount of this venous blood loss. The potential exists for a symptomatic air embolus in this semi-sitting position, although this has not been observed in the authors' series to date. The use of a precordial Doppler can help in identifying an air embolus and the appropriate treatment can be performed.

▪ The vertebral artery runs immediately anterior to the cervical nerve root. When manipulating the cervical nerve root and osteophytes that may exist in this space, the surgeon should carefully monitor for an increase in venous bleeding. Because the vertebral artery is surrounded by a rich venous plexus, this venous bleeding is a good indicator of the proximity to the artery itself.

▪ Cervical instability following surgery can be avoided by preserving at least 50% of the facet complex during the bony decompression. When drilling the superomedial quadrant of the pedicle, careful attention must be paid to drill only the volume necessary to allow a nerve hook access behind the cervical nerve root.

REFERENCES

1. Howe JF, Loeser JD, Calvin WH. Mechanosensitivity of dorsal root ganglia and chronically injured axons: a physiological basis for the radicular pain of nerve root compression. Pain 1977;3(1):25–41.
2. Ratliff JK, Cooper PR. Cervical laminoplasty: a critical review. J Neurosurg 2003;98(3 Suppl):230–238.
3. Bailey RW, Badgley CE. Stabilization of the cervical spine by anterior fusion. J Bone Joint Surg Am 1960;42-A:565–594.
4. Henderson CM, Hennessy RG, Shuey HM Jr, et al. Posterior-lateral foraminotomy as an exclusive operative technique for cervical radiculopathy: a review of 846 consecutively operated cases. Neurosurgery 1983;13(5):504–512.
5. Smith GW, Robinson RA. The treatment of certain cervical-spine disorders by anterior removal of the intervertebral disc and interbody fusion. J Bone Joint Surg Am 1958;40-A(3):607–624.
6. Bohlman HH, Emery SE, Goodfellow DB, et al. Robinson anterior cervical discectomy and arthrodesis for cervical radiculopathy. Long-term follow-up of one hundred and twenty-two patients. J Bone Joint Surg Am 1993;75(9):1298–1307.
7. Grieve JP, Kitchen ND, Moore AJ, et al. Results of posterior cervical foraminotomy for treatment of cervical spondylitic radiculopathy. Br J Neurosurg 2000;14(1):40–43.
8. Klein GR, Vaccaro AR, Albert TJ. Health outcome assessment before and after anterior cervical discectomy and fusion for radiculopathy: a prospective analysis. Spine 2000;25(7):801–803.
9. Fessler RG, Khoo LT. Minimally invasive cervical microendoscopic foraminotomy: an initial clinical experience. Neurosurgery 2002;51 (5 Suppl):S37–S45.
10. Hosono N, Yonenobu K, Ono K. Neck and shoulder pain after laminoplasty. A noticeable complication. Spine 1996;21(17):1969–1973.
11. Zeidman SM, Ducker TB. Posterior cervical laminoforaminotomy for radiculopathy: review of 172 cases. Neurosurgery 1993;33(3):356–362.
12. Woertgen C, Holzschuh M, Rothoerl RD, et al. Prognostic factors of posterior cervical disc surgery: a prospective, consecutive study of 54 patients. Neurosurgery 1997;40(4):724–728; discussion 728–729.

Chapter 11

Lumbar Discectomy

Bradley K. Weiner and Aristidis Zibis

DEFINITION

- Clinically significant lumbar disc herniations are characterized by a focal distortion of the normal anatomic configuration of discal material resulting in compression *and* subsequent dysfunction of the lumbar nerve roots.

ANATOMY

- The functional components of the intervertebral disc are the annulus fibrosus (fibrous concentric rings, type I collagen) enclosing the central nucleus pulposus (gelatinous, type II collagen, proteoglycans), and the vertebral endplates (hyaline cartilage).
- The anatomic unit of the lumbar spine is the vertebral body with its attached posterior elements and the disc below (**FIG 1A**).
- The nerve roots travel within the common dural sac (the cauda equina) and then exit at each level. They are numbered according to the pedicle beneath which they pass.
- The spinal canal is divided into zones from medial to lateral: central canal, subarticular zone, foraminal zone, and extraforaminal (far-lateral) zone (**FIG 1B**).
- Disc herniations are best classified based in the following ways:
  - Based on the integrity of the annulus fibrosus and whether there is a connection of herniated discal material with the disc space (**FIG 2**)
  - Based on the anatomic location of the herniated material relative to the disc space, the canal, and the compressed nerve root using the nomenclature above (**FIG 3**)
- Accurate anatomic classification of disc herniations facilitates preoperative planning and can minimize the risk of surgical complications such as missed pathology and iatrogenic nerve root injury.
- The importance of a complete knowledge of spinal anatomy and understanding of the particular patient's pathoanatomy cannot be overstated.

PATHOGENESIS

- In the normal disc, the nucleus pulposus imbibes and releases water to balance mechanical loads. The annulus fibrosus converts these loads to hoop stresses, thereby containing the nuclear material. The endplates allow diffusion of nutrition into, and waste products out of, the nucleus.
  - Together, they allow for the three basic spinal segmental functions: mobility, stability, and protection of the nearby neurologic structures.
- With early or intermediate disc degeneration (natural aging with or without minor repetitive trauma), the endplates fail to allow adequate diffusion, the nucleus fails to replace degraded proteoglycans, and annular support weakens (failure of cross-linking, development of clefts). Biomechanical dysfunction occurs, with possible herniation of nuclear material.
- Many disc herniations do not cause pain or neurologic symptoms. A combination of herniation, nerve root compression, and an inflammatory interface is required for nerve root dysfunction and associated radiculopathy and sciatica.

NATURAL HISTORY

- Many studies have shown that with time and nonoperative treatment, over 90% of patients with a first-time lumbar disc herniation will get better without surgery. Accordingly, to propose surgery requires clear indications.
  - Absolute indications
    - Bladder or bowel involvement secondary to a massive disc herniation and cauda equina syndrome: immediate surgical intervention

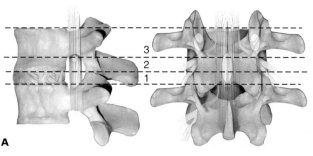

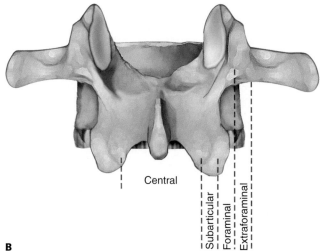

Central

Subarticular

Foraminal

Extraforaminal

FIG 1 • A. Anatomic unit. The first floor is the disc level, the second floor is the foraminal level, and the third floor is the pedicle level. **B.** Regions of the canal.

A

B

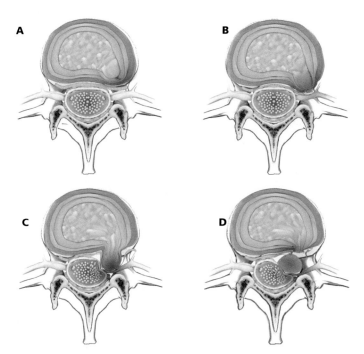

FIG 2 • Classification of disc herniations based on relation to outer annulus: (**A**) protrusion, (**B**) subannular extrusion, (**C**) transannular extrusion, (**D**) sequestration.

- Progressive (ie, worsening) neurologic deficit: the earlier the better prognostically
- Relative indications
  - Failure of conservative measures greater than 6 weeks to 3 months
  - Multiply recurrent sciatica
  - Significant neurologic deficit
- In each case, the properly informed patient must clearly understand the current best evidence: long-term (5-year) outcomes are similar between surgery and nonoperative treatment, but surgery can afford more rapid resolution of symptoms.

HISTORY AND PHYSICAL FINDINGS

- The most common complaint is pain with or without associated paresthesias or weakness in a specific monoradicular anatomic distribution.

IMAGING AND OTHER DIAGNOSTIC STUDIES

- MRI is the imaging study of choice for the diagnosis and anatomic classification of lumbar disc herniations. It is highly

sensitive and specific and provides, along with the clinical picture, adequate information for detailed preoperative planning.
- CT-myelography is invasive and less specific than MRI but provides excellent sensitivity when MRI is unavailable or contraindicated.
- Plain radiographs may show disc space narrowing, early formation of osteophytes, or a "sciatic scoliosis." While providing no direct evidence of a herniated disc, they may be helpful to rule out unexpected destructive pathology (eg, infection, tumor, fracture) in patients who have failed to respond to nonoperative intervention or those with red flags. They also allow excellent delineation of bony anomalies that may prove vital to preoperative planning and intraoperative localization, such as transitional lumbosacral articulations or spina bifida occulta.

DIFFERENTIAL DIAGNOSIS

- Intraspinal, extrinsic compression or irritation at the level of the nerve root: spinal stenosis, osteomyelitis or discitis, neoplasm, epidural fibrosis (scar)
- Intraspinal, extrinsic compression or irritation proximal to the nerve root: conus and cauda lesions such as neurofibroma or ependymoma
- Intraspinal, intrinsic nerve root dysfunction: neuropathy (diabetic, idiopathic, alcoholic, iatrogenic [chemotherapy]), herpes zoster, arachnoiditis, nerve root tumor
- Extraspinal sources distal to the nerve root: pelvic or more distal neoplasms with associated sciatic or femoral nerve compression, sacroiliac disease (eg, infection, osteoarthritis), osteoarthritis of the hip, peripheral vascular disease

NONOPERATIVE MANAGEMENT

- The evidence base is still a bit unclear, but the following are commonly recommended.
- Rest: bed rest (no more than 2 or 3 days), activity or job modification, weight loss
- Medication: analgesics, nonsteroidal anti-inflammatories, tapered doses of oral steroids
- Exercise: physical therapy (McKenzie program)
- Injections: epidural or selective root blocks (may provide some temporary relief while the natural history takes over)
- Time: 6 weeks to 3 months (unless absolute indications for surgery exist as noted above)

SURGICAL MANAGEMENT

- The evidence base is clear: open discectomy and microdiscectomy are the operative techniques with the best-documented long-term outcomes and are the gold standards of surgery for lumbar disc herniations.

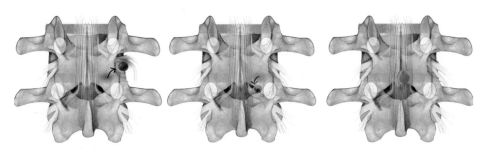

FIG 3 • The patterns of disc migration can be characterized relative to the structures of the anatomic unit (eg, at the disc level or at the pedicle level). The area of root compression can be described relative to the nerve root anatomy (eg, at the shoulder of the traversing root, in the axilla of the exiting root).

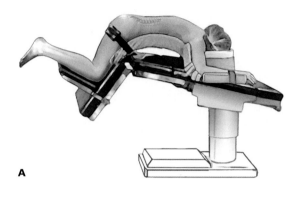

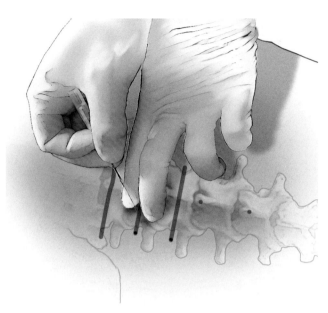

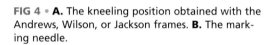

FIG 4 • **A.** The kneeling position obtained with the Andrews, Wilson, or Jackson frames. **B.** The marking needle.

Preoperative Planning

▪ This is *vital* and should aim to answer three questions:
  ▪ What nerve root is involved (answered by history and physical examination)?
  ▪ Where is the herniated material relative to the disc space, the canal, and the nerve root (answered by MRI)?
  ▪ What approach will afford the best visualization and access to the herniated material while minimizing injury to tissues not directly involved in the pathologic process?

Positioning

▪ A "kneeling" position is generally used, with the patient stabilized on an Andrews frame, a Wilson frame, or the Jackson table (**FIG 4A**).
  ▪ Some hip and knee flexion will decrease lumbar lordosis and facilitate an approach through the interlaminar window.
  ▪ The abdomen must be free to decrease intra-abdominal pressure and venous backflow through the plexus of Batson into the spinal canal.
▪ Shoulders should be abducted less than 90 degrees and with some flexion. The neck should be neutral or gently flexed.
▪ Eyes must be protected and elbows, knees, and feet well padded.

▪ A needle is passed between and lateral to the spinous processes at the involved level and C-arm imaging is used to confirm that the proper level will be approached (Fig 4B). The needle is removed and the level marked and labeled on the skin.
▪ The involved side will be determined preoperatively by patient complaint and location of herniation on MRI but should also be marked on the patient's skin at this point.

Approach

▪ The interlaminar window approach is used in about 90% of lumbar disc herniations requiring surgery. It is appropriate for herniations within the central canal or subarticular zones from L1 to S1 and for herniations within the foramen at L5–S1.
▪ The intertransverse window approach is used in about 10% of lumbar disc herniations requiring surgery. It is appropriate for herniations within the foraminal and extraforaminal zones from L1 to L5.
▪ For each step in the procedure, incision, excision, and retraction of tissues should be minimized. The goal is to *get the job done completely and safely with minimal trauma to tissues not directly involved in the pathologic process.*

INCISION AND DISSECTION

▪ The skin incision is made directly midline posteriorly and extends from the top of the cephalad spinous process to the bottom of the caudal spinous process, about 1.5 inches for single-level pathology.
▪ The subcutaneous tissues are then gently and bluntly mobilized and retracted to allow visualization of the dorsolumbar fascia.

▪ From here, one of two windows of approach will be undertaken based on the location of the disc herniation: the interlaminar window or the intertransverse window.

INTERLAMINAR WINDOW

- The dorsolumbar fascia is incised just off the midline in a gentle curvilinear fashion on the involved side at a length to match the skin incision.
- A Cobb elevator is used to gently elevate the muscle (multifidus) from the spinous processes to the midportion of the facet joint laterally.
  - The degree of muscle elevation should be limited to what is necessary to allow adequate laminar exposure for laminotomy.
- A retractor is then placed. We prefer a retractor with a medial hook for the interspinous ligament and a blade for gentle lateral muscular retraction (**TECH FIG 1A**).
  - An intraoperative C-arm image is then obtained to confirm the level. Alternatively, a lateral radiograph can be taken.

- A cylindrical retractor, placed transmuscularly using a sequential dilation technique, is a reasonable alternative as long as great care is taken to expose the correct portion of the interlaminar window (there is a tendency to be "pushed" too far laterally).
- At this point, illumination and magnification are gained by the use of the operative microscope (our preference) or a headlamp and loupes.
  - Outcomes are similar for the two when used properly, and the surgeon should decide on his or her preference based on experience and comfort level.
- A laminotomy on the undersurface of the cephalad lamina and minimal medial facetectomy is then performed using a Kerrison rongeur (**TECH FIG 1B**).

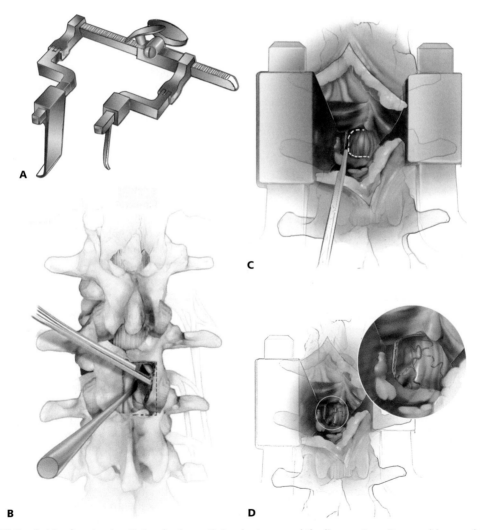

TECH FIG 1 • A. Muscle retractor. **B.** Laminotomy. **C.** Laminotomy and the ligamentum. Bony excision used for the "typical disc herniation" in the canal or subarticular zones. It may need to be extended cephalad for herniations extending upward into the second story or may need to include the upper portion of the caudal lamina for herniations extending downward into the third story of the level below. The ligamentum is either freed from its insertions on the undersurface of the lamina above and the undersurface of the facet capsule laterally using a sharp curette, creating a flap, or is incised and split as depicted. **D.** Identifying the lateral edge of the root. The traversing root is readily identified by vessels that travel along its lateral edge longitudinally, rise up onto its shoulder, and form a plexus in its axilla. Further caudally, the root is closely associated with the medial border of the pedicle.

- The degree of laminotomy and facetectomy should be enough to allow full visualization of the underlying nerve root at the area of compression and to allow access for excision of herniated disc material—no more and no less.
  - For small disc herniations in the canal or subarticular zones (the "typical disc herniation"), minimal bony excision is required at lower lumbar levels.
  - For larger disc herniations and those extending cephalad into the second story, a larger laminotomy or even hemilaminectomy may be required. The key in these situations is to preserve at least 5 mm of the lateral pars interarticularis and at least 50% of the medial facet.
- Laminotomy of the upper surface of the caudal lamina is generally not needed unless the herniated material has migrated caudally to the third story of the level below adjacent to the pedicle.
- The ligamentum flavum is then addressed. One of two techniques is used: the Rick Delamarter and John McCulloch flap or the Rob Fraser split (**TECH FIG 1C**).
  - The former preserves the ligamentum flavum as a complete barrier to minimize scar formation from posterior, while the latter offers a little less coverage but preserves the ligament's biomechanical integrity.
- The lateral edge of the traversing nerve root is then identified.
  - This is readily identified by consistent lateral veins and the root's association with the pedicle (**TECH FIG 1D**).
  - These veins can then be gently mobilized to allow exposure of the underlying annulus.
  - Occasionally, anomalous roots lateral to the traversing root may be present. Again, safety is ensured by identifying the veins directly overlying the annulus and using these to provide a window to access.

Herniation Exposure

- For herniations within the canal or subarticular zones and in the first or second story (85% of encountered discs), the traversing nerve root is gently mobilized medially, allowing exposure of the herniated disc.
  - If the root is immobile, the surgeon should excise more bone within the subarticular region (medial facetectomy) to afford visualization and palpation of the medial border of the pedicle associated with the traversing root.
  - Access to the disc cephalad to this will be within a safe zone lateral to the traversing root and within the axilla of the exiting root.
  - Once larger fragments are teased out, the traversing root will become mobile, allowing greater access.
  - Retraction should be minimal at upper levels (L1–L3 due to presence of the conus) and limited to about 40%—that is, to less than half the width of the unilateral hemilaminotomy below this (**TECH FIG 2**).
    - Retraction should be relaxed during periods in which no active work is undertaken in or near the disc space: the nerve is rested while the pituitary rongeur is being cleaned, and gently re-retracted

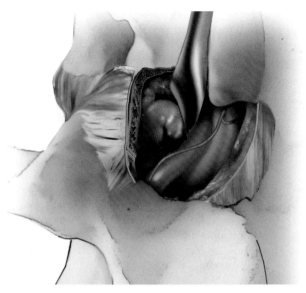

TECH FIG 2 • Root retraction is minimal and intermittent.

  when it returns. This will minimize trauma to the root.
  - Hemostasis is then obtained by gently tucking small pieces of Gelfoam or thrombin cephalad and caudally to the exposed disc space. These are to be removed at the end of the case.
    - If bipolar cautery is used, it should be done with caution to avoid root injury.
- Herniations extending caudally to the third story of the level below (uncommon, 5%) are most often within the "axilla" of the traversing root. Retraction of the root is not used; rather, the herniation (usually sequestered) is gently teased out.

Discectomy

- Once visualized, any free disc material is removed with a pituitary rongeur. A ball-tipped probe is used to tease out any additional free fragments hiding further out in the subarticular zone or under the common dural sac or root.
- The disc space is then entered (this will be the first step in "contained" herniations) by annulotomy. A long-handled no. 15 blade facing away from the traversing root is used, preferably with a longitudinal orientation.
- Within the disc space, any loose fragments are removed with the pituitary rongeur (**TECH FIG 3**), and the disc space is irrigated.
  - More aggressive excision ("complete discectomy") may slightly decrease the risk of recurrence, but at the price of increased back pain and a potential for accelerating the degenerative process.
  - Depth of work should be limited to avoid anterior perforation and potential vascular injury. The surgeon should respect the anterior portion of the annulus and avoid perforating it with an instrument.
  - Discectomy is complete when no additional loose fragments can be removed from the disc space and free mobility of the nerve root is confirmed.

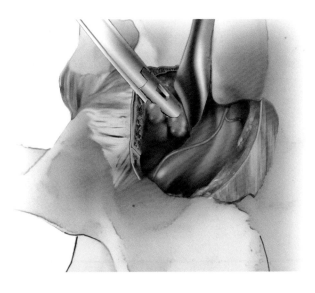

- The root retractor is then removed, along with the pieces of Gelfoam.
- The wound is thoroughly irrigated. This "washing," coupled with removing the root retractor, is usually adequate to stop any epidural bleeding.
  - If it persists, temporarily placing Gelfoam again is almost always adequate.
- Unless there is still a bit of oozing, drains are generally not indicated, and the wound is closed in three layers (fascia, subcutaneous tissue, and skin [absorbable, subcuticular]).

TECH FIG 3 • Discectomy. After annulotomy, the pituitary rongeur is used to remove the herniation and loose fragments within the disc space.

INTERTRANSVERSE WINDOW

- The dorsolumbar fascia is incised 1.5 fingerbreadths off the midline longitudinally (**TECH FIG 4A**).
- The plane between the multifidus medially and the longissimus laterally is freed by finger dissection, allowing palpation of the facet joint.
- A retractor is placed within this plane (**TECH FIG 4B**) and an intraoperative C-arm image is obtained to confirm the level.
- The tip of the superior articular process and the lateral pars interarticularis are exposed with electrocautery and partially resected (**TECH FIG 4C,D**).
- The intertransverse membrane is gently retracted laterally using a ball-tipped probe.
- Gentle blunt dissection is used to identify the exiting nerve root and the underlying herniated material.

Gentle technique, patience, and really good lighting and magnification are required here (again, we prefer the operative microscope, but outcomes are similar regardless). There is plenty of adipose tissue and a venous plexus surrounding the dorsal root ganglion of the root that must be identified before introducing the pituitary rongeur.
- A ball-tipped probe and pituitary rongeur are used to gently tease out the loose fragment, with minimal to no retraction applied to the root. This can be traced back into the disc space as necessary and any loose fragments removed.
- The wound is irrigated, hemostasis is obtained, and closure is performed as described above.

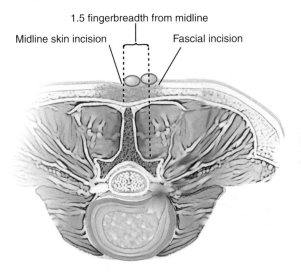

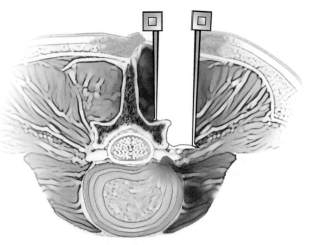

A
B

TECH FIG 4 • **A.** The fascial incision is made 1.5 fingerbreadths from the midline. **B.** Retraction. *(continued)*

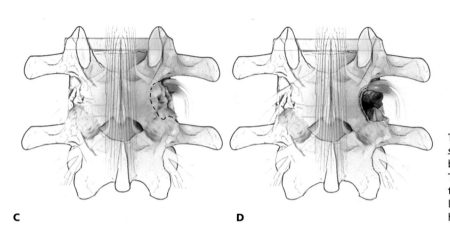

C   D

TECH FIG 4 • *(continued)* **C.** The *shaded areas* represent the area of bony excision during discectomy. **D.** The intertransverse membrane is then gently mobilized laterally, allowing exposure and excision of the herniated disc.

PEARLS AND PITFALLS

Wrong-level exposure, exploration, or surgery is always a risk. The level is marked preoperatively and intraoperatively as noted above.	■ The surgeon should beware of obese patients with a significant lumbar lordosis. It is very common to expose the wrong level despite proper localization of the skin incision. Thus, the correct level must be ensured radiographically before entering the spinal canal. ■ The surgeon should also beware of patients with "transitional" lumbar vertebrae (sacralization or lumbarization). Here it is often best to correlate the level on intraoperative images with the preoperative MRI, which will clearly show the disc herniation as well as the immobile, uninvolved transitional levels (narrow disc space with maintained bright signal intensity on T2 with or without poorly developed facet joints).
Certain differences exist between revision discectomy via the interlaminar window and primary surgery.	■ In revision surgery, the laminotomy and facetectomy should be extended cephalad and laterally to allow exposure of "normal" dura (above and lateral to areas of epidural fibrosis [scar]). ■ Identification of the traversing root may be difficult (scar, loss of characteristic veins), but it will still *always* be associated with its pedicle. The medial border of the pedicle is readily identified, and tissues medial to it (scar, root) are gently mobilized to identify the fragment and disc space. ■ If the root is completely immobile, further medial facetectomy will be required and the disc space should be entered in line with the subjacent pedicle to ensure being lateral to the traversing root and medial to the exiting root.
Revision discectomy via the intertransverse window for foraminal or extraforaminal disc herniations is not recommended as the planes will be distorted and safe surgery is difficult.	■ Using the interlaminar window instead, with resection of the inferior articular process of the cephalad vertebra with or without arthrodesis, is safer and affords excellent visualization.
Anomalous neural anatomy can be best identified preoperatively on MRI.	■ The surgeon should beware of large, perfectly round soft tissue masses within the foramen on parasagittal imaging or in the canal on axial imaging. If it does not look like the other roots (mimicking a large round disc herniation) but has their signal intensity, it is likely an anomalous or conjoined root.

POSTOPERATIVE CARE

■ After surgery, patients may be fitted with a light lumbar corset if desired and are encouraged to walk once anesthesia has worn off and pain permits. About 85% are discharged as outpatients. Fifteen percent will be older (less mobile) or have nausea and vomiting requiring an overnight stay and 23-hour observation.

■ Once home, patients engage in a program of progressive walking, stretching, and corset use for comfort. For those progressing slowly, physical therapy may be introduced. Heavy lifting and excessive bending and twisting should be avoided in the first few weeks.

■ If all is well, they may drive in about a week and return to light work once they feel up to it. Heavy labor should be avoided for 6 to 12 weeks to ensure proper soft tissue healing (skin, muscle, annulotomy). Long-term activities are not restricted.

OUTCOMES

■ There is an 85% likelihood of an excellent or good outcome 5 years postoperatively.
■ Patients with significant medical or social comorbidities (eg, diabetes, heavy smoking), worker's compensation or litigation, and psychological problems (depression) are less likely to do well.
  ■ Each factor is associated with a 15% reduction in the likelihood of an excellent or good outcome.
  ■ Truly informed consent is recommended.

COMPLICATIONS

■ Surgeon-dependent: wrong level, wrong side, missed pathology, iatrogenic instability, "battered root syndrome," dural tear, hemorrhage, positioning (eg, eyes, ulnar nerve)
■ Operative environment or patient-dependent: wound infection, disc space infection, urinary retention, thrombophlebitis or pulmonary embolism

REFERENCES

1. Atlas SJ, Deyo RA, Keller RB, et al. The Maine Lumbar Spine Study, Part II: 1-year outcomes of surgical and non-surgical management of sciatica. Spine 1996;21:1777–1786.
2. Boden SD, Davis DO, Dian TS, et al. Abnormal MR scans of the lumbar spine in asymptomatic subjects. J Bone Joint Surg Am 1990; 72A:403–408.
3. McCulloch JA. Microdiscectomy. In: JW Frymoyer, ed. The Adult Spine: Principles and Practice. New York: Raven Press, 1991: 1765–1783.
4. McCulloch JA, Weiner BK. Microsurgery in the lumbar intertransverse interval. AAOS Instr Course Lect 2002;51:233–241.
5. Spangfort EV. The lumbar disc herniation: a computer-aided analysis of 2,504 operations. Acta Orthop Scand 1972;142:1–95.
6. Weber H. Lumbar disc herniation: a controlled prospective study with ten years of observations. Spine 1983;8:131–140.
7. Weiner BK, Dabbah M. Lateral lumbar disc herniations: an independent assessment of longer-term outcomes. J Spinal Disord Tech 2005;18:519–521.

Chapter 12

Lumbar Decompression

Bradley K. Weiner and Aristidis Zibis

DEFINITION

- Degenerative changes that are part of the aging process may lead to compression of neurologic tissues within the spinal canal or subarticular zones (with or without the foraminal zone) of the lumbar spine.
- This *spinal canal stenosis* may lead to neurogenic claudication or a monoradiculopathy.

ANATOMY

- The functional vertebral unit is depicted in **FIGURE 1**. More details are given in the anatomy section of Chapter SP-12.
- Spinal canal stenosis is best classified based on vertical extent of compression, regions of the canal involved, and severity of the involvement.
- Accurate anatomic classification facilitates preoperative planning and can minimize the risk of surgical complications such as missed pathology and iatrogenic root injury.

PATHOGENESIS

- Degenerative changes can affect the disc, the soft tissues, and the facet joints of the spinal unit.
- Annular bulging of the disc, ligamentum flavum hypertrophy and infolding, and osteophyte formation on the facet joints can contribute to neurologic compression. Occasionally, epidural lipomatosis also contributes to spinal stenosis, especially in the presence of insulin-dependent diabetes mellitus (IDDM).
- This compression occurs slowly and gradually affects the blood supply (arterial inflow and venous outflow) of traversing nerve roots and the free flow of cerebrospinal fluid within the common dural sac. When increased demands are placed, as in walking, the nutritional needs of the nerve roots cannot be met and noxious byproducts of metabolism cannot be removed, resulting in neurophysiologic malfunction characterized clinically by paresthetic and cramping symptoms in the legs.
- As in lumbar disc herniations, many patients with spinal stenosis are asymptomatic, suggesting that other factors intrinsic to nerve root function and adaptability are equally important (eg, smoking, vascular disease, diabetes).

NATURAL HISTORY

- Patients with mild to moderate symptoms and mild to moderate neurologic compression may respond to conservative care. Unless the compression increases, symptoms generally remain stable, with minimal resolution and minimal worsening.
- The more severe the symptoms and the more severe the neurologic compression, the more likely symptoms will progress, the less likely they will respond to conservative measures, and the more likely patients will seek surgical intervention.

HISTORY AND PHYSICAL FINDINGS

- Symptomatic patients with spinal canal stenosis generally present with neurogenic claudication (70%), monoradiculopathy (15%), or a combination of the two.
- Foraminal stenosis (10% to 15% of cases) is best diagnosed clinically by a severe monoradiculopathy of an exiting nerve root, and radiographically on parasagittal MRI imaging or CT sagittal reconstruction (**FIG 2**).

IMAGING

- As described in Chapter SP-12, MRI is the imaging study of choice for the diagnosis and anatomic classification of spinal canal stenosis.
- CT myelography is invasive and can better resolve the bony component of stenosis compared to MRI. Myelograms taken in flexion-extension may demonstrate a dynamic component to the stenosis. CT myelograms may be particularly useful in patients who have had prior surgery (where MRI may be difficult to interpret due to scarring) and in those with associated spinal deformity (eg, scoliosis).
- Plain radiographs are useful in demonstrating instability in the coronal (lateral listhesis) or sagittal (spondylolisthesis) planes that may need to be addressed with fusion in addition to decompression. Upright anteroposterior, lateral, and flexion-extension views can be obtained.

DIFFERENTIAL DIAGNOSIS

- Vascular claudication, bilateral hip osteoarthritis, peripheral neuropathy, and "pump problems" such as congestive heart failure or coronary artery disease resulting in poor peripheral vascular flow.

NONOPERATIVE MANAGEMENT

- Patients with mild or moderate claudicant symptoms *or* a monoradiculopathy may respond to physical therapy, nonsteroidal anti-inflammatories, and epidural or root sleeve steroid injections. While some patients may relapse into symptoms, many in this group are content to repeat these efforts or to live with their symptoms.
- Patients with significant claudication generally do not respond to nonoperative measures, or they respond only temporarily. Most will elect to undergo operative decompression. Similar to disc herniations, absolute surgical indications include a cauda equina syndrome and progressive neurologic deficits.

SURGICAL MANAGEMENT

- The evidence base is clear: decompressive laminectomy or laminotomy is the operative technique with the best-documented long-term outcomes and is the gold standard of surgery for spinal canal stenosis.

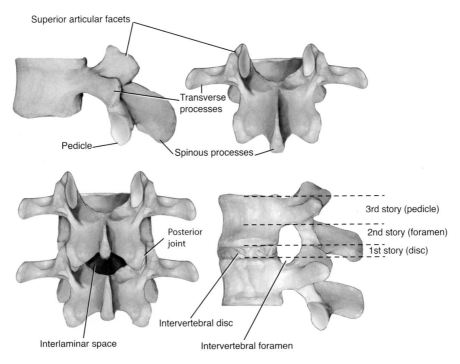

Superior articular facets

Transverse processes

Pedicle

Spinous processes

3rd story (pedicle)

2nd story (foramen)

1st story (disc)

Posterior joint

Interlaminar space

Intervertebral disc

Intervertebral foramen

FIG 1 • Functional vertebral unit.

Preoperative Planning

■ Planning is *vital* and should aim to answer several questions:
  ■ What is the patient's clinical syndrome?
  ■ What levels are involved?
  ■ Is the involvement "intersegmental"?
  ■ Are the foramina involved?
  ■ Is there associated pathology: disc herniation, synovial cyst, or degenerative spondylolisthesis or lateral listhesis?
■ The answers to these questions will direct the surgical approach, with the goal being complete and safe decompression of compressed neurologic tissue while minimizing damage to tissues not directly involved in the pathologic process.

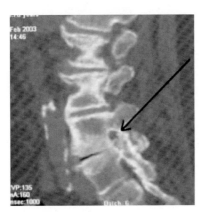

FIG 2 • Classic foraminal stenosis due to osteophyte formation on the tip of the superior articular facet demonstrated on CT sagittal reconstruction.

Positioning

■ Prone positioning on a well-padded frame is used (generally the Andrew's, Wilson, or Jackson). The hips and knees are gently flexed to decrease lumbar lordosis and to facilitate the interlaminar approach. The abdomen is free to decrease intra-abdominal pressure and venous backflow into the canal.
■ Shoulders should be gently flexed and abducted to less than 90 degrees; eyes, elbows, knees, and feet need to be well padded.
■ A needle is passed between and lateral to the spinous processes at the involved level or levels and C-arm imaging used to confirm the level. The needle is removed and the level or levels are marked and labeled on the skin.

Approach

■ After initial dissection, one of two windows will be undertaken based on the location of stenosis: the interlaminar window or the intertransverse window.
■ The traditional interlaminar approach of laminotomy or laminectomy is used in about 90% of cases of spinal canal stenosis requiring operative intervention.
  ■ It is used to decompress soft and bony tissues that compress the neurologic structures within the central canal and subarticular zones throughout the lumbar spine.
■ Two less invasive approaches may also be used and have outcomes similar to those seen with the more traditional approach: microdecompression via a unilateral approach and microdecompression via spinous process osteotomies.
  ■ Both techniques afford bilateral decompression of spinal canal stenosis via a unilateral approach.

INCISION

- The skin incision is made directly midline posteriorly and extends from the top of the most cephalad involved spinous process to the bottom of the most caudally involved spinous process (about 1.5 inches for single-level pathology).
- The subcutaneous tissues are gently mobilized and retracted to allow visualization of the dorsolumbar fascia.

Traditional Interlaminar Window for Decompression

- The dorsolumbar fascia is incised in the midline along the length of the skin incision, allowing exposure of spinous processes at each level.
- A Cobb elevator is then used to gently elevate the muscles (multifidus) from the spinous processes and laminae to the midportion of the facet joints bilaterally.
- A retractor is then placed and an intraoperative fluoroscopic image obtained to confirm the levels.
- At this point, illumination or magnification, based upon surgeon preference and experience, is gained by the use of the operative microscope or headlamp or loupes.
- A midline laminotomy is performed on the undersurface of the cephalad lamina to above the level of the insertion of the ligamentum flavum.
    - The insertion point is invariably in line with the most cephalad portion of the facet joint.
- This laminotomy is then continued into the subarticular zone laterally (medial facetectomy) and then to include the superior surface of the caudal lamina (**TECH FIG 1**).
- This bony work allows for exposure and excision of soft and hard tissues compressing the common dural sac and nerve roots and should be enough to get the job done safely and completely while avoiding iatrogenic injury.
    - The surgeon should aim to limit the medial facetectomies to less than 50% bilaterally and to preserve at least 5 mm of the lateral pars intra-articularis.
- In cases with concomitant congenital stenosis (involvement in the anatomic "third story"; about 15% of cases), complete midline laminectomy may be needed because the lamina itself is part of the pathologic compressive process.
- In the absence of congenital stenosis or deformity, a decompressive procedure that spans the distance from the top to the bottom of the facet joint will adequately decompress the central portion of the canal in most cases. This is because in most cases central stenosis occurs where the disc, ligamentum flavum, and facets converge to impinge upon neural structures.
- Soft and hard compressive tissue is then excised, allowing for decompression of the common dural sac and nerve roots.
    - This includes the ligamentum flavum in its entirety (in the midline—decompression of the central canal; its insertion on the undersurface of the capsule; a trumpeted decompression within the subarticular zone via medial facetectomy) and undercutting of the tip of the superior articular process and osteophytes from the facet joints.

- Generally, no retraction of the underlying dura and roots is needed since most pathology is visible and accessible posteriorly.
- Concomitant pathology will also need to be addressed if present.
    - Degenerative spondylolisthesis should be treated by spinal fusion with or without instrumentation, as discussed in following chapters.
    - Synovial cysts will need to be completely excised and the pseudocapsule gently peeled from the dura.
    - Disc herniation should be addressed as described in Chapter SP-12.
- The process is repeated at each clinically involved level. Generally, a residual laminar bridge is maintained at each level for routine decompression for degenerative stenosis (laminotomy). Cases of congenital stenosis require midline laminectomy given the compression within the "third story."
- The wound is then irrigated and hemostasis obtained. The use of a drain is optional, depending on the degree of oozing. The wound is then closed in three layers (fascia, subcutaneous tissue, skin in running subarticular fashion).

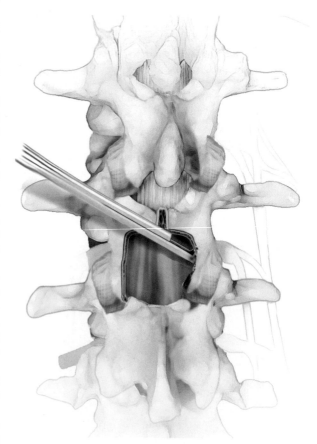

TECH FIG 1 • Laminotomy or laminectomy is performed to allow access to the ligamentum flavum, which is excised in its entirety in a trumpeted fashion throughout the segment. Medial facetectomy is included to address any bony stenosis in the subarticular zones.

MICRODECOMPRESSION VIA THE INTERLAMINAR WINDOW

Unilateral Approach

- Microdecompression via a unilateral approach may be used for patients with a predominant monoradiculopathy with or without neurogenic claudication and degenerative stenosis with minimal to no spondylolisthesis.
    - In other words, it is a good option in any case that may be adequately decompressed via laminotomy.
- A unilateral approach and decompression similar to that described above is undertaken on the ipsilateral side.
- The contralateral side is decompressed via excision of the inferior half of the spinous process and laminar junction, allowing exposure and excision (by working underneath the interspinous ligament) of the contralateral ligamentum flavum via progressive angulation of the microscope, progressive resection of the contralateral laminae (covering the entire area where the ligamentum inserts), and ligamentum resection in its entirety (**TECH FIG 2**).
- This operation is technically demanding but affords a recovery similar to that seen with microdiscectomy.

Spinous Process Osteotomy Approach

- Microdecompression via spinous process osteotomies may be used as a less invasive alternative for surgeons more comfortable with the traditional approach.
    - It affords the visualization of traditional midline approaches while preserving the spinous process and interspinous and supraspinous ligaments.
- A unilateral approach is used, similar to typical discectomy.
- The spinous processes are then osteotomized just posterior to their junction with the laminae.
- When the retractor is placed, the typical bilateral interlaminar window is exposed and decompression as described above is undertaken (**TECH FIG 3**).
- Once the retractor is removed, the spinous processes fall back into place and generally heal back to the residual laminar ring.

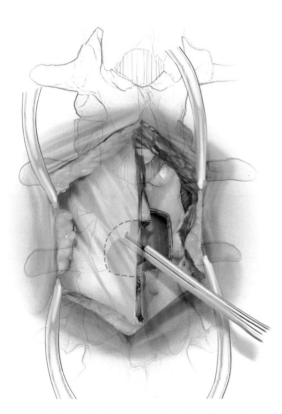

TECH FIG 2 • Microdecompression. A unilateral approach is used and a unilateral decompression performed. The contralateral side is decompressed by angulating under the interspinous ligament in a trumpeted fashion.

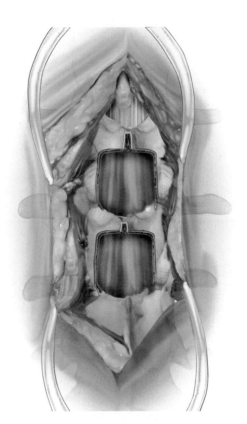

TECH FIG 3 • Spinous process osteotomies. A unilateral approach is used and the spinous processes are osteotomized near their base. The spinous processes are then retracted, allowing exposure of the "usual" interlaminar window. After decompression, the spinous processes fall back into place and generally heal to the residual laminar bridge.

TECHNIQUES

FORAMINAL DECOMPRESSION VIA THE INTERTRANSVERSE WINDOW

- Foraminal stenosis may be present with or without associated stenosis within the central canal and subarticular zone (addressed separately as above). With the exception of L5–S1, where it is accessible via an interlaminar window, it will need to be addressed via the intertransverse window.

- Adequate decompression of foraminal stenosis via an interlaminar approach requires resection of the lateral pars and results in potential instability at the level. The intertransverse window is a less morbid and easier approach to the foraminal zone and requires minimal resection of the lateral pars.

- The multifidus is taken medially and the longissimus is taken laterally by finger dissection, allowing placement of a retractor in this intermuscular–nervous plane.

- The tip of the superior articular process and the lateral pars interarticularis are exposed with electrocautery.

- Staying within the capsule of the facet joint to protect the underlying exiting root, the surgeon excises the tip of the superior articular process entirely, affording a bony decompression of the foramen (**TECH FIG 4**). Concomitant soft tissue stenosis (ligamentum flavum insertion in the subarticular zone or lateral disc herniation) can then be easily addressed if present.

- Irrigation, hemostasis, and closure are performed as described above.

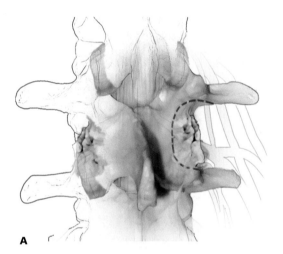 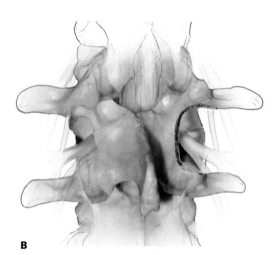

TECH FIG 4 • Foraminal decompression. Excision of the tip of the superior articular process and part of the pars interarticularis via a paraspinal approach (**A**) affords decompression of the exiting root in the foramen (**B**).

PEARLS AND PITFALLS

Revision decompression is difficult due to significant midline scar formation.	■ The goals should be to find residual lamina and to excise this cephalad and laterally, allowing exposure of previously undisturbed dura and roots. The decompression can then be carried caudally and medially using this normal dura as a guide.

POSTOPERATIVE CARE

■ After surgery, patients are fitted with a light lumbar corset and are encouraged to walk once anesthesia has worn off and pain permits. About 25% will be ready for discharge as 23-hour observation patients. The others (older patients and those with comorbidities) are discharged once they are medically stable and can mobilize adequately.

■ Once home, patients engage in a program of progressive walking, stretching, and corset use for comfort. For those progressing slowly, physical therapy may be introduced.

■ If all is well, they may drive in about a week and return to light work once they feel up to it. Heavy labor should be avoided for 6 to 12 weeks to ensure proper soft tissue healing. Long-term activities are not restricted.

OUTCOMES

■ In most patients, there is an 80% likelihood of an excellent or good outcome 2 years after surgery.

■ Patients with significant medical comorbidities (eg, diabetes, heavy smoking, peripheral vessel disease, coronary artery disease) are less likely to do well; these comorbidities reduce the likelihood of an excellent or good result by an estimated 15% to 20%.

■ Truly informed consent is recommended, as these procedures are not benign in this population.

COMPLICATIONS

■ Dependent on the surgeon: wrong level, wrong side, missed pathology, iatrogenic instability, root injury, dural tear, hemorrhage, positioning (eg, eyes, ulnar nerve)
■ Dependent on the operative environment and patient: wound infection, urinary retention, thrombophlebitis or pulmonary embolism

REFERENCES

1. Herkowitz HN, Kurz LT. Degenerative lumbar spondylolisthesis with spinal canal stenosis: a prospective study comparing decompression with decompression and intertransverse process arthrodesis. J Bone Joint Surg Am 1991;73A:802–808.
2. Johnsson KE, Rosen I, Uden A. The natural course of lumbar spinal stenosis. Clin Orthop Relat Res 1992;279:82–86.
3. Katz JN, Lipson SJ, Chang LC, et al. 7 to 10 year outcome of decompressive surgery for degenerative lumbar spinal stenosis. Spine 1996; 21:92–98.
4. Weinstein JN, et al. Initial results of 'SPORT': operative and nonoperative treatment of lumbar spinal canal stenosis. Reported at the International Society for the Study of the Lumbar Spine Annual Meeting, 2006.
5. Weiner BK, Fraser RD, Peterson M. Spinous process osteotomies to facilitate lumbar decompressive surgery. Spine 1999;24:62–66.
6. Weiner BK, Walker M, Brower RS, et al. Microdecompression for lumbar spinal canal stenosis. Spine 1999;24:2268–2272.

Chapter 13

Posterolateral Thoracolumbar Fusion With Instrumentation

Mark Dumonski, Thomas Stanley, Michael J. Lee, Bart Wojewnik, and Kern Singh

ANATOMY

- Pedicle morphology is detailed in Table 1.

IMAGING AND OTHER DIAGNOSTIC STUDIES

- Standing posteroanterior and lateral radiographs should be obtained whenever possible.
- Additional flexion–extension views may provide insight into subtle instabilities (**FIG 1**).
- Full-length posteroanterior and lateral radiographs are obtained in cases of spinal deformity to assess for global balance (coronal or sagittal).
- Lateral bending views can help determine the flexibility of the curve and levels for fusion.
- Axial computed tomography (CT) images can provide invaluable information about pedicle morphology, particularly in the setting of deformity.

SURGICAL MANAGEMENT

Indications

- Degenerative
  - Spondylolisthesis
  - Iatrogenic instability
  - Discogenic back pain
  - Pseudarthroses
- Adult deformity
  - Curve progression
- Neurologic deficit
  - Back pain refractory to nonoperative care
  - Pulmonary compromise secondary to deformity
  - Coronal or sagittal imbalance
- Pediatric deformity
  - Progressive scoliosis more than 50 degrees
  - Kyphosis more than 75 degrees
  - Curve progression despite bracing in a skeletally immature individual
  - Isthmic spondylolisthesis more than 50%

Preoperative Planning

- Pedicle anatomy can be best assessed on CT (**FIG 2**).
- A general assessment as to whether a pedicle is instrumentable can be gained by examining its size on an anteroposterior radiograph of the pedicle.
- Pedicle width and length and starting points can be determined from the axial image.

Positioning

- Patients should be placed in the prone position on a radiolucent table (**FIG 3**).
- Care is taken to ensure that the neck is in a neutral position and is not hyperextended.
- The arms are positioned at 90 degrees or less of abduction to minimize the likelihood of rotator cuff impingement. The arms are allowed to hang down slightly in a forward-flexed position about 10 degrees. The axilla should be clear from any padding to prevent brachial plexus palsy.

Table 1	Pedicle Morphology			
Region	**Thoracic**	**Lumbar**	**Sacral**	**General Points**
Size	Width increases cephalad and caudad to T5. T5 is the smallest pedicle (mean 4.5 mm).	Width decreases moving cephalad.	S1 pedicle is the widest of all pedicles (mean 18 mm).	Narrowest in mediolateral dimension
Horizontal angulation	Medial angulation increases gradually to 30 degrees at T1. T12 is angled laterally; T11 is neutral.	Medial angulation increases to 30 degrees at L5. Angulation is 10 degrees medial at L1.		Angulation is medial at all levels except T12.
Vertical angulation	Angulation increases gradually to T2, then slightly decreases. There is a large increase in superior angulation between L1 (2 degrees) and T12 (10 degrees).	L5 is angled slightly inferior. L3 and L4 are neutral. L1 and L2 are angled slightly superior.		
Length	Pedicles become shorter cephalad and caudad to T8. Longest pedicle is at T8 (45 mm).	Average length is 50 mm throughout the lumbar spine.		There is a high standard deviation in the length of T12 pedicle.

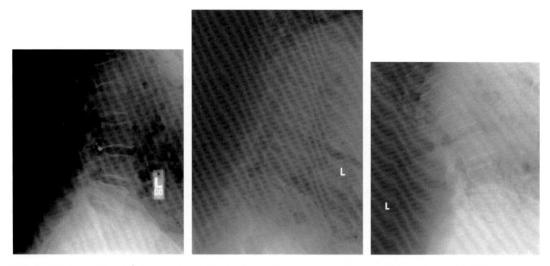

FIG 1 • Flexion and extension lumbar lateral spine radiographs can show evidence of spondylolisthesis as seen here at the L4–5 level.

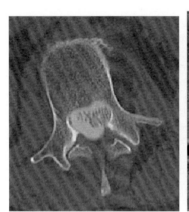
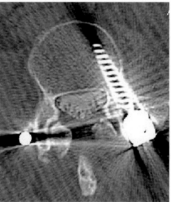

FIG 2 • Pedicle anatomy for screw placement can be assessed with CT scan.

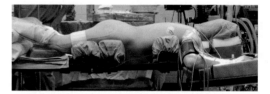

FIG 3 • The patient is positioned prone on the Jackson frame.

- Elbow pads are placed along the medial epicondyle to protect the ulnar nerve.
- The chest pad is placed just proximal to the level of the xiphoid process and distal to the axilla. In women, care is taken to tuck the breasts and ensure that the nipples are pressure-free.
- The iliac pads are placed two fingerbreadths distal to the anterior superior iliac spine, allowing the abdomen to hang free and reducing any unnecessary epidural bleeding.
- Proper placement of the chest and iliac pads allows for optimal restoration of sagittal alignment via gravity.

Approach

- Two approaches are used: the midline approach and the paraspinal approach.
- The midline approach is used for most spinal procedures as it allows direct access to the spinal canal.
- The paraspinal approach, also known as the Wiltse approach, was initially described for spondylolisthesis but is also used for far-lateral discectomies and minimally invasive muscle-sparing techniques (eg, minimally invasive pedicle screw instrumentation or transforaminal lumbar interbody fusion).
- Specific screw entry points are detailed in Table 2.

Table 2	Pedicle Screw Starting Points
Region	**Starting Point**
Proximal thoracic (T1–T3)	Junction of the midpoint of the transverse process and the lateral pars
Midthoracic (T4–T9)	Junction of the proximal transverse process and the lateral third of the superior articular process
Distal thoracic (T10–T12)	Junction of the midpoint of the transverse process and the lateral pars
Lumbar	Junction of the midpoint of the transverse process and 2 mm lateral to the pars
Sacral	At the inferolateral aspect of the L5–S1 facet joint

THORACOLUMBAR PEDICLE SCREW PLACEMENT

Pedicle Start Point

- Once the bony anatomy of the dorsal elements is meticulously exposed, the proper position of the pedicle entry point is defined. Anatomic landmarks include the lateral edge of the facet joint, the pars interarticularis, and the transverse processes (TECH FIG 1A).
- The actual pedicle starting point may vary significantly from the commonly quoted "norms" in many patients. What follows are general guidelines. Preoperative imaging studies (such as CT scan, or even the relationship between the pedicle and the lateral aspect of the pars on an anteroposterior radiograph) can provide clues about anatomic variations in a given patient or level.
- In both the lower (T10–12) and upper (T1–3) thoracic spine, the entry point is at the junction of the bisected transverse process and the lateral edge of the pars interarticularis.
  - In the midthoracic region (T5–9), the starting point is more medial and cephalad. Here, it is at the junction of the superior margin of the transverse process and the lateral third of the superior articular process (TECH FIG 1B).
- In the lumbar spine, the entry point is at the midpoint of the transverse process and 2 mm lateral to the pars interarticularis.
- The sacral entry point is at the inferolateral aspect of the L5–S1 facet joint.
- Using a 4-mm high-speed burr, the posterior cortex is breached to a depth of about 5 mm (TECH FIG 1C).
- Alternatively, fluoroscopic imaging may be used with the bull's-eye technique to identify the correct starting point, particularly when patient anatomy is distorted (TECH FIG 1D).

Cannulating the Pedicle

- A 3.2-mm hand drill is placed into the starting hole and advanced along the axis of the pedicle (TECH FIG 2A,B).

The drill is advanced under fluoroscopic guidance into the vertebral body to an ultimate depth of 35 to 40 mm in the lumbosacral spine, 25 to 30 mm in the lower and upper thoracic spine, and 30 to 35 mm in the midthoracic spine.

- Measurements of pedicle length can be made on axial CT or MRI scans and used to guide screw length.
- The advantage of using a hand drill is that cortical violations are lessened. When resistance is met (cortex), the drill fails to advance, and consequently the angle is adjusted.
- Alternatively, a "gearshift" type of device can be used to sound the pedicle. The gearshift should be rotated or wiggled as it is advanced with only gentle pressure. This technique allows the instrument to seek the proper path within cancellous bone rather than being pushed forcefully through a cortical wall. The process is analogous to feeding a guidewire into a vein during central line placement: the idea is to provide guidance, not force, to the instrument as it navigates a path within the cortical margins of the bone.
- For the S1 pedicle, the drill is directed 25 degrees medially and 10 degrees inferiorly toward the sacral promontory. A lateral fluoroscopic image is used to identify the sacral promontory (TECH FIG 2C).
  - Ideally, the screw tip should achieve tricortical purchase (engaging the anterior and posterior cortex and superior endplate of S1) (TECH FIG 2D).
- A flexible ball-tipped probe is then advanced down the pedicle tract. Bone should be encountered at the base of the tract as well as along all four walls of the pedicle. Medial and lateral cortical breaching is most common as the pedicle is narrowest in this plane.
  - A medial pedicle breach is most likely to occur at a depth between 15 and 20 mm ventral to the transverse process, which is the depth at which the spinal canal is encountered in most levels.

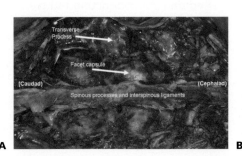
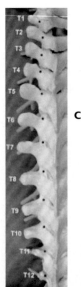
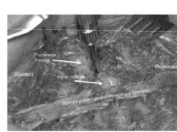
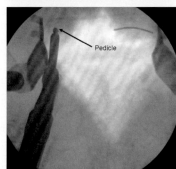

TECH FIG 1 • **A.** Posterior anatomy of the lumbar spine. **B.** Starting points for pedicle screws in the thoracic spine. **C.** The posterior cortex is breached with a 4-mm burr. **D.** The "bull's-eye" technique with fluoroscopy can be used to correctly identify the starting point.

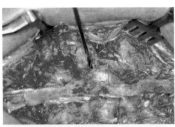

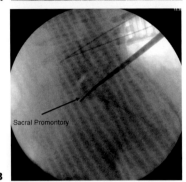

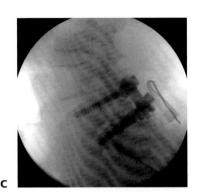

TECH FIG 2 • A. The hand drill is advanced into the pedicle. **B.** Path for the tricortical sacral pedicle screw. **C.** L5–S1 instrumentation with tricortical sacral fixation.

■ If a proper start site is selected, lateral breaches are more likely to occur deeper than 20 mm due to failure to medialize and follow the proper trajectory as the pedicle transitions into the vertebral body. However, if the start site is too lateral, a lateral breach may occur more superficially.

Pedicle Screw Sizing

■ With the ball-tipped probe advanced along the length of the pedicle tract, the surgeon measures the tract depth using a hemostat and a ruler (**TECH FIG 3A**).

■ In general, pedicles are tapped 1 mm smaller than the diameter of the screw to be used to optimize screw purchase. If the pedicle is sclerotic, "line-to-line" tapping should be performed. If the patient is osteoporotic, tapping is not necessary.

■ After tapping, the ball-tipped probe is again advanced through the pedicle tract to confirm that the pedicle cortices and anterior vertebral body are intact.

■ A Kirschner wire is then placed into the pedicle while the remaining pedicle tracts are cannulated.

■ All Kirschner wires are confirmed to be positioned properly via fluoroscopy. At this point, fusion bed preparation may occur (**TECH FIG 3B,C**).

Fusion Bed Preparation

■ The wound is copiously irrigated before decortication to preserve the local bone graft generated with high-speed burring.

■ Using a high-speed burr, the transverse process, the pars interarticularis, and the lateral wall of the facet joint of each level to be fused are decorticated.

■ Bone graft is placed over the decorticated areas. The fusion bed can be prepared with any combination of autogenous iliac crest bone graft, autogenous local bone graft (from the spinous processes and lamina), allograft, demineralized bone matrix, or bone morphogenic protein (**TECH FIG 4**).

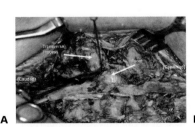

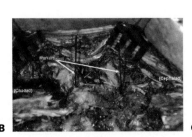

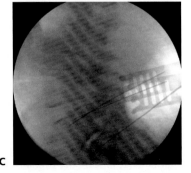

TECH FIG 3 • A. With the ball-tipped probe inserted in the pedicle path, a hemostat marks the length probe inserted. **B,C.** Pedicle marker positions are confirmed with fluoroscopy.

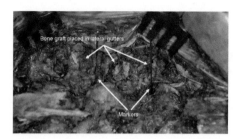

TECH FIG 4 • After decortication, bone graft is placed over the decorticated areas.

- Decorticating and bone-grafting the intertransverse, lateral pars, and lateral facet regions are performed before placing the screws to optimally prepare the fusion bed without the instrumentation getting in the way.
- Once the bone graft has been placed, the Kirschner wires serve as identifying landmarks for pedicle screw cannulation. Care is taken to advance the screw slowly in the same angulation noted with the Kirschner wire in place.

PELVIC FIXATION

- Sacropelvic fixation can be used in the setting of long-deformity reconstructions and tumor and in traumatic settings involving the lower lumbosacral spine.
- Modern pelvic fixation is most easily accomplished via modular iliac screw placement.
- After dissection of the posterior superior iliac spine, a starting point is identified 1.5 cm distal to the tubercle.
- A burr or rongeur is used to create a recessed defect such that the iliac screw head will lie recessed within the posterior superior iliac spine.
- A gearshift is then inserted into the starting point and advanced between the inner and outer tables of the pelvis, with the medial point of the probe scraping along the medial wall.
    - The trajectory should generally aim toward the hip joint.
    - The cortex of the medial wall is thicker than the lateral, and thus lateral violations are more likely than medial violations.
- A ball-tipped probe is used to assess the inner and outer tables.
- Depth is measured and the screw is inserted. The screw is typically 7.5 to 8.5 mm in diameter and roughly 60 to 80 mm long (**TECH FIG 5**).

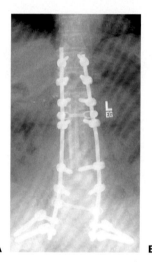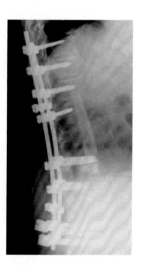

A   **B**

TECH FIG 5 • Fusion to pelvis with iliac screws.

CROSS-CONNECTORS

- Cross-connectors can significantly increase the rotational and bending stiffness of a multilevel construct.
- One, two, or three cross-links can be used, depending on

the length of the construct. If multiple cross-connectors are used, they should be spread as far apart as possible from each other for maximal construct rigidity.

HOOK INSERTION

- Hooks can be placed about the pedicle, transverse process, or lamina.
- Fixation is increased with a claw configuration.
- A claw figuration is composed of two hooks directed toward each other, separated by one or two levels. Claws are primarily used at the ends of a construct (**TECH FIG 6A**).
- Pedicle hooks provide the strongest fixation of all hook constructs. Always oriented cephalad, the pedicle hook is placed between the lamina of the superior vertebra and

the superior articular process of the inferior vertebra (**TECH FIG 6B**). The U-shaped tip fits around the pedicle and allows for increased stability.

- The inferior facet of the vertebra can be removed with an osteotome. It is helpful to resect enough of the facet so that the lateral edge of the spinal canal is identified so that it can be avoided during implant placement. The cartilage of the superior facet is removed with a curette. A pedicle hook developer is

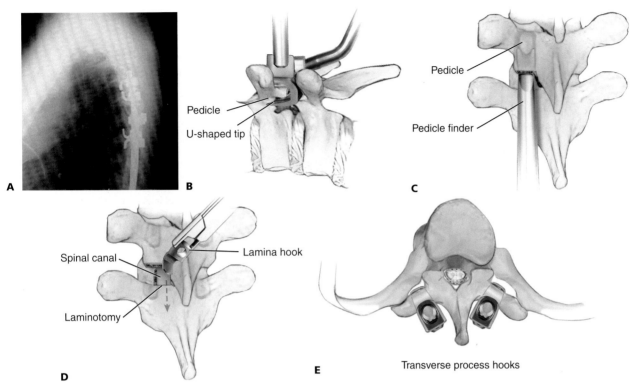

TECH FIG 6 • **A.** Thoracic hooks oriented in the claw configuration. **B.** Placement of a thoracic pedicle hook. **C.** A pedicle hook developer developing a plane for the pedicle hook. **D.** Placement of an upgoing laminar hook. **E.** Upgoing and downgoing transverse process hooks.

placed within the facet to develop the plane before placing the hook itself (**TECH FIG 6C**).

- Laminar hooks can be placed on the superior (downgoing) or inferior (upgoing) laminae (**TECH FIG 6D**). They should be used with caution as a portion of the implant is placed within the spinal canal. Generally, placing two laminar hooks into the canal at the same level (eg, two downgoing hooks or two upgoing hooks on the same lamina) should be avoided to minimize implant volume in the canal unless canal volume is capacious.

- The ligamentum flavum is dissected off the lamina, and the laminar surface receiving the hook is prepared with a Kerrison rongeur so the hook will be flush against the bone.

- Transverse process hooks can be used when sublaminar or pedicle hooks are not possible (**TECH FIG 6E**). They can be oriented either cephalad or (more commonly) caudad. A transverse process hook developer is used to create a plane for the implant. Although weaker than sublaminar or pedicle hooks, they avoid violation of the spinal canal.

PEARLS AND PITFALLS

Careful assessment of preoperative imaging (CT) allows for more accurate pedicle screw placement.	▪ Breaching the medial or inferior pedicle cortex endangers the exiting nerve root. Medial pedicle breaches are typically identified at a depth of 15 to 20 mm.
Fluoroscopy can be used to identify proper pedicle starting points when patient anatomy is distorted.	▪ Too medial a starting point for pedicle screw entry may injure the supra-adjacent facet joint.

POSTOPERATIVE CARE

- With secure multilevel pedicle screw fixation, it is probably not necessary to brace patients postoperatively, although that decision should be individualized based on the patient's pathology.

COMPLICATIONS

- Infection
  - The incidence of infection for posterior spine surgery is increased with the addition of an instrumented fusion.
  - A 1% infection rate has been noted for discectomies, a 6% infection rate for discectomies and fusion.

- Although there is a wide range reported for instrumented posterior fusions, the overall infection rate appears to be around 5% to 6%.
- Pseudarthrosis (nonunion rates, particularly crossing the lumbosacral junction)
  - The incidence of nonunion after posterior lateral inter-transverse fusion ranges from 3% to 25%.
  - Smoking has been shown to be a risk factor for nonunion.
  - A wide range of fusion rates across the lumbosacral junction has been reported (22% to 89%).
  - A 92.5% fusion rate is reported across the L5–S1 junction when using iliac screws.
- Neurologic and vascular injury
  - Although there is potential for severe vascular injury with pedicle screws in the thoracolumbar spine, vascular complications are rare, outside of a few reports.
  - The risk of nerve root irritation has been reported to be very low (0.2%) from pedicle screw instrumentation.

REFERENCES

1. Ali RM, Boacjie-Adjei O, Rawlins BA. Functional and radiographic outcomes after surgery for adult scoliosis using third-generation instrumentation techniques. Spine 2003;28:1163–1169.
2. Bernard TN Jr, Seibert CE. Pedicle diameter determined by computed tomography: its relevance to pedicle screw fixation in the lumbar spine. Spine 1992;17:S160–S163.
3. Bernhardt M, Swartz DE, Clothiaux PL, et al. Posterolateral lumbar and lumbosacral fusion with and without pedicle screw internal fixation. Clin Orthop Relat Res 1992;284:109–115.
4. Bridwell KH, Lewis SJ, Edwards C, et al. Complications and outcomes of pedicle subtraction osteotomies for fixed sagittal imbalance. Spine 2003;28:2093–2101.
5. Brown CW, Orme TJ, Richardson HD. The rate of pseudarthrosis (surgical nonunion) in patients who are smokers and patients who are nonsmokers: a comparison study. Spine 1986;11:942–943.
6. Brox JI, Sorensen R, Friis A, et al. Randomized clinical trial of lumbar instrumented fusion and cognitive intervention and exercises in patients with chronic low back pain and disc degeneration. Spine 2003;28:1913–1921.
7. Fischgrund JS, Mackay M, Herkowitz HN, et al. Degenerative lumbar spondylolisthesis with spinal stenosis: a prospective, randomized study comparing decompressive laminectomy and arthrodesis with and without spinal instrumentation. Spine 1997;22:2807–2812.
8. Fritzell P, Hagg O, Wessberg P, et al. Chronic low back pain and fusion: a comparison of three surgical techniques: a prospective multicenter randomized study from the Swedish lumbar spine study group. Spine 2002;27:1131–1141.
9. Horowitch A, Peek RD, Thomas JC Jr, et al. The Wiltse pedicle screw fixation system: early clinical results. Spine 1989;14:461–467.
10. Horwitz NH, Curtin JA. Prophylactic antibiotics and wound infection following laminectomy lumbar disc herniation. J Neurosurg 1997;86:975–980.
11. Keller A, Brox JI, Gunderson R, et al. Trunk muscle strength, cross-sectional area, and density in patients with chronic low back pain randomized to lumbar fusion or cognitive intervention and exercises. Spine 2004;29:3–8.
12. Kornblum MB, Fischgrund JS, Herkowitz HN, et al. Degenerative lumbar spondylolisthesis with spinal stenosis: a prospective long-term study comparing fusion and pseudarthrosis. Spine 2004;29:726–733.
13. Leufven C, Nordwall A. Management of chronic disabling low back pain with 360 degrees fusion: results from pain provocation test and concurrent posterior lumbar interbody fusion, posterolateral fusion, and pedicle screw instrumentation in patients with chronic disabling low back pain. Spine 1999;24:2042–2045.
14. Lonstein JE, Denis F, Perra JH, et al. Complications associated with pedicle screws. J Bone Joint Surg Am 1999;81A:519–528.
15. Lynn G, Mukherjee DP, Kruse RN, et al. Mechanical stability of thoracolumbar pedicle screw fixation: the effect of crosslinks. Spine 1997;22:1568–1572.
16. Matsunaga S, Sakou T, Morizono Y, et al. Natural history of degenerative spondylolisthesis: pathogenesis and natural course of the slippage. Spine 1990;15:1204–1210.
17. Molinari RW, Bridwell KH, Lenke LG, et al. Complications in the surgical treatment of pediatric high-grade isthmic dysplastic spondylolisthesis: a comparison of three surgical approaches. Spine 1999;24:1701–1711.
18. Moore KR, Pinto MR, Butler LM. Degenerative disc disease treated with combined anterior and posterior arthrodesis and posterior instrumentation. Spine 2002;27:1680–1686.
19. Parker LM, Murrell SE, Boden SD, et al. The outcome of posterolateral fusion in highly selected patients with discogenic low back pain. Spine 1996;21:1909–1916.
20. Rechtine GR, Sutterlin CE, Wood GW, et al. The efficacy of pedicle screw/plate fixation on lumbar/lumbosacral autogenous bone graft fusion in adult patients with degenerative spondylolisthesis. J Spinal Disord 1996;9:382–391.
21. Sato H, Kikuchi S. The natural history of radiographic instability of the lumbar spine. Spine 1993;18:2075–2079.
22. Steinmann JC, Herkowitz HN. Pseudarthrosis of the spine. Clin Orthop Relat Res 1992;284:80–90.
23. Suk SI, Kim WJ, Lee SM, et al. Thoracic pedicle screw placement in deformity: is it safe? Spine 2001;26:2049–2057.
24. Weinstein SL, Dolan LA, Spratt KF, et al. Health and function of patients with untreated idiopathic scoliosis: a 50-year natural history study. JAMA 2003;289:559–567.
25. Weinstein SL, Ponseti IV. Curve progression in idiopathic scoliosis. J Bone Joint Surg Am 1983;65A:447–455.
26. Zindrick MR, Wiltse LL, Doornik A, et al. Analysis of the morphometric characteristics of the thoracic and lumbar pedicles. Spine 1987;12:160–166.

Chapter 14

Transforaminal and Posterior Lumbar Interbody Fusion

Mitchell F. Reiter and Saad B. Chaudhary

DEFINITION

- Several types of lumbar arthrodesis have been developed to address the various pathologic processes that occur.
- Each of these fusion techniques offers certain advantages and disadvantages that provide the surgeon with a range of options for addressing each patient's condition.
- The standard lumbar arthrodesis techniques include:
  - Anterior lumbar interbody fusion (ALIF)
  - Posterior spinal fusion (PSF), which includes two subtypes:
    - Posterior interlaminar and facet fusion
    - Posterior lateral intertransverse fusion
  - Combined anterior and posterior fusion (AP fusion or 360-degree fusion)
  - Posterior lumbar interbody fusion (PLIF) and its variant the transforaminal lumbar interbody fusion (TLIF)
- The PLIF procedure uses a posterior approach to the spine that involves radical discectomy and endplate preparation combined with an interbody fusion using a structural graft or cage with or without supplemental posterior instrumentation.
- The TLIF procedure is similar to PLIF with the modification that the interbody region is accessed unilaterally via a more lateral approach in conjunction with pedicle screw instrumentation.
- PLIF and TLIF are versatile techniques that offer several advantages over the other fusion methods.[2]
  - They allow for pathology in all three columns of the spine to be addressed and for a circumferential fusion to be achieved through a single posterior approach.
  - They directly address the disc as a potential pain generator in patients with discogenic pain syndromes.
  - They have demonstrated a high rate of fusion that approximates the arthrodesis rate achieved with a more extensive combined anterior and posterior fusion procedure.
  - They allow for direct decompression of the spinal canal if necessary.
  - They permit some correction of spinal deformities, including asymmetric disc space collapse, spondylolisthesis, and mild kyphosis.
- PLIF and TLIF procedures also avoid some of the drawbacks inherent to anterior lumbar interbody fusion procedures, such as:
  - There is a reduced risk of the complications associated with an anterior approach, including vascular injury, higher rates of thromboembolic disease, and retrograde ejaculation in males.
  - They preserve a virgin anterior approach should revision surgery become necessary or should an adjacent segment arthroplasty become an option in the future.
- PLIF and TLIF have the disadvantage, however, of potential nerve root injury from preparation and instrumentation of the disc space through a posterior approach.

ANATOMY

- The standard posterior approach to the lumbar spine is used for posterior interbody fusion techniques.
- Applied surgical anatomy considerations for TLIF and PLIF are nearly identical, with both techniques using a midline incision and standard posterior exposure.
- Both PLIF and TLIF techniques require that the interbody region be accessed via posterior annulotomy.
- The major difference is that the PLIF procedure uses a bilateral and more-medial approach to access the interbody region, whereas the TLIF technique involves a unilateral approach with complete removal of one facet joint to allow more lateral access to the disc space (**FIG 1**).
  - As a result, the exiting root is in greater danger when performing a TLIF, whereas the traversing root is in greater danger with a PLIF.
- Gaining access to the posterior annulus and interbody region during TLIF and PLIF procedures is a critical step that requires an understanding of the local neurologic anatomy and the triangular working window to the annulus. The triangular working window consists of the following:
  - The traversing nerve root and thecal sac form the medial border of the triangle.
  - The exiting nerve root from the proximal vertebral level forms the lateral border (eg, L4 for an L4–5 TLIF or PLIF).
  - The superior aspect of the pedicle of the distal vertebra forms the base of the triangle.
- A confluence of epidural veins traveling longitudinally and transversely drapes the floor of the spinal canal and neuroforamen.
- With careful exposure, a triangular working window measuring up to 1.5 cm wide and of slightly greater height can be created.
- A noncollapsed disc space of an adult lumbar spine averages between 12 and 14 mm in height, with an anteroposterior diameter of about 35 mm.[4]

PATHOGENESIS

- The PLIF and TLIF procedures allow for fusion of the anterior column of the spine in the interbody region, which offers several biologic and biomechanical advantages over posterior spinal fusions:
  - The anterior column of the spine is known to support 80% of the body's compressive load; consequently, intervertebral structural grafts are subjected to compressive loading, which facilitates arthrodesis.
  - Since interbody structural grafts are load-sharing, they significantly reduce the cantilever bending forces applied to posterior spinal implants, thus protecting them from failure.
  - The interbody space has been shown to provide an optimal milieu for promoting arthrodesis for several reasons:
    - A large surface area of highly vascular cancellous bone is available.

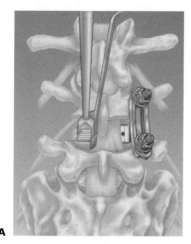

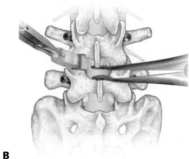

FIG 1 • **A.** PLIF technique, demonstrating the bilateral approach to the interbody region with complete facetectomies. Medial retraction of the neurologic elements is necessary to facilitate access to the disc space. **B.** TLIF technique, demonstrating the more lateral approach to the disc space with unilateral facetectomy. With the TLIF technique, medial retraction of the neurologic elements is frequently not needed. (**A**, Courtesy of Medtronic; **B**, Courtesy of Synthes Spine.)

- The disc space represents a relatively shorter gap to span when compared to intertransverse fusion.
- The outer annulus serves as a barrier that reduces fibrous tissue ingrowth into the fusion mass during healing of an interbody arthrodesis.

INDICATIONS

- Discogenic pain syndromes due to internal disc disruption or degeneration as well as postdiscectomy chronic low back pain are well suited to PLIF or TLIF for several reasons:[9,12]
  - These procedures directly address the disc as the pain generator and have been shown to have superior clinical outcomes in treating discogenic pain compared to isolated posterior spinal fusions, which do not remove and fuse the painful disc.
  - They allow for restoration of interbody height and some correction of local kyphosis without putting undue stress on the posterior implants.
  - They permit decompression of the exiting and traversing nerve roots indirectly by restoring foraminal height and directly via open laminectomy and foraminotomy. Because of this, PLIF and TLIF are ideally suited to patients with discogenic pain syndromes occurring in conjunction with radicular symptoms caused by herniated disc pathology or stenosis (**FIG 2**).

- Low-grade isthmic spondylolisthesis can also be treated successfully with PLIF and TLIF procedures as an alternative to performing a combined anterior and posterior fusion.[10]
  - PLIF and TLIF allow for direct decompression of the spinal canal and exiting nerve roots as well as indirect foraminal decompression through restoration of disc space height.
  - Addition of the interbody fusion raises the arthrodesis rate over stand-alone posterior fusion.
  - When clinically indicated and with proper instrumentation, PLIF and TLIF allow for reduction of the spondylolisthesis and slip angle, with some restoration of lordosis. In experienced hands and in conjunction with a wide decompression and intraoperative neurologic monitoring, some higher-grade spondylolistheses can be successfully reduced and stabilized with the PLIF and TLIF procedures.
- PLIF and TLIF procedures can be a useful adjunct to adult deformity surgeries such as degenerative scoliosis and spondylolisthesis and offer several advantages:
  - They can be used to provide anterior column support at the caudal end of fusion constructs and the lumbosacral junction without requiring an additional anterior approach to the spine.
  - They improve the arthrodesis rate, which can be helpful when an interlaminar fusion is not possible because a midline decompression was necessary to address spinal stenosis.

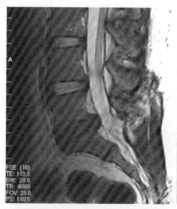

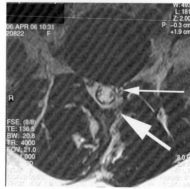

FIG 2 • **A.** T2-weighted sagittal MRI image demonstrating L5–S1 disc degeneration with a recurrent disc herniation in this patient who had undergone a previous L5–S1 discectomy. **B.** T2-weighted axial image of the same patient. Note the dorsal displacement of the traversing left S1 nerve root (*thin arrow*) by the disc and the previous left-sided laminotomy defect (*thick arrow*).

■ They allow for some additional deformity correction by releasing asymmetrically collapsed disc spaces and providing interbody structural support.

■ Several recent presentations (not yet published) have found that routine cases of degenerative spondylolisthesis may not benefit from the addition of an interbody arthrodesis and may be best managed with standard posterior laminectomy and fusion procedures.

■ PLIF and TLIF can also help raise the fusion rate in arthrodesis procedures in which clinical conditions pose a challenge to spinal fusion, such as:

■ Patients unwilling or unable to quit smoking

■ Patients with diabetes mellitus or on systemic corticosteroids

■ Patients on chemotherapy or with an irradiated fusion bed

■ Revision spinal fusion procedures in which the posterolateral fusion bed is fibrotic and hypovascular

■ Any other situations in which the clinician feels that the addition of an interbody arthrodesis is justified because conditions exist that may impede the formation of a posterior arthrodesis

CONTRAINDICATIONS

■ PLIF should not usually be attempted at the level of the conus medullaris (typically L1–2) or above, and great caution must be taken using the TLIF procedure at the level of the cord or conus.

■ Severe osteoporosis is a relative contraindication to these procedures as disc space preparation can result in major endplate violations with subsequent implant subsidence.

■ Anomalous neural anatomy such as a conjoined nerve root can make the performance of a PLIF or TLIF procedure impossible.

■ Even in some cases of "normal" nerve root anatomy, local variations in take-off angles of the exiting and traversing roots can place the roots at risk during interbody approaches. Caution should be exercised in such cases and interbody fusion abandoned if not felt to be safe.

■ Severe focal kyphosis is poorly addressed with a PLIF or TLIF procedure and is usually better treated with an anterior procedure that allows for release of the anterior longitudinal ligament and annulus fibrosus.

■ Irreducible higher-grade spondylolistheses are not well treated with the PLIF and TLIF procedures as the surface area of the opposing vertebral endplates is minimized.

NONOPERATIVE MANAGEMENT

■ Before considering PLIF and TLIF surgeries, standard nonoperative management options for the pathologic conditions being addressed should typically be exhausted.

■ Nonsurgical treatment usually involves a combination of analgesic medications, physical therapy, and activity and lifestyle modification. When applicable, interventional pain management techniques such as trigger point injections, facet blocks, or epidural steroid injections should be considered.

■ Surgical intervention is usually reserved for patients who remain symptomatic despite several months of nonoperative treatment and whose symptoms are severe enough to justify the risks associated with operative care.

SURGICAL MANAGEMENT

■ As mentioned earlier, PLIF and TLIF procedures are capable of addressing a wide variety of pathologic conditions and in specific situations offer several compelling advantages.

■ Given their versatility, the well-trained spinal surgeon needs to be aware of the indications for these procedures and must be capable of executing them properly.

■ While the usefulness of the PLIF and TLIF procedures is clear, one must remain mindful that these procedures are technically demanding and should be undertaken only after careful training and preoperative planning and with meticulous surgical technique.

Preoperative Planning

■ Preoperative imaging studies should be reviewed to determine the appropriate size and trajectories necessary for pedicle screw insertion as well as the anteroposterior diameter of the disc space.

■ Disc space height as well as adjacent disc height and overall lumbar alignment should be measured to help determine optimal interbody implant size.

■ An assessment should be made as to whether direct or indirect neurologic decompression will be necessary.

■ When using the TLIF technique, the interbody approach should be performed on the patient's symptomatic side if he or she has radicular complaints or from the side of maximal neurologic compression if the lower extremity symptoms are of equal severity.

■ Although sometimes difficult to assess, the patient's MRI needs to be studied carefully to identify anomalous neural anatomy such as a conjoined nerve root.

■ If a conjoined nerve root is suspected, the TLIF should be performed from the opposite side and the patient should be counseled preoperatively that the interbody portion of the procedure may not be possible because the contralateral side may demonstrate intraoperative nerve root anomalies as well.

■ For the PLIF procedure, the presence of a conjoined nerve root usually necessitates a unilateral PLIF. If identified preoperatively, conversion to a TLIF should be strongly considered.

■ Deformity at the level of the planned fusion needs to be assessed so that intraoperative measures can be taken to provide for correction.

Positioning

■ The patient should be positioned prone on an operating room table that allows for fluoroscopic imaging, such as a Jackson spine table (**FIG 3**).

■ The abdomen should be free to decompress the vena cava. This maneuver has been found to reduce epidural venous engorgement and bleeding.

■ A Foley catheter and lower extremity sequential compression devices should be used routinely.

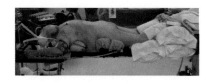

FIG 3 • Prone positioning with the abdomen free of compression, lower extremity compression devices in place, knees flexed, and all bony prominences padded. All tubes and wires are secured so that the area under the patient is free of obstruction, which facilitates later use of the fluoroscopy unit.

- Pillows should be used to keep the knees slightly flexed to minimize tension on the lumbar nerve roots.
- Intraoperative physiologic monitoring with somatosensory evoked potentials and "free run" electromyographic monitoring should be considered. Physiologic monitoring will also allow for pedicle screw stimulation testing to help detect any inadvertent pedicle wall breaches.

Approach

- The standard posterior approach to the lumbar spine is used, including exposure out to the tips of the transverse processes so that an adequate intertransverse fusion can be performed.
  - Some surgeons choose to perform a more limited dissection and do not perform the posterolateral portion of the fusion, hoping that by preserving the blood supply and muscular attachments in the intertransverse region there will be reduced erector muscle dysfunction and fibrosis with improved outcomes.

- True minimally invasive TLIF options have been developed. With these techniques, the procedure is modified so that it can be carried out through cannulas and with percutaneous instrumentations. These modifications will not be discussed in this chapter. The surgeon should be adept at open interbody fusions before considering minimally invasive approaches.
- For the standard TLIF procedure, the spinous processes and interspinous ligaments can usually be left intact. Preserving these structures minimizes epidural scarring and provides a larger surface area for the posterior fusion.
  - If decompression of the contralateral side of the spinal canal is required, the TLIF procedure can be modified to include a central laminectomy.
- Two exposure options exist for the PLIF procedure, each of which will be discussed in more detail later in the chapter:
  - Extensive resection including wide laminectomy with bilateral facetectomies
  - Limited resection using bilateral laminotomies and medial facetectomies

TRANSFORAMINAL LUMBAR INTERBODY FUSION

Pedicle Screw Insertion

- After exposure, pedicle entry points are identified at the junction of the transverse process with the superior articular process of each vertebra.
- A high-speed burr or awl is then used to access each pedicle, followed by use of a pedicle probe and tap to create a proper path for the screws.
- Polyaxial pedicle screws are then placed bilaterally in the standard fashion.
- Fluoroscopy or image guidance systems, electromyographic responses, or both can be used to aid in proper screw positioning.
- If desired, the transverse processes can be decorticated using a high-speed burr or curette before screw insertion. This is recommended to facilitate the posterior arthrodesis as access to the transverse processes becomes somewhat limited once the pedicle screws are in place.

Disc Space Distraction

- After screw placement, the next step is to provide posterior distraction to open the posterior portion of the disc space.
  - Lumbar disc spaces are normally lordotic, which can make insertion of an appropriate-sized interbody cage through the narrow posterior portion of the disc space difficult.
  - With distraction, the disc space alignment can be neutralized, thereby facilitating access to the interbody region with minimal bony resection.
- Several methods of achieving interbody distraction exist, and these can be combined as needed to achieve the desired alignment. The choice of distraction technique is largely based on surgeon preference, as all three methods have been found to be effective.
- Distraction option 1: Use of rods and screws
  - Rods are loaded bilaterally into the pedicle screws, followed by provisional placement of the system's locking nuts.

- Distraction is then carried out using the rods on both sides and a standard distractor (**TECH FIG 1A–C**).
- To allow for the distraction, the rods need to be slightly longer than will ultimately be necessary.
- The polyaxial screw heads should be angled as laterally as possible to maximize the volume of space medial to the rods. This maneuver facilitates later access to the disc space without requiring rod removal.
- Alternatively, several systems have pedicle screw distractor instruments that provide distraction off the screws without requiring rods to be inserted.
- Distraction instruments obviate the need to use longer rods and allow for unimpeded access to the facet and disc space during interbody preparation and implant insertion.
  - Lateral fluoroscopy should be used to judge the amount of distraction obtained at the posterior margin of the disc space.
  - Once adequate alignment is obtained, the system's locking nuts are tightened to maintain the distraction.
  - Care should be taken not to excessively distract off the screws in osteoporotic patients, as this could lead to screw loosening.
- Distraction option 2: Spinous process distraction
  - Distraction can also be achieved by using a lamina spreader placed between the spinous processes (**TECH FIG 1D**).
  - Distracting off the spinous process can reduce the risk of screw loosening that might occur with excessive distraction on the pedicle screws.
- Distraction option 3: Interbody dilators
  - Another option available to facilitate interbody distraction is to use interbody dilators, which are placed into the disc space and rotated to restore disc space height (**TECH FIG 1E**).
- This technique minimizes stress applied to the posterior implants and provides the most powerful method of vertebral body distraction.

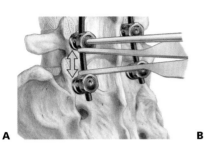
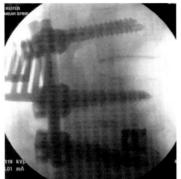
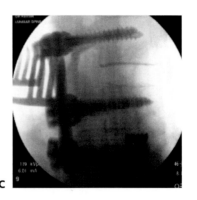
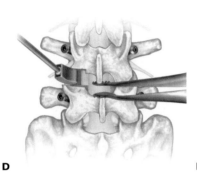
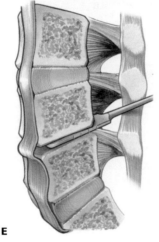

TECH FIG 1 • Interbody distraction techniques. **A.** A distractor is placed over the rod between the pedicle screws. **B.** A two-level TLIF procedure. The upper-level disc space remains slightly lordotic before distraction using the rods and screws. **C.** Distraction has neutralized the upper disc space, which facilitates access for endplate preparation and graft insertion. **D.** Lamina spreader placed between the spinous processes. **E.** A dilator or shaver is placed into the disc space. (**A,** Courtesy of Depuy Spine; **D,** Courtesy of Synthes Spine; **E,** Courtesy of Aesculap.)

- Use of interbody distractors is not possible until access to the disc space has been achieved, so this technique is not an option until the disc space has been accessed.

Complete Unilateral Facetectomy

- The inferior articular process of the cephalad vertebra should be exposed and removed using an osteotome or rongeurs (**TECH FIG 2A**).
- The superior articular process of the caudal vertebra is then dissected free of the ligamentum flavum with curettes and removed using Kerrison rongeurs. To maximize access to the disc space, the entire superior articular process down to the cephalad aspect of the pedicle should be removed so that the top of the pedicle can be easily seen and palpated (**TECH FIG 2B**).
- The lateral aspect of the hemilamina and the caudal portion of the pars interarticularis are resected using Kerrison rongeurs to provide access to the neural foramen and posterolateral annulus.
- The triangular working zone between the exiting and traversing nerve roots and the superior aspect of the pedicle should be identified (**TECH FIG 2C**).
  - The exiting nerve root is present just below the pedicle of the cephalad vertebra.
    - The exiting nerve can be identified visually or palpated but should not be deliberately manipulated as the sensitive dorsal root ganglion is in this region.
    - While it is critical to identify the location of the exiting nerve root, care should be taken not to unnecessarily dissect the nerve out of its sleeve

of fatty tissue; in some cases the nerve will be located and palpated but never fully visualized.
  - The traversing nerve root and the lateral aspect of the thecal sac will be present in the medial portion of the triangle. Nerve root retractors can be used to mobilize the neurologic elements medially to provide additional access to the posterolateral annulus (**TECH FIG 2D**).
  - As in all lumbar spinal surgical procedures, if trouble is encountered locating a nerve root, the surgeon should find or palpate the associated pedicle and look along the medial and inferior pedicle wall.
- With the neurologic elements accounted for, the posterolateral annulus can be accessed through the previously described triangular working zone by carefully coagulating and dividing the obstructing epidural veins using bipolar cautery (**TECH FIG 2E**).
  - Significant bleeding can be encountered at this stage, and the use of cottonoids in conjunction with hemostatic agents such as Gelfoam, Floseal, or Surgiflo can be helpful.
  - If the surgeon is not careful, the exiting or traversing nerve roots can be damaged while dealing with the bleeding arising from the epidural venous plexus. Working methodically while remaining constantly aware of the location of these neural structures is critical.

Disc Space Preparation

- A nerve root retractor is used to mobilize the thecal sac and traversing nerve root medially to improve exposure

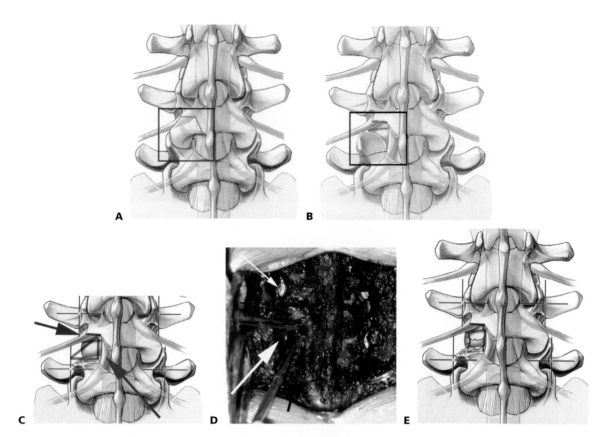

TECH FIG 2 • **A.** Removal of inferior articular process. **B.** Removal of superior articular process. **C.** Exposure after unilateral facetectomy, with the triangular working zone outlined in gray. The exiting nerve root (*red arrow*) forms the lateral border and the traversing nerve root and thecal sac (*blue arrow*) form the medial border of the working zone. **D.** Intraoperative picture following facetectomy and discectomy. Pedicle screws at L4 and L5 are marked by the small and large white arrows, respectively. The exiting L4 nerve root (*small black arrow*) and the traversing L5 nerve root (*large black arrow*) are both being gently retracted, with the annular window into the interbody region (*blue arrow*) seen between them. **E.** Posterolateral annulus with overlying epidural veins. To avoid inadvertent injury while obtaining hemostasis, one must constantly be aware of the location of the neurologic elements when working in the epidural space. (**C** and **E**, Courtesy of Aesculap.)

of the posterolateral annulus. An advantage of the TLIF procedure is that minimal neural retraction is necessary to access the interbody region. Depending on the local nerve root anatomy, however, retraction of the traversing root may be necessary even with a TLIF.

- A scalpel is then used to incise a rectangular region of the annulus lateral to the traversing nerve root to create a window into the disc space (**TECH FIG 3A**).
- It is extremely important to have proper instruments available to facilitate the critical step of disc space preparation. These instruments are frequently provided by the vendor of the graft or implants to be used in the interbody region and should include (**TECH FIG 3B**):
  - Interbody paddle scrapers to dilate and prepare the endplates
  - Offset curettes to facilitate access to the contralateral side of the disc space
  - Rasps, ring curettes, and reverse curettes to assist in endplate preparation
  - Osteotomes or box chisels to improve access to the interbody region when the disc space is narrowed posteriorly
  - Long straight and upbiting pituitary rongeurs for débridement of the interbody region

- After creation of the annular window, typically shavers or dilators of increasing size are serially introduced into the disc space and rotated (**TECH FIG 3C,D**).
  - Lateral fluoroscopy can be helpful in determining the proper depth of penetration into the disc space. The anterior and anterolateral annulus should be palpated by the instrument and never violated, or catastrophic vascular injury could occur.
  - Instruments used within the disc space are typically marked so that they are not overinserted to avoid potentially catastrophic violation of the anterior annulus. It is helpful to preoperatively estimate disc space length (posterior to anterior) on MRI or CT scan to have an idea of how far the instruments can be inserted.
- After dilation and shaving, a combination of curettes and rongeurs is used to perform a thorough discectomy and endplate preparation down to bleeding bone (**TECH FIG 3E,F**).
  - Care should be taken not to violate the endplates in regions expected to load share with the interbody implant as this can make implant placement difficult and lead to settling of the structural graft.
  - Several TLIF techniques do call for perforation of the endplates to expose cancellous bleeding bone in

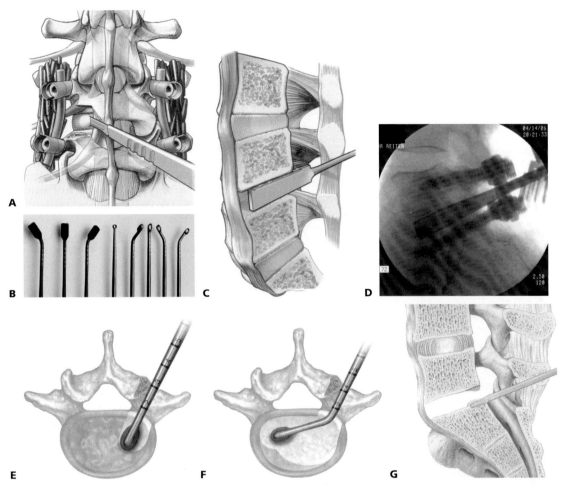

TECH FIG 3 • **A.** With the TLIF's lateral approach, annular incision is frequently possible without neurologic retraction. **B.** Disc space preparation instruments (from left to right): left offset, straight, and right offset rasps, ring curette, reverse curette, straight, left, and right offset curettes. Other instruments not shown may include dilators, shavers, osteotomes, and straight and angled pituitary rongeurs. **C.** Schematic of a shaver introduced into a disc space. Rotation of the shaver should remove endplate cartilage to facilitate arthrodesis. **D.** Lateral fluoroscopic image of a shaver within the disc space at L5–S1. To avoid violation of the endplates, care must be taken when working in the interbody region to maintain a parallel trajectory to the disc space. Straight (**E**) and offset (**F**) curettes maximize the area of the disc space that can be accessed and facilitate proper endplate preparation. **G.** Access to concave disc spaces can be facilitated by removal of posterior endplate osteophytes. (**A,C,** Courtesy of Aesculap; **B,** Courtesy of Biomet Spine; **E,F,** Courtesy of Synthes Spine; **G,** Courtesy of Depuy Spine.)

non-load-sharing interbody regions, using osteotomes for the anterior portion of the disc space or curettes and awls for other areas.

- Because of the concave nature of the endplates, it is sometimes necessary to use osteotomes or box chisels to remove a rim of bone from the posterior aspect of the vertebral bodies to improve access to the disc space and allow for placement of a properly sized graft (**TECH FIG 3G**). The surgeon should remember that aggressive removal of the posterior lip may lead to a greater risk of implant backout with root compression.
- On completion of the discectomy and endplate preparation, exposed bony endplates should be visible on the cephalad and caudal vertebral bodies.
- To minimize the risk of neurologic injury and postoperative dysesthetic pain, several recommendations should

be followed during the disc space preparation and graft insertion:

- Retraction on the neurologic elements should be minimized, and it should be released intermittently throughout the procedure.
- The thecal sac should never be retracted across the midline of the spinal canal.
- Particularly in revision cases, the neurologic elements should be carefully mobilized off the floor of the canal and disc space before retraction.
- Implants should be selected that can be inserted without excessive neural retraction.
  - This can be an issue with use of threaded cylindrical cages because the height and width of the device must be equal; consequently, a cage of the appropriate height might be too wide to be safely inserted.

TECHNIQUES

Graft Placement

- A variety of interbody grafting techniques have been described for use in the TLIF procedure:
  - Placement of two vertical fibular allografts or vertical titanium mesh cages posteriorly in the disc space with cancellous graft packed anteriorly (**TECH FIG 4A**)
  - Use of an oblique threaded cylindrical cage or machined cortical allograft bone dowel (**TECH FIG 4B**)
  - Use of an obliquely placed rectangular PEEK cage or bullet-shaped cortical allograft
  - Placement of a curved titanium cage, PEEK cage, or machined cortical allograft anteriorly and as centrally as possible within the disc space, with cancellous graft placed behind the device (**TECH FIG 4C**)
- While it has been shown that anterior cage placement is biomechanically superior to posterior cage placement, studies comparing the clinical efficacy of these various techniques do not exist.
- When choosing an interbody graft and grafting technique, surgeons should consider several factors:
  - Ability to insert the device without requiring excessive neurologic retraction
  - Volume of cancellous graft that can be packed within and around the cage or allograft
  - The effect of the graft's position and shape on the ability to restore lordosis with later compression of the posterior instrumentation[6]
- The remainder of this section will describe the technique in which a single curved titanium or PEEK cage or allograft is placed anteriorly and centrally within the disc space.
- After endplate preparation, graft trials should be used to determine the proper size for the interbody spacer

(**TECH FIG 4D**). Fluoroscopic imaging should be used to confirm proper sizing of the trial.
- The anterior and lateral aspects of the disc space should then be tightly packed with morselized graft material.
  - Several options are available for use as morselized graft material, including autogenous iliac crest bone graft, local bone graft from the removed facet and lamina, allograft corticocancellous bone, allograft demineralized bone matrix, ceramic bone graft extenders, and bone-inducing substances such as bone morphogenetic protein.
  - The choice of graft should depend on surgeon experience, host factors that may affect fusion, patient preference, cost, and availability.
- Graft impactors should be used to maximize the amount of bone that can be placed into the interbody space. For the technique using a central and anteriorly placed cage, the anterior 25% of the disc space should be filled initially with tightly packed morselized graft material.
- Before inserting the actual cage or graft, the trial should be reinserted to confirm that the morselized graft has not blocked the pathway for insertion of the structural graft.
- The implant should then be inserted into the interbody space and placed anteriorly and as centrally as possible.
  - Implant position should be confirmed with AP and lateral fluoroscopy during insertion.
  - Straight and offset impactors can be used to facilitate proper cage positioning.
- Additional morselized graft material should then be packed into the posterior aspect of the disc space behind the implant (**TECH FIG 4E,F**).

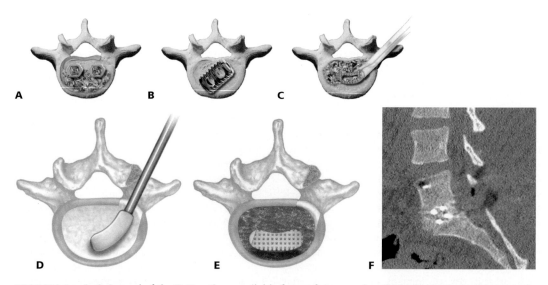

TECH FIG 4 • A–C. Several of the TLIF options available for graft type and position. **A.** Vertical cages or grafts placed posteriorly within the disc space with cancellous graft packed anteriorly. **B.** A single oblique threaded cage or graft. **C.** An anteriorly and centrally placed cage with cancellous graft placed posteriorly. **D.** Trial insertion to ensure that the appropriately sized device will fit and that cancellous graft packed into the disc space has not obstructed the pathway. **E.** Structural graft in place anteriorly with cancellous graft packed in the remaining portion of the disc space. **F.** Postoperative sagittally reconstructed CT scan demonstrating bone graft anteriorly, posteriorly, and within a titanium TLIF cage. (**D–F**, Courtesy of Synthes Spine.)

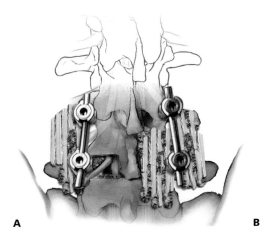
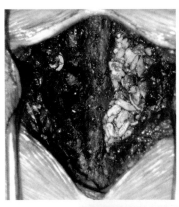
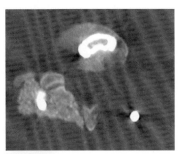
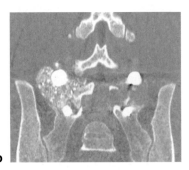
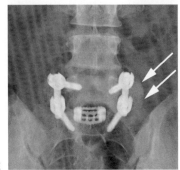

TECH FIG 5 • **A.** Schematic demonstrating posterolateral and interlaminar bone grafting. **B.** Intraoperative photograph with unilateral posterior morselized graft in place on right. Axial (**C**) and coronal (**D**) CT images demonstrating posterolateral and interlaminar graft in place. **E.** Postoperative radiograph demonstrating a solid unilateral arthrodesis (*white arrow*) in the posterolateral region. Assessment of fusion status in the posterolateral region is sometimes easier than assessing fusion within the interbody space.

Compression and Posterolateral Grafting

- With the implant in place, distraction is released from the spinous processes or pedicle screws. Compression is then applied to the pedicle screw construct and the locking nuts are finally tightened.
- Compression both loads the anterior implant and restores lordosis to the spine.
- The contralateral spinous processes, lamina, facet joint, and transverse processes should then be decorticated (ideally the transverse processes were decorticated at the time of screw insertion).
- Morselized graft can then be placed into the contralateral interlaminar, facet, and intertransverse regions (**TECH FIG 5**).

- The interspinous ligament, if preserved, will serve to prevent graft migration into the exposed portion of the spinal canal and foramen.
- Some surgeons may also wish to place graft on the ipsilateral side in the intertransverse region, but care must be taken to avoid allowing graft to enter the spinal canal or compress the exiting nerve root.
- Final AP and lateral fluoroscopic images should be obtained.

Closure

- Before closure, final hemostasis should be obtained and the neurologic elements inspected to ensure that no graft material has fallen into the spinal canal.
- A Valsalva maneuver can also be performed to confirm the integrity of the dural sac.
- A standard layered closure over a drain is then carried out.

POSTERIOR LUMBAR INTERBODY FUSION

- Most of the technique for PLIF is similar to that described above for TLIF, except that a bilateral and more medial approach to the interbody space is used.
- This section describes the PLIF procedure by highlighting the differences between the TLIF and PLIF techniques.

- As noted in the exposure section, two PLIF exposure options are available (**TECH FIG 6**):
  - Extensive resection including wide laminectomy with bilateral complete facetectomies
  - Limited resection using bilateral laminotomies and medial facetectomies

TECHNIQUES

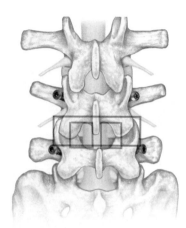

TECH FIG 6 • Bony resections necessary for each of the two PLIF exposures. Wide laminectomy and complete facetectomies are demonstrated by the gray line. Laminotomy and partial facetectomies are shown by the red line.

- The decision to use the wide laminectomy with total facetectomies is affected by several considerations:
  - It provides maximal exposure and minimizes the amount of neural retraction necessary to place the interbody grafts or implants. This is essentially a bilateral TLIF.
  - It should be strongly considered when fusing levels with a smaller interpedicular distance, such as in patients of short stature and in the upper lumbar spine.
  - It results in iatrogenic instability and therefore must be supplemented with pedicle screw instrumentation. Even with pedicle screws, a bilateral PLIF represents a more unstable situation. In patients with poor bone quality, the pedicle screws can loosen and lead to instability of the construct, with possible cage migration.
  - It eliminates the ability to fuse the facet joints posteriorly and reduces the host bone contact area available for the posterolateral fusion.
- Limited resection using bilateral laminotomies and medial facetectomies:
  - Preserves the segment's biomechanical stability by preserving the spinous processes, the interspinous ligaments, and most importantly the lateral half of the facet joints and associated pars interarticularis
  - Must be employed for cases in which posterior instrumentation is not being used
  - May be difficult in patients with a tall disc space as there may not be enough room for passage of the larger interbody graft required without more extensive resection of the facets
  - Should only be attempted by surgeons very familiar with the PLIF procedure as additional neural retraction is necessary, with a consequent higher risk of neurologic injury
- After the exposure, pedicle screws are inserted and disc space distraction is applied as described for the TLIF procedure.

- The PLIF procedure can be performed without pedicle screws if one uses the limited resection technique during exposure and care is taken not to destabilize the segment.

Laminotomy and Partial Facetectomy

- If the partial resection technique is being used, a laminotomy is performed by using curettes to detach the ligamentum flavum from each of the adjacent lamina as well as the superior articular process of the caudal vertebra.
- Kerrison rongeurs are then used to remove lateral portions of the adjacent lamina and the medial half of the superior and inferior articular processes.
- This process should be repeated bilaterally and should result in working windows for approaching the disc space on each side of spinal canal.
  - When using the limited resection technique, care should be taken to preserve the spinous process, interspinous ligaments, lateral pars, and lateral half of the facet joints.
- As in the TLIF procedure, the exiting and traversing nerve roots need to be identified and appropriate caution used to avoid traumatizing these sensitive neurologic structures during the procedure. To minimize root injury, one should remove enough lateral bone to be able to access the disc space without major retraction of the traversing root.
- The wide laminectomy and bilateral facetectomy technique simply involves enlarging the above approach.
  - Resection of the spinous process and interspinous ligaments medially will improve the ability to retract the thecal sac toward the midline.
  - For a maximally sized working window, total facetectomies can be performed to allow for more lateral access to the disc space (see Fig 1A).
- After exposure, the posterolateral annulus can be accessed through the previously described triangular zone cephalad to the pedicle of the inferior vertebra, medial to the exiting nerve root, and lateral to the traversing nerve root and thecal sac (see Tech Fig 2C).
- Epidural veins are carefully coagulated and divided in the same way as described for the TLIF procedure.

Disc Space Preparation

- Disc space preparation is performed in an identical fashion as described above for the TLIF procedure except that bilateral annular windows are created somewhat more medially than for a TLIF.
- The thecal sac and traversing nerve root are mobilized medially, and a combination of shavers, curettes, and rongeurs is used to perform a thorough discectomy down to exposed endplate.
- In noninstrumented PLIF procedures, achieving adequate interbody graft contact area is critical to reduce the risk of graft subsidence.
  - Closky et al[1] demonstrated that in patients of average bone density and size, interbody graft contact area should exceed 6.2 cm^2 or an area roughly 2.5 × 2.5 cm.

- Instrumentation reduces the risk of subsidence but has not been shown to improve the clinical outcome when compared to properly performed noninstrumented PLIF procedures.

Graft Placement

- The PLIF procedure requires the placement of structural interbody grafts inserted from each side of the spinal canal (TECH FIG 7).
- As in the TLIF, many graft options exist, including structural autograft or allograft bone as well as threaded or rectangular titanium or PEEK implants.
- Dr. Lee[4,8] has cautioned that most commercially available implants typically do not meet the surface area requirements for noninstrumented PLIF and should be used only when supplemented with pedicle screws.
- Regions of the interbody space not filled with structural graft should be packed as tightly as possible with morselized graft material.
- Fluoroscopy can be used to assess interbody implant position.

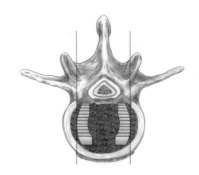

TECH FIG 7 • Bilateral PLIF grafts surrounded by cancellous bone. (Courtesy of Medtronic.)

Compression, Posterolateral Grafting, and Closure

- Compression (when pedicle screw instrumentation has been used), posterolateral grafting, and closure are all accomplished in a fashion similar to that described for the TLIF procedure.

PEARLS AND PITFALLS

Indications	■ As in all lumbar fusion surgeries, clinical success will depend largely on proper patient selection.
	■ Fusions performed primarily for discogenic back pain have a limited success rate, and realistic expectations will enhance patient satisfaction with the procedure.
	■ Revision procedures with extensive epidural scarring are technically challenging and benefit from a more lateral approach to the disc space to minimize retraction of neurologic elements typically surrounded by fibrous tissue.
Interbody access and preparation	■ Distraction techniques are used to neutralize the alignment of the adjacent endplates as much as technically feasible.
	■ Concave endplates may require use of an osteotome or box chisel to facilitate access to the disc space and allow for placement of a properly sized graft.
	■ An array of interbody preparation instruments, including offset curettes, must be available to facilitate comprehensive removal of endplate cartilage and disc material.
	■ Since achieving an interbody fusion is critical to the success of the procedure, adequate time and effort must be spent in disc space preparation. The surgeon must not rush interbody preparation.
	■ To avoid serious endplate violation, care must be taken to maintain a parallel trajectory to the disc space when working with instruments in the interbody region.
Neurologic injury	■ Identifying the location of the exiting nerve root is a vital step in the procedure and should occur before incising the annulus.
	■ Insufficient laminectomy can result in poor visualization and excessive neural retraction with inadvertent neurologic injury.
	■ Exiting nerve roots with a more acute angle of takeoff from the thecal sac can result in a smaller triangular working zone and should be gently retracted laterally.
	■ Medial retraction of the thecal sac and traversing nerve root should be minimized and must never cross the midline.
	■ Neurologic retraction should be released frequently to allow for reperfusion of these sensitive structures.
	■ Free run electromyographic monitoring can provide live feedback and help reduce the risk of neurologic injury from overzealous neurologic retraction.
	■ Great care must be taken to account for the dura and neurologic elements every time that an instrument or graft is inserted into the disc space.
	■ Should significant difficulties arise such as obstructing anomalous neural anatomy, major epidural bleeding, or a complex dural tear, one must be willing to abandon the interbody portion of the fusion rather than risk causing a catastrophic injury.

Epidural bleeding	▪ Epidural bleeding can be troublesome in the posterior annular region, and use of hemostatic agents such as Gelfoam, Floseal, or Surgiflo should be strongly considered. ▪ Great care must be taken to identify the neurologic structures when using bipolar cautery. ▪ Should a dural tear occur, it should be repaired as soon as technically possible, as reduced intrathecal pressure will produce engorgement of the epidural veins with significantly more bleeding.
Graft placement	▪ Bony resection must allow sufficient access to the interbody region to allow placement of an adequately sized graft. ▪ Graft type should be chosen carefully in situations where access to the disc is limited or a tall disc space exists. ▪ Due to their narrower widths, rectangular grafts or cages can be inserted more easily into a tall disc space than cylindrical grafts, which require a larger transverse exposure. ▪ Fluoroscopy and offset impactors should be used during graft insertion to facilitate optimal final implant position.

POSTOPERATIVE CARE

▪ The patient is typically mobilized out of bed the day after surgery.

▪ Postoperative bracing is typically not required for the TLIF or instrumented PLIF procedures but can be used according to surgeon preference.

▪ Most physicians prefer to use a thoracolumbosacral orthosis during the postoperative period for noninstrumented PLIF procedures.

▪ Serial radiographs are used to assess for fusion.

OUTCOMES

▪ Fusion rates for the PLIF and TLIF procedures are similar, with studies finding rates of obtaining a solid arthrodesis varying between 89% and 100%. Several recent larger studies have reported fusion rates above 95%.[7,10,11]

▪ While clinical success rates vary between studies, most series report similar outcomes with PLIF and TLIF as for anterior interbody and combined anterior and posterior fusion procedures.

▪ Most of the studies on PLIF and TLIF using visual analog scale (VAS) and Oswestry Disability Index (ODI) scores as outcome measures demonstrate an overall patient satisfaction rate of about 80% with the procedure.[3,7,8,14]

▪ Longer-term studies indicate that the results of PLIF and TLIF procedures tend to be durable once a solid arthrodesis has been achieved.

COMPLICATIONS

▪ Neurologic injury is an uncommon complication of PLIF and TLIF and has been reported to occur in between 0% and 4% of patients. Many of these injuries represent a neuropraxia due to excessive nerve root retraction and resolve spontaneously.[13,15]

▪ Dural tears are a more common complication and have historically been reported to occur in 0.5% to 18% of PLIF and TLIF procedures.

▪ The dural tear rate appears to be significantly lower with the TLIF procedure compared to the PLIF, likely related to the fact that less neural retraction is necessary when using the TLIF's more lateral approach to the disc space.[5]

▪ More recent studies demonstrate a trend toward much lower rates of dural tears in both PLIF and TLIF procedures, with a reported incidence in the range of 1% to 5%.

▪ Implant migration or failure is a rare complication in the TLIF procedure but has been reported to occur in up to 2.4% of cases in which a noninstrumented PLIF is performed.

Properly sizing the interbody implants and fully packing the disc space with graft material can help reduce the risk of this complication.

▪ Other complications of posterior lumbar fusions that are not specific to the PLIF and TLIF procedure include wound infection, excessive bleeding, pedicle screw malposition, and epidural hematoma.

REFERENCES

1. Closkey RF, Parsons JR, Lee CK, et al. Mechanics of interbody spinal fusion: analysis of critical bone graft area. Spine 1993;18:1011–1015.
2. Enker P, Steffee AD. Interbody fusion and instrumentation. Clin Orthop Relat Res 1994;300:90–101.
3. Hackenberg L, Halm H, Bullmann V, et al. Transforaminal lumbar interbody fusion: a safe technique with satisfactory three- to five-year results. Eur Spine J 2005;14:551–558.
4. Herkowitz HN, Rothman RH, Simeone FA, eds. The Spine, ed 5. Philadelphia: Saunders Elsevier; 2006.
5. Humphreys SC, Hodges SD, Patwardhan AG, et al. Comparison of posterior and transforaminal approaches to lumbar interbody fusion. Spine 2001;26:567–571.
6. Kwon BK, Berta S, Daffner SD, et al. Radiographic analysis of transforaminal lumbar interbody fusion for the treatment of adult isthmic spondylolisthesis. J Spinal Disord Tech 2003;16:469–476.
7. Lauber S, Schulte TL, Liljenqvist U, et al. Clinical and radiologic 2- to 4-year results of transforaminal lumbar interbody fusion in degenerative and isthmic spondylolisthesis grades 1 and 2. Spine 2006;31:1693–1698.
8. Lee CK, Vessa P, Lee JK. Chronic disabling low back pain syndrome caused by internal disc derangements: the results of disc excision and posterior lumbar interbody fusion. Spine 1995;20:356–361.
9. Lin PM. Posterior lumbar interbody fusion (PLIF): past, present, and future. Clin Neurosurg 2000;47:470–482.
10. McAfee PC, DeVine JG, Chaput CD, et al. The indications for interbody fusion cages in the treatment of spondylolisthesis: analysis of 120 cases. Spine 2005;30:S60–S65.
11. Miura Y, Imagama S, et al. Is local bone viable as a source of bone graft in posterior lumbar interbody fusion? Spine 2003;28:2386–2389.
12. Moskowitz A. Transforaminal lumbar interbody fusion. Orthop Clin North Am 2002;33:359–366.
13. Okuda S, Miyauchi A, et al. Surgical complications of posterior lumbar interbody fusion with total facetectomy in 251 patients. J Neurosurg Spine 2006;4:304–309.
14. Potter BK, Freedman BA, Verwiebe EG, et al. Transforaminal lumbar interbody fusion: clinical and radiographic results and complications in 100 consecutive patients. J Spinal Disord Tech 2005;18:337–346.
15. Villavicencio AT, Burneikiene S, Bulsara KR, et al. Perioperative complications in transforaminal lumbar interbody fusion versus anterior-posterior reconstruction for lumbar disc degeneration and instability. J Spinal Disord Tech 2006;19:92–97.

Chapter **15**

Iliac Crest Bone Graft Harvesting

Michael J. Lee, Thomas Stanley, Mark Dumonski, Patrick Cahill, Daniel Park, and Kern Singh

DEFINITION

- The use of autogenous bone graft is considered by most surgeons to be the gold standard for achieving fusion in the spine.
- Autogenous bone graft can be used at any spinal level, anterior or posterior.
- The posterior ilium is most frequently harvested for nonstructural, cancellous bone graft.
- Tricortical, structural bone grafts for cervical interbody fusions are typically harvested from the anterior ilium.

ANATOMY

- Anterior ilium
  - The anterior ilium has a concave anterosuperior surface.
  - The anterior iliac crest becomes its thickest (iliac tubercle) 2 to 3 cm posterior to the anterior superior iliac spine (ASIS) (**FIG 1A**).

- The lateral femoral cutaneous nerve typically courses medial to the ASIS; however, it can infrequently cross lateral to the ASIS and be at risk for injury (**FIG 1B**).
- Posterior ilium
  - The posterior iliac crest thickness ranges from 14 to 17 mm.
  - The superior cluneal nerve passes over the iliac crest 7 to 8 cm lateral to the posterior superior iliac spine (PSIS) and is at risk for injury with a lateral incision (**FIG 1C**).
  - The superior gluteal artery exits the pelvis from the greater sciatic notch and can be injured if bone harvesting approaches the sciatic notch (**FIG 1D**).

SURGICAL MANAGEMENT

Positioning

- A roll or bump of towels or a blanket beneath the ipsilateral ischial tuberosity can facilitate access to the anterior iliac crest.

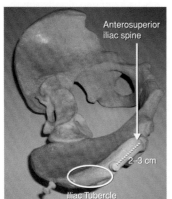

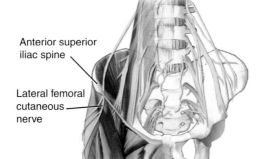

FIG 1 • **A.** Ideal anterior iliac crest bone graft is obtained 2 to 3 cm posterior to the anterior superior iliac spine. **B.** The lateral femoral cutaneous nerve generally traverses medial to the anterior superior iliac spine. **C.** The superior cluneal nerves cross the posterior iliac crest 8 cm anterior to the posterior superior iliac spine. **D.** The superior gluteal artery exits from the greater sciatic foramen.

Anterosuperior iliac spine

Anterior superior iliac spine

Lateral femoral cutaneous nerve

2–3 cm

Iliac Tubercle

A

B

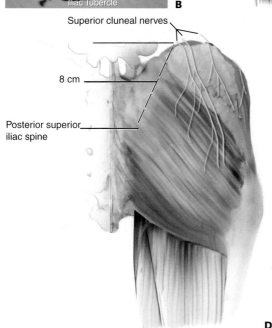

Superior cluneal nerves

8 cm

Posterior superior iliac spine

Superior gluteal artery

Piriformis muscle

C

D

TECHNIQUES

SURGICAL APPROACH

Anterior Iliac Crest

- A skin incision is made parallel to the iliac crest and is centered over the iliac tubercle.
- The incision is carried down to the bone of the crest and the muscles are elevated subperiosteally to expose the wing of the ilium (**TECH FIG 1**).
  - The tensor fascia latae, gluteus medius, and gluteus minimus originate from the lateral aspect of the ilium. These muscles are innervated by the superior gluteal nerve.
  - The abdominal muscles are also attached to the iliac crest and are segmentally innervated. The incision over the crest is, therefore, internervous and safe.

Posterior Iliac Crest

- The posterior superior iliac crest is palpable under the skin dimple in the superomedial aspect of the gluteal region.

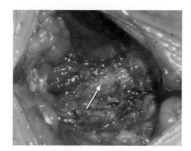

TECH FIG 1 • The anterior iliac crest (*arrow*).

- A vertical incision over the PSIS is made to minimize injury to the cluneal nerves.
- An oblique or curved incision may be made over the posterior iliac crest. The cluneal nerves cross the iliac crest 7 to 12 cm anterolateral to the PSIS; therefore, the incision should be made medial to this cutaneous innervation.
- The subcutaneous tissue is divided to the level of the iliac crest.
- Using Bovie cautery, the iliac crest is incised.
- The muscles are elevated subperiosteally from the posterolateral surface of the ilium.
  - The gluteus maximus, medius, and minimus originate from the lateral surface of the ilium. The superior gluteal nerve innervates the gluteus medius and minimus and the inferior gluteal nerve innervates the gluteus maximus.
  - The paraspinal musculature is innervated segmentally.

Posterior Iliac Crest: Midline Skin Incision

- A midline spine incision may be extended distally and the posterior iliac crest approached laterally under the skin and subcutaneous fat. This avoids the use of a second skin incision.
- The fascia overlying the PSIS is incised on the medial surface, where it is more robust; this facilitates fascial closure upon completion of the bone graft harvesting.
- The PSIS is exposed on its outer surface with the aid of electrocautery via a subperiosteal dissection.

ANTERIOR TRICORTICAL ILIAC CREST BONE GRAFT

- After exposure of the anterior iliac crest, an oscillating saw can be used to make parallel cuts through the inner and outer table (**TECH FIG 2A**).
- Curved osteotomes can be used to make longitudinal cuts in the inner and outer tables to complete the tricortical bone graft harvesting (**TECH FIG 2B,C**).

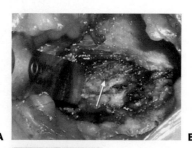

A

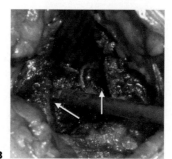

B

C

TECH FIG 2 • **A.** An oscillating saw is used to make two parallel cuts in the anterior iliac crest (*arrow*). **B.** The void left by anterior iliac crest harvest (*arrows*). **C.** Resected tricortical anterior iliac crest bone graft.

POSTERIOR ILIAC CREST BONE GRAFT

Corticocancellous Strips

- After exposure of the posterior iliac crest, adequate visualization can be obtained with the use of a Taylor retractor.
- Caution should be taken to avoid penetrating the sciatic notch and potentially injuring the superior gluteal artery.
- The removal of bone in the vicinity of the sciatic notch can weaken the thick bone that forms the notch, resulting in pelvic instability.
  - It is important to stay cephalad to the sciatic notch and remove bone only from the false pelvis. The false or greater pelvis is the portion of pelvis that lies cephalad to the pelvic brim, which defines the inner diameter of the pelvis.
  - For a landmark, an imaginary line dropped anteriorly from the PSIS with the patient in the prone position

can be used as the caudal limit of bone removal (**TECH FIG 3A**).

- Using a straight osteotome, multiple corticocancellous vertical strips can be cut from the iliac crest edge. A curved osteotome can be used to complete the cuts distally (**TECH FIG 3B,C**).
- After removal of the corticocancellous strips, gouges or curettes can be used to harvest additional cancellous bone (**TECH FIG 3D**).

Uncapping the Posterior Superior Iliac Spine

- With a rongeur, an osteotome, or both, the cap of the PSIS can be removed, allowing for harvesting of the cancellous bone between the two tables (**TECH FIG 4A**).
- Using a curette or gouge, the cancellous graft is then harvested through this window (**TECH FIG 4B**).

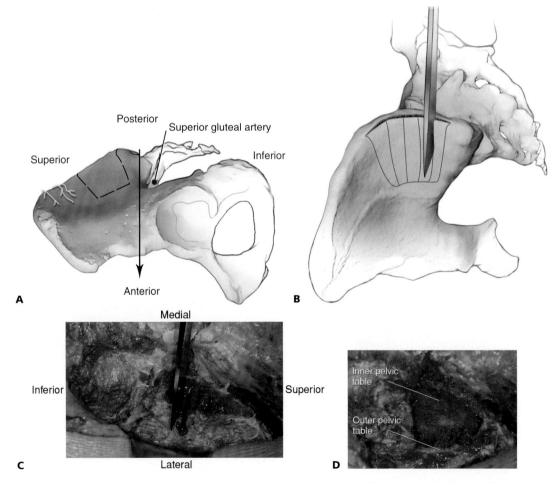

TECH FIG 3 • A. Line directed anteriorly from the posterior superior iliac spine marks the caudal safe zone for bone grafting to avoid injury to the contents of the sciatic notch. **B,C.** Using osteotomes, several corticocancellous strips can be created from the posterior iliac crest. **D.** The void left after posterior bone graft harvesting.

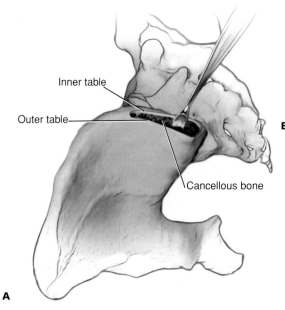

Inner table

Outer table

Cancellous bone

A

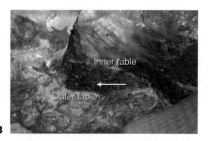

Inner table

Outer table

B

TECH FIG 4 • **A.** The cap of the posterior superior iliac spine can be removed to expose cancellous bone. **B.** After removal of the cap of the posterior superior iliac spine, cancellous bone is exposed for harvesting (*arrow*).

ILIAC CREST GRAFT SITE RECONSTRUCTION

- Several graft site techniques have been described to improve cosmesis and function and to potentially reduce the onset of chronic dysesthesias.
- Malleable bone cement contoured to the void can be used, particularly when structural bone graft has been harvested (**TECH FIG 5A**).

- Crushed allograft bone chips can also be packed into the ilium between the inner and outer table, allowing for bone reconstitution.
- After filling the defect with allograft or demineralized bone matrix, malleable polymerized lactide sheets can be contoured to the defect to allow for reconstitution of the external iliac anatomy (**TECH FIG 5B**).

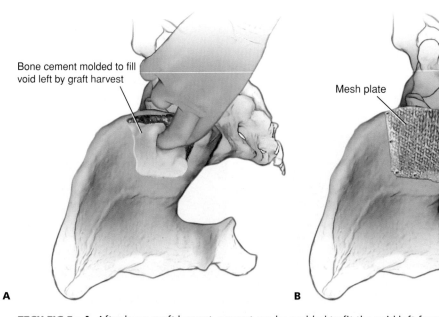

Bone cement molded to fill void left by graft harvest

A

Mesh plate

B

TECH FIG 5 • **A.** After bone graft harvest, cement can be molded to fit the void left from the harvest. **B.** A mesh sheet can be used to traverse the bone graft void to restore the crest.

PEARLS AND PITFALLS

Posterior iliac crest exposure	■ Preservation of the outer table spares the nociceptors located in the posterior periosteum. Also, preserving the most distal portion of the iliac crest can allow for placement of iliac screws ipsilateral to the site of harvest if desired.
Lateral femoral cutaneous nerve	■ The lateral femoral cutaneous nerve passes 2 to 3 cm medial to the anterior superior iliac spine. Avoiding this area can minimize the risk of injury and meralgia paresthetica.
Superior cluneal nerves	■ The superior cluneal nerves cross the posterior cortex 8 cm lateral to the posterior iliac spine. Injury to these nerves can cause numbness to the posterior buttocks and occasionally painful neuromas. Vertical incisions are preferred.
Superior gluteal artery	■ Special care should be taken when working near the sciatic notch. The superior gluteal artery exits the sciatic notch and can be injured if graft is taken too close to the notch. If injured, this vessel may retract into the pelvis and cause significant hemorrhage.

COMPLICATIONS

■ Donor site pain is common after bone graft harvesting.
  ■ Most symptoms resolve within 3 months.
  ■ Chronic donor site pain persists beyond 3 months and can be debilitating.
■ Anteriorly, nerves at risk for injury include the lateral femoral cutaneous, ilioinguinal, and iliohypogastric.
  ■ Injury to the lateral femoral cutaneous nerve may give rise to meralgia paresthetica (paresthesias along the lateral thigh).
  ■ The ilioinguinal nerve may be injured when the abdominal wall is retracted medially from the anterior iliac crest. The nerve may be compressed beneath the retractor on the inner part of the wall of the ilium. Ilioinguinal neurologic injury is characterized by pain radiating from the iliac toward the inguinal and genital areas.
■ Posteriorly, nerves at risk for injury include the cluneal, superior gluteal, and sciatic.
  ■ The sciatic nerve may be injured when the dissection is extended down to the sciatic notch. A surgical instrument such as an osteotome may be passed deep to the sciatic notch to cause this injury. The bony rim of the notch should be palpated before the dissection is carried to this area.
  ■ Injury to the cluneal nerves gives rise to numbness to the buttocks or, more rarely, painful cluneal neuromas.
■ Injury to the superior gluteal artery is rare but may occur with bone graft harvesting too close to the sciatic notch, or via inappropriate placement of retractors or elevators.
  ■ If cut, the superior gluteal artery may retract into the pelvis.
  ■ If the superior gluteal vessel is lacerated, it can be compressed locally and exposed for ligation or clipping. A finger may be used to apply direct pressure to the vessel, against the bone.
  ■ If the bleeding vessel is still not accessible, the area should be packed and then accessed anteriorly via a retroperitoneal or transperitoneal approach.
  ■ Arterial occlusion by embolization or by use of a Fogerty catheter is another option.
■ The deep circumflex iliac artery, the iliolumbar artery, or the fourth lumbar artery may cause troublesome bleeding when working on the inner table of the ilium.
■ A hernia through the iliac bone graft donor site may occur after the removal of a full-thickness bone graft from that site.

Symptoms may appear as an iliac swelling, sometimes associated with pain or symptoms of bowel obstruction. Strangulated hernia and valvulae are very rare occurrences.
■ Fracture
  ■ Removal of a large quantity of bone graft from the posterior ilium may disrupt the mechanical keystone effect of the sacroiliac joint and the posterior sacroiliac ligament, causing instability.
  ■ The ensuing instability transfers the stress forces to the pelvic ring, causing fractures of the superior and inferior pubic rami.
  ■ Patients with such instability may develop symptoms indistinguishable from other spinal disorders. History of clicking or thudding, as well as pain in the thigh and gluteal region, is characteristic.
  ■ Anteriorly, bone resection less than 3 cm from the ASIS may result in an avulsion fracture of the ASIS from the attached muscle groups (sartorius, tensor fascia lata).
■ The incidence of infection of the bone graft site ranges from 1% to 5%.
■ Careful subperiosteal dissection can limit hematoma formation. Hemostasis after bone graft harvesting with clotting agents (Gelfoam) should be used to limit hematoma formation.
■ The harvesting of tricortical grafts, particularly in thin patients, can result in a cosmetic deformity. Careful closure of fascial attachments should be performed to minimize soft tissue defects.

REFERENCES

1. Cowley SP, Anderson LD. Hernias through donor sites for iliac crest bone grafts. J Bone Joint Surg Am 1983;65A:1032–1035.
2. Ebraheim NA, Yang H, Lu J, et al. Anterior iliac crest bone graft: anatomic considerations. Spine 1997;22:847–849.
3. Kurtz LT, Garfin SR, Booth RE. Harvesting autogenous iliac crest bone grafts: a review of complications and techniques. Spine 1989; 14:1324–1332.
4. Robertson PA, Wray AC. Natural history of posterior iliac crest bone graft donation for spinal surgery: a prospective analysis of morbidity. Spine 2001;26:1473–1476.
5. Schnee CL, Freese A, Weil RJ, et al. Analysis of harvest morbidity and radiographic outcome using autograft for anterior cervical fusion. Spine 1997;22:2222–2227.
6. Silber JS, Anderson DG, Daffner SD, et al. Donor site morbidity after anterior iliac crest bone harvest for single-level anterior cervical discectomy and fusion. Spine 2003;28:134–139.

Chapter 16

Anterior Lumbar Interbody Fusion, Disc Replacement, and Corpectomy

P. Justin Tortolani, Paul C. McAfee, and Matthew N. Scott-Young

DEFINITION

- Lumbar disc degeneration is an age-related process heralded by a loss of disc height and gradual changes to the biochemical structure and biomechanical behavior of the intervertebral disc.
- Disc degeneration is not painful in most individuals, but in some patients, the degenerative changes do become painful and lead to the clinical entity known as degenerative disc disease (DDD). It is unclear why disc degeneration is painful in some but not in most.
- The etiology of DDD is multifactorial, including genetic and environmental determinants.
- "Discogenic pain" is the term used to describe pain due to a degenerative disc.

ANATOMY

- The intervertebral disc is composed of the outer annulus fibrosus and the inner nucleus pulposus (**FIG 1A**).
- The vertebral endplate is composed of cancellous bone in the center and strong, dense, cortical bone along the periphery.
- MRI provides information about the extent of hydration within the disc nucleus. The degenerated disc nucleus will have low signal characteristics (appear dark) on T2-weighted MRI images (**FIG 1B**).
- Dark discs on MRI do not necessarily correlate with symptomatic low back pain.[3]

PATHOGENESIS

- Various mechanisms have been proposed to explain disc degeneration with age:
  - Reduced nutrition and waste transport
  - Decreased concentration of viable cells
  - Loss of matrix proteins, proteoglycans, and water
  - Degradative enzyme activity
  - Fatigue failure of the matrix
  - Herniated nucleus pulposus
- Alterations to the vertebral endplate microenvironment such as venous pooling and reduced oxygen tension are additional factors.
- Nicotine has known detrimental effects on the intervertebral disc, perhaps via these mechanisms.
- Several factors have been implicated in the generation of discogenic pain: altered disc structure and function, release of inflammatory cytokines, and nerve ingrowth into degenerated discs, which under normal conditions are only minimally innervated in the outermost portion of the annulus.

NATURAL HISTORY

- Radiographic findings of disc degeneration typically appear around age 30.
- Posttraumatic disc herniations, vertebral endplate injuries, and genetic factors may predispose patients to earlier presentation.
- As structural changes occur within the intervertebral disc, associated changes in the vertebral body endplate become apparent:
  - Anterior, lateral, or posterior osteophyte formation
  - Schmorl nodes, cystic cavities, along the endplate can be visualized
  - Endplate sclerosis
- The degenerative changes at the level of the disc, bony endplate, and ultimately the posterior facet-joint complex ultimately restrict motion at the affected level or levels. At this stage, patients will typically complain more of back stiffness and soreness rather than pain. Neurogenic claudication due to narrowing of the spinal canal and spinal stenosis typically becomes more limiting than complaints of back pain.
- The final stage in the natural history of disc degeneration is autofusion.
- Patients should be counseled that disc degeneration itself is an inevitable process of aging and that any back pain experienced could, but may not necessarily, be associated with the disc degeneration.
- The overwhelming majority of patients have only occasional episodes of low back pain. Long-term disability resulting from DDD is rare.

PATIENT HISTORY AND PHYSICAL FINDINGS

- No pathognomonic history or physical examination findings exist for the diagnosis of lumbar DDD.
- Discogenic back pain is typically worst in situations in which an axial load is applied to the lumbar spine, as in prolonged sitting or standing with a forward-bent posture (ie, washing dishes, vacuuming, shaving, or brushing teeth).
- Conversely, positions such as side-lying (ie, the fetal position) or floating erect in water place the least amount of strain across the intervertebral disc and should therefore provide some pain relief.
- Leg pain (in the absence of neural compression), if present, is nonradicular and "referred" in that it does not follow lumbar dermatomes into the lower leg and is not typically associated with loss of motor power, reflex changes, numbness, or tingling.
- Patients will occasionally describe a discrete traumatic disc injury in which they first experienced back pain. Imaging studies that depict an old endplate fracture above or below a degenerative disc help corroborate this history.
- Loss of truncal musculature fitness from abdominal wall hernias, obesity, and prior abdominal wall surgery (ie, rectus

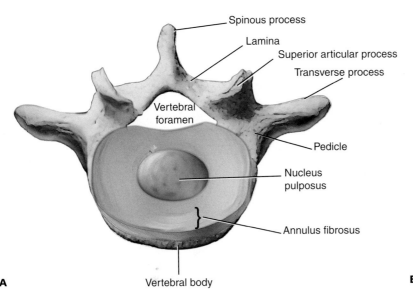

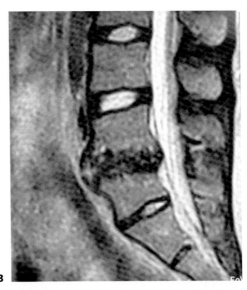

FIG 1 • A. The intervertebral disc is composed of the outer annulus fibrosus (radial orientation of collagen fibers) and the inner nucleus pulposus (relatively higher water content and proteoglycans). The cancellous center of the lumbar vertebral body is surrounded by a peripheral rim of relatively strong cortical bone. **B.** T2-weighted sagittal MRI showing degenerative disc disease at the L4-5 disc space. The nucleus pulposus is low signal intensity (dark) compared to the adjacent discs, which are high signal intensity (bright) due to relatively higher water concentration. The vertebral body endplates are irregular, with anterior vertebral osteophytes.

muscle transfer procedures) may worsen discogenic back pain.
- Other causes of back pain should be sought in the history, physical examination, and imaging studies, including muscular strain, spondylolysis or spondylolisthesis, herniated nucleus pulposus, compression fracture, pseudarthrosis, tumor, and discitis.
- Patients with isolated DDD by definition should have a normal neurologic examination.

IMAGING AND OTHER DIAGNOSTIC STUDIES
- Standing plain radiographs
  - Lateral radiographs allow for measurement of the intervertebral disc height and allow comparison to other lumbar intervertebral discs (**FIG 2A**).
  - Anteroposterior (AP) radiographs allow for determination of asymmetric, coronal plain disc degeneration, which may be a precursor to lumbar degenerative scoliosis.
  - Flexion-extension radiographs may be helpful in diagnosing an occult spondylolisthesis or spondylolysis.
- MRI provides excellent visualization of the discs, the degree to which they have degenerated, and the relationship of the discs to the adjacent endplate and surrounding neurologic structures (**FIG 2B**).
- Provocative discography attempts to reproduce the patient's typical back pain by pressurizing the disc with normal saline. The patient needs to be awake to provide subjective feedback as to the quality and intensity of the pain. Architectural changes to the disc are inferred by contrast administered with the saline.
- CT discography provides more detailed information about the disc morphology after contrast administration (**FIG 2C**).
- Normal laboratory tests, including complete blood count, erythrocyte sedimentation rate, and C-reactive protein, can

help rule out a disc space infection; severe disc degeneration can sometimes mimic infection radiologically.

DIFFERENTIAL DIAGNOSIS
- DDD
- Discitis
- Pyogenic vertebral osteomyelitis

NONOPERATIVE MANAGEMENT
- DDD is analogous to hip and knee osteoarthritis in that the intervening cartilage (in the case of the disc: collagen, water, and proteoglycans) fails under compressive loads.
- Weight reduction and activity modification (avoidance of exacerbating activities) may be effective first-line treatments.
- Nonsteroidal anti-inflammatory medications
- Acupuncture or massage therapy
- Physical therapy with aquatic or dry land exercises
- Gentle pelvic traction
- Methylprednisolone (Solu-Medrol) taper
- Epidural injections
- Narcotic medications for severe episodes of pain

SURGICAL MANAGEMENT
- Indications
  - Discogenic back pain refractory to nonoperative management
  - Discitis with pyogenic vertebral osteomyelitis refractory to nonoperative management
  - Spinal deformity requiring radical discectomy
- A thorough and complete discectomy improves the effectiveness of anterior interbody fusion by creating a wide surface area of exposed bone.
- Interbody reconstruction and fusion can be accomplished by a variety of methods, including structural autogenous bone

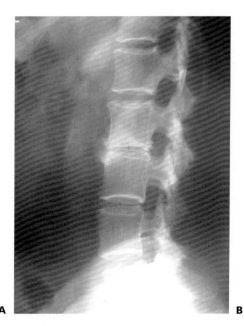 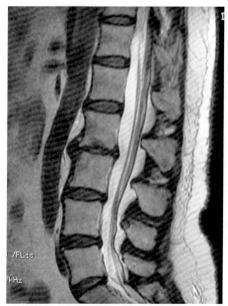 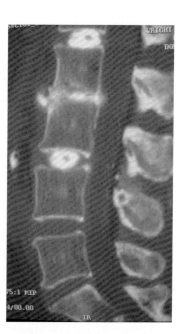

A   B   C

FIG 2 • A. Lateral radiograph showing degenerative disc disease at the L2-3 level. **B.** Sagittal T2-weighted MRI of the same patient with low signal intensity in the nucleus of the L2-3 disc. Anterior and posterior disc bulges are present. **C.** Sagittal CT discogram of the same patient showing dramatic loss of integrity of the L2-3 nucleus and annulus with leakage of contrast anteriorly. The patient's pain was concordant at the L2-3 disc level. The L1-2 and L3-4 discs served as negative controls with regard to both disc architecture and pain.

graft (iliac crest or fibula), structural allograft (ie, femoral or humeral ring, femoral head, machined bone dowel), or synthetic device (titanium, PEEK, carbon-fiber, composite) packed with cancellous bone or collagen sponges impregnated with bone morphogenic protein 2 (BMP-2).

■ Regardless of the method used, prerequisites are that the interbody spacer be strong enough to resist intervertebral compressive loads and provide an appropriate biologic environment for healing.

■ The particular interbody fusion device of choice (eg, Bagby-Kuslich [BAK; Zimmer Spine, Warsaw, IN], lumbar-tapered [LT] cage [Medtronic Sofomor Danek, Memphis, TN], Bengal carbon fiber cages [DePuy Spine, Raynham, MA]) is inserted with instruments designed for proper implantation.

■ BMP-2 has been approved by the U.S. Food and Drug Administration for anterior interbody application and has been shown to increase the fusion rate when compared to iliac crest bone graft.[5]

Preoperative Planning

■ Plain radiographs, MRI, or CT scans should be carefully evaluated for undiagnosed spondylolysis or spondylolisthesis, which may alter the surgical plan.

■ Templates can be used with plain radiographs or MRI scans to gauge the size of the final implant to be used.

■ Oversized implants can lead to undesired stretch on neurologic structures and reduced motion of lumbar disc replacements.

■ The level of the confluence of the common iliac veins into the inferior vena cava and the bifurcation of the aorta can be located on the axial MRI scans.

■ At L5-S1 the pubic symphysis occasionally precludes appropriate visualization and instrumentation of the disc space in patients with a deep-seated L5-S1 relative to the pelvis. Evaluation of the lateral radiograph with the pubis on the film is critical to visualize the trajectory into the disc space and avoid this miscalculation.

Positioning

■ The patient is placed over an inflatable pillow over a 1-inch-thick foam pad, which is placed on the mattress of the operating table. The pillow allows for modulation of lordosis throughout the procedure and the foam pad props the patient up, allowing the arms to be tucked posteriorly, out of the plane of the spine during imaging.

■ Positioning over the break in the table allows for increased lordosis if needed.

■ The use of fluoroscopic C-arm imaging is crucial for appropriate patient and implant positioning. It is helpful to verify that adequate fluoroscopic imaging of operative landmarks can be achieved after the patient is positioned but before the incision is made.

Approach

■ Anterior retroperitoneal approaches will typically allow access to the lumbar discs from L2-3 to the sacrum.

■ The renal vessels limit more proximal extension of the exposure.

■ Lateral exposures to the lumbar spine are required for access to the L2 vertebra and above.

ANTERIOR LUMBAR RADICAL DISCECTOMY

Exposure

- Identify the intervertebral disc and mark the midline with a spinal needle or screw placed into the vertebral body (we prefer not to place a needle into the disc space because this may create unwanted disc injury) (**TECH FIG 1A**).
- Use AP and lateral fluoroscopic imaging to check the midline. The midline marker also serves to verify the spinal level.
- At L5-S1, retract the left common iliac artery and vein to the patient's left and the right common iliac artery and vein to the right. At levels above L5-S1, the aorta and inferior vena cava must be mobilized to the patient's right.
- The great vessels can be held in their retracted position using handheld Hohmann retractors, custom-designed pins, or K-wires, all of which can be advanced directly into the vertebral bodies (virtually eliminating the risk of vessel migration into the field of interest) (**TECH FIG 1B**).
  - Alternatively, stainless-steel vein retractors or radiolucent retractors can be fixed to the arms of an abdominal retractor system (Omni) or floating, Endo-ring-type retractor system. These blade retractors have the disadvantage of allowing vessel migration into the field by sliding under the retractor blades as motion occurs during the procedure. The advantage of the radiolucent retractors is that better visualization of the operative field is possible with fluoroscopy. In addition, blade-type retractors can be easily manipulated during the procedure without having to reinsert into the vertebral body.
- Attempt to retract the vessels as far lateral as you can to allow for the widest possible view of the intervertebral disc. Poor visualization at this stage will compromise the quality of the discectomy and any ensuing interbody device placement.

Removing the Disc

- Using a 10-blade on a long handle, incise the intervertebral disc starting laterally along the superior endplate and

move toward midline. Always move away from the vessels to avoid an accidental lateral plunge into the great vessels. The blade should be inserted between the cartilage endplate and bone if possible, and we use both hands on the knife shank for optimal control and coordination (**TECH FIG 2A,B**).

- A large, sharp Cobb elevator is then used to release as much of the cartilaginous endplate as possible from the superior and inferior endplates. By angling the Cobb blade toward the bone and pronating and supinating the hand, almost the entire disc (annulus and nucleus) can be removed, as if peeling an orange in one large piece (**TECH FIG 2C**).
- Long-handled no. 2 and no. 3 Cobb curettes are used to remove the remaining disc, taking the dissection all the way to the posterior longitudinal ligament (**TECH FIG 2D**). Systematic removal of endplate cartilage enhances thorough removal. Thus, start anteriorly on the superior endplate and move posteriorly. Then start anteriorly on the inferior endplate and move posteriorly.
  - The curette will function much more effectively if it is used as a cutting instrument rather than a scraper. For this reason, we prefer that curettes be sharp, nonangled, and used with a pronating–supinating motion with the edge of the curette between the cartilage endplate and the endplate bone.
- The posterior longitudinal ligament is not routinely removed, but the posterolateral corners of the disc space must be thoroughly débrided of disc material for several reasons:
  - Periphery of the endplate is the strongest bone and therefore provides the most stable support of an interbody device.
  - Disc material that is left over can be pushed posteriorly into the epidural space, causing an iatrogenic disc herniation during implant insertion.
  - If anterior decompression of the neural foramen is one of the goals of surgery, visualization and removal of a herniated disc or disc–osteophyte complex will not be possible without proper visualization in this region.

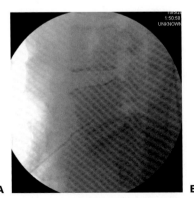
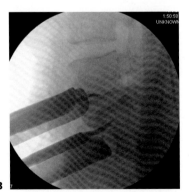

A   **B**

TECH FIG 1 • A. Lateral radiograph showing the spinal needle inserted into the L4 vertebral body above the L4-5 disc to be removed. **B.** Lateral radiograph showing sharp Hohmann retractors placed into the L4 vertebral body above and L5 vertebral body below. Blade-type retractors can be left in place lateral to the Hohmann retractors for additional visibility, as shown.

- The lateral extent of the discectomy is determined by the width of the device to be inserted, but care must be taken to maintain the width of the discectomy posteriorly as the natural tendency is to remove less disc laterally in the posterior portion of the disc space.
- A lamina spreader can be gently distracted in the anterolateral interbody region to gain enhanced visibility of the posterior disc space (**TECH FIG 2E**).

- Removal of a posterior or foraminal disc herniation can be accomplished by passing an angled Kerrison rongeur posteriorly and into the neuroforamen. Identification of the ventral aspect of the dura enhances the safety of this maneuver (**TECH FIG 2F**).
- Epidural bleeding can be brisk during posterior disc removal, but thrombin-soaked Gelfoam gauze and removal of intervertebral distraction can be used to control it.

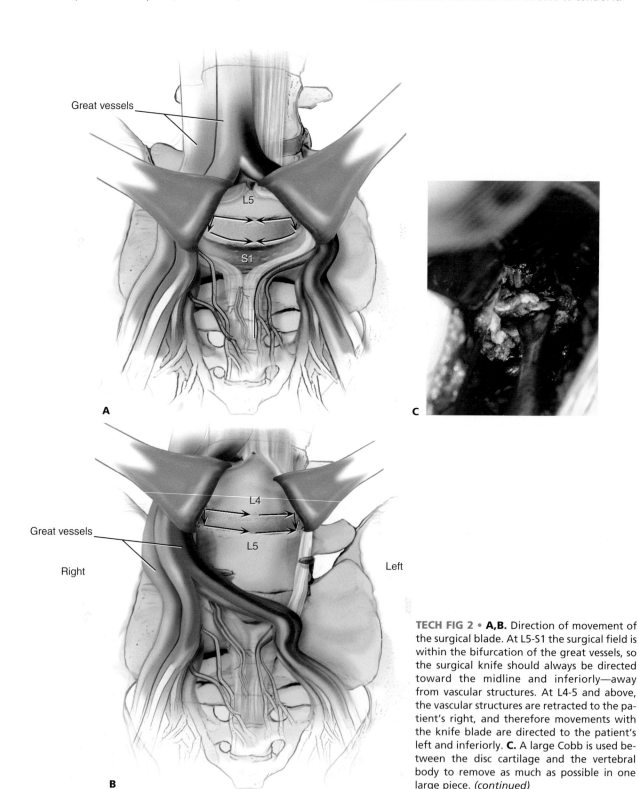

Great vessels

L5

S1

A

C

L4

L5

Great vessels

Right

Left

B

TECH FIG 2 • A,B. Direction of movement of the surgical blade. At L5-S1 the surgical field is within the bifurcation of the great vessels, so the surgical knife should always be directed toward the midline and inferiorly—away from vascular structures. At L4-5 and above, the vascular structures are retracted to the patient's right, and therefore movements with the knife blade are directed to the patient's left and inferiorly. **C.** A large Cobb is used between the disc cartilage and the vertebral body to remove as much as possible in one large piece. *(continued)*

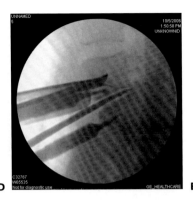
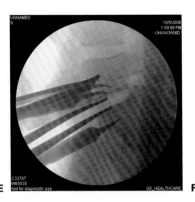
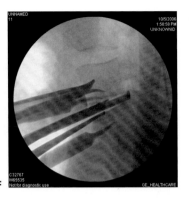

TECH FIG 2 • *(continued)* **D.** Lateral radiograph showing a no. 2 Cobb curette used to remove the cartilaginous disc endplate. **E.** Lateral radiograph demonstrating a lamina spreader creating distraction within the disc space. The distractor enhances visualization of the posterior portion of the disc space. Care should be taken to make sure that the distractor is seated anteriorly and laterally on strong endplate bone to avoid damage to the central cancellous region. **F.** Lateral radiograph showing the use of a 4-mm-long Kerrison rongeur to decompress the neural foramen.

ANTERIOR LUMBAR INTERBODY FUSION

- Once the discectomy has been completed, disc space distractors are inserted to gauge the size of the final implant (**TECH FIG 3A**). Appropriate distractor size can be gauged by comparing the operative level with a normal disc above or below. In addition, the interface between the distractor and the bony endplate should be less than 1 mm. This ensures good interference fit of the final device.
- For threaded devices such as the LT cage, a cannulated guide channel is inserted over the disc distractors. This working channel serves to prevent inadvertent migration of the great vessels into the disc space.
- Endplate reamers are then inserted to appropriate depth as determined by lateral fluoroscopic imaging (**TECH FIG 3B**). Care should be taken to aim the reamer

for the midportion of the disc space posteriorly on lateral fluoroscopy rather than through one endplate or the other.
  - Asymmetric reaming will result in excessive removal of one endplate compared to another and the final implant will be more likely to fail in subsidence. Because the reamer tends to follow the path of least resistance, an exceptionally sclerotic endplate will predispose one to asymmetric reaming by this mechanism.
- Final threaded implants are then screwed into the appropriate depth and orientation (**TECH FIG 3C,D**). The first cage (in a dual-cage system) is inserted in the same trajectory as the reamers, and lateral fluoroscopic imaging during cage placement ensures that the cage is not placed too anteriorly or posteriorly. The cage should not

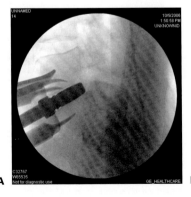
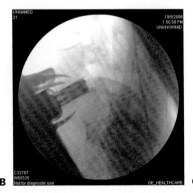
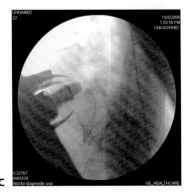

TECH FIG 3 • **A.** Lateral radiograph showing a radiopaque disc distractor within the intervertebral disc. The distractor approximates the height of the disc space above (L3-4), and there is at most 1 mm of space between the intervertebral endplate and the distractor. **B.** Lateral radiograph showing reaming of the intervertebral channel for the anterior interbody device. Because the vertebral body is shallower in the AP plane away from the midline, reaming should stop shy of the posterior vertebral body line, as shown. **C.** Lateral radiograph showing threaded cage entry into the disc space. The cage is directed parallel to the vertebral endplates. *(continued)*

TECHNIQUES

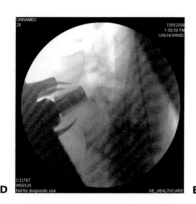 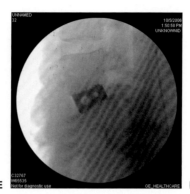 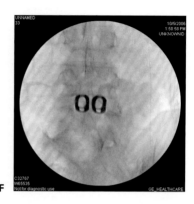

TECH FIG 3 • *(continued)* **D.** Final cage placement should not extend beyond the depth of the reamer. **E.** Lateral radiograph showing final cage placement. The overlapping pedicles confirm true lateral positioning. **F.** AP radiograph showing parallel positioning of paired cages.

be inserted beyond the depth of the reamer or else the threads will strip and the cage will lose a large percentage of its fixation strength.
- Saving the C-arm image of the final reamer depth allows the surgeon to reference this image when inserting the cage.

- The second cage is inserted using the first cage as a reference for trajectory and depth. Final images should be true AP and lateral projections showing the cage devices to be in good position. Overlapping pedicles on the lateral image will appear sharp, confirming true lateral positioning (**TECH FIG 3E,F**).

LUMBAR TOTAL DISC REPLACEMENT

Determining Implant Size

- Determine midline and the appropriate spinal level by inserting a bone screw, which will serve as a reference throughout the case. Obtaining true AP and lateral images is critical to ensure that the remainder of the instruments and devices can be referenced off these radiographic landmarks (**TECH FIG 4A**).
- Once the discectomy is completed, a sizing guide, or "lollipop," is used to ascertain the size of the implant to be used (**TECH FIG 4B**). These guides vary in depth and width to conform to the size of the vertebral endplate.

The endplate of S1 is often more shallow in the AP dimension than L5, and this may necessitate the use of a smaller implant at this level.
- The largest footprint that is still covered by the vertebra is chosen. This helps to ensure that the final device will be supported by the greatest percentage of peripheral cortical bone.
- The height and lordosis of the final implant are determined by trial wedges that fit into the interbody location (**TECH FIG 4C–E**). The vertebral endplates should be flush with the trials.

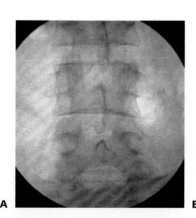 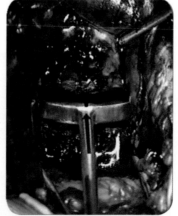 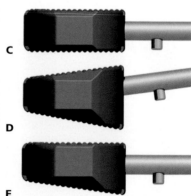

TECH FIG 4 • A. True AP fluoroscopic image. The distance between the midpoint of the vertebra and the pedicles should be the same. The cortical margins of the pedicles themselves should be the same size (ensuring the spine is not rotated). Finally, the spinous processes should bisect the vertebra. The spinous processes are the least reliable landmark, as they can be malformed, especially at L5 and S1. **B.** A sizing guide, or "lollipop," demonstrates how well the endplate will be covered by the final implant. The largest size that allows good peripheral endplate coverage in both the sagittal and coronal planes is desired. **C–E.** Using radiolucent trial wedges of varying height and lordosis allows the final device to be individualized to the patient's anatomy. (**B–E:** Courtesy of DePuy Spine, Raynham, MA.)

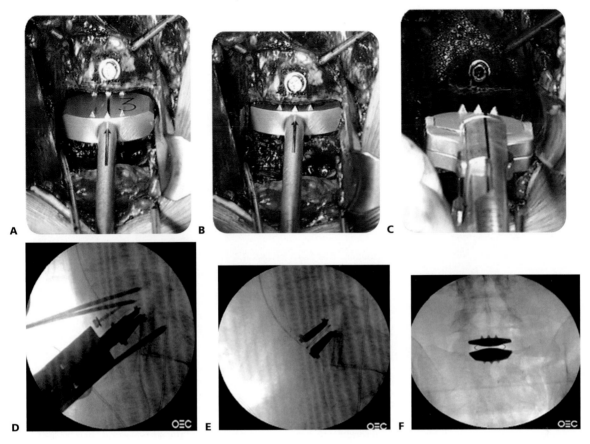

TECH FIG 5 • A. Intraoperative photograph showing introduction of the channel cutter into the disc space. **B.** Care is taken to ensure that the cutting channels are centered on the midline marking screw and are directed straight posterior. **C.** Intraoperative photograph showing prosthesis insertion into the grooves created by the channel cutter. **D.** Lateral fluoroscopic image showing implant insertion. The insertion instruments are still connected, which allows for fine adjustment to the final positioning. **E,F.** Lateral and AP fluoroscopic images of the final TDR placement with all of the instruments removed. The final implant should be in the center of the vertebral body on the AP image and in the center (sagittal midline) or just posterior to the center of the vertebral body on the lateral image.

Implant Placement

- Grooves for a central keel or for fixation teeth are then cut. Make sure the central groove is in the midline and that the trajectory for the grooves is directly posterior and not angled (**TECH FIG 5A,B**).
- The final implant is then inserted (**TECH FIG 5C,D**). Double-check that the implant is the correct size and is inserted in the correct orientation regarding lordosis.
- It can be helpful to break the bed or inflate the lumbar pillow to get the disc implant started in a particularly collapsed disc. Once the implant is halfway into the disc space, the lordosis should be removed so that the implant will move easily into the posterior portion of the disc (**TECH FIG 5E,F**).

ANTERIOR LUMBAR CORPECTOMY

Vertebra Removal

- The indications for anterior corpectomy in the lumbar spine are lumbar burst fracture, catastrophic failure of lumbar disc replacement or interbody device (ie, vertebral fracture), lumbar vertebral osteomyelitis, correction of kyphosis, and vertebral body malignancy.
- In cases of corpectomy for vascular tumors, preoperative embolization should be performed (**TECH FIG 6A**).
- In cases of corpectomy, lumbar radical discectomies are performed above and below the vertebral body to be removed (see discectomy technique above).

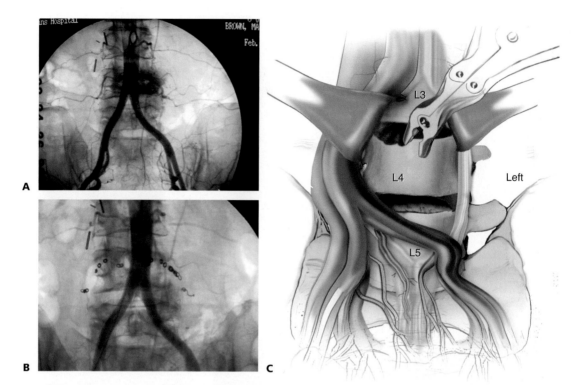

TECH FIG 6 • A. Pre-embolization angiogram depicting the aortic bifurcation in a 65-year-old patient with metastatic renal cell carcinoma to the L4 vertebra. Note the degree of vascularity of the L4 vertebral body. **B.** Postembolization angiogram depicting a striking reduction in contrast entering the L4 vertebral body. Small embolization coils are seen in the vascular network surrounding the vertebral body. **C.** Anterior discectomy enables the surgeon to use a large rongeur to gain access to the edge of the vertebra and thereby remove the vertebral body bone.

- This enables the surgeon to become oriented to the midline and also to judge the depth and width of the corpectomy to be performed.
  - The discectomy space also allows the surgeon to use a large rongeur efficiently to remove the vertebral body (**TECH FIG 6B**).
- Retractors should be placed above and below the entire vertebra to be removed so there is an unobstructed view for the surgeon and the assistants. The vertebral body bleeds more rapidly than the endplates, so the assistants need to be able to visualize the operative field to suction effectively.
- A Leksell rongeur can be used to remove all of the vertebral body back to the level of the posterior cortex. If this needs to be removed, angled curettes are used to develop the plane behind the vertebra, starting at the disc space. Kerrison punches or angled curettes are then used to lift the posterior cortex off the ventral dura.
  - Healthy vertebral body bone should be saved for interbody fusion.

Filling the Interbody Space

- Once the corpectomy is completed, bone graft or an interbody device is contoured to fit into the defect. The wooden end of a cotton-tipped applicator can be cut to the length of the defect and can then be used as a size gauge for the final interbody device. This is particularly useful when cutting and contouring a bone graft because calipers and rulers do not always fit easily into the

central portion of the corpectomy defect to give an accurate height measurement.
- Check the height of the corpectomy defect with the wooden applicator throughout its entire depth, from anterior to posterior. Keep in mind that the shape of the corpectomy site may be lordotic, and thus the bone graft or implant needs to be fashioned appropriately.
- Allograft strut grafts such as femoral head, humerus, or femoral shafts can be cut using an oscillating saw to fit snugly into the interbody space. The advantages of allograft are it can be packed with morselized autogenous bone, it has a similar modulus of elasticity to host vertebral bone, and it will become osseointegrated over time.
- Autogenous tricortical iliac crest and autogenous fibula have the greatest healing potential but are also associated with significant harvest site morbidity.
- Metal cages generally are the easiest to fashion to fit the corpectomy space and can be packed with morselized corpectomy bone (**TECH FIG 7A**). The disadvantages are their expense and relatively reduced surface area at the endplate for fusion compared to bone.
- The width of the corpectomy should be kept as narrow as possible without compromising decompression or removal of pathologic bone (**TECH FIG 7B**).
  - Allows bone ingrowth from the corpectomized vertebral body into the interbody bone graft
  - Enhances the stability of the interbody strut
- A bone screw with a washer can be used above and below large defects as an "anti-kickout" buttress for allografts (**TECH FIG 7C**).

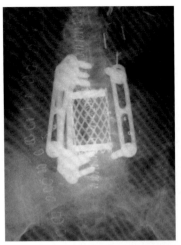
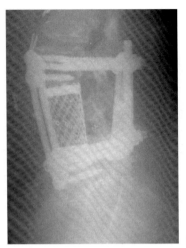
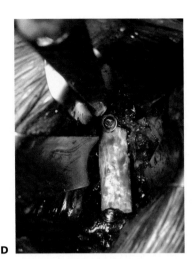

A B D

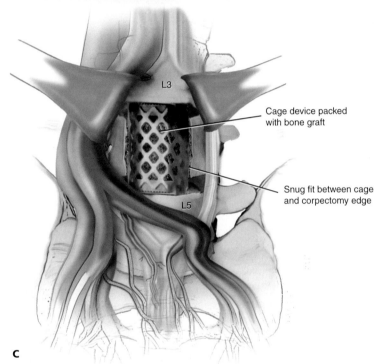

L3

Cage device packed
with bone graft

Snug fit between cage
and corpectomy edge

L5

C

TECH FIG 7 • A,B. AP and lateral postoperative radiographs of a patient in whom posterior element resection followed by fusion and instrumentation with pedicle screws was performed as a first stage, followed by complete anterior corpectomy and reconstruction with a cylindrical titanium mesh cage packed with autogenous bone graft. An anterior side plate was applied as the lateral vertebral body wall was completely removed. **C.** The corpectomy strut device should fit snugly against the cut edge of the vertebral body to promote side-to-side fusion from host bone to strut graft. **D.** Intraoperative image of anterior allograft reconstruction after corpectomy, irrigation, and débridement of the L3 vertebra in a 62-year-old man with L3 vertebral body destruction from pyogenic vertebral osteomyelitis. 4.5-mm cortical screws with washers are used to prevent allograft kickout.

PEARLS AND PITFALLS

Use of a pulse oximeter on the left great toe provides real-time feedback to the surgeon about perfusion to the distal extremity during great vessel retraction.	■ There should be a low threshold for prophylactic inferior vena cava filter placement in patients with venous injuries requiring repair, as pulmonary embolism, although rare, carries potentially catastrophic consequences.
Perforation of the cancellous vertebral body endplates with Cobb curettes or the lamina spreader increases the likelihood of implant subsidence.	■ Early (less than 2 weeks) implant malpositions or migrations can be easily revised as the anterior tissue planes are still preserved.
Epidural bleeding can be effectively controlled quickly with thrombin-soaked Gelfoam gauze and release of any disc space distractors.	■ Overdistraction of the disc space with a lumbar disc replacement implant will result in compromised motion and may be associated with new postoperative leg pain related to stretch injury to the lumbosacral nerve trunks.
Marking the location of the dorsalis pedis and posterior tibial pulses with a marking pen facilitates reassessment of pulses in the postoperative setting when lower extremity swelling is more prevalent.	

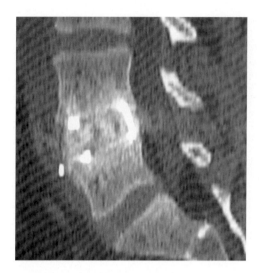

FIG 3 • Sagittal fine-cut CT image depicting trabecular bone bridging across the disc space 3 months after anterior interbody fusion with a threaded titanium cage packed with collagen sponges impregnated with bone morphogenic protein 2.

POSTOPERATIVE CARE

■ As soon as the patient emerges from anesthesia, a complete neurologic examination and brief history should be performed. Specifically, patients should be asked if they have any new leg pain. If present, CT myelography or plain CT scans should be obtained to ensure that no bone, disc material, or portion of an implanted device is impinging on the lumbar nerve roots.

■ Nasogastric tubes for the first 12 to 24 hours help to minimize abdominal wall distention and postoperative ileus.

■ Patients are encouraged to walk on postoperative day 1.

■ Lumbar corsets or abdominal binders are prescribed at the discretion of the surgeon and may reduce the tension on the abdominal incision in the early postoperative period.

■ Return to heavy manual labor is restricted in patients undergoing anterior interbody fusion until the fusion is solid. Fine-cut CT scans are useful in documenting solid fusion if there is doubt on AP, lateral, or flexion-extension radiographs (**FIG 3**).

■ Manual labor should be restricted in patients undergoing disc replacement until the bone–prosthesis interface is judged to be stable. In nonkeeled total disc replacement devices requiring porous ingrowth for definitive fixation, such as the Charite (DePuy Spine, Raynham, MA), at least weeks out of work is recommended.

OUTCOMES

■ Level IV evidence reported by Tropiano et al showed significant improvements in back pain, radiculopathy, and disability at mean of 8.7 years after insertion of the Prodisc lumbar disc replacement.[10]

■ Anterior lumbar interbody fusion with titanium cages and iliac crest bone graft has been shown to yield significantly greater fusion rates (97%) versus allograft dowels packed with iliac crest bone graft (48%).[8]

■ Patients undergoing anterior lumbar fusion with the titanium cages packed with BMP-2-impregnated collagen sponges have significantly improved fusion rates and clinical outcomes compared to patients in whom the cages were packed with iliac crest bone graft.[5]

■ In a prospective, randomized trial comparing Charite lumbar disc replacement to stand-alone anterior lumbar interbody fusion with titanium cages and iliac crest bone graft (control group), a significantly greater percentage of patients undergoing disc replacement were satisfied with their procedure versus the control group at 2-year follow-up.

   ■ Hospital stay was significantly shorter in the disc replacement group compared to controls.

   ■ However, at 2 years there was no statistical difference between the disc replacement group and the control group with respect to pain or disability.[2]

■ Clinical outcomes and flexion-extension range of motion correlate with surgical technical accuracy of lumbar disc replacement.[6]

COMPLICATIONS

■ Most complications associated with anterior lumbar discectomy, interbody fusion, disc replacement, and corpectomy are approach-related.[1,2,4,7,10]

■ The most common complications of anterior lumbar interbody fusion are pseudarthrosis and device failures such as migration or breakage.

■ The complications of lumbar disc replacement depend on the exact type of device being inserted but generally can be categorized as follows:[9,11]

   ■ Device failures: metal endplate breakage, core dislodgement or fracture, polyethylene degradation

   ■ Bone-implant failures: subsidence, vertebral body fracture, implant migration or dislocation

   ■ Iatrogenic deformity: kyphosis, scoliosis

   ■ Host response: osteolysis, heterotopic ossification

   ■ Infection

■ Revision approaches to the anterior lumbar spine carry six times the risk of major bleeding or thromboembolic complications.[7] Preoperative intravenous filter insertion, ureteral stenting, and percutaneous venous access wires are critical to reduce these risks.

REFERENCES

1. Bertagnolli R, Zigler J, Karg A, et al. Complications and strategies for revision surgery in total disc replacement. Orthop Clin North Am 2005;36:389–395.
2. Blumenthal SL, McAfee PC, Guyer RD, et al. A prospective, randomized, multi-center FDA IDE study of lumbar total disc replacement with the CHARITE™ Artificial Disc vs. lumbar fusion: part I: evaluation of clinical outcomes. Spine 2005;30:1565–1575.
3. Boden SD, McCowin PR, Dina TS, et al. Abnormal magnetic resonance scans of the lumbar spine in asymptomatic subjects: a prospective investigation. J Bone Joint Surg Am 1990;72A:403–408.
4. Brau SA, Delamarter RB, Schiffman ML, et al. Vascular injury during anterior lumbar surgery. Spine J 2004;4:409–412.
5. Burkus JK, Heim SE, Gornet MF et al. Is INFUSE bone graft superior to autograft bone? An integrated analysis of clinical trials using the LT-CAGE lumbar tapered fusion device. J Spinal Disord Tech 2003;16:113–122.
6. McAfee PC, Cunningham BW, Holtsapple G, et al. A prospective, randomized, multi-center FDA IDE study of lumbar total disc replacement with the CHARITE™ Artificial Disc vs. lumbar fusion: part II: evaluation of radiographic outcomes and correlation of surgical technique accuracy with clinical outcomes. Spine 2005;30:1576–1583.

7. McAfee PC, Geisler FH, Saiedy SS, et al. Revisability of the CHARITE Artificial Disc Replacement: analysis of 688 patients enrolled in the U.S. IDE study of the CHARITE Artificial Disc. Spine 2006;31:1217–1226.

8. Sasso RC, Kitchel SH, Dawson EG. A prospective, randomized controlled clinical trial of anterior lumbar interbody fusion using a titanium cylindrical threaded fusion device. Spine 2004;29: 113–122.

9. Tortolani PJ, McAfee PC, Saiedy S. Failures of lumbar disc replacement. Semin Spine Surg 2006;18:78–86.

10. Tropiano P, Huang RC, Girardi FP, et al. Lumbar disc replacement: seven to eleven year follow-up. J Bone Joint Surg Am 2005;87A: 490–496.

11. van Ooij A, Oner FC, Verbout AJ. Complications of artificial disc replacement: a report of 27 patients with the SB CHARITE disc. J Spinal Disord Tech 2003;16:369–383.

DEFINITION

- Anterior thoracic approaches provide a means of decompression, stabilization, and fusion for a variety of spinal pathologies, such as deformity, trauma, infection, tumors, and disc herniations.

ANATOMY

- The thoracic vertebral bodies are heart-shaped in the anteroposterior plane.
  - The thoracic pedicles are oval and are larger superoinferiorly than mediolaterally.
  - The average height is 8 to 15 mm and the average width is 3 to 10 mm.
- The medial cortex is the thickest; however, there is no epidural space between the medial cortical edge and the dura.[16]
- The facet joints are situated more anteriorly and articulate superiorly and inferiorly with a rib. As the transition from the thoracic to lumbar spine occurs, the thoracic vertebrae begin to resemble the lumbar vertebrae and the facets change from a frontal orientation to one that is more lateral.

PATHOGENESIS

Intervertebral Disc Herniation

- Seventy-five percent of thoracic disc herniations occur between T8 and L1. They are classified as central, centrolateral, lateral, or paramedian.
  - Most herniations occur central or centrolateral and are often calcified.
- The spinal canal in the thoracic spine is relatively small.
  - Neurologic consequences occur from direct anterior compression of the spinal cord from a herniated disc. There can be posterior displacement of the cord and local vascular insufficiency.

Infection

- The mechanism of spinal infections is controversial. Proposed routes of infection include hematogenous spread from other infected foci, local extension from nearby infections, and direct inoculation.
  - The two proposed routes of hematogenous spread are venous and arterial.
  - Advocates of venous hematogenous spread argue that organisms are carried to the spine via the plexus of Batson, similar to the mechanism of tumor metastasis.[2]
  - Proponents of arterial hematogenous spread note that the metaphyseal bone near the anterior longitudinal ligament is an area where infections typically begin. This region has an end-arteriole network that is susceptible to bacterial seeding.[19]

Tumor

- Most spine tumors are of metastatic origin. The spinal column is the most frequent site of skeletal metastasis.[18]
- Malignant cells are carried to the spine through the valveless extradural venous plexus of Batson.[2,8] A recent anatomic model suggests that malignant cells can also metastasize through the segmental arteries.[20]

Trauma

- The articulation of the vertebral column, ribs, and sternum makes the thoracic spine relatively stable.[1]
- High-energy injuries are frequently required to produce injury to the thoracic spine.
- Forces associated with injury are axial compression, flexion, lateral compression, flexion–rotation, shear, flexion–distraction, and extension.

NATURAL HISTORY

Intervertebral Disc Herniation

- Wood et al described 20 patients with asymptomatic thoracic disc protrusions followed by magnetic resonance imaging (MRI).[21] All patients remained asymptomatic at an average of 26 months, and most disc herniations were smaller or unchanged on repeat MRI.
  - It is unknown how often asymptomatic thoracic herniations become symptomatic.
- Brown et al reported on 55 patients with 72 thoracic disc herniations.[3] Fifty-four were treated initially with conservative therapy and 15 eventually required surgery. Nine of 11 patients with lower extremity complaints went on to have surgery. Two patients had myelopathy and were treated surgically. All 55 patients ultimately returned to their previous level of activity.
  - Patients with lower extremity symptoms and myelopathy are likely to require surgical intervention.

Infection

- Vertebral osteomyelitis is rare and accounts for 2% to 4% of all cases of osteomyelitis.
- *Staphylococcus aureus* is the most common organism, accounting for almost 50% of pyogenic infections.[5]
- The incidence is rising as a result of a growing immunocompromised and elderly patient population, increased intravenous drug abuse, and an increase in invasive diagnostic and therapeutic procedures.
- Before medical and surgical treatment, spinal osteomyelitis carried a mortality rate of greater than 70%.[10] The advent of antibiotics and anterior spinal débridement techniques has reduced mortality to less than 15%.[6,13]
- Carragee reported on 72 patients were treated nonoperatively with antibiotics.[6] Over 33% of them required surgical débridement. Results related to patient age and immune status.

Tumor

- Over 90% of spinal tumors are metastatic lesions with a distant primary source.
- Primary tumors from the breast, prostate, lung, kidney, and thyroid are most likely to metastasize to the vertebral column.[18]
- Tumors that affect the anterior elements of the spine can be benign or malignant.
- Benign primary tumors that have a predilection for the anterior elements include giant cell tumors and hemangiomas. Malignant tumors that commonly affect the anterior elements include osteosarcomas, chondrosarcomas, myelomas, and lymphomas.[15]
- Improved diagnostics have allowed for more accurate diagnosis and improved staging.[9]
- Chemotherapy and radiotherapy have improved survival and local control.[14]
- Treatment goals include preservation of neural function, spinal stability, margin-free tumor resection, and correction of deformity.

Trauma

- Fractures of the thoracolumbar spine are the most common spinal injuries.
- The thoracic spine configuration of vertebrae, sternum, and ribcage confers an inherent stability.[1]
- Injuries to this region require significant force, and unstable injuries are usually a result of high-energy injuries such as motor vehicle accidents, falls from heights, and crush injuries.
- Patients can have associated injuries such as pneumothoraces, pulmonary contusions, and vascular injuries.
- Although most thoracic injuries do not involve neurologic deficit, complete neurologic deficits are more common with thoracic spine injuries due to the small neural canal, the tenuous blood supply, and the high energy needed to cause injury.[4]

PATIENT HISTORY AND PHYSICAL FINDINGS

- Neurologic status is examined.
  - Manual motor testing
  - Pin-prick and light touch sensory examination may help to localize the cord level of injury based on dermatome.
  - Babinski reflex and clonus are upper motor neuron signs.
  - Reflex examination of the patellar and Achilles tendons: hyperactivity is an upper motor neuron sign.

IMAGING AND OTHER DIAGNOSTIC STUDIES

- It is often useful to obtain an MRI and a CT-myelogram preoperatively. MRI is the key radiologic study to confirm the diagnosis and localize pathology. Plain CT scans are helpful in delineating bony anatomy.
- A plain CT scan should be obtained in concert with MRI on every patient with a destructive bony process, such as tumor or infection, to preoperatively assess the degree of bony loss and determine the optimal strategy for reconstruction.
- CT-myelography may be needed if MRI scans cannot be obtained or if quality of the MRI is suboptimal due to patient movement, metal artifact from prior implants, or other factors.

- CT can detail ossification of the posterior longitudinal ligament or ligamentum flavum.
- CT-myelography can also clarify whether cord compression is primarily anterior secondary to a disc fragment, or circumferential due to stenosis.

DIFFERENTIAL DIAGNOSIS

- Spinal tumors
- Infections
- Transverse myelitis
- Ankylosing spondylitis
- Fractures
- Intercostal neuralgia
- Herpes zoster
- Cervical and lumbar herniated discs
- Disorders of thoracic and abdominal viscera
- Amyotrophic lateral sclerosis
- Multiple sclerosis
- Arteriovenous malformations

NONOPERATIVE MANAGEMENT

Intervertebral Disc Herniation

- In the absence of myelopathy, most patients can be treated conservatively.
- A conservative treatment plan should include nonsteroidal anti-inflammatories, rest, activity modification, and physical therapy focusing on trunk stabilization.[3]
- Other options include intercostal nerve blocks and pharmacotherapy such as narcotics, tricyclic antidepressants, serotonin-reuptake inhibitors, and certain antiepileptics.

Infection

- Vertebral infections should be treated nonoperatively with culture-specific antibiotics and spinal immobilization.
- Open or CT-guided biopsy can aid in targeting appropriate antibiotic treatment.
- Treatment frequently involves 6 weeks of parenteral antibiotics followed by a course of oral antibiotics.
- An infectious disease consultant can help guide the antibiotic regimen.
- External immobilization with an orthosis can help stabilize the spine, decrease pain, and prevent deformity.
- Bracing is particularly important in patients with greater than 50% destruction of the vertebral body since they are at greater risk for deformity.[7]
- Response to treatment can be followed clinically with erythrocyte sedimentation rate, C-reactive protein, and a complete blood count.

Tumor

- A multidisciplinary approach including a neuroradiologist, pathologist, oncologist, and spine surgeon is used to treat spinal tumors.
- A CT-guided biopsy can help establish a diagnosis in 76% to 93% of lesions.[9,18]
- Metastatic lesions that do not compromise spinal stability and without rapid neurologic progression can be managed nonoperatively.[18]
- Nonoperative treatment can include radiation, chemotherapy, embolization, and bracing.

- Most primary spinal tumors cannot be treated non-operatively.

Trauma

- Most thoracic and thoracolumbar spine injuries can be effectively treated nonoperatively.
- Conservative treatment can include recumbency, bracing, and pain management for patients without neurologic deterioration and with a structurally stable injury.[11,17]
- Decubitus ulcers, thromboembolism, urinary tract infections, and late pain are complications reported with nonoperative treatment.[12]

SURGICAL MANAGEMENT

- Indications for discectomy
  - Progressive myelopathy due to anterior compressive lesions
  - Lower extremity weakness or paralysis
  - Radicular pain refractory to conservative therapy
  - Deformity correction
- Indications for corpectomy
  - Fractures with anterior spinal cord compression
  - Metastatic or primary thoracic tumors
  - Osteomyelitis
  - Sequestered disc herniations that have migrated behind the vertebral body
  - Ossification of the posterior longitudinal ligament

- Indications for bone grafting and cage or allograft placement
  - Infection
    - Although somewhat counterintuitive, anterior spinal infections can be successfully managed with allograft, cage, or instrumentation reconstruction if a thorough débridement of infected tissues is performed and postoperative antibiotics are administered
  - Tumor
  - Trauma
  - Degenerative disease
  - Deformity correction (scoliosis, kyphosis)
- Indications for polymethylmethacrylate (PMMA) use
  - Anterior column reconstruction of tumors in patients with a life expectancy of less than 1 year
  - Patients in whom the use of radiation or chemotherapy is anticipated
- Indications for plate fixation
  - Anterior and middle column instability
  - Revision of failed posterior fusion
  - Pseudarthrosis
- Indications for use of solid rod instrumentation
  - Patient under 30 years of age
  - Thoracic and thoracolumbar curves of less than 65 degrees (Cobb angle)
  - Thoracic or lumbar compensatory curves that correct to less than 20 degrees with side bending
  - Hypokyphosis (less than 20 degrees from T5 to T12)

THORACIC DISCECTOMY

- After elevating the articular ligaments of the costotransverse and costovertebral articulations, the remaining rib head is excised (**TECH FIG 1**).
- The superior edge of the pedicle of the caudal vertebra is resected with a rongeur to expose the dural tube.
- To find the disc herniation, the surgeon follows the superior edge of the pedicle to the vertebral body and disc space.
- The disc herniation is removed using small angled curettes and pituitary rongeurs.
- Discectomy can be facilitated by removing a small portion (1 to 2 cm) of the adjacent vertebral bodies. If the disc is extremely calcified or has migrated behind the vertebral body, it is helpful to perform hemicorpectomies of the adjacent vertebral bodies.

- The portion of the disc that lies away from the ventral aspect of the spinal cord should be removed first. Once a cavity is created by removing this initial disc and bone, the rest of the disc can be removed into this cavity, ensuring that all forceful maneuvers are directed anteriorly away from the thecal sac.
- We prefer to keep the posterior longitudinal ligament (PLL) intact whenever possible, as its removal often results in substantial epidural bleeding. We will pass an elevator or nerve hook through a rent in the PLL if one is present to ensure adequate decompression from pedicle to pedicle. If the PLL needs to be removed, we use bipolar cautery to cauterize the PLL and then carefully remove it with either a Kerrison or a combination of pituitary rongeur and curette.

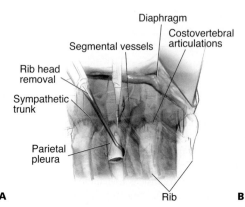
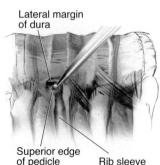

TECH FIG 1 • The rib head can be removed with a high-speed burr once the costotransverse and costovertebral articulations are excised.

THORACIC OR THORACOLUMBAR CORPECTOMY

- The posterior aspect of the vertebral body is identified.
  - Discectomy is performed above and below the level of the corpectomy.
  - The lateral annulus is incised using a no. 10 blade to the anterior midline.
  - An elevator is then used to separate the disc from the endplates.
  - Discectomy is completed using curettes and rongeurs.
- Attention is turned to the vertebrectomy. Using a 4-mm burr, the surgeon removes most of the bone from the vertebral body.
  - Corpectomy is completed by removing the remaining bone with a rongeur (**TECH FIG 2**).
  - Depending on the nature of the pathology, the PLL may need to be removed for the purposes of decompression.
- For retropulsed fracture fragments, the fragments are first thinned using a high-speed 4-mm ball-tipped burr.

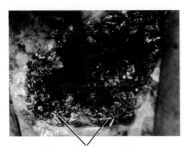

Ligated segmental
vessels

TECH FIG 2 • Corpectomy site.

- Then a thin, sharp curette is used to peel the fragments away from the dura and into the created trough.
  - It is important to work quickly but carefully at this point as there can be a significant amount of epidural bleeding.
- The posterior cortical fragments are removed from the contralateral (deep) side of the canal first so that the bulging dura will not obscure the rest of the fragments.
- Decompression is adequate when the dura can be seen bulging into the corpectomy trough and the spinal canal has been decompressed throughout its complete width.

Plating

- A flat surface is prepared for the plate by removing lateral endplate prominences and rib heads with a high-speed burr.
- Using an awl insertion guide, a posterior bicortical thoracic bolt is placed at the cephalad and caudad fixation levels.
- The trajectory should be parallel to the endplate and angled slightly anteriorly to avoid penetrating the canal (**TECH FIG 3A**).
- If sagittal correction or interbody graft placement is needed, distraction is performed on the endplates using a lamina spreader.
- A correct-length plate is applied over the bolts without extending into the adjacent disc spaces (**TECH FIG 3B,C**). Nuts are applied loosely to secure the plate to the posterior bolts.
- Using a drill or awl, correct-length anterior screws are placed angling slightly posteriorly.
  - In general, bicortical screws are preferred because the cancellous bone of the vertebral body provides relatively weak purchase, especially in patients with tumors or infections.

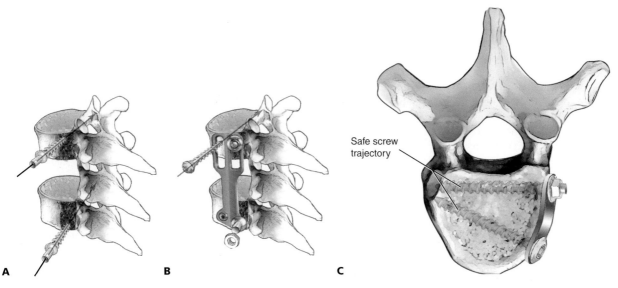

Safe screw
trajectory

A   B   C

TECH FIG 3 • Application of plate and screws. **A.** Osteophytes are removed, and a trajectory is planned parallel to the endplate and angled slightly anteriorly to avoid penetration of the canal. **B.** Nuts secure the posterior bolts, and screws are applied anteriorly. **C.** It is important for the screws to be a safe distance from the dural covering of the spinal cord.

SCREW–ROD INSTRUMENTATION

- Use of an anterior screw–rod construct allows for correction of coronal plane deformity through fusion of fewer spinal motion segments compared with posterior instrumentation.
- The entry position for the anterior vertebral screws is determined based on the location of the vertebral foramen, as this identifies posterior body cortex.
- The surgeon inserts the most cephalad and caudad

- screws first in the midlateral vertebral body at the same distance from the posterior cortex (**TECH FIG 4**).
- The screw tips should engage the far cortex of each vertebra and should be directed toward the posterolateral corner of the vertebra.
- The rest of the screws are placed in similar fashion.
- The rods are inserted as directed by the particular system, and alignment is corrected before tightening.

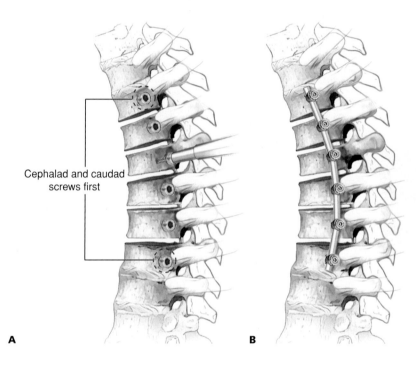

Cephalad and caudad
screws first

A   B

TECH FIG 4 • Application of screw–rod instrumentation.

BONE GRAFTING AND CAGES

- It is of utmost importance to prepare an adequate fusion bed.
- A thorough decortication is performed.
- Although placement of the graft on preserved bleeding subchondral endplates is preserved, creating a slot or peg hole in the adjacent vertebral bodies can help to prevent graft extrusion.
- Before graft placement, kyphotic deformity can be corrected by distracting adjacent vertebrae.
  - Extreme care must be taken to avoid injury to the adjacent endplates during distraction, especially in patients with osteoporosis or other states with compromised bone quality (tumors, infections).
- After the graft has been anchored, compression locks the graft in position.
- If tricortical iliac crest bone is used, we prefer to have the cortical smooth surface face the spinal canal.
- Single-level corpectomy defects can be supported with tricortical iliac crest grafts, whereas larger defects are

better stabilized with autogenous fibular strut grafts or shaft allografts.
  - Depending on the size of the patient, humeral shafts often provide the best fit in the thoracic spine.
- For cage placement, the ends of the cage can be trimmed to create the necessary cage configuration (**TECH FIG 5A**).
  - Alternatively, stackable cages (eg, those made of PEEK) can be measured to fit the space.
- The packed cage is implanted between the distracted adjacent endplates (**TECH FIG 5B**).
- The cage is stabilized when the distraction is released.
- Bone graft should be packed in and around the cage.

Polymethylmethacrylate

- PMMA may be used in patients with spinal tumors who have poor life expectancy, or who are unlikely to heal anterior bone grafts due to poor bone quality or healing potential.

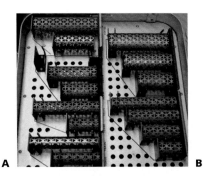
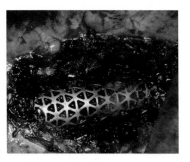

TECH FIG 5 • A. Titanium mesh cages. **B.** Cage placement.

- It provides immediate spinal stability and is strongest in compression.
- The PMMA can be reinforced and anchored with Steinmann pins drilled into the adjacent vertebral bodies.

- Bends in the Steinmann pins can prevent pin migration.
- To increase interdigitation of the cement, multiple drill holes are placed in the adjacent vertebral bodies.

PEARLS AND PITFALLS

Thoracic corpectomy	▪ By keeping the posterior longitudinal ligament intact until the end of procedure, epidural bleeding can be minimized.
Choice of graft	▪ Patients with short life expectancies and those who will need adjuvant chemotherapy or radiation should be reconstructed with PMMA to provide the maximal short-term stability.
Graft sizing	▪ It is important not to undersize the graft, as it is more prone to migration.
Thoracic discectomy	▪ When removing herniated disc fragments, the surgeon should always direct the angled curettes away from the dura.

POSTOPERATIVE CARE

- Chest tubes remain until output is less than 150 mL over 24 hours.

COMPLICATIONS

- The exiting nerve root can be injured while removing the pedicle.
- Vascular injury
- Intercostal neuralgia
- Atelectasis
- Neurologic injury
- Wrong-level surgery
- Significant bleeding can be encountered when entering the epidural space.

REFERENCES

1. Andriacchi TP, Schultz A, Belytschko T, et al. A model for studies of mechanical interactions between the human spine and rib cage. J Biomech 1974;7497–7507.
2. Batson OV. The role of the vertebral veins in metastatic processes. Ann Intern Med 1942;16:38–45.
3. Brown CW, et al. The natural history of thoracic disc herniation. Spine 1992;17:S97–S102.
4. Burke DC, Murray DD. The management of thoracic and thoraco-lumbar injuries of the spine with neurological involvement. J Bone Joint Surg Br 1976;58B:72–78.
5. Butler JS, Shelly MJ, Timlin M, et al. Nontuberculous pyogenic spinal infection in adults: a 12-year experience from a tertiary referral center. Spine 2006;31:2695–2700.
6. Carragee EJ. Pyogenic vertebral osteomyelitis. J Bone Joint Surg Am 1997;79A:874–880.
7. Frederickson B, Yuan H, Olans R. Management and outcomes of pyogenic vertebral osteomyelitis. Clin Orthop Relat Res 1978;131:160–167.
8. Harada M, Shimizu A, Nakamura Y, et al. Role of the vertebral venous system in metastatic spread of cancer cells to the bone. Adv Exp Med Biol 1992;324:83–92.
9. Lis E, Bilsky MH, Pisinski L, et al. Percutaneous CT-guided biopsy of osseous lesion of the spine in patients with known or suspected malignancy. AJNR Am J Neuroradiol 2004;25:1583–1588.
10. Makins GH, Abbott FC. On acute primary osteomyelitis of the vertebrae. Ann Surg 1896;23:510–539.
11. Mumford J, Weinstein JN, Spratt KF, et al. Thoracolumbar burst fractures: the clinical efficacy and outcome of nonoperative management. Spine 1993;18:955–970.
12. Rechtine GR II, Cahill D, Chrin AM. Treatment of thoracolumbar trauma: comparison of complications of operative versus nonoperative treatment. J Spinal Disord 1999;12:406–409.
13. Rezai AR, et al. Contemporary management of spinal osteomyelitis. Neurosurgery 1999;44:1018–1025.
14. Simmons ED, Zheng Y. Vertebral tumors: surgical versus nonsurgical treatment. Clin Orthop Relat Res 2006;443:233–247.
15. Simon MA, Springfield D. Surgery of Bone and Soft-Tissue Tumors. Philadelphia: Lippincott-Raven, 1998.
16. Vaccaro AR, et al. Placement of pedicle screws in the thoracic spine. 1. Morphometric analysis of the thoracic vertebrae, J Bone Joint Surg Am 1995;77A:1193–1199.
17. Weinstein JN, Collalto P, Lehmann TR. Long-term follow-up of non-operatively treated thoracolumbar spine fractures. J Orthop Trauma 1987;1:152–159.
18. White AH, Kwon B, Lindskog D, et al. Metastatic disease of the spine. J Am Acad Orthop Surg 2006;14:587–598.
19. Wiley AM, Trueta J. The vascular anatomy of the spine and its relationship to pyogenic vertebral osteomyelitis. J Bone Joint Surg Br 1959;41B:796–809.
20. Willis TA. Nutrient arteries of the vertebral bodies. J Bone Joint Surg Am 1949;31A:538–540.
21. Wood KB, et al. Magnetic resonance imaging of the thoracic spine: evaluation of asymptomatic individuals. J Bone Joint Surg Am 1995;77A:1631–1638.

Chapter 18

Lateral Approaches to Interbody Fusion

Keith W. Michael and S. Tim Yoon

DEFINITION

- Lateral approach to interbody fusion.
- Many different names including extreme lateral interbody fusion (XLIF) or direct lateral interbody fusion (DLIF). This approach is often called the transpsoas approach because approaches to lumbar levels require traversing the psoas muscle. The lateral approach can also be used to access thoracic spine as well.
- Typically, this technique relies on a combination of neuromonitoring and direct visualization to safely navigate through the lateral lumbosacral neurologic plexus.

ANATOMY

- After the superficial dissection, the lateral abdominal wall muscles are traversed to approach the lumbar spine. This leads directly into the retroperitoneal space.
- The psoas muscle flanks the lateral lumbar spine and is covered by a thin slippery fascia.
- Within the psoas muscles traverse the lumbosacral plexus, genitofemoral nerve, and lateral cutaneous nerve (**FIG 1**).[1,2]
- The frequency of lumbosacral nerves found on various different locations of the lateral projection of the lumbar spine is indicated in **FIG 2**. Although there are general trends from disc level to disc level and anterior to posterior, each individual has significant variability that can be different from the "typical" situation.[3]
- As one progresses distally in the lumbar spine, the lumbosacral plexus covers more of the lateral aspect of the lumbar spine and more often covers the ventral aspect of the spine.

- The lateral iliac crests are typically slightly below or at the level of the L4-5 disc space. However, there is variability between patients, and at times high iliac crest (or deep seated L4-5 disc space) may prevent parallel access to the L4-5 disc space from a direct lateral approach (**FIG 3**).
- When approaching the upper lumbar levels, the ribs may interfere with direct lateral approach to the spine. This may require choosing an incision that is not perfectly lateral to the disc space or excising a rib to improve access (**FIG 3**).
- Lateral lumbar radiographs are useful to assess the rib and iliac crest position relative to the level that needs to be approached.
- Aorta, inferior vena cava, and common iliac vessels run on the ventral surface of the anterior longitudinal ligament (ALL) (**FIG 4**). Axial imaging allows preoperative localization of these structures to understand the safe zone for each patient.

SURGICAL MANAGEMENT

Indications

- Spondylolisthesis low grade
  - Isthmic
  - Degenerative
- Deformity
  - Scoliosis
  - Kyphosis
  - In combination with pedicle subtraction osteotomy (PSO)
- Foraminal stenosis with vacuum disc and instability
- Adjacent segment disease with instability
- Discitis after failure of medical management
- Other situations when interbody fusion is necessary

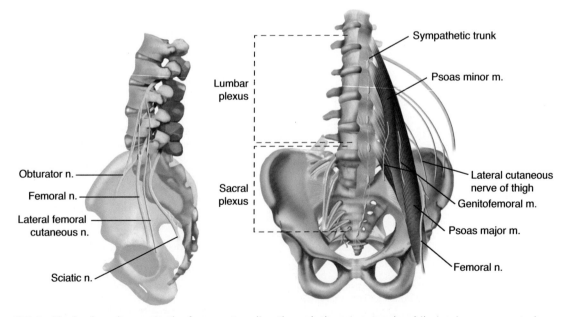

FIG 1 • The lumbar plexus exits the foramen traveling through the psoas muscle while moving more ventral as it progresses caudally. n, nerve; m, muscle.

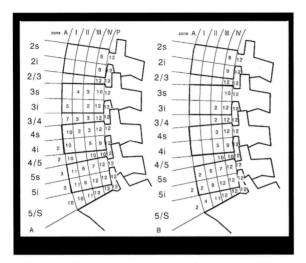

FIG 2 • Moro et al. identified and counted the location of the lumbar plexus and genitofemoral nerve relative to each disc space in 12 cadavers. (From Moro T, Kikuchi S, Konno S, Yaginuma H. An anatomic study of the lumbar plexus with respect to retroperitoneal endoscopic surgery. Spine 2003;28:423–428, with permission.)

Preoperative Planning

■ Anteroposterior (AP) and lateral standing radiographs allow assessment of accessibility of each disc level relative to the iliac crest and ribs.

■ Determine side of approach. Typically the disc is approached from the convex side (ie, the more open side of the disc) to facilitate intradiscal work. However, in scoliosis cases when the approach to the L4-5 level (the convex side) dictates the side of the approach, this may place the other levels on the concave side. Surgeons have the choice of going forward with performing surgery on the same side (convex at L4-5 and concave at the other lumbar levels) and work around the inconvenience of working in the concavity (**FIG 5**). In flexible curves, bending the patient can alleviate this problem significantly. Rarely, some surgeons may choose to flip the patient to work on the convex side for the rest of the curve.

■ Establish a neuromonitoring plan. Typically electromyography (EMG) monitoring is performed. This can consist of both free-running EMG as well as stimulated proximity sensing. EMGs help to monitor the motor branches of the lumbosacral plexus; however, sensory nerves cannot be monitored. The genitofemoral and lateral cutaneous nerves cannot be monitored.

■ Ensure the anesthetic plan is compatible with the neuromonitoring plan. The patient must have muscle twitches during the surgery to allow for EMG monitoring.

Positioning

■ Positioning on the operative table is extremely important in lateral interbody fusion.

■ Typically, the procedure is performed on a regular operative bed with the capacity to break or flex in the middle. Usually, the table's orientation is reversed such that the base is attached to the feet allowing the C-arm to pass freely underneath the thoracolumbar spine.

■ The patient is positioned in a true lateral position, as close to vertical as possible. This can be fine tuned under fluoroscopy by tilting the bed.

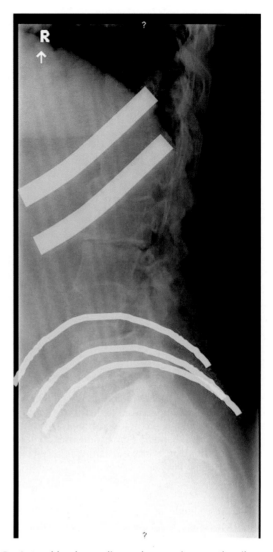

FIG 3 • Lateral lumbar radiographs superimpose the ribs and iliac crest over the disc spaces to determine which levels are accessible with a lateral approach.

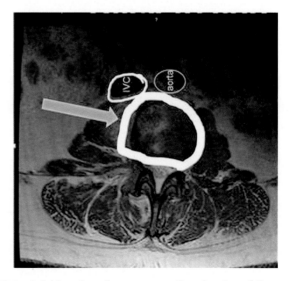

FIG 4 • Axial imaging allows preoperative planning of the working window, including evaluating the proximity of the aorta and inferior vena cava.

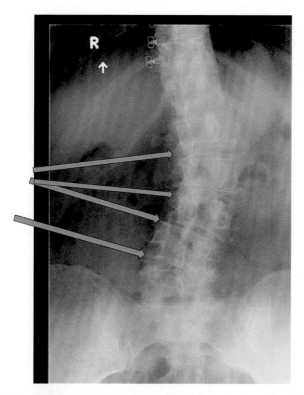

FIG 5 • Anteroposterior lumbar radiographs help determine the best approach side in preoperative planning. The approach side is often determined by the orientation of the L4-5 disc or by the convexity of the curve. Bending films can be used to determine the flexibility of the curve, which is often reproduced by flexing the operating room table.

■ The iliac crest should be position approximately 4 inches cephalad to the center of the break in the table. This allows the flexion of the table to open the disc space while still giving enough room for the C-arm to pass underneath the table to provide a perfect lateral of the L4-5 disc space (**FIG 6**).
■ Hips are flexed approximately 30 degrees to take tension off the iliopsoas. Knees are flexed approximately 30 degrees to compensate for the hip flexion and to keep the feet in a good position on the bed.

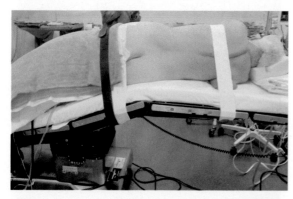

FIG 6 • The iliac crest is positioned approximately 4 inches cephalad of the break in the table. This allows the disc space to be opened by flexing the table while allowing the C-arm to pass freely underneath the table.

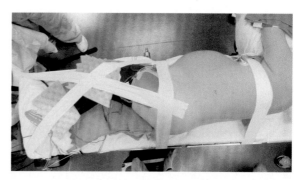

FIG 7 • Horizontal tape straps are placed at the hip and the chest followed by a crossing pattern of tape on the lower extremities to secure them while the table is tilted during surgery.

■ Once positioned and prior to flexing the table, the patient is taped to the table. First, tape the patient horizontally at the hip (just inferior to the iliac crests) and at the chest (just below the axilla). Next, a crossing pattern of tape holds the legs in position because the table will be tilted throughout the case (**FIG 7**).
■ After taping, flex the table. Flexing typically requires reverse Trendelenburg at the base while flexing the long end of the table. The goal is to have the involved disc space perpendicular to the floor. Feel the tension of the abdominal oblique muscles on the convex side to determine when sufficient flexion has been achieved, then use reverse Trendelenburg to make the lumbar spine parallel with the floor. Another round of taping of the hip area may be necessary.

Approach[4]

■ The approach technique in the lumbar spine can be divided into the "one incision" or "two incision" techniques. With the one incision technique, a single incision is created directly lateral to the disc space in a position that is as parallel as possible to the two endplates of the disc (**FIG 8**). With the two incision technique, an initial incision is made posterior to the direct lateral position. Then a second incision is made directly lateral to the spine in a manner similar to the one incision technique. The addition of the posterior incision allows

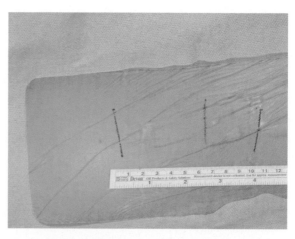

FIG 8 • Three incisions are planned, each parallel to the respective disc space. This is the one incision technique as the posterior incision is omitted.

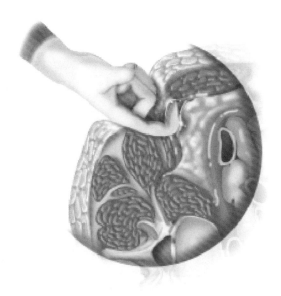

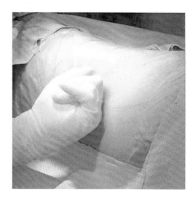

FIG 9 • The posterior incision allows finger localization of the disc space and direct finger-guided delivery of instruments to the lateral disc space.

finger localization of the retroperitoneal space prior to incising the lateral abdominal musculature and facilitates finger-guided (through the posterior incision) placement of the instruments to the lateral disc space (**FIG 9**). The "single incision" technique can also be used safely, but extra care must be taken to identify the retroperitoneal space, and a larger incision may be necessary to allow a finger to be placed through the direct lateral incision as opposed to through the posterior incision.

- If multiple levels are involved a single longitudinal incision or multiple small transverse incisions paralleling each of the involved disc spaces can be used. Multiple well-localized transverse incisions at each disc space have the advantage of ensuring one is able to work directly aligned over each disc space without undue soft tissue tension.
- The single transverse incision for each disc space is described in the technique section; however, the two incision technique is detailed in the Pearls and Pitfalls section.

LOCALIZING THE INCISION[4,7]

- First turn the C-arm parallel to the floor (ie, beam is horizontal). Then make adjustments to the table to obtain a perfect AP view of the disc space. The body, pedicles, and spinous processes are used as guides.
- Once the true AP is obtained (ie, beam is horizontal in orientation), arc the C-arm 90 degrees into the lateral position. Then adjust the bed angle to get a parallel view of the endplates. Although these steps to align the disc space to the vertical and horizontal planes are not

absolutely necessary, it can be very helpful for the surgeon to maintain orientation and help the surgeon stay within the safe zone throughout the case.

- Using a guidewire or other radiopaque instrument, mark the anterior and posterior border of the involved disc on the skin while the C-arm captures a true lateral of the disc space. Mark the incision such that it exactly parallels the orientation of the disc, which may change at each level based on the changes in lordosis or kyphosis (**TECH FIG 1**).

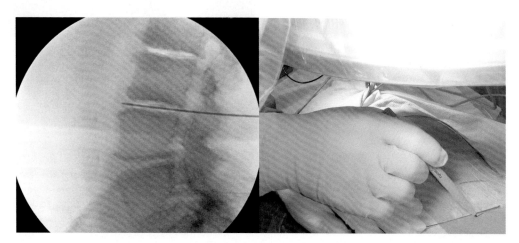

TECH FIG 1 • The guidewire is used to localize the incision parallel to the disc space using fluoroscopy at each surgical level.

APPROACH/DISSECTION

- After incising the skin sharply, dissect through the subcutaneous tissue to the fascia overlying the external oblique muscle.
- Dissect through the external oblique, internal oblique, and transversus muscles and fascia to enter the retroperitoneum. Sharp, blunt, or electrocautery dissection can be performed through the external layers of the abdominal muscles, but careful blunt dissection is recommended beyond that to minimize chances of damage to the peritoneum.
- Characteristic features of the retroperitoneum include the presence of retroperitoneal fat causing a very slippery feel to the tissues and the ability to feel striations in the psoas musculature. In many situations it is possible to directly palpate the disc and vertebral body undulations (**TECH FIG 2**).

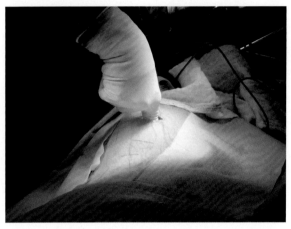

TECH FIG 2 • Gentle finger sweeps allow localization of the retroperitoneal space, psoas, and lateral disc space.

PLACING THE GUIDEWIRE

- After ensuring the approach is retroperitoneal, a small dilator is then placed through the psoas into the disc space. Neuromonitoring during this step will alert the surgeon to proximity of motor nerves and redirection of the dilator may be necessary. Once the dilator is docked on the lateral aspect of the disc and neuromonitoring is safe, then place the guidewire into the disc space.
- If the incision was localized correctly, the guidewire will be oriented perfectly vertical and centered in the incision in order to fall in the center of the disc.
- Care should be taken to pass the initial dilator to the lateral aspect of the disc by shuttling it with a finger (either through the same incision or the second posterior incision). This will prevent inadvertent bowel injury.
- The ideal position for the guidewire varies from level to level. Although it is more convenient to place the guidewire slightly posterior to midpoint, because of the lumbar plexus it is advisable to start at the midpoint or slightly anterior at L4-5 or any level at which neuromonitoring warning is present at the more posterior position. The orientation of the guidewire should be inline with the fluoroscopy beam resulting in a single superimposed circle (**TECH FIG 3**).

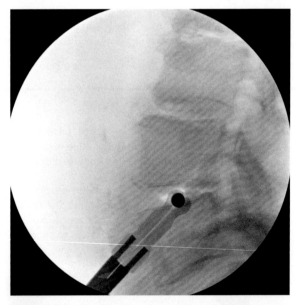

TECH FIG 3 • Under fluoroscopy the guidewire is positioned on the lateral disc space just posterior to the midpoint of the disc parallel with the fluoroscopy beam.

EXPOSURE

- Once the guidewire is in position, a series of larger soft tissue dilators are used to bluntly spread the soft tissue and psoas muscle. Each dilator connects to the EMG neuromonitoring system to help localize the motor nerves of the lumbosacral plexus.
- Starting with the smallest dilator, slide it over the guidewire. Rotate the dilator clockwise and counterclockwise with gentle pressure to advance to the lateral aspect of the disc. Attach the neuromonitoring system during dilation to determine if it is safe to proceed. Ensure the EMG electrode is oriented posteriorly, typically marked by a line on the dilator probe, as this is where the lumbosacral plexus and exiting nerve roots are most likely to be encountered.

- Repeat this step until the largest dilator is passed to the lateral disc space and reveals safe monitoring parameters.
- Many surgeons prefer the "dock shallow" approach where the dilators are placed on the psoas muscle instead of through the muscle. Once the retractor is placed on the psoas, the dissection can occur under direct visualization. This reduces the risk of neurological injury, especially to sensory nerves that are not detected by EMG neuromonitoring.

DOCKING AND OPENING THE RETRACTOR

- Attach the retractor arm to the mount affixed to the anterior side of the bed.
- Connecting the neuromonitoring clip to the retractor will allow for neuromonitoring during the placement of the retractor.
- Connect the retractor arm to the retractor (**TECH FIG 4**).
- Depending on where you attach the retractor arm, the blades will open anteriorly or posteriorly. Typically in the lumbar spine, it is often more favorable to dock posteriorly and open the blades anteriorly.[3]
- Open the blades anteriorly, cephalad, and caudad. Affix the light sources. At this time, using a combination of direct visual inspection and the neuromonitoring probe tip, explore the remaining soft tissue over the lateral disc space. When "shallow docking" dissection through the psoas may be necessary. Remember the neuromonitoring system will not detect sensory nerves. It is important to check for nervous structures before proceeding with the discectomy or using bipolar electrocautery.
- Once the wound bed is confirmed to be free of nervous structures, the posterior blade can be affixed with the docking blade into the disc space. This should be done under direct vision to avoid entry to adjacent nervous structures. An optional anterior retractor can be placed over the ALL to help retract anterior soft tissues and provide a reference to prevent disruption of the ALL during discectomy.

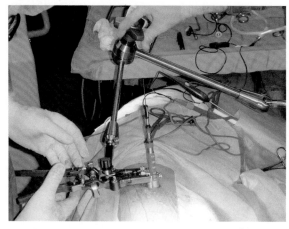

TECH FIG 4 • Once the dilator is in place, the blades are oriented so as to open inline with the disc space prior to locking the position with the holding arm.

DISCECTOMY

- With the lateral annulus exposed, perform a rectangular annulotomy and remove the nucleus pulposus with a pituitary rongeur.
- Pass a Cobb elevator along the cartilaginous surface of the superior and inferior endplate with special care not to violate the bony endplate. Use AP fluoroscopy to ensure the Cobb takes down the annulus at both the superior and inferior endplate on the far lateral side. This step allows the disc space to open and allows the cage to pass to the far lateral cortex. Depending on the level, orientation and shape of the disc endplate, an angled or straight Cobb may be preferred.
- Using a combination of curettes and pull shavers, perform a complete discectomy. Rotary shavers can facilitate discectomy; however, judicious use is encouraged as they can result in a high incidence of endplate violation.
- Kerrison rongeur is used to debride any overlying annulus or osteophyte at the opening of the discectomy to improve visualization.

TRIALING AND SIZING

- Once a complete discectomy is performed, size the interbody cage using the sizing trials. In addition to choosing the appropriate height, select the depth and width.
- Placing a cage that extends to both lateral rims of the endplates, improves coronal plane correction and reduces the potential for cage collapse through the endplate. This can be confirmed on AP fluoroscopy images (**TECH FIG 5**).
- Choosing AP cage size depends on the anatomical situation. Larger cages are biomechanically superior, but the bigger footprint requires more dissection and hence more chance of encountering neurological structures (**TECH FIG 6**).

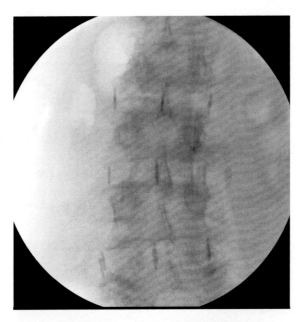

TECH FIG 5 • Use anteroposterior fluoroscopy to confirm the cage covers both lateral cortices to reduce the chance of collapse.

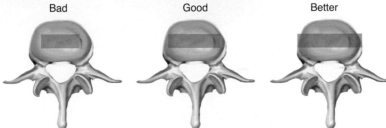

Bad   Good   Better

TECH FIG 6 • Increased anteroposterior width provides increased contact surface area to prevent collapse without compromising fusion surface area. The cage should be centered in the antero-posterior direction.

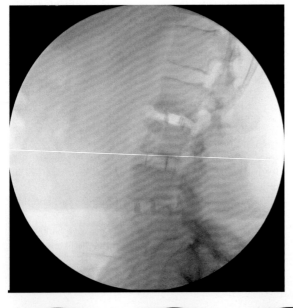

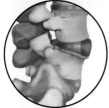 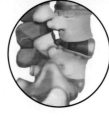 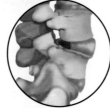

GRAFT PREPARATION AND DELIVERY

- Most available cages are made of PEEK (poly-ether-ether-ketone). The cage should be filled with bone graft material. This can be held in place with circumferential sutures during delivery or by using a graft slider.
- The graft can be delivered by impacting it into place; however, there is a risk for endplate violation. The graft

slider can safely deliver the graft without the chance for endplate violation (**TECH FIG 7**). Graft delivery should be checked on AP fluoroscopy to ensure the radiographic markers in the graft extend to or slightly beyond the lateral body cortex.

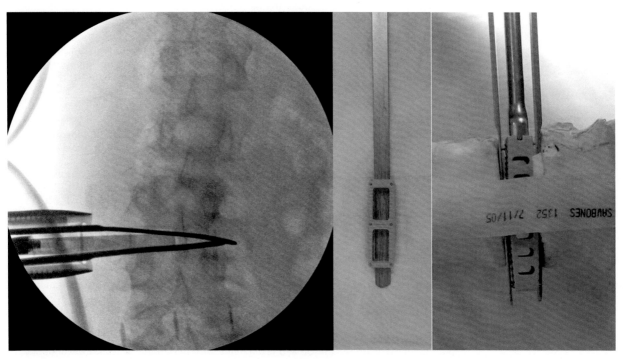

TECH FIG 7 • The graft slider delivers the graft while preventing endplate violation.

CLOSURE

- Confirm graft location on with final AP and lateral fluoroscopic images.
- Obtain hemostasis prior to retractor removal. Partially collapse the retractor and gently remove while inspecting for bleeding along the walls.

- Layered closure is then performed, including the external abdominal fascia.
- If the thoracic cavity was entered, a chest tube may be indicated.

ADDITIONAL FIXATION

- When posterior instrumentation is planned, additional anterior fixation is not required.
- Percutaneous pedicle screws, either unilateral or bilateral, are commonly used to augment the lateral interbody graft. This is usually performed in the prone position following the lateral interbody fusion. Refer to the section on percutaneous pedicle screw instrumentation for additional information.

- If the ALL is disrupted intraoperatively, there is a marked increase in the risk of graft dislodgement. In this case, additional anterior fixation may be indicated.
- In some instances, vertebral body screw fixation with rod, plate, or through the cage itself can be performed to improve biomechanics. However, this typically requires more dissection of the psoas and increases morbidity.

PEARLS AND PITFALLS

Maintain vertical orientation	■ Rotating and tilting the bed rather than the C-arm to fine tune images improves the surgeon's sense of orientation. This method keeps the retractor vertical. This is more important in multilevel cases and with cases that have rotational malalignment. ■ Working vertically within the confines of the retractor will prevent excessive anterior dissection that may threaten the ALL or posterior dissection that may encroach on the posterior longitudinal ligament (PLL) and dura. ■ It will also help place the graft perfectly lateral.
Cage size	■ Cages that have undersized footprints increase the risk of collapse, especially in osteoporotic patients. ■ Passing the Cobb elevator through the far side of the annulus, on both the superior and inferior endplate, will allow placement of a cage that spans the entire width of the body lateral rim to lateral rim.
Endplate violation	■ Passing the Cobb elevator too aggressively across the endplate can cause a disruption. ■ The rotatory shavers commonly violate the endplate if they are used too aggressively. ■ Delivery of a large cage that is not perfectly parallel with the disc space risks endplate violation. This can be avoided with use of the graft slider.
Preservation of the ALL	■ The ALL serves as an anterior tension band that allows the cage to distract the foramina and the posterior structures enabling indirect decompression. ■ Furthermore, ALL incompetence dramatically increases the risk of graft dislodgement, especially if the plan includes prone lordotic positioning that may open up the disc space further. ■ If the ALL disruption is recognized intraoperatively, it is prudent to fix the graft either with direct screw fixation or anterior compression plating to minimize the risk of graft dislodgement. ■ Understanding where the anterior blade of the retractor is docked relative to the ALL, localizing the ALL, and protecting it with additional retractors may reduce the risk of disruption.
Two-incision technique	■ A longitudinal 4 cm incision is made approximately 5 to 8 cm posterior to the planned transverse incision overlying the disc space. ■ Dissection is carried through the fascia and abdominal muscles into the retroperitoneal space, which is confirmed by feel. ■ Approach is made through the skin and subcutaneous tissue down to the level of the fascia through the standard transverse incision. ■ A finger is passed into the retroperitoneal space via the posterior incision and used to push up underneath the muscle and fascia inline with the transverse incision. Monopolar electrocautery can then be used to safely divide the abdominal muscles and fascia to enter the retroperitoneal space.

POSTOPERATIVE CARE

■ No additional postoperative protocols or restrictions are required after lateral interbody fusion than is standard for posterolateral or anterior fusion.

■ With both anterior and posterior column support (assuming posterior augmentation is performed), postoperative bracing is typically not necessary.

■ Generally, because of the minimally invasive retroperitoneal approach, patients typically mobilize quickly and with less pain than open posterolateral fusions.[5]

OUTCOMES

■ Less intraoperative blood loss compared with open posterior fusion.[6]

■ No significant difference in outcomes or complication profile in obese patients.[5]

■ Early outcome data for the treatment of adult degenerative scoliosis suggests less morbidity, blood loss, and overall complication rate compared with open posterior fusion historical cohorts.[7]

COMPLICATIONS[5,6,8]

■ Psoas palsy
■ Lumbosacral plexus injury
■ Quadriceps palsy
■ Meralgia paresthetica (lateral femoral cutaneous nerve)
■ Genitofemoral nerve injury
■ Implant subsidence
■ Broken cage
■ Cage displacement
■ Endplate violation
■ ALL disruption
■ Vascular injury
■ Bowel injury

REFERENCES

1. Benglis DM, Vanni S, Levi AD. An anatomical study of the lumbosacral plexus as related to the minimally invasive transpsoas approach to the lumbar spine. J Neurosurg Spine 2009;10: 139–144.
2. Park DK, Lee MJ, Lin EL, et al. The relationship of the intrapsoas nerves during a transpsoas approach to the lumbar spine, anatomic study. J Spinal Disorder Tech 2010;23(4):223–228.

3. Moro T, Kikuchi S, Konno S, et al. An anatomic study of the lumbar plexus with respect to retroperitoneal endoscopic surgery. Spine 2003;28(5):423–428.

4. Ozgur BM, Aryan HE, Pimenta L, et al. Extreme Lateral Interbody Fusion (XLIF): a novel surgical technique for anterior interbody fusion. Spine J 2006;6(4):435–443.

5. Rodgers WB, Cox CS, Gerber EJ. Early complications of extreme lateral interbody fusion in the obese. J Spinal Disord Tech 2010; 23(4):393–397.

6. Knight RQ, Schwaegler P, Hanscom D, et al. Direct lateral lumbar interbody fusion for degenerative conditions: early complication profile. J Spinal Disord Tech 2009;22(1):34–37.

7. Dakwar E, Cardona RF, Smith DA, et al. Early outcomes and safety of the minimally invasive, lateral retroperitoneal transpsoas approach for adult degenerative scoliosis. Neurosurg Focus 2010; 28(3):E8

8. Tonetti J, Vouallat H, Kwon BK, et al. Femoral nerve palsy following mini-open extraperitoneal lumbar approach: Report of three cases and cadaveric mechanical study. J Spinal Disord Tech 2006;19(2):135–141.

9. Rodgers WB, Cox CS, Gerber EJ. Experience and early results with a minimally invasive technique for anterior column support through extreme lateral interbody fusion: XLIF. Musculoskeletal Review 2007;1:28–32.

Chapter 19

Minimally Invasive Transforaminal Interbody Fusion

Reginald S. Fayssoux and Choll W. Kim

DEFINITION

■ Minimally invasive transforaminal interbody fusion (MIS TLIF) is a modification of the Wiltse exposure for decompression and interbody fusion of the motion segment using specialized retractor and instrumentation systems and fluoroscopic guidance to minimize the surgical corridor.

■ Standard TLIF is a well-established technique for decompression and fusion of a vertebral motion segment which utilizes a midline exposure to perform a unilateral facetectomy and exposure of Kambin's triangle to access the disc space for interbody fusion.

■ TLIF, in comparison to standard posterolateral fusion, allows for improved fusion rates, indirect decompression via restoration of intervertebral disc height, and anterior column support without the need for an anterior retroperitoneal /transperitoneal exposure. The increased risk of neurologic injury to the exiting and traversing nerve roots with TLIF must be weighed against these advantages.

■ MIS TLIF, in comparison to standard open TLIF, is performed through small paramedian incisions and is typically coupled with minimally invasive posterior (ie, facet) fusion and instrumentation.[1] Typically, formal posterolateral fusion is not done, consequently, MIS TLIF relies heavily on the interbody fusion for avoidance of pseudarthrosis and successful outcomes.

■ MIS TLIF has been shown to have less blood loss, earlier postoperative recovery and decreased rates of infection in comparison to standard surgery.[1–3] MIS TLIF may potentially have improved long-term outcomes as a result of the preservation of important musculotendinous attachments and the maintenance of integrity of the dorsolumbar fascia.[4]

■ MIS TLIF is much more reliant on fluoroscopic imaging guidance in comparison to standard TLIF, thus there is increased radiation exposure to the surgeon, staff, and patient. The amount of radiation exposure lessens with surgeon experience. Navigation with fluoroscopic or CT imaging may allow for decreased radiation exposure to the surgeon and staff.

ANATOMY

Paraspinal Anatomy

■ The lumbar multifidus muscle is a key stabilizer of the lumbar spine.[4]

  ■ Largest and most medial of the deep lumbar paraspinal musculature

  ■ Originates from the spinous process and inserts on the superior articular process of the vertebra one to two levels caudally (**FIG 1**)

  ■ Designed for short, powerful movements with maximum force generated during lumbar flexion to optimize its ability to stabilize the lumbar spine motion segments during movement

  ■ Detachment of the multifidus tendon with traditional midline laminectomy compromises multifidus function.

  ■ A paramedian approach, in contrast, preserves the multifidus tendon attachments.

Discectomy

■ Kambin's triangle is an anatomic safe corridor to the intervertebral disc space bounded medially by the dural tube/ traversing nerve root, laterally by the exiting nerve root, and caudally by the pedicle (**FIG 2**).

■ Exposure of Kambin's triangle is accomplished by facetectomy. In the technique we describe, a total facetectomy is performed. The inferior articular process is removed; however, the pars is maintained (to protect the dorsal root ganglion on cage insertion). The superior articular process is removed up to the cranial aspect of the pedicle.

■ The exiting nerve root hugs the medial and inferior border of its associated pedicle. The sensitive dorsal root ganglion typically lies inferior to the pedicle.

Pedicle Screw Placement

■ Percutaneous pedicle screw placement requires understanding the topographic anatomy of the posterior elements as well as the radiographic projection of the pedicle on various radiographic views.

■ The anatomic starting point for pedicle screw placement is typically at the intersection of a horizontal line that bisects the transverse process and a vertical line at or just lateral to the lateral aspect of the pars. The upslope of the facet-transverse process junction is a palpable anatomic landmark.

  ■ The more lateral the starting point, the more medial angulation is needed. This can be problematic in a patient with a narrow pelvis as the posterior iliac crests can limit the ability to medialize pedicle screw tracts.

  ■ The more medial the starting point, the greater the risk of facet violation.

■ The radiographic starting point for pedicle screw placement is typically at the lateral aspect of the radiographic pedicle. At the low lumbar spine, because of medial pedicle angulation, an anatomic starting point may be preferred that may not necessarily coincide with the lateral aspect of the radiographic pedicle.

■ The radiographic pedicle correlates with the anatomic isthmus of the pedicle for hourglass-shaped pedicles. In the lower lumbar spine, where the pedicles are more cylindrical (ie, without an isthmus) and medially angulated, the anatomic correlate of the radiographic pedicle is less clear.

■ Pedicles are oriented sagittally at the thoracolumbar junction and angulate progressively medial as one moves caudal. At S1, the pedicles typically project more than 20 degrees medial.

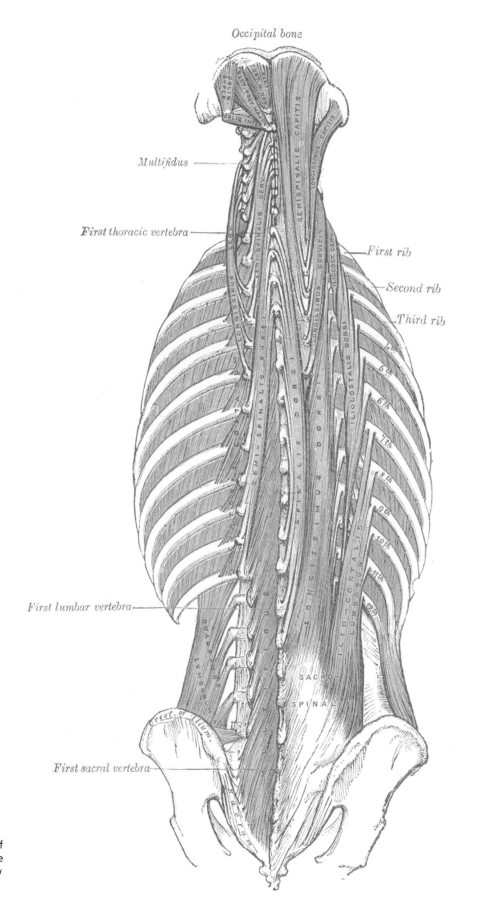

FIG 1 • The multifidi are the deepest and most medial of the lumbar paraspinal musculature. They originate from the spinous process and insert on the superior articular process of the vertebra one to two levels caudally. They are unique among the lumbar paraspinal muscles in that they generate a significant amount of force despite their limited excursion. These characteristics suggest that they play a key role in motion segment stability.

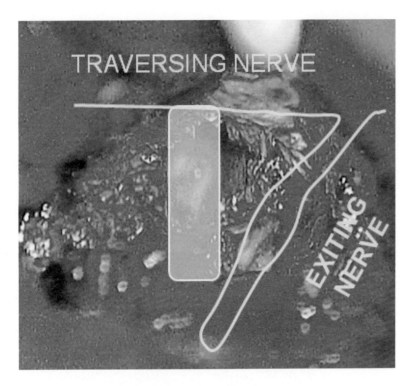

FIG 2 • Kambin triangle is a safe corridor to the disc space bounded medially by the traversing nerve root, superiorly by the exiting nerve root, and inferiorly by the pedicle.

PATIENT HISTORY AND PHYSICAL FINDINGS

▪ Earlier postoperative recovery with MIS TLIF is advantageous in elderly patients.

▪ Patients with severe osteoporosis are not ideal candidates for MIS TLIF because of the difficulty in avoiding endplate violation and subsequent graft subsidence.

▪ MIS TLIF is challenging in obese patients because of the difficulty in obtaining good radiographic imaging and the difficulty in manipulating instruments through a long working corridor. The advantages in terms of postoperative recovery, however, are most apparent in obese patients as the difference in the extent of soft tissue dissection between MIS and standard techniques is greatest.

▪ MIS TLIF can be a useful consideration in patients with previous midline surgery as dissection through scar tissue can be avoided. However, scar tissue from intracanal epidural bleeding at levels adjacent to previous surgery can complicate the exposure of Kambin triangle and extension of previous pedicle screw instrumentation can be challenging.

IMAGING AND OTHER DIAGNOSTIC STUDIES

▪ Pedicles should be evaluated radiographically prior to surgery to ensure that pedicle screw placement is feasible. If not, alternative means of fixation should be considered (eg, spinous process plate fixation).

▪ A narrow pelvis (decreased distance between the posterior iliac crests) can make medial angulation of lower lumbar pedicle screws challenging. A more medial starting point with a straightforward pedicle screw trajectory or alternative means of fixation may need to be considered in these situations.

▪ CT and MRI axial sections can be used to identify pedicle screw starting points and to approximate screw diameters and lengths.

▪ Nerve root anomalies can be identified on preoperative imaging and, if unilateral, should prompt consideration for MIS TLIF exposure on the contralateral side. Alternative techniques that do not require nerve root retraction can also be considered (eg, standard posterolateral fusion without interbody, anterior fusion through an anterior, or lateral retroperitoneal exposure with posterior MIS fusion and instrumentation, etc).

▪ TLIF, in general, should be pursued with care at the level of the cord or conus medullaris as the risk of significant neurologic injury is increased.

SURGICAL MANAGEMENT

▪ Indications
  ▪ One or two level lumbar pathology in the presence of:
    ▪ Spinal stenosis with instability (eg, degenerative or isthmic spondylolisthesis)
    ▪ Symptomatic degenerative disc disease
▪ Relative contraindications
  ▪ High-grade spondylolisthesis (Meyerding grade 3 or 4)
  ▪ Severe osteoporosis
  ▪ Nerve root anomalies
▪ There are multiple methods of performing an MIS TLIF. The different techniques are similar with respect to the decompression and discectomy but can differ with respect to the method used for distraction of the disc space, the fusion technique used to supplement the interbody fusion, and the instrumentation used for stabilization of the motion segment.
  ▪ The technique we describe involves subtotal discectomy using interbody spacer trials to sequentially distract the disc

space and contralateral facet fusion with bilateral pedicle screw placement.
■ Other methods using alternative techniques can be equally successful in properly selected patients.
  ■ The disc space can be distracted via the pedicle screws.
  ■ Posterior interlaminar or posterolateral bone graft can be used to supplement the interbody fusion.
  ■ Alternative means of posterior instrumentation/stabilization include unilateral pedicle screw placement, unilateral pedicle screw placement with a contralateral facet screw, unilateral pedicle screw placement with a spinous process plate, and isolated spinous process plate fixation.

Preoperative Planning

■ Patients should be evaluated for:
  ■ Osteoporosis
  ■ Potential issues with bone healing (nicotine use, diabetes mellitus, etc)
  ■ Previous surgery and the potential for epidural scarring
  ■ Obesity and retractor blade depth requirements
  ■ Need for contralateral decompression
■ Imaging should be evaluated for:
  ■ Mobility of the motion segment
  ■ Extent and nature of canal stenosis
    ■ Determines cranial/caudal extent of decompression
    ■ Need for osteophyte removal at the contralateral recess
  ■ Nerve root anomalies—best seen on T1-weighted axial imaging
  ■ Pedicle orientation, diameters, and pedicle screw lengths

Positioning

■ Patients are positioned prone on a radiolucent spine table. We prefer to position our patients using a Wilson frame attachment for the Jackson table to aid exposure of the

interlaminar window and distraction of the motion segment. With release of the disc space and careful attention to the radiographic alignment, we have not found inadvertent fusion in kyphosis to be an issue.
■ Upper limbs are carefully positioned to avoid iatrogenic injury (eg, brachial plexus palsy, ulnar nerve compression, rotator cuff tendinitis, etc).
■ Extension of the hips aids in obtaining lordotic alignment of the motion segment.
■ Flexion of the knees reduces root tension for the lower lumbar levels.
■ Room setup (**FIG 3**)
  ■ C-arm from opposite side of TLIF
    ■ This is a key point. With the C-arm coming in from the opposite side of the exposure, the C-arm base can be locked and the boom can be "wagged" in and out of the field. This allows for frequent imaging and decreases the need for the surgeon to step out of the surgical field. This is especially critical in the initial phases of the learning curve when frequent imaging is prudent.
  ■ Table mount on opposite side of TLIF at level of hip
  ■ Light source on same side of TLIF

Imaging

■ Consistent terms for intraoperative fluoroscopic imaging help in obtaining reproducible imaging. We use:
  ■ PUSH in/out
  ■ LEAN or TILT north/south (ie, toward the head/toward the feet)
  ■ RAINBOW over/under
  ■ MOVE north/south
  ■ WAG north/south
■ Properly aligned anteroposterior (AP) and lateral images are crucial for the MIS TLIF technique. The best method for identifying the "perfect" image, in our opinion, is to sequentially image from "imperfect" to "perfect" back to "imperfect."

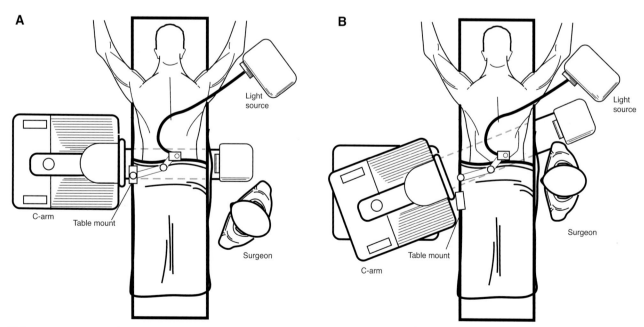

FIG 3 • Room Setup. The C-arm should come from the side opposite the surgeon. This allows the C-arm to be easily moved to the side ("wagged") allowing the surgeon access to the surgical exposure (3B). The C-arm can be brought back into position to expedite frequent imaging (3A).

PATIENT POSITIONING AND PLANNING OF INCISION SITES

- AP positioning
    - The C-arm should start in a direct upright position ("90-90").
    - The table should be rotated ("airplaned") until a perfectly rotated image is obtained. The C-arm should then be "tilted" until level endplates are obtained. The C-arm should not be "rainbowed."
    - A properly aligned AP image of the vertebral body should show the superior endplate as a single, dense line. The pedicles should be symmetric and located just below the superior endplate. The spinous process should be in the midline (although this can be misleading in the presence of scoliosis because of deformity of the spinous processes) (**TECH FIG 1**).
    - A horizontal line on the back marking the disc space can be used to guide the orientation of the C-arm for a properly aligned lateral image.
- A properly aligned lateral image should show the superior endplate as a single, dense line. The pedicles should be superimposed.
- For discs with significant angulation to a vertical plumb line (eg, L5–S1), the patient can be placed into reverse Trendelenburg to ease access to the disc.
- Planning incisions
    - Mark the center line on a properly aligned AP image (**TECH FIG 2**).
    - Mark two parallel paramedian lines approximately 4 cm lateral to the center line.
    - Using lateral imaging, mark the point in line with the disc space on the paramedian skin markings (**TECH FIG 3**).
    - This point will be the center of a 3-cm incision.

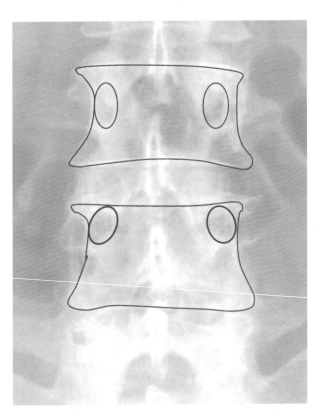

TECH FIG 1 • A "perfect" anteroposterior image of the vertebra should have the spinous process in the midline, the pedicles should be symmetric and just inferior to the superior endplate, and the superior endplate should be a single, dense line. The inferior vertebra (L4) in this image is a "perfect" anteroposterior image. The superior vertebra (L3) in this image is rotated—note the asymmetric pedicles.

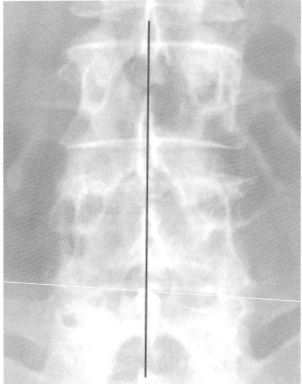

TECH FIG 2 • After a perfect anteroposterior image is obtained of the surgical levels, the midline is marked. Parallel lines 4 cm lateral to the midline are marked. Paramedian incisions (2.5 cm) will be made on these paramedian lines, with the midpoint of these incisions at a point in line with the disc space (on lateral imaging).

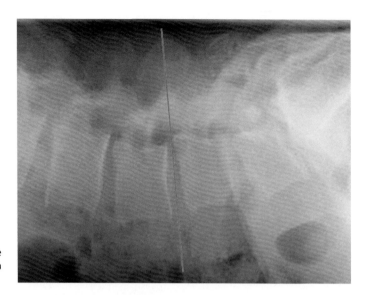

TECH FIG 3 • The point in line with the disc space marks the midpoint of the 2.5 cm paramedian skin incision.

EXPOSURE OF THE IPSILATERAL TLIF TARGET SITE

- The skin incision is made with a no. 11 blade followed by a fascial incision in line with skin incision. Finger dissection proceeds along the interval between the multifidus and longissimus to the lateral aspect of the facet joint (**TECH FIG 4**).
- The multifidus tendinous attachments at the target facet joint are released with a Cobb elevator using C-arm for localization. Because the facet joints at the lower lumbar levels are in close proximity due to the lordotic alignment of the lower lumbar spine, it is easy to inadvertently release the tendons from the wrong facet joint. This leads to increased bleeding and increased muscle

creep and can be avoided by careful fluoroscopic localization prior to tendon release.
- Release of the tendinous attachments at the facet joint allows the serial dilator tubes to "surround" the facet joint (**TECH FIG 5**). Twisting the dilators as they are placed aids in the release of the tendinous attachments.
- Blade lengths are measured at the lateral aspect of the dilator tube and the retractor with appropriately sized blades is placed over the dilators. Rotating the retractor back and forth as they are placed over the dilating tubes can be helpful—similar to the twisting motion used when pulling a tight ring off of one's finger.

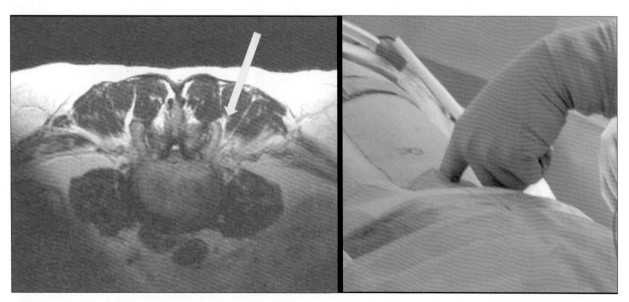

TECH FIG 4 • After the skin is incised, the paraspinal fascia is incised in line with the skin incision. Finger dissection then proceeds between the multifidus and longissimus muscles to the lateral aspect of the facet joint.

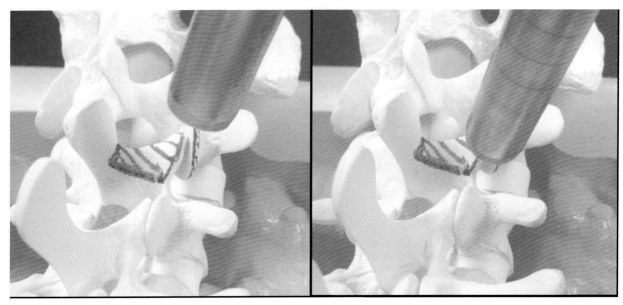

TECH FIG 5 • After the multifidus tendinous attachments are released from the facet joint, dilators are used to expand the surgical corridor and encircle the facet joint.

- The retractor blades should be positioned so that they are in line with the disc space and are directed medially toward the facet joint and base of the spinous process (**TECH FIG 6**).
- Key landmarks (**TECH FIG 7**)
  - Medially: base of spinous process
  - Laterally: facet joint line

- Minimizing retractor opening decreases amount of muscle creep.
- We prefer retractors with gaps between the retractor blades which allows for angulation of instrumentation (**TECH FIG 8**).

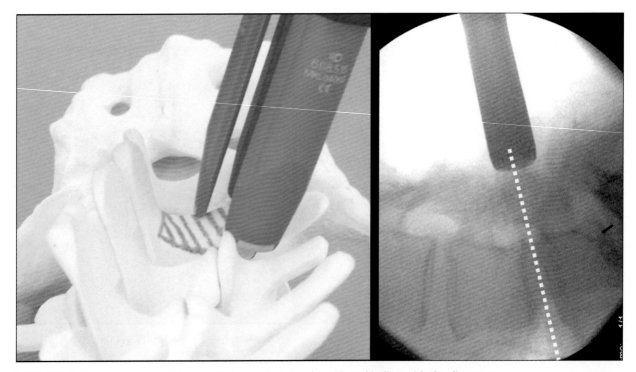

TECH FIG 6 • The retractor should be medially angulated and positioned in line with the disc space.

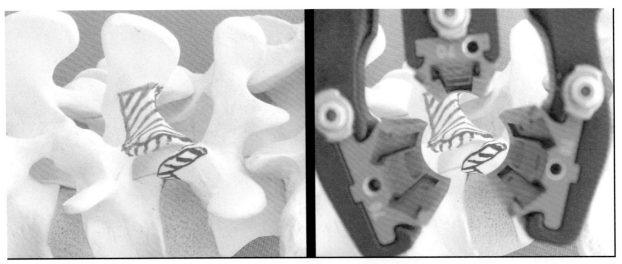

TECH FIG 7 • The key anatomic landmarks are the base of the spinous process medially and the facet joint line laterally. The amount of retractor blade distraction should be sufficient to visualize these landmarks but should be minimized as much as possible to avoid muscle creep.

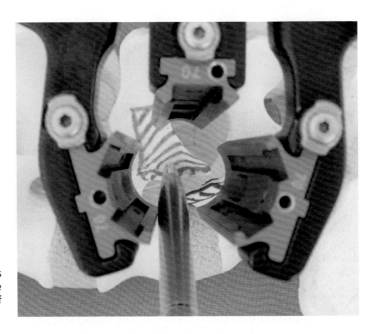

TECH FIG 8 • We prefer retractor with gaps between the retractor blades (as opposed to tube retractor systems) as they allow angulation of instruments within the working corridor.

FACETECTOMY AND CONTRALATERAL DECOMPRESSION

- Paraspinal muscle fibers within the surgical field are gently cauterized to expose the base of the spinous process and the facet joint.
- The facet joint line is identified (**TECH FIG 9**).
- The cranial limit of bony resection is sufficient to allow the residual pars to be inline with the inferior endplate of the cranial vertebra (**TECH FIG 10**).
- The ligamentum flavum is maintained for protection of the dural tube during removal of the inferior articular process.

- Ligamentum flavum is released with a curved curette and resected with Kerrison rongeurs to expose the dural tube.
- The contralateral ligamentum flavum and joint capsule are resected to achieve contralateral decompression (**TECH FIG 11**). Additional bone at the base of the spinous process can be removed if more access is needed to the contralateral side. The angulation of the retractor is the key to obtaining a surgical corridor that allows access to the contralateral lateral recess (**TECH FIG 12**). Alternatively, contralateral exposure can be used to decompress the contralateral lateral recess.

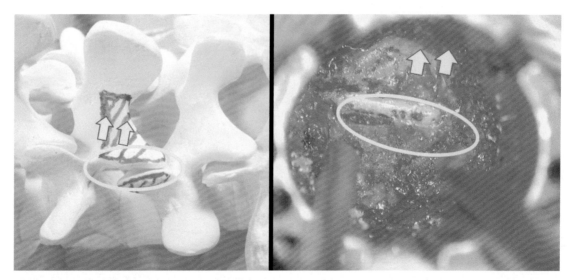

TECH FIG 9 • The facet joint line is a key anatomic landmark demarcating the lateral extent of exposure. The burr is used to remove bone from the inferolateral edge of the inferior articular process to the base of the spinous process.

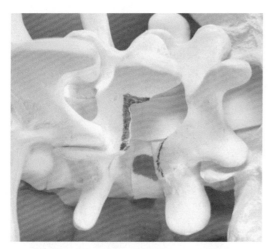

TECH FIG 10 • The inferior articular process and pars is resected, leaving a residual amount of pars sufficient to protect the dorsal root ganglion. Bone cranial to the pedicle (superior articular process) is completely resected.

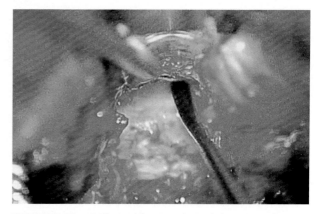

TECH FIG 11 • A thorough contralateral decompression can be performed via a unilateral exposure with appropriate angulation of the retractor.

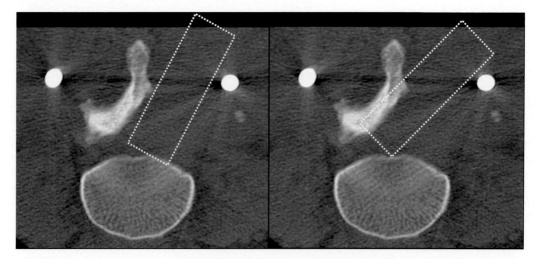

TECH FIG 12 • The retractor is angulated and bone resected from the base of the spinous process to allow adequate visualization of the contralateral lateral recess for decompression.

DISCECTOMY

- The retractor blades are maintained in line with the disc space but are redirected laterally towards Kambin triangle (**TECH FIG 13**).
- The superior articular process is removed up to the cranial aspect of the pedicle. Care must be taken to remove *all* bone cranial to the pedicle within the corridor used for interbody cage placement. Residual bone (typically at the lateral aspect of the SAP cranial to the pedicle) will cause the larger size cages to migrate medially into the traversing nerve root. When all bone cranial to the pedicle has been removed, retraction of the dural tube is not typically necessary for safe cage placement.
- The dural tube should be released from the posterior vertebral body to allow the traversing nerve root to move out of the way of the spacers/cage. This is especially important in revision settings when the dural tube is commonly adherent to the posterior vertebral bodies as a result of previous epidural bleeding and scarring and thus at increased risk for injury.
- The disc within Kambin triangle is exposed.
- Epidural veins are cauterized with bipolar electrocautery. The location of the traversing and exiting nerve roots should be assessed at all times to prevent inadvertent neural injury.
- A horizontal slit annulotomy is made with a no. 15 blade scalpel and is subsequently opened with a rotary shaver.

- Posterior disc osteophytes are removed with rongeurs/osteotomes. Removal of the posterior lips can ease access to the disc space (**TECH FIG 14**). We typically maintain the posterosuperior lip to decrease the chance for impingement of the exiting nerve root by the cage and the chance for cage migration posteriorly.
- Subtotal discectomy and endplate preparation is accomplished using a combination of straight and angled curettes and rasps.
  - Smooth rotating paddle sizers and spacer trials can be used to dilate and release disc space. We prefer to avoid use of the rotary shaver, especially in osteoporotic bone, because of the risk of endplate violation.
  - Fluoroscopic guidance can be used to ensure thorough discectomy. The most commonly missed portions of the disc are the ipsilateral lateral disc and the contralateral posterior disc.
  - Concave endplates can make discectomy challenging unless posterior osteophytes/lips are removed and/or the curettes are appropriately bent to accommodate the concavity.
  - Thorough release of the disc space and restoration of disc height aids in reduction of spondylolisthesis.

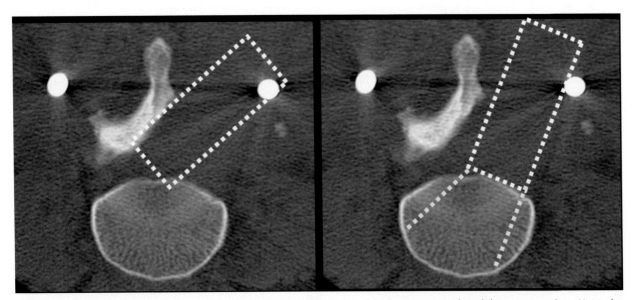

TECH FIG 13 • The retractor is then redirected to Kambin triangle for discectomy and endplate preparation. Note the difficult to access areas for discectomy: the ipsilateral lateral disc space and the contralateral posterior disc space.

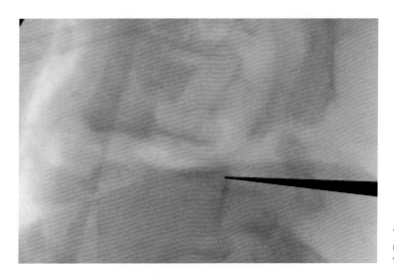

TECH FIG 14 • An osteotome can be used to remove the posterosuperior osteophyte from the caudal level to ease access to the disc space.

CAGE SELECTION AND INSERTION

- Trial spacers are sequentially trialed until good purchase is obtained. Undersizing the cage can increase the stress on posterior instrumentation, risking failure. Oversizing the cage risks endplate compromise and subsequent graft subsidence.
- Options for cage selection include oblique and banana-shaped cages.
  - Oblique cages are easier to insert but can have suboptimal purchase in the presence of concave endplates if the implant is not appropriately contoured.
  - Banana-shaped cages are more difficult to place but are more biomechanically sound. They are less likely to migrate posteriorly.
  - Bulleted cages (a modification for ease of insertion) should be used with caution as violation of the anterior annulus is possible with aggressive insertion.
  - A recent innovation is an expandable oblique cage that allow for cage insertion at a contracted height,

to minimize the risk of nerve root impingement, with the ability to expand once inserted into the disc space (**TECH FIG 15**).
- Bone graft is packed anteriorly within the disc space. A combination of local autograft bone together with allograft bone graft extender is used to fill the disc space.
- The cage is inserted with care taken to avoid impingement of both the traversing and exiting nerve root. The residual pars protects the exiting nerve root during cage insertion (**TECH FIG 16**).
- If endplate violation occurs and the cage settles into an endplate defect, there is a risk for graft subsidence. In this situation, the cage can be "pushed" to the contralateral side of the disc space using the trial spacers and a second cage can be inserted into the location of the endplate defect to prevent migration of the initial cage back into the defect.
- The annulotomy window is sealed with fibrin sealant.

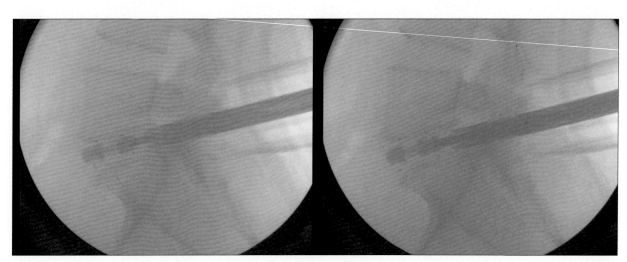

TECH FIG 15 • Expandable cage options are inserted at a contracted height to allow safer entry into the disc space with less chance for impingement of the traversing and exiting nerve roots. The cage is then expanded in the interbody space to restore disc height and obtain interbody cage purchase.

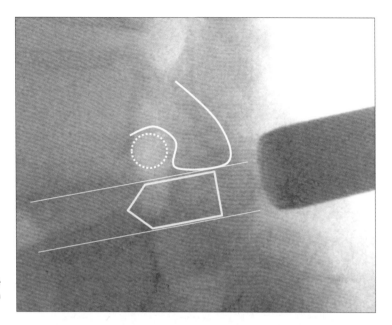

TECH FIG 16 • Maintaining the pars protects the exiting nerve root and dorsal root ganglion during cage insertion.

PEDICLE SCREW TRACT CANNULATION

- Bilateral pedicle screw placement is the most stable construct. A unilateral construct may be acceptable in a young patient with normal bone density and excellent pedicle screw purchase.
- Properly aligned AP images are obtained at the target vertebrae. This is the most crucial step for safe percutaneous pedicle screw placement. We prefer to cannulate all pedicles under AP imaging before moving to lateral imaging.
- A Jamshidi needle is docked at the appropriate starting point at the lateral margin of the pedicle. The anatomic starting point identified through palpation should match the radiographic starting point on imaging. If not, ensure that true AP imaging has been obtained (**TECH FIG 17**).
- The needle is gently tapped to seat the needle tip into the bone. A line is drawn on the needle shaft 20 mm above the skin. This represents the length of the pedicle, from the starting point to the base of the pedicle.

- The needle is aligned parallel to the endplate and held in the appropriate amount of mediolateral angulation for the level being performed. The needle is advanced toward the medial border of pedicle using gentle taps with the mallet. The tip should be just medial to the medial border of the pedicle when the 20 mm mark reaches the skin. On lateral imaging, the tip should be just past the posterior vertebral line (**TECH FIG 18**).
- Oblique imaging (bullseye imaging) is useful and is especially helpful for cannulating medially angulated L5 and S1 pedicles and checking for medial and lateral breaches.
  - Starting with the AP view, the C-arm is angulated 15 degrees in the axial plane ("rainbowed") to line the beam up with the pedicle axis.

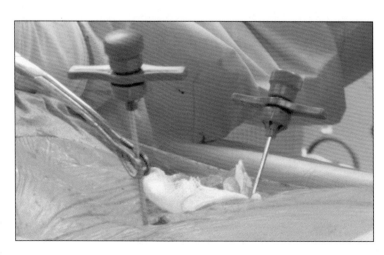

TECH FIG 17 • Jamshidi needles are docked on the radiographic pedicle starting points and their positions checked on anteroposterior fluoroscopy.

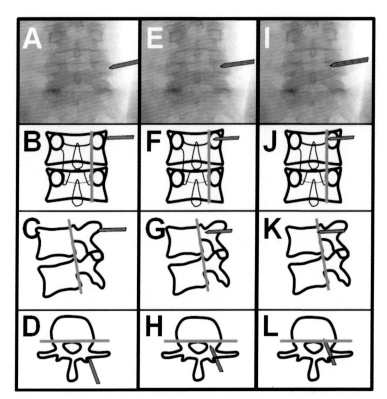

TECH FIG 18 • Traversing the pedicle with a Jamshidi needle radiographically requires an understanding of the anatomic correlates to radiographic imaging findings. Once the Jamshidi needle has approached the medial pedicle wall on anteroposterior imaging, it should be just ventral to the posterior vertebral body wall on lateral imaging.

- The needle should be advanced down the center of the radiographic pedicle, keeping the needle shaft in line with the C-arm beam.
- Guidewires are placed after ensuring that there is an adequate fascial incision to accommodate placement of the pedicle screw (muscle/fascia can become entrapped underneath the head of the pedicle screw). Guidewires are inserted past the tip of the Jamshidi needle into "crunchy" cancellous bone. If the bone is too hard to manually insert the guidewire, a needle driver clamped to the guidewire 5 mm above the top of the Jamshidi needle can be gently tapped with a mallet (**TECH FIG 19**). After checking guidewire positioning on lateral imaging, screw lengths can be determined.

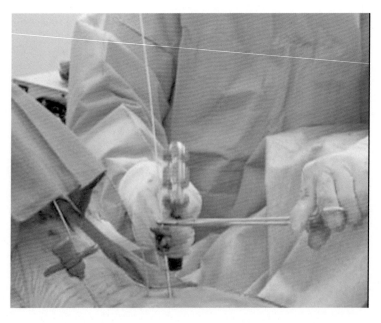

TECH FIG 19 • Uncontrolled advancement of the guidewire risks catastrophic vascular or visceral injury. Grasping the guidewire with a needle driver 5 to 10 mm above the Jamshidi needle followed by gentle tapping of the needle driver allows for controlled insertion of the guidewire.

TAPPING AND INSERTION OF SCREWS

- Cannulas are used to dilate the muscle around the guidewire.
- The pedicle is tapped over the guidewire. We typically undertap by 1 mm. Tapping should be done under fluoroscopic imaging to prevent potentially catastrophic advancement of the guidewire.
- The tap can be tested for pedicle breach with triggered electromyography.
  - Threshold values (8 to 10 mA) should prompt placement of a screw with the same diameter as the tap to avoid breaching the pedicle.
  - Electrodiagnostic evidence of pedicle breach should prompt careful radiographic assessment of the pedicle

screw tract with AP and oblique imaging. Redirecting the guidewire or aborting screw placement should be considered if there is concern for pedicle breach.
- Screws are placed over the guidewire, again, under fluoroscopic imaging to prevent inadvertent guidewire advancement (**TECH FIG 20**). The guidewire can be removed once the screw tip is past the posterior vertebral body wall.
- Insert screws deep to avoid prominent hardware. The radiographic projection of the transverse process can aid in proper placement with regard to depth (**TECH FIG 21**). If two levels are being performed and segmental fixation is desired, care must be taken to properly align screw heights to achieve a smooth contour for rod seating.

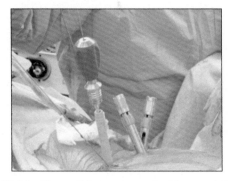

TECH FIG 20 • The pedicles are tapped with cannulated taps, neuromonitoring is checked, and then screws are inserted. This should be done under lateral imaging to monitor for inadvertent advancement of the guidewire.

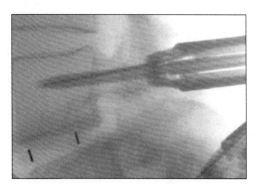

TECH FIG 21 • Guidewires should be removed once the screw tip is 5 mm past the posterior vertebral body wall to minimize the chances of the guidewire binding within the screw cannula and inadvertently advancing. Screws should be inserted deep to avoid prominent hardware; the radiographic transverse process can be a useful guide. For multilevel fusions with segmental instrumentation, screws should be inserted to a depth where the polyaxial motion of the screw head is maintained to ease rod insertion and capture.

ROD PASSAGE

- The rod length is determined with MIS calipers.
- If necessary, the rod should be contoured after attachment to its holder to prevent issues with the attachment mechanism.
- The rods are passed under the fascia and through the rod sleeves under lateral fluoroscopic imaging (**TECH FIG 22**).

Entrapment of fascia underneath the screw heads/rod must be avoided as this can result in severe postoperative pain.
- Confirm rods are seated within the sleeves, visually or with a tester.

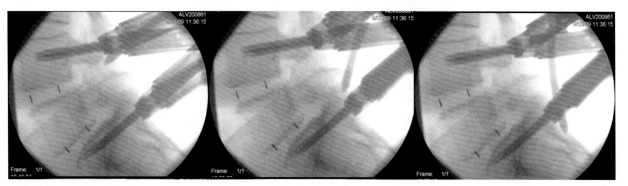

TECH FIG 22 • Appropriate length rods are contoured and then introduced into the screw sleeves, reduced into the screw heads, and captured with set screws.

ROD REDUCTION

- A rod reducer can be used to reduce the rod to the screw heads. If this is difficult, ensure that polyaxial motion of the screw heads is present. This may necessitate slight backing out of the screw.
- Screw caps are placed and compression or distraction can then be performed as needed.

- The rod sleeves are removed and a final check for entrapment of the muscle/fascia is done prior to closure.
- If reduction of a spondylolisthesis is desired, the rods can be fixed into the caudal vertebrae and the pedicle screws from the cranial vertebra can be reduced to the rod. This technique is dependent on good screw purchase to prevent pullout (**TECH FIG 23**).

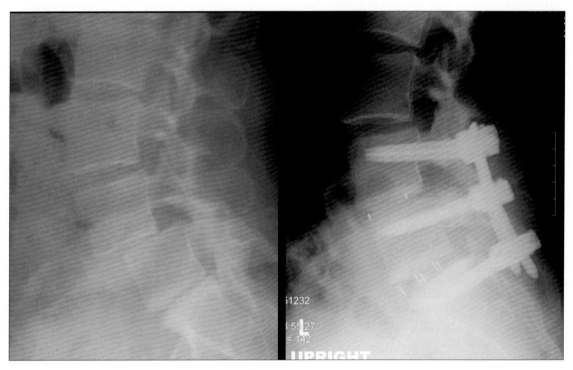

TECH FIG 23 • Reduction of spondylolisthesis at L4–5 using rod reduction technique after thorough discectomy and minimally invasive interbody cage placement.

CLOSURE

- The surgical sites are compressed for 2 to 3 minutes to tamponade muscle bleeders.
- The epidural space is checked. We typically do not find it necessary to use a subfascial drain.
- Muscle fascia is closed with 0 Vicryl on a tapered needle.

- The surgical sites are compressed again for 2 to 3 minutes.
- The dermis is closed with 2-0 Vicryl on a tapered needle.
- A topical skin adhesive (eg, Dermabond) is used to seal the skin.

INCIDENTAL DUROTOMY

- The patient can be placed into Trendelenburg to minimize leakage.
- A suture repair is performed, if possible.
- If suture repair is not possible, for small durotomies (less than 5 mm), we have found a layered patch to be effective. A collagen matrix patch (eg, Duragen) is sealed with fibrin glue (eg, Tisseel). This is repeated with

progressively larger collagen matrix patches. We typically use three layers (ie, patch, fibrin glue, second patch, fibrin glue, third patch, fibrin glue).

- Cerebrospinal fluid leakage is rarely a problem because of the minimal dead space.
- Patients are placed supine with the head of bed flat postoperatively for 24 hours.

PEARLS AND PITFALLS

Patient selection	■ As with all spinal surgery, proper patient selection is the key to successful outcomes. Osteoporotic patients, obese patients, and patients with isthmic spondylolisthesis are challenging and should be avoided during the initial learning curve for this minimally invasive technique.
C-arm placement	■ The C-arm should be placed on the opposite side of the TLIF exposure to ease use of frequent imaging.
Retractor positioning for contralateral decompression	■ The angulation of the retractor is the key to obtaining adequate exposure to perform a contralateral decompression. Removal of the base of the spinous process can aid in obtaining adequate visualization.
Preservation of pars	■ Preserving the pars helps avoid impingement of the exiting nerve root during cage placement.
Removal of bone superolateral to pedicle	■ Ensuring removal of ALL bone superolateral to the pedicle clears the corridor for cage placement and prevents medial migration of the cage into the traversing root during insertion.
Removal of posterior lip	■ Lessens the risk of endplate disruption from discectomy instrumentation and eases graft sizing and placement.
Endplate violation	■ Avoid aggressive use of discectomy instruments, especially in osteoporotic patients. If an endplate defect occurs, placement of a second cage may be helpful to avoid graft subsidence.
Pedicle cannulation	■ Properly aligned AP and lateral imaging is crucial to safe pedicle screw placement. Serial imaging going from "imperfect" to "perfect" back to "imperfect," improves identification of "perfect" imaging. Oblique imaging is useful for medially angulated pedicles.
Inadvertent guidewire advancement	■ Images should be taken frequently during tapping and screw placement.
Muscle/fascia entrapment	■ Entrapment of muscle/fascia should be checked for prior to closure.

POSTOPERATIVE CARE

■ Perioperative antibiotic prophylaxis.

■ Patients are mobilized early (ie, day of surgery, if possible)

■ Antispasmodic medications are a useful addition to the postoperative pain control regimen.

■ Oral steroids can be used for postoperative radiculitis. This should be a diagnosis of exclusion; new or unexpected postoperative neurologic symptoms or signs should be investigated with imaging.

OUTCOMES

■ The literature supports earlier postoperative recovery, less blood loss, and decreased rates of infection in comparison to standard TLIF. Fusion rates are comparable to open posterior interbody fusion techniques.

COMPLICATIONS

▫ Infection
  ▫ The risk of infection with MIS TLIF appears to be decreased in comparison to standard techniques.
▫ Bleeding
  ▫ Bleeding is rarely enough to require transfusion.
  ▫ Epidural bleeding can lead to epidural hematoma. Risk of epidural hematoma is minimized with judicious use of subfascial drains.
▫ Nerve injury
  ▫ Releasing the dural tube from the posterior vertebral body minimizes the risk of injury to the traversing nerve root during cage insertion.

▫ Maintaining the pars minimizes the risk of injury to the exiting nerve root during cage insertion.

▫ The procedure may need to be aborted or done on the contralateral side if conjoined or anomalous nerve root anatomy is identified.

▫ New or unexpected postoperative neurologic deficit should be worked up expeditiously. Re-exploration to evacuate epidural hematoma and ensure there is no neural entrapment should be considered in the perioperative period as necessary.

▫ Cerebrospinal fluid leakage
  ▫ Suture is usually not necessary. Most durotomies tend to be small and can be sealed with layered collagen matrix patch and fibrin sealant.

▫ Hardware issues
  ▫ Graft subsidence can occur with endplate violation and can subsequently lead to pedicle screw failure. Care must be taken to avoid endplate violation, especially with elderly osteoporotic patients.
  ▫ Pedicle screw breach is possible. Medial breaches may occur more frequently in comparison to standard techniques because of the ease of medial angulation through the paramedian exposure. Accurate radiographic views are crucial. Neuromonitoring is a useful adjunct. Neuromonitoring of the tap does not preclude breach by the screw.
  ▫ Adjacent segment deterioration
  ▫ May be minimized in comparison to standard techniques as a result of the preservation of adjacent segment musculotendinous attachments. Compromise of the cranial facet during screw placement must be avoided.

REFERENCES

1. Dhall SS, Wang MY, Mummaneni PV. Clinical and radiographic comparison of mini-open transforaminal lumbar interbody fusion with open transforaminal lumbar interbody fusion in 42 patients with long-term follow-up. J Neurosurg Spine 2008;9(6):560–565.
2. Karikari IO, Isaacs RE. Minimally invasive transforaminal lumbar interbody fusion: a review of techniques and outcomes. Spine (Phila Pa 1976) 2010;35(26)(suppl):S294–S301.
3. McGirt MJ, Parker SL, Lerner J, et al. Comparative analysis of perioperative surgical site infection after minimally invasive versus open posterior/transforaminal lumbar interbody fusion: analysis of hospital billing and discharge data from 5170 patients. J Neurosurg Spine 2011;14(6):771–778.
4. Kim CW, Garfin SR, Fessler RG. Rationale of minimally invasive spine surgery. In: Herkowitz HN, Garfin SR, Eismont FJ, et al, eds. *Rothman-Simeone The Spine*. 6th ed. Philadelphia, PA: Elsevier Saunders; 2011:998–1006.

Chapter 20

Minimally Invasive Lumbar Microdiscectomy and Laminectomy

David Greg Anderson, Christopher K. Kepler, and Victor M. Popov

DEFINITION

▪ Lumbar microdiscectomy is the most common spinal operation.[1]

▪ Lumbar spinal stenosis is the most common indication for spinal surgery in elderly patients.[1]

▪ The pathology of lumbar spinal stenosis is a combination of degenerative changes involving the disc space, facet joints, and ligamentum flavum, which ultimately leads to compression of the neural elements and in some cases neurogenic symptoms.[2]

▪ Studies have shown favorable outcomes from surgery for patients with herniated disc disease and lumbar stenosis.[1,3,4]

▪ Minimally invasive surgical decompression has been shown to decrease perioperative morbidity and quicken patient recovery.[2,5,6]

▪ This chapter reviews the technique of performing lumbar decompressions for herniated disc disease and lumbar stenosis using a minimally invasive approach.

HISTORY AND PHYSICAL FINDINGS

▪ Although the exact clinical presentation varies from person to person, most patients with herniated disc disease and lumbar stenosis present with pain radiating into the lower extremities.

▪ The classic presentation of herniated disc disease involves pain radiating into a single extremity along a specific dermatomal distribution. There are often associated neurologic findings, including changes in strength, sensation, and reflexes.

▪ The classic presentation of lumbar stenosis is neurogenic claudication which involves crampy pain radiating into one or both extremities when standing and walking. The pain commonly progresses from proximal to distal and is improved or relieved by spinal flexion (ie, leaning forward or sitting down). This is in contrast to vascular claudication which is relieved by standing still. Significant neurologic deficits in lumbar stenosis are uncommon; however, those with herniated disc disease will commonly show changes in reflexes, motor, and sensory functioning. Acute loss of bowel or bladder control in the setting of significant compression of the cauda equina is a surgical emergency.

▪ Nonsurgical measures that may be considered for both herniated disc disease and lumbar stenosis include nonsteroidal anti-inflammatory drugs, epidural steroids, and physical therapy.

SURGICAL MANAGEMENT

Preoperative Planning

▪ Surgical intervention may be considered for patients with severe, ongoing symptoms of leg pain that are unresponsive to nonsurgical therapy.

▪ It is important to demonstrate anatomic compression of lumbar nerve roots in a distribution that correlates to the clinical symptoms. This is usually done with either MRI or CT myelography.

Setup

▪ The procedure is typically done under general anesthesia, although epidural or spinal anesthesia may be used according to surgeon preference.

▪ Prior to surgery, prophylactic antibiotics and lower extremity compression stockings are administered.

▪ The patient is positioned prone on a spinal frame which allows fluoroscopic imaging of the spine (**FIG 1**).

▪ Care should be taken to ensure no compression of the abdominal region.

▪ Care should be taken to ensure accessibility for fluoroscopic imaging.

▪ A standard sterile prep and drape of the lumbar region is performed.

Localization of the Incision

▪ Palpable landmarks including posterior superior iliac spine, intercrestal line, and spinous processes are demarcated and used to determine the approximate level for the skin incision.

▪ A spinal needle is introduced lateral to the midline in the proposed location of the surgical incision and directed to avoid penetration of the spinal canal (to minimize inadvertent penetration of the dura) (**FIG 2**).

▪ The C-arm is used to obtain a lateral projection of the spine and spinal needle so the location and trajectory of the needle can be used to plan the incision.

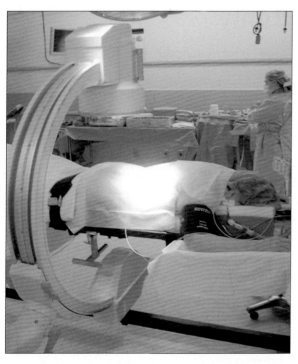

FIG 1 • Positioning of the patient in the prone position on a radiolucent operative table.

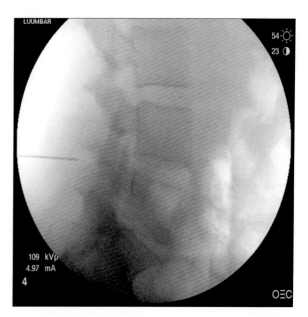

FIG 2 • Spinal needle is used to demarcate the proposed location for the surgical incision.

Placement of the Tubular Retractor

- A skin incision equal in length to the diameter of the tubular retractor is made through the skin and underlying fascia. The incision is placed lateral to the spinous process.
- In cases of herniated disc disease, the incision is made on the side of the herniation.
- In cases of lumbar stenosis, the incision is positioned on the side that will give the best access to both sides of the spinal canal or will allow decompression of the region of symptomatic stenosis without sacrificing excessive facet joint or over thinning the pars interarticularis region.
- For ipsilateral decompression, the skin incision is generally positioned about 1.5 to 2 cm from the midline.

- For bilateral decompression, the skin incision is generally positioned 3 to 4 cm lateral to the midline to allow angulation of the tubular retractor across the midline to reach the contralateral side of the spinal canal.
- A small Cobb elevator is used to elevate the periosteum at the site of the operative exposure (**TECH FIG 1**). The authors prefer to use this rather than dilation over a K-wire which has the risk of penetrating the dura and is less effective in creating the working space adjacent to the lamina.
- Dilators are placed through the incision to expand the operative portal (**TECH FIG 2**).

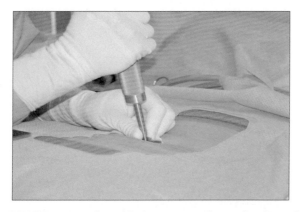

TECH FIG 1 • Use of a Cobb elevator to perform subperiosteal dissection.

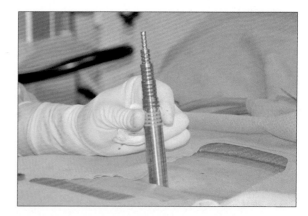

TECH FIG 2 • Serial dilators are placed to allow placement of the tubular retractor.

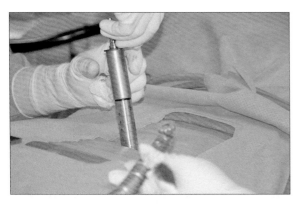

TECH FIG 3 • Placement of the tubular retractor.

■ A tubular retractor of appropriate length is selected and placed over the dilators to the level of the spine (**TECH FIG 3**).

■ The diameter of the tubular retractor used depends on the nature of the planned surgical procedure. As a general rule, a 14- to 18-mm diameter tubular retractor is used for a microdiscectomy procedure, whereas an 18- to 20-mm tubular retractor is used for spinal stenosis cases.

■ The tubular retractor is secured to the table-mounted retractor holder and the position of the retractor is verified with lateral fluoroscopy (**TECH FIG 4**).

■ If necessary, the position of the tubular retractor is adjusted to allow optimal access to the spinal pathology.

■ Use of a sharp K-wire prior to sequential dilation is avoided as an incidental dural puncture can occur.

■ An appropriate length of the tubular retractor should reach from the skin edge to the spine to minimize soft tissue creep at the base of the retractor.

Visualization Through the Tubular Retractor

■ An operative microscope is focused on the tissue at the base of the tubular retractor (**TECH FIG 5**).

■ The residual soft tissue at the base of the tubular retractor should be resected with electrocautery to allow good visualization of the bony elements (**TECH FIG 6**).

■ Care should be taken to avoid injury to the facet joint capsule during soft tissue clearance.

Ipsilateral Decompression

■ Prior to beginning the decompression, the inferior edge of the lamina, underlying ligamentum flavum, and medial portion of the facet joint should be identified

■ It is helpful to palpate the lateral edge of the pars intra-articularis to avoid excessive resection of bone which could result in an iatrogenic pars fracture.

■ The ligamentum flavum is released from the undersurface of the lamina using a curved curette

■ The medial lamina is removed using a Kerrison rongeur.

■ The ligamentum flavum is traversed with a straight curette by dividing the ligamentum inline with its fibers.

■ The ligamentum flavum is resected as necessary to visualize and remove the spinal pathology.

■ The pedicle is identified by palpation within the spinal canal and used as a landmark for identification of the spinal pathology.

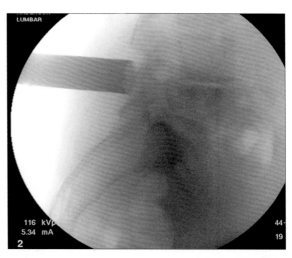

TECH FIG 4 • Lateral fluoroscopic image to confirm appropriate level and position of the tubular retractor.

■ The ventral surface of the spinal canal and intervertebral discs can be visualized by gentle retraction of the dura.

■ Any sequestered disc material is removed by "sweeping" the free disc fragments into the laminotomy site using a ball-tipped probe.

■ Extruded disc material is generally removed by breaking the thin, inflammatory membrane over the herniation with a Penfield no. 4 instrument and working through the existing annular tear.

■ The use of large annular incisions is discouraged as they may predispose to recurrent disc herniation.

■ If lateral recess stenosis is present, the medial portion of the superior articular process is trimmed using a curved tip Kerrison rongeur.

■ Ipsilateral foraminal stenosis can also be addressed by using a curved tip Kerrison rongeur to trim the superior tip of the superior articular process.

■ After an adequate decompression of the neural elements has been achieved and confirmed with palpation using a ball-tipped probe, hemostasis of the wound should be achieved prior to closure.

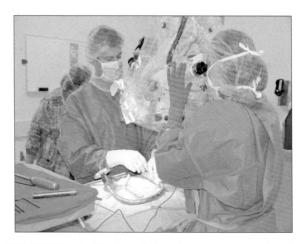

TECH FIG 5 • Positioning of the microscope to visualize the tissue at the base of the tubular retractor.

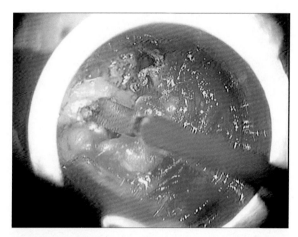

TECH FIG 6 • Use of the electrocautery to clear soft tissue and expose the bony anatomy.

- Avoid over thinning the inferior articular process or pars interarticularis which may fracture leading to instability or persistent pain.
- If the high-speed burr (drill) is to be used to thin the bone prior to resection, leave the ligamentum flavum intact during drilling to protect the dura (**TECH FIG 7**). The authors prefer to use a 3-mm round burr rather than a matchstick style of burr, as it is felt to be more controllable, especially when "end cutting."
- Palpate between the dura and the overlying bone to ensure that an adequate plane exists prior to resection of the bone, as this will lessen the risk of an iatrogenic dural laceration.
- Neovascularization around the nerve root can easily be appreciated while working under the microscope and is a good clinical sign of a symptomatic lesion.

Bilateral Decompression Through a Unilateral Tubular Approach

- When stenotic changes affect both sides of the spinal canal and cause bilateral neurogenic symptoms, a bilateral decompression of the neural elements should be performed (**TECH FIG 8**).

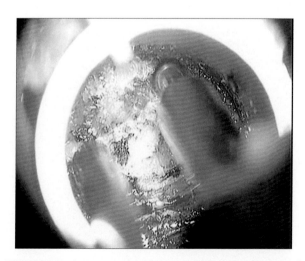

TECH FIG 7 • Intraoperative photograph depicting the use of a high-speed burr/drill to thin the lamina.

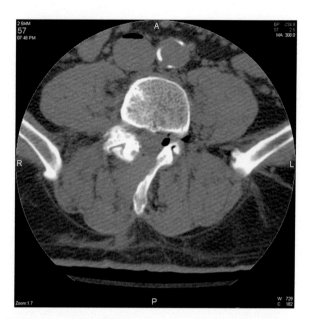

TECH FIG 8 • Bilateral decompression of the spinal canal is accomplished by drilling away the base of the spinous process and traversing to the contralateral side of the spinal canal. The contralateral facet is trimmed as needed to decompression the spinal canal. The tube is then redirected and the ipsilateral side of the spinal canal is decompressed until the dura is free of any compression.

- The side of the incision is generally chosen to allow optimal access to the pathology, remembering that foraminal stenosis is often easiest to decompress on the contralateral side.
- The incision is localized in a fashion similar to the unilateral decompression, but is placed 3 to 4 cm lateral to the midline to allow the tubular retractor to be angulated to reach the contralateral side of the spinal canal.
- After docking the tubular retractor on the lamina and confirming the localization of the tubular retractor with fluoroscopy, an ipsilateral bony laminotomy is performed leaving the ligamentum in place.
- The tubular retractor is then angled toward the contralateral side of the spinal canal and the operating table is tilted to provide the most direct microscopic visualization of the contralateral side.
- Drilling is carried out to provide access to the contralateral side of the spinal canal by removal of the base of the spinous process and the undersurface of the contralateral lamina.
- As the drilling proceeds, the surgeon will notice the cancellous bone of the inferior articular process.
- The drilling should continue until the facet joint is thin enough that it can be trimmed (medial facetectomy) with a Kerrison rongeur.
- Throughout drilling, the ligamentum flavum should be preserved to protect the underlying dura.
- On the contralateral side, the ligamentum flavum is released ventral to the facet joint and the thickness of the residual facet joint can be palpated and assessed.
- After the facet joint is sufficiently thinned and drilling is completed, a curette is used to release the bony attachments of the ligamentum flavum which is then removed.

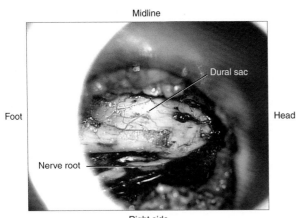

Midline

Dural sac

Foot

Head

Nerve root

Right side

- The contralateral pedicle is identified by palpation.
- The exiting and traversing nerve roots are identified.
- Bone and ligament decompression is achieved as needed to decompress the neural structures (**TECH FIG 9**).
- After completion of the contralateral decompression, the tubular retractor is wanded back to the ipsilateral side. Decompression of the ipsilateral side is then achieved in a similar manner as described.
- Meticulous hemostasis is performed, followed by tube withdrawal and wound closure.

TECH FIG 9 • Adequate decompression is achieved when no further compression of the dura is present.

WOUND CLOSURE

- Deep tissue (thoracolumbar fascia, if possible) is closed with interrupted suture followed by closure of the subcutaneous tissue and skin. The subcutaneous incision is infiltrated with a long-acting local anesthetic agent and a surgical dressing is placed.

POSTOPERATIVE CARE

- Routine postanesthesia recovery is performed. The patient is then mobilized for ambulation and activities of daily living.
- Discharge is generally performed on the day of surgery. A 30-minute per day walking program is recommended.
- Pain management is achieved with either a mild oral narcotic or an over-the-counter medication, such as ibuprofen or acetaminophen, depending on the patient's individual pain control requirements.
- An office visit and wound check is performed 10 to 14 days after surgery.
- Early outpatient physical therapy to assist in rehabilitation is often recommended.

OUTCOMES

- Studies have reported improved outcomes with surgery when compared to nonoperative modalities with respect to walking, endurance, and pain control.[1,3,4]
- Minimally invasive procedures have been shown to provide symptomatic relief at least equivalent to open procedures and are associated with reduced blood loss and shorter hospital stays.[7–12]
- With a minimally invasive approach, less blood loss, less postoperative pain, and a shorter hospitalization are anticipated.[2,5,10]

COMPLICATIONS

- As with all surgical procedures, complications occur with minimally invasive decompression procedures.
- The incidence of problems can be minimized, with careful technique and experience with these procedures.
- The incidence of dural tear varies but has been reported to be as high as 16% in one study. No long-term sequelae were noted in these patients.[2] When using a tubular retractor, very little soft tissue dead space is created and thus the incidence of pseudomeningocele or dural-cutaneous fistula is very low even if formal dural suture repair is not utilized.
- Small dural tears with no nerve rootlet extrusion may be successfully treated with a small pledget of Gelfoam followed by dural sealant.[4]
- Larger tears or those with exposed nerve roots should undergo a formal dural repair with suture in a water tight fashion.
- Suture repair should be accomplished working through the tubular retractor using a micropituitary instrument as a needle holder and using double armed 6-0 Gore-Tex suture. An arthroscopic knot pusher is used to tie knots during the repair.
- Infection rates from tubular decompression surgery are very low. In the rare event of a wound infection, treatment with debridement and appropriate antibiotic therapy should be employed.

CONCLUSION

- Minimally invasive surgery for lumbar spinal stenosis is an effective and safe procedure with many advantages compared with traditional open lumbar decompression.
- One of the major drawbacks with this approach is the need for the surgeon to overcome the learning curve.

REFERENCES

1. Atlas SJ, Keller RB, Robson D, et al. Surgical and nonsurgical management of lumbar spinal stenosis: four-year outcomes from the Maine Lumbar Spine Study. Spine 2000;25(5):556–562.
2. Khoo LT, Fessler RG. Microendoscopic decompressive laminotomy for the treatment of lumbar stenosis. Neurosurgery 2002;51(suppl 5): S146–S154.

3. Atlas SJ, Keller RB, Wu Y, et al. Long-term outcomes of surgical and nonsurgical management of lumbar spinal stenosis: 8–10 year results from the Maine Lumbar Spine Study. Spine 2005;30(8):936–943.

4. Turner JA, Ersek M, Herron L, et al. Surgery for lumbar spinal stenosis, attempted meta-analysis of the literature. Spine 1992;17(1):1–8.

5. Asgarzadie F, Khoo LT. Minimally invasive operative management for lumbar spinal stenosis: overview of early and long-term outcomes. Orthop Clin N Am 2007;38(3):387–399.

6. Palmer S, Turner R, Palmer R. Bilateral decompression of lumbar spinal stenosis involving a unilateral approach with microscope and tubular retractor system. J Neurosurg (Spine 2) 2002; 97(2 suppl):213–217.

7. Guiot BH, Khoo LT, Fessler RG. A minimally invasive technique for decompression of the lumbar spine. Spine 2002;27(4):432–438.

8. Benz RJ, Garfin SR. Current techniques of decompression of the lumbar spine. CORR 2001;(384):75–81.

9. Rosen DS, O'Toole JE, Eichholz KM, et al. Minimally invasive lumbar spinal decompression in the elderly: outcomes of 50 patients aged 75 years and older. Neurosurgery 2007;60(3):503–508.

10. Podichetty VK, Spear J, Isaacs RE, et al. Complications associated with minimally invasive decompression for lumbar spinal stenosis. J Spinal Disord Tech 2006;19(3):161–166.

11. Riew KD, Rhee JM. Microsurgical techniques in lumbar spinal stenosis. Instr Course Lect 2002;51:247–253.

12. Park P, Foley KT. Minimally invasive transforaminal lumbar interbody fusion with reduction of spondylolisthesis: technique and outcomes after a minimum of 2 years' follow-up. Neurosurg Focus 2008; 25(2):E16.

Chapter 21

Percutaneous Pedicle Screw Fixation and Fusion for Trauma

David H. Wei, Kelley Banagan, and Steven C. Ludwig

DEFINITION

- The advancement of minimally invasive techniques in spinal surgery, specifically percutaneous pedicle screw fixation, has reduced approach-related morbidity.
- These techniques have been shown to be advantageous in patients with spine tumors and deformities and have become increasingly applicable for managing complex spinal trauma, including thoracolumbar trauma.
- The goals of treatment of traumatic spine fracture remain the same whether an open or percutaneous approach is used: stabilize the spine to facilitate rehabilitation, enhance neurological recovery, and prevent neurological deterioration, delayed pain, and postoperative deformity.

ANATOMY

- Traditional open posterior surgical approaches can result in extensive soft tissue damage, muscle denervation, and ischemia, with subsequent paraspinal muscular atrophy and decreased strength.
- In addition, open approaches can lead to increased blood loss, protracted postoperative pain, and higher infection rates.
- In contrast, minimally invasive procedures involve less extensile and thus less disruptive dissection. Important relevant anatomy and anatomic landmarks are discussed in following text.

PATHOGENESIS

- The most common mechanisms of traumatic injury to the thoracolumbar spine are motor vehicle accidents, falls from height, and domestic violence.
- When traumatic injury results in spinal cord injury, the loss of neurological function is attributed to both a primary and a secondary injury process.
- The primary injury is sustained when the spinal cord and column absorb energy from the trauma, with resultant spinal deformation, and persistent postinjury compression.
- A cascade of secondary effects ensue, including vascular changes, cell membrane lipid peroxidation, free radical formation, electrolyte shifts, neurotransmitter accumulation, and inflammation. This cascade results in expansion of the initial area of injury in a rostrocaudal fashion, leading to further gray matter loss and white matter degeneration.

IMAGING AND OTHER DIAGNOSTIC STUDIES

- Preoperative advanced imaging is a critical tool for understanding the patient's pathoanatomy and preoperative planning.
- Commonly, CT scans and MRIs are obtained to assess bony and spinal cord injury, respectively.
- Additionally, MRIs can be used to assess the competency of the posterior ligamentous structures, which can assist in determining the overall stability of the injury.

- Using preoperative images as a guide, the fluoroscope can then be precisely rotated in the axial plane to the degree of medial angulation seen on axial view CT scans or MRIs at the respective level.

NONOPERATIVE MANAGEMENT

- Thoracolumbar trauma has historically been managed with conservative treatment in the form of traction, casting, and bed rest.
- However, nonoperative treatment can be complicated by the morbidities associated with prolonged immobilization.
- With the development of minimally invasive spine surgery (MISS), we have learned that decreased surgical time, decreased blood loss, and a reduction in postoperative surgical site infection can decrease surgical morbidity in patients with multiple traumatic injuries.[2]
- The application of these principles in the setting of spine trauma offers the patient earlier mobilization and rehabilitation.
- Recent evidence suggests that benefits of MISS include decreased incidence of pneumonia, decreased length of stay in the intensive care unit, shorter number of ventilator-dependent days, and decreased hospital charges.[3–6]

SURGICAL MANAGEMENT

- Indications for minimally invasive percutaneous pedicle screw fixation continue to be established.
- Multiple variables are important when considering surgical intervention, including fracture morphology, neurological involvement, and the status of the posterior ligamentous complex.
- The Thoracolumbar Injury Classification and Severity Score can be used to help guide the surgeon's decision-making process for operative versus nonoperative fracture management.
- Once the decision for surgical intervention has been made, the relative indications for minimally invasive techniques include unstable thoracolumbar burst fractures, stable burst fractures for which conservative treatment has failed, flexion-distraction injuries, extension-distraction injuries, unstable sacral fractures requiring lumbopelvic stabilization, and fracture-dislocations.

Preoperative Planning

- Before the surgical procedure, a thorough understanding of the patient's surgical anatomy is essential because traditional visual and tactile landmarks for pedicular fixation are not present. Thus, without optimal preoperative flouroscopic visualization, the surgeon must keep in mind the potential risk for screw malposition.
- In addition, corrective maneuvers for fracture reduction need to be planned. Fracture reduction can be accomplished with a mini-open technique at the fracture level (**FIG 1**), through patient positioning, or with more standardized compression-distraction forces through the pedicular implants.

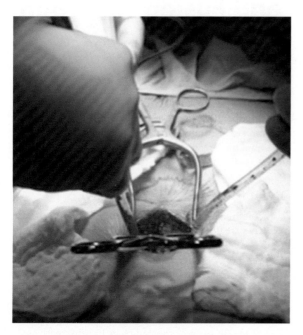

FIG 1 • Intraoperative photograph of a mini-open technique to achieve biological fusion in addition to percutaneous pedicle screw placement.

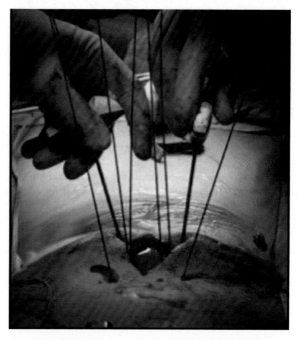

FIG 2 • Intraoperative photograph of a patient with spine trauma being treated with a minimally invasive technique.

■ Achieving biological fusion is challenging in multilevel traumatic cases, and the benefit of doing so is not entirely clear. If necessary, the fusion procedure can be performed in a staged fashion through a standardized midline approach when the patient is physiologically stable ("damage control").

■ Alternatively, in cases in which anterior reconstruction or decompression is indicated, fusion can be achieved anteriorly with stabilization performed posteriorly with minimally invasive percutaneous pedicle screw placement.

■ Other options for achieving fusion include the use of a posterior cannula through a midline posterior approach to the facet joint. **FIG 2** shows a hybrid approach to facet fusion, combining percutaneous fixation and a mini-open technique.

Positioning

■ The operative setup and positioning for minimally invasive spine procedures are the same as for conventional open posterior procedures.

■ The patient is positioned prone on a radiolucent table with care being taken to pad the entire body in a systematic fashion.

■ Ensure that the eyes are well protected, the cervical spine is in a neutral position, the arms are positioned in 90 degrees of abduction and 90 degrees of elbow flexion, the bony prominences are well padded, and vital structures and distal extremities are protected from incidental injury during the operation. Additionally, the abdomen must be free of compression to improve venous return.

Approach

■ Percutaneous pedicle instrumentation can be performed by one of four methods: true anteroposterior (AP) targeting, Magerl (or owl's eye) technique, image-guided navigation, and biplanar fluoroscopy.

■ We describe the first two methods because these are the authors' preferred techniques for the following reasons:

  ■ By using only a true AP view, the setup is more time-efficient.

  ■ Sterility is maintained when not alternating between AP and lateral views.

  ■ Two surgeons can operate simultaneously on both sides, thereby reducing procedure time and radiation exposure. However, this technique might not be feasible for every patient. Obesity, severely deformed anatomy, and osteopenia are factors that might preclude acceptable imaging of vertebral landmarks.

■ When performing MISS, fluoroscopic imaging is essential. Therefore, the surgeon must be able to obtain a clear image and identify each vertebral body that requires treatment in both the AP and lateral views.

■ After the patient is positioned, the surgeon should obtain a true AP view with the center of the X-ray beam parallel to the superior endplate of the vertebra. This will produce a single superior endplate shadow as the anterior and posterior margins are superimposed on each other.

■ Furthermore, the pedicle shadows should be just inferior to the superior endplate shadow and the spinous process will lie equidistant between the pedicles (**TECH FIG 1**).

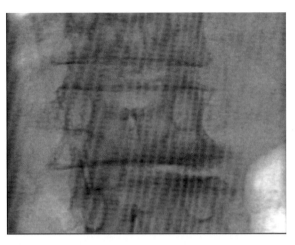
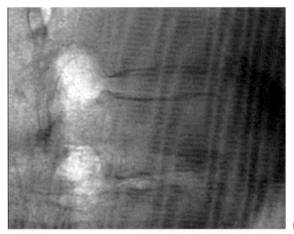

TECH FIG 1 • True anteroposterior view (**A**) and lateral view (**B**) fluoroscopic images obtained before commencing percutaneous pedicle screw placement.

MARKING PEDICLE STARTING POINTS ON THE SKIN

- After a true AP fluoroscopy view is obtained, the surgeon defines the starting points on the patient's skin by placing a Kirschner wire (K-wire) longitudinally over the lateral border of the pedicles on either side of the spine.
- This position is marked, and the K-wire is then placed transversely across the pedicles of each targeted vertebra.
- A second line is marked to intersect the first two longitudinal lines.
- Next, skin incisions are marked 1 cm lateral to the intersection of the skin marks. This accounts for the divergent trajectory of the pedicles and helps to better align the skin and fascial incisions with the bony target (**TECH FIG 2**).

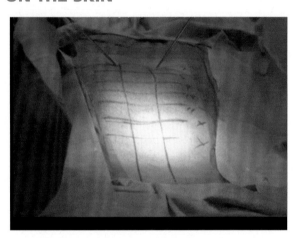

TECH FIG 2 • Preoperative skin markings show the minimally invasive screw starting points.

TRUE AP VIEW METHOD

- The skin and fascia are incised, and the muscular tissues are dissected bluntly until the transverse process is palpated. Jamshidi needles are inserted into the incisions and are docked at the correct starting point for each pedicle.
- This point is the intersection of the lateral border of the upgoing facet, the midline of the transverse process, and the upslope of the pars interarticularis.
- A true AP view image is obtained to verify this location, and the needle tip should overlie the midlateral wall of the pedicle. If the pedicle is imagined to be a clock face, this is is the 3 o'clock position for the patient's right pedicle and the 9 o'clock position for the patient's left pedicle.
- The craniocaudal direction of the needle can be simultaneously verified on fluoroscopy. Once the proper position of the Jamshidi needle is confirmed, it is tapped with a mallet to penetrate a few millimeters into the cortex.

- At that time, the needle shaft can be realigned to be parallel to the superior vertebral endplate.
- The shaft of the Jamshidi needle is then marked 2 cm above the skin to track the depth of penetration into the pedicle. The depth is confirmed by checking the preoperative imaging studies and measuring the length of the pedicle at each level.
- Then, with the needle shaft parallel to the endplate on the true AP view and with 10 to 12 degrees of lateral to medial angulation, the needle is tapped to the depth of the mark on the shaft.
- The tip of the needle should then be at the base of the pedicle, anterior to the posterior wall (**TECH FIGS 3** and **4**). A blunt-tipped guidewire is driven through the needle into the cancellous bone and advanced 10 to 15 mm past the tip of the needle.

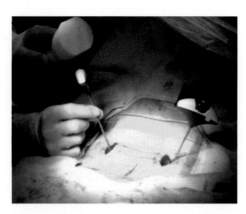

TECH FIG 3 • Intraoperative photograph of the Jamshidi needle being advanced into the pedicle.

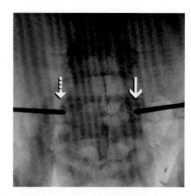

TECH FIG 4 • Anteroposterior view fluoroscopic image confirms appropriate placement of the Jamshidi needles within the pedicles.

■ The needle is removed as the guidewire is held in position, the pedicle is tapped, and a cannulated pedicle screw is placed. A true lateral view radiograph

can be used to confirm the appropriate depth of the screw. All the aforementioned steps are performed at each vertebral level to be instrumented.

MAGERL, OR OWL'S EYE, TECHNIQUE

■ This method involves a fluoroscopic view along the axis of the pedicle. To obtain the owl's eye (or en face) view, the X-ray beam is positioned directly inline with the pedicle axis.
■ First, a true AP view of the vertebra of interest is obtained. The C-arm is then rotated until the X-ray beam is parallel to the pedicle (typically 10 to 30 degrees oblique to the true AP view) (**TECH FIG 5**).
■ Once a proper view has been obtained, the skin incision should be made directly over the pedicle.
■ Placement of the Jamshidi needle, K-wire exchange, and pedicle cannulation or screw placement should then be performed in the same manner as with other techniques.
■ Intermittent lateral view fluoroscopic images or preoperative images can aid in determining the depth of instrument positioning.
■ Obtaining an en face view of the S1 pedicle is achieved in a slightly different manner. Because the pedicle is not cylindrical at the S1 level, only the medial wall is visible on its projection.
■ The surgeon must first align the C-arm in the sagittal plane such that the superior sacral endplate

appears as a single line. The C-arm is then rotated axially to obtain the maximum resolution of the medial pedicle wall.
■ As with the lumbar spine, determination of the medial angulation of the pedicle can be aided with preoperative axial view CT scans or MRIs.

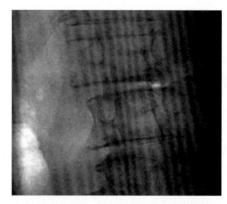

TECH FIG 5 • Fluoroscopic image shows the Magerl technique of screw insertion.

ROD PLACEMENT

■ A few basic principles allow the successful and efficient percutaneous placement of rods. Of primary importance is screw positioning, with special attention paid to align the screw heads in the coronal and sagittal planes.
■ Screw depth is determined by advancing the screws to a position at which they meet slight resistance against the lateral border of the facet joint.

■ The tops of the screw extensions and cannulae should demonstrate a smooth transition between levels and symmetric angulation.
■ The tops of the screw extensions can be used to assess rod contouring in the appropriate coronal and sagittal planes.
■ Once contoured, the rod should be inserted in a cranial to caudal manner because of the protective, shingling effect of the thoracic and lumbar lamina.

- An example of the workflow for rod insertion during a multilevel procedure is as follows.
  - First, rod length is estimated and precontoured before passage.
  - Second, to maximize sensory feedback, a two-handed technique should be used (**TECH FIG 6**). The surgeon's dominant hand is placed on the rod holder, and the nondominant hand remains free to manipulate the screw heads.

- While pushing the rod, the surgeon can rotate each screw head to allow passage. To confirm successful placement, the surgeon can attempt to rotate the screw heads.
- If rotation of the screw head is possible, the rod passage must be reattempted.
- Alternatively, the surgeon can use another instrument, such as a screwdriver, for tactile feedback as the rod passes through each screw head.

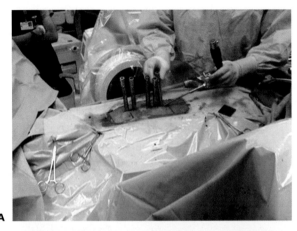

A

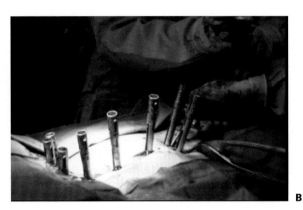

B

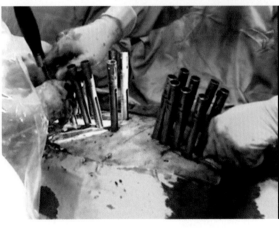

C

TECH FIG 6 • A–C. Intraoperative photographs show three different angles and stages of rod placement and passage and technique.

PEARLS AND PITFALLS

- The owl's eye technique can provide an excellent view of the pedicle, but certain disadvantages are associated with the technique.
  - First, this technique precludes working simultaneously on either side of the patient, requiring realignment of the C-arm twice per level. This increases radiation exposure to the patient and the surgical team.
  - Second, this technique is associated with a higher rate of medial pedicle wall violation, likely secondary to the more medial starting position of the pedicle screws. Because the spinal canal is not well visualized with the en face projection, a medial violation might not be recognized. Therefore, it is critical that pedicle cannulation is started in a lateral position at the junction of the transverse process and facet.
- When longer or curved rods are needed, insertion and positioning of these rods can be challenging.
- Precise and careful positioning of the pedicle screws is essential and should not be overlooked. It is important to remain deep to the fascia and to use the rod's bend to steer the tip and facilitate the passage.
- Furthermore, the development of more advanced implant systems has made multilevel procedures easier to perform.
- Determining proper rod length for multilevel constructs can also be challenging. Although most implant manufacturers have equipment to aid in this process, multiple inspections should be performed using lateral view fluoroscopy to confirm that the rod length is correct.

- Percutaneous pedicle fixation of the upper thoracic spine deserves special consideration because of the inherent magnitude of upper thoracic kyphosis.
- Adequate fluoroscopic images might be difficult to obtain because of patient positioning and body habitus.
- To aid in fluoroscopic imaging, placing the patient's head into a skeletal pin headrest and simultaneously flexing the cervical spine and translating the spine anteriorly might facilitate the process.
- Positioning the head in this fashion also enables the rod and the rod holder to be manipulated through the upper screw extensions without maneuvering around the patient's head.
- Percutaneously placed multilevel constructs that cross the thoracolumbar junction can also present a challenge.
- Although the lordotic portion of the rod might pass easily across the thoracic kyphosis, passage of the rod from the upper thoracic region toward the lumbosacral junction generally becomes more difficult as the kyphotic portion of the rod is passed across the thoracic apex.
- Manipulation of the kyphotic portion of the rod into a more coronal plane or a frank lordotic position usually assists the passage of the rod across the thoracic spine. Rod inserters that allow in situ rotation of the rod can help to overcome these challenges.

POSTOPERATIVE CARE

- Standard postoperative care should be delivered to all patients after percutaneous pedicle fixation, including pain control, deep vein thrombosis prophylaxis, and progressive physical therapy.

OUTCOMES

- The literature evaluating the results of MISS with percutaneous pedicle fixation continues to evolve. Several studies have examined the rates of postoperative surgical infection associated with minimally invasive techniques.
- O'Toole et al.[7] reported three surgical site infections among 1338 minimally invasive spinal procedures in 1274 patients with a mean age of 55.5 years. The surgical site infection rate was 0.10% for simple decompressive procedures, 0.74% for fusion and/or fixation procedures, and 0.22% overall.
- The authors compared their rate with the 2% to 6% reported rates in large clinical series of open spinal procedures and concluded that minimally invasive techniques might reduce postoperative wound infections by nearly tenfold.
- Rodgers et al.[8] examined a retrospective cohort of 313 patients treated with minimally invasive extreme lateral interbody fusion and found no surgical site infections.
- Wang et al.[9] compared 20 patients with type A thoracolumbar fractures treated with traditional open pedicle screw fixation with 17 patients treated with percutaneous pedicle screw techniques.
- The authors found that the percutaneously treated cohort had significantly smaller incisions, less estimated blood loss, shorter intraoperative time, decreased lengths of stay, and less postoperative pain.
- Poelstra et al.[10] conducted a retrospective review of 10 patients managed with damage control orthopedics and minimally invasive techniques for unstable thoracolumbar fractures associated with life-threatening injuries.
- Nonoperative brace treatment was not possible because of fracture type, associated injuries, or body habitus (>300 lb), and all patients were too hemodynamically unstable to undergo open spinal stabilization.
- Patients were followed for a minimum of 1 year. Postoperative CT scans confirmed that a total of 82 screws in 10 patients were placed without pedicle breaches. Blood loss was an average of 177 mL, and the average length of surgery from time of incision to transfer of the patient to the intensive care unit was 95 minutes.
- All patients underwent minimally invasive spinal stabilization within 48 hours after injury, all patients survived their trauma, and no revision surgery was performed.

- The authors concluded that damage control spinal stabilization via a minimally invasive technique is appropriate for patients who have suffered multisystem trauma and complex unstable spinal injuries. However, further studies are needed to assess whether immediate patient survival and eventual functional outcomes are truly improved with an MISS damage control approach.
- In a patient with multiple traumatic injuries, minimally invasive spinal fixation might play an important role in allowing early stabilization of thoracolumbar spinal fractures and could consequently minimize the morbidities associated with delayed fixation.
- McHenry et al.[13] retrospectively reviewed risk factors of respiratory failure in 1032 patients at a level 1 trauma center after operative stabilization of thoracolumbar spinal fractures.
- They found the following five independent risk factors for respiratory failure: age older than 35 years, Injury Severity Score of >25 points, Glasgow Coma Scale score of <12 points, blunt chest injury, and surgical stabilization performed more than 2 days after admission.
- They concluded that early operative stabilization of thoracolumbar fractures—the only risk factor that can be controlled by the physician—might decrease the risk of respiratory failure in multiply injured patients.

COMPLICATIONS

- As with any surgical intervention, the benefits of operative stabilization must be weighed against the risks of surgery, especially in a critically ill patient suffering from multiple systemic traumatic injuries.
- Although the risk of blood loss is less compared with conventional open techniques, care should be coordinated among the entire medical team to optimize preoperative risks in cases of hemodynamic instability, coagulopathy, hypothermia, or elevated serum lactate levels.
- Compared with open surgical techniques, postoperative infection rates associated with minimally invasive techniques are substantially reduced. Implant malpositioning, loss of reduction, and failure of fusion are other potential pitfalls of minimally invasive techniques that are yet to be determined.

CONCLUSIONS

- The purported benefits of MISS are reduction of blood loss, reduced postoperative pain, lower complication rates, fewer days spent in the hospital, and quicker return to work.
- These benefits have been shown to be true when looking at degenerative conditions of the spine treated in this fashion.

However, when looking at applying minimally invasive solutions for traumatic injuries of the spine, these benefits are yet to be proven.

■ The greatest benefit, however, of the minimally invasive procedure in a traumatically injured patient is reduction in the postoperative infection rate. Thus, when a surgeon is deciding whether to use minimally invasive techniques for traumatic thoracolumbar disorders, he or she needs to establish the proper indications for the procedure, offer the procedure for those cases in which it is superior to performing a conventional open procedure, establish revision strategies if the technique is not effective, and minimize complications.

ACKNOWLEDGMENT

The authors thank Senior Editor and Writer Dori Kelly, MA, for invaluable assistance with the manuscript.

REFERENCES

1. Scalea TM, Boswell SA, Scott JD, et al. External fixation as a bridge to intramedullary nailing for patients with multiple injuries and with femur fractures: damage control orthopedics. J Trauma 2000;48(4):613–621.
2. Kerwin AJ, Frykberg ER, Schinco MA, et al. The effect of early surgical treatment of traumatic spine injuries on patient mortality. J Trauma 2007;63(6):1308–1313.
3. Pakzad H, Roffey DM, Knight H, et al. Delay in operative stabilization of spine fractures in multitrauma patients without neurologic injuries: effects on outcomes. Can J Surg 2011;54(4):270–276.
4. Croce MA, Bee TK, Pritchard E, et al. Does optimal timing for spine fracture fixation exist? Ann Surg 2001;233(6):851–858.
5. Cengiz SL, Kalkan E, Bayir A, et al. Timing of thoracolomber[sic] spine stabilization in trauma patients; impact on neurological outcome and clinical course. A real prospective (rct) randomized controlled study. Arch Orthop Trauma Surg 2008;128(9):959–966.
6. O'Toole JE, Eichholz KM, Fessler RG. Surgical site infection rates after minimally invasive spinal surgery. J Neurosurg Spine 2009; 11(4):471–476.
7. Rodgers WB, Cox CS, Gerber EJ. Early complications of extreme lateral interbody fusion in the obese. J Spinal Disord Tech 2010; 23(6):393–397.
8. Wang HW, Li CQ, Zhou Y, et al. Percutaneous pedicle screw fixation through the pedicle of fractured vertebra in the treatment of type A thoracolumbar fractures using Sextant system: an analysis of 38 cases. Chin J Traumatol 2010;13(3):137–145.
9. Poelstra KA, Gelb D, Kane B, et al. The feasibility of damage control spinal stabilization (MISS) in the acute setting for complex1 thoracolumbar fractures. Presented at the 23rd Meeting of the North American Spine Society, October 14–18, 2008, Toronto, Canada.
10. McHenry TP, Mirza SK, Wang J, et al. Risk factors for respiratory failure following operative stabilization of thoracic and lumbar spine fractures. J Bone Joint Surg Am 2006;88(5):997–1005.

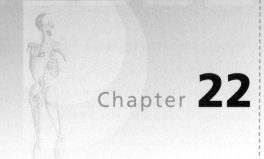

Chapter 22

Costotransversectomy for Canal Decompression and Anterior Column Reconstruction via a Posterior Approach

Yu-Po Lee, Charles C. Chang, Ankur D. Patel, and Steven R. Garfin

DEFINITION

Posterolateral (Costotransversectomy) Approach to the Thoracic Spine

▪ The costotransversectomy uses a posterolateral approach to the thoracic spine. This approach provides access to the posterior spine, the lateral spinal canal, and also to the anterolateral portion of the vertebral body.

▪ This approach was originally employed as a means to drain tuberculosis abscesses.[1,2] Other indications now include biopsy and removal of neoplastic tissue(s), resection of fractured bone fragments, spinal cord decompression, and to facilitate various spinal fusions (**FIG 1A–D**).[2–6]

▪ In comparison to the formal anterior thoracotomy, the costotransversectomy approach allows extrapleural access to the thoracic spine. Because the pleural cavity is not violated, this reduces the risk of pulmonary complications.[7,8] Additionally, although anterior thoracotomy provides limited access in the regions of the thoracic inlet and the levels near the diaphragm, the costotransversectomy approach can expose any level of the entire thoracic spine.

▪ Limitations of the costotransversectomy approach center around its poor visualization of the anterior canal. This makes addressing midline pathology such as broad-based calcified discs or central herniation more difficult via the costotransversectomy approach. Furthermore, a transthoracic approach may be advantageous in situations of multilevel involvement in order to avoid operative blood loss and thoracic cage instability from rib resection.

ANATOMY

▪ The thoracic vertebrae are chiefly distinguished from the adjacent cervical and lumbar spinal regions by the presence of complex osteoligamentous articulations with the ribs.[9–11]

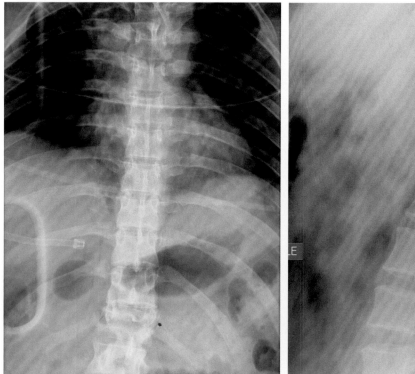
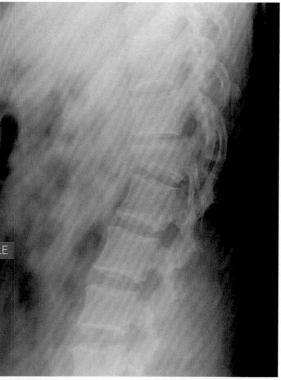

FIG 1 ▪ **A:** Anteroposterior (AP) view of T12 fracture dislocation. **B:** Lateral view of T12 fracture dislocation. The decision was made to perform a costotransversectomy to avoid taking down the diaphragm. *(continued)*

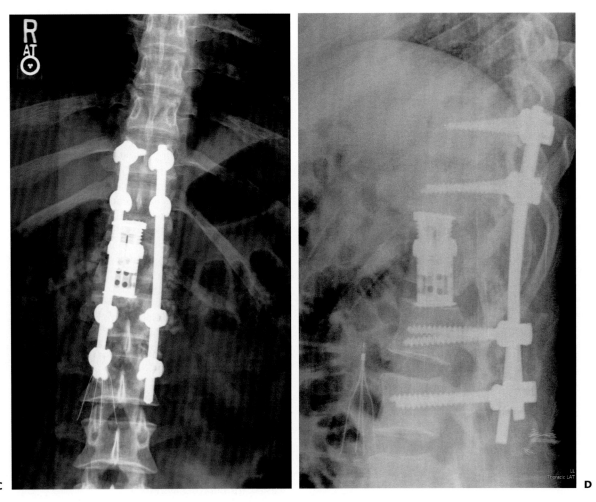

FIG 1 • *(continued)* **C:** Postoperative AP view of T12 corpectomy and posterior T10–L2 spinal fusion. **D:** Lateral view of T12 corpectomy and reconstruction with lateral expandable cage.

■ Two major articulations account for the costovertebral joint.

■ Ventrally, each thoracic rib articulates with the adjacent vertebral body and rostral intervertebral disc by the anterior costovertebral ligament, also known as the radiate ligament. Dorsolaterally, the costotransverse ligaments support the costal articulation with the transverse process.

■ The superior costotransverse ligament extends from the inferior edge of the transverse process to the superior margin of the caudally adjacent vertebrae.

■ The medial costotransverse ligament, also known as the capsular ligament, attaches the posterior neck of the rib with the anterior margin of the transverse process.

■ Finally, the lateral costotransverse ligament attaches the transverse process to the posterior costal tubercle.

■ The osseous variability along the length of the spine adds to the complex three-dimensional anatomy of the region, making thoracic spine surgery a technical process requiring a thorough understanding and proper preoperative planning.

■ There are 12 thoracic vertebrae, each with slight variations in measurable dimensions. Specifically, variations exist between vertebral body diameter, facet positioning, pedicle dimensions, and transverse process and spinous process dimensions.[9–11]

■ Pedicle widths gradually decrease from T1 to T4, and increase from T4 to T12. Pedicle width is approximately 4.5 mm at T4, whereas pedicle width at T12 is approximately 7.8 mm. Pedicle height and length tend to increase from T1 to T12. Medial orientation and transverse pedicle angle tend to decrease from T1 to T12.[9–11]

NATURAL HISTORY

■ The natural history of the disease depends on the underlying pathology.

PATIENT HISTORY AND PHYSICAL FINDINGS

■ A thorough history and physical exam is the basis of complete preoperative planning. The history should include medical and surgical history, social history addressing functional disability and socioeconomic issues, and history of pain or neurologic symptoms.

- The physical exam should consist of observation of deformity and gait, palpation for tenderness or masses, range of motion of the spine and joints, assessment of intact neurologic function with a sensory/motor exam, and rectal examination.

IMAGING AND OTHER DIAGNOSTIC STUDIES

- As previously mentioned, safe preoperative planning relies on understanding the complex three-dimensional anatomy of the costovertebral articulations, vertebrae dimensions, and locations of the neurovascular bundles.
- Proper imaging including radiographs and/or advanced imaging modalities is essential to preoperative planning.
- MRI is the imaging modality of choice for most pathologies to characterize the soft tissue of the involved region, especially cases involving spinal cord compression.
- CT myelography may offer comparable visualization of the neural elements and is especially beneficial in cases where spinal instrumentation has been used previously.
- For bony anatomy, CT is the preferred modality. Sagittal reconstruction and three-dimensional CT imaging may be useful supplements to axial sequences.
- Frequently, both MRI and CT imaging are obtained for preoperative planning to characterize both the regional soft tissue and bony anatomy, respectively.

DIFFERENTIAL DIAGNOSIS

Indications for costotransversectomy include:
- Anterolateral spinal decompression of infection/abscess
- Vertebral body biopsy or partial resection (neoplastic, traumatic)
- Anterior intraspinal tumor
- Removal of paracentral herniated disc
- Congenital kyphosis or kyphoscoliosis
- Sympathectomy
- Various fusions, including limited anterior spinal fusion
- Rib pain

NONOPERATIVE MANAGEMENT

- The decision to treat a patient operatively or nonoperatively is dependent on the underlying disease. With some tumors, radiation may be the first line of treatment. With most thoracic disc herniations and other degenerative diseases, nonoperative treatment is often tried prior to consideration for surgery unless there is neurologic deterioration.
- Nonoperative treatment is dependent on the underlying disease.

SURGICAL MANAGEMENT

- In thoracic disc resection, the costotransversectomy approach should be performed on the affected side. This is usually the side with greater deficit on neurologic exam, which should correlate with imaging studies obtained preoperatively.
- In cases of central herniations without lateralizing deficits or root pain, the right-sided approach has been favored to avoid injury to the artery of Adamkiewicz, which usually originates from the left intercostal arteries from T8 to L2.
- The side of approach for other pathologies depends on the location of the lesion

Preoperative Planning

- A thorough history and physical exam is essential. In cases where a tumor or infection is suspected, the history may provide clues as to the origin of the tumor or infection.
- Appropriate laboratory values should be obtained. These include a basic metabolic panel, complete blood count (CBC), prothrombin time (PT), and partial thromboplastin time (PTT). In cases where tumors or infections are suspected, an erythrocyte sedimentation rate (ESR) and C-reactive protein (CRP) are also recommended. In cases where infections are suspected, blood cultures may be helpful in identifying an organism.
- Arranging for appropriate blood products is recommended. In the case of tumors and infections, there can be considerable blood loss and hemostasis may be difficult to achieve. In addition to packed red blood cells, fresh frozen plasma and platelets may also need to be called for ahead of time.
- Appropriate imaging including radiographs and MRI and CT are essential.
- If time permits, a biopsy is recommended in the cases where tumors are suspected and a primary is not known. Embolization of tumors that have a propensity to bleed (renal cell carcinoma, hemangioma, hemangiosarcoma) is recommended.
- Discussion with anesthesia regarding maintaining mean arterial pressure above 70 mm Hg to ensure adequate perfusion to the spinal cord.

Positioning

- Various positioning techniques are available depending on the surgeon's preference. It is the authors' preference to use a prone position on the operating table. Longitudinal chest rolls with the arms tucked in on a radiolucent table is our preferred method to maintain stability during the corpectomy and allow access for fluoroscopy (**FIG 2**).
- After desired positioning is achieved, the patient should be draped wide enough to allow adequate exposure of the ribs laterally. Additionally, the posterior iliac crests are commonly prepped and draped in the field on both sides in the event bone graft is necessary.

Approach

- The spinous process of the level desired should be palpated and confirmed using a lateral radiograph. Be aware that the

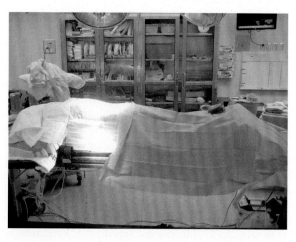

FIG 2 • Position of the patient. We prefer a radiolucent table to facilitate the use of fluoroscopy.

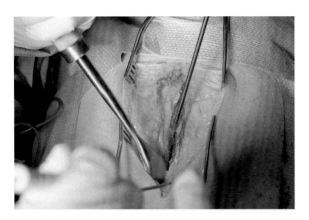

FIG 3 • We prefer a standard midline approach. Following skin incision through the subcutaneous fat, the trapezius is cut in a longitudinal direction inline with the incision to expose underlying muscles.

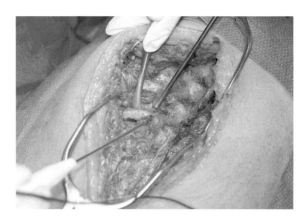

FIG 5 • The anterior surface of the rib can then be elevated subperiosteally with caution not to disrupt the neurovascular bundle nestled under the inferior aspect of the rib.

thoracic spinous processes are relatively long and thin and tend to overlap adjacent levels. The incision should span over two to three levels above and below the level where the costotransversectomy is going to be performed.

- Depending on the level of the lesion and extent of exposure required, various incisions may be used. Incisions vary from a straight midline incision, a midline incision with a "T" over the rib to be resected, a paramedian incision made midway between the spinous process, and medial scapular border for proximal lesions above T7 or a curvilinear incision. It is the authors' preference to use a midline incision that can be extended as needed to allow adequate exposure to resect the ribs. The importance of draping widely is emphasized here again.

- Following skin incision through the subcutaneous fat, the trapezius is cut in a longitudinal direction inline with the incision to expose underlying muscles (**FIG 3**). Depending on the region of thoracic spine, the rhomboid muscles, latissimus dorsi, and thoracodorsal fascia are divided next to access the paraspinal muscles.

- The paraspinal muscles are elevated off of the spinous processes and laminae to gain access to the spine. A subperiosteal

dissection will minimize blood loss. The muscles are then elevated off of the transverse processes and ribs to expose the costotransverse articulation (**FIG 4**).

- Pedicle screw fixation may be performed at this point if a fusion a planned and a rod can be placed on the side opposite from the costotransversectomy. This will provide stability during the corpectomy.

- The anterior surface of the rib can then be elevated subperiosteally with caution not to disrupt the neurovascular bundle nestled under the inferior aspect of the rib (**FIG 5**). Take care not to enter the pleural cavity.

  - In cases where the pleural cavity is violated, the pleura may be repaired with 6-0 or 4-0 Prolene in running locked fashion. To ensure adequate closure of the pleural cavity, immerse the wound in saline and perform a Valsalva maneuver. If bubbles persist, a chest tube can be placed at the end of the procedure.

- The rib is cut approximately 6 to 10 cm from the costovertebral articulation (**FIG 6**). The transected rib can be elevated and the pleura swept away from the undersurface of the rib. Any remaining muscle attachments to the rib should be cleared to visualize the costotransverse ligament, which can

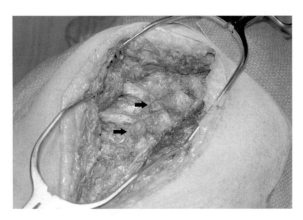

FIG 4 • The muscles are then elevated off of the transverse processes and ribs to expose the costotransverse articulation (*black arrows*).

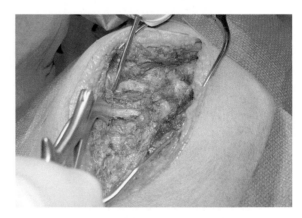

FIG 6 • The rib is cut approximately 6 to 10 cm from the costovertebral articulation. The transected rib can be elevated and the pleura swept away from the undersurface of the rib.

be removed. With careful reflection of the pleura from the anterolateral surface of the vertebral body, the costovertebral joint can be disarticulated by dissecting the anterior costovertebral ligament to free the rib.

▪ Once disarticulation of the rib is complete, the transverse process can be removed to visualize the disc space.

▪ The intercostal artery and nerve should be ligated or retracted to avoid significant bleeding during rib resection.

▪ If a corpectomy is planned, a laminectomy can be useful to improve visualization and resection of the vertebral body. A laminectomy can be performed to visualize the spinal cord in standard fashion.

▪ To gain access to the discs above and below the vertebra and to avoid retraction on the spinal cord, the nerve roots above and below the pedicle may need to be tied off and transected. We generally use 2-0 silk ties (**FIG 7**). This is generally well tolerated without significant side effects.

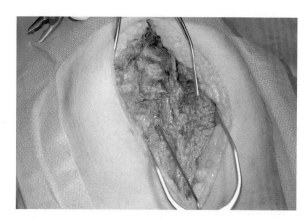

FIG 7 • To gain access to the discs above and below the vertebra and to avoid retraction on the spinal cord, the nerve roots above and below the pedicle may need to be tied off and transected. Figure of the nerve root passing underneath the pedicle.

CORPECTOMY

▪ Using a high-speed burr, the center of the pedicle can be burred down into the vertebral body.

▪ Then, the lateral portion of the pedicle may be removed with a rongeur and the medial portion may be removed by pushing the pedicle wall laterally to avoid injury to the spinal cord.

▪ In cases of infection, purulent drainage should be encountered at this point and the cavity should be irrigated and debrided. In tumors cases, lytic or solid tumor masses may be encountered. With lytic lesions, the tumor may be debrided from the cavity and hemostasis obtained. With solid tumors, it might be possible to resect the tumor en bloc. These specimens may be sent to pathology for the appropriate tests.

  ▪ Use of thrombin and Gelfoam and other hemostatic agents may be necessary, and preparation of these materials is recommended prior to entering the cavity.

  ▪ Use of a Cell Saver can be considered, but in cases of tumor or infection, the use of an autogenous blood recovery system is not recommended.

▪ Next, a Penfield no. 1 may be used to elevate the periosteum off of the vertebral body and separate the pleura away from the vertebra if more exposure is needed (**TECH FIG 1**). To avoid injury to the segmental vessels, try to get the Penfield no. 1 under the periosteum and elevate the soft tissues subperiosteally from the lateral and anterior portions of the vertebral body.

  ▪ If the segmental vessels are injured, clamp the vessels to obtain hemostasis. Then tie them with 2-0 silk ties or vessel clips.

▪ Then, the vertebra may be removed posterolaterally with curettes and pituitary rongeurs (**TECH FIG 2**). Be careful not to retract the spinal cord as this could lead to neurologic injury. With tumors or infections, there is often a cavity. Clean this cavity out using curettes and pituitaries.

▪ Once the tumor or pus has been excavated from this cavity, the lateral wall of the vertebral body may be removed with a rongeur. If you need more exposure, knock the posterior wall of the vertebral body into the cavity that you have created with a downward facing curette and remove the pieces with a pituitary. This reduces the risk of spinal cord injury.

TECH FIG 1 • Elevate the periosteum off of the vertebral body with a Penfield no. 1 or periosteal elevator and separate the pleura away from the vertebra if more exposure is needed. The *thin arrow* is pointing at the dura. The *larger arrow* is pointing at the pedicle.

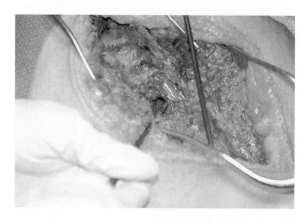

TECH FIG 2 • Figure of the cavity created from resection of bone from the costotransversectomy approach.

- Always be cognizant of the integrity of the anterior wall of the vertebral body because the aorta and vena cava are just anterior to the anterior wall of the vertebral body. If the anterior wall has been destroyed by tumor or infection, elevate the periosteum off of the anterior wall of the vertebral body or define the anterior border of the vertebra prior to performing the corpectomy to reduce the risk of vessel injury.
  - If further exposure is necessary, removal of another rib may provide better visualization and access.
- Once the tumor, pus, and granulation tissue have been adequately resected, remove enough of the vertebral body to allow space for a strut or cage.

DISCECTOMY AND APPLICATION OR INTERBODY CAGE

- Remove the disc at each end of the cavity to expose the endplates of the vertebrae above and below.
- Tying and ligating the exiting nerve roots will improve visualization of the discs and facilitate the discectomy. Make a box annulotomy with a no. 15 scalpel blade and remove the disc above and below the corpectomy site. Start with a pituitary and remove as much of the disc as you can.
- Use curettes to thoroughly remove the cartilaginous endplates. Remove the endplate in a posterolateral direction to avoid sending any material into the ventral portion of the spinal cord. Angled curettes and scrapers can be useful here to avoid injury to the spinal cord. Scrape the endplates in a mediolateral direction versus anteroposterior (AP) direction to avoid injury to the vessels anteriorly or the spinal cord posteriorly.

Cage Placement

- Place an allograft strut or cage posterolaterally to sit securely on the endplates. Our preference is to use an expandable cage. An expandable cage can be helpful in these cases to avoid retraction on the spinal cord and potential neurologic injury because it is smaller than standard cages or allograft struts when it is initially inserted.
- The resected ribs provide an excellent source of graft material. If necessary, iliac crest may be obtained for additional graft. Demineralized bone matrix or other extenders may be necessary to obtain a fusion.
- Calipers and trials are used to get the exact size of the cage. Evaluation of radiographs of the disc and vertebral body above and below the corpectomy site should give a rough estimation of the size of the cage.
- Fill the expandable cage with the harvested graft. Insert the cage in a posterolateral direction to avoid injury to the spinal cord.
- Expand the cage to secure the cage in place and get AP and lateral fluoroscopic views to check for good positioning of the cage. Leave the handle on the cage when taking the radiographs in case the cage must be repositioned. Expand the cage to obtain a good interference fit. You should be able to pull on the cage with a Kocher clamp without it moving.
- Decorticate and pack the remaining graft in the posterolateral gutters and place the ipsilateral rod.
- After the appropriate procedure is completed, closure is performed in routine fashion.
- Use of a drain is recommended especially in the case of tumors or infections to continue evacuation of infected material or tumor cells. Closure with unbraided, nonabsorbable suture is recommended to decrease the risk of infection or wound dehiscence.

POSTOPERATIVE CARE

- Management of the patient after spinal surgery of any region depends greatly on the pathology, level of surgery, and general health of the patient. It is the authors' normal practice to drain cavities created by costotransversectomy using bulb suction drainage.
- Pain management: Proper pain management is necessary to alleviate pain during respiratory movements, decreasing incidence of atelectasis or other respiratory problems.
- Prophylaxis: Pulsatile compression stockings may be continued postoperatively.
- Positioning in bed: During the first 12 postoperative hours, the patient is allowed to lie supine, as pressure on the wound discourages hematoma development. The patient is rolled every 2 hours to prevent wound maceration and pressure ulcers. Dressings are changed at 48 hours and daily thereafter as needed. Sutures are removed after 14 to 17 days and the wound is not soaked during this time. In patients who have had radiation to the area, the sutures are left longer to allow the wound to heal completely.

- Ambulation: Patients are encouraged to ambulate on postoperative day 1. Those with residual neurologic deficits can be mobilized to chair with assistance when possible, otherwise repositioning with log rolling every 2 hours to prevent skin breakdown is necessary. Patients with neurologic deficits begin physical rehabilitation 48 hours after surgery, with both passive and active exercises performed in bed.
- Bracing: Bracing is not usually required. However, if fixation is a concern, thoracolumbar orthosis with or without thigh extension may be instituted until radiographs suggest adequate osseous support.

OUTCOMES

- The outcomes for surgical procedures involving costotransversectomy vary depending on the type of pathology, preoperative extent of the lesion, and anatomical location.
- Bohlman and Zdeblick described the results of 19 patients who underwent excision of herniated discs.[3] Eleven of the patients had the costotransversectomy approach, whereas the remaining eight patients underwent an anterior transthoracic

disc resection. After 5 years, five were freed from pain with normal neurologic exam, three suffered mild residual weakness or mild pain requiring occasional analgesics, one had continued debilitating back pain requiring workers compensation, and two suffered poor results with remaining paraplegia. Fusion was not performed in every patient. The authors' methods left the anterior disc space and anterior longitudinal ligament intact after remaining disc resection.

■ In another study, Smith et al. used a single posterior midline incision and a costotransversectomy in the management of 16 patients with congenital kyphosis and acquired kyphoscoliosis.[4] Thirteen patients had a satisfactory outcome, with no clinically important postoperative complications; two suffered substantial postoperative complications not requiring secondary surgery (including lower extremity dysesthesia and residual pelvic obliquity caudad to fusion); and one patient had poor results requiring revision surgery for failed instrumentation. Overall, the authors claimed costotransversectomy to be a useful approach for anterior spinal fusion when used in conjunction with a posterior approach in the management of kyphoscoliosis.

■ Similar results were noted in a study by Sciubba et al. The authors reviewed seven cases where a costotransversectomy was used in conjunction with an expandable cage to correct thoracolumbar kyphosis resulting from spinal tumors, osteomyelitis, or fractures.[12] A costotransversectomy was chosen in these cases because a transthoracic approach was deemed too risky due to medical comorbidities. The authors noted a 53% kyphosis correction. None of the patients had a decline in neurological function, and pain management consisted of minimal use of oral narcotics.

■ Lastly, the costotransversectomy approach for tumor resection has also been studied. In a study by Cybulski et al., the authors performed a retrospective review of 15 patients who had a modified costotransversectomy to treat metastatic tumors causing impinging on the thoracic spine.[13] Ten of these patients also had a concurrent posterior spinal fusion. The authors noted adequate decompression of the spinal canal in all cases. Also, all patients who were ambulating preoperatively maintained the ability to ambulate postoperatively. Improvements in pain and/or further neurologic improvement were noted in 75% of the patients.

■ Hence, the costotransversectomy approach can be a very useful method to treat pathologies of the thoracic spine. As noted in the studies cited, there are many risks associated with this procedure, and a thorough discussion with the patient regarding the risks and benefits of the surgery is recommended prior to surgery. However, it can have very good results when used for the right indications. It seems to have maximum benefit when a transthoracic approach is deemed too risky or morbid for the patient to tolerate.

COMPLICATIONS

■ Possible complications following costotransversectomy are those typical of spine surgery. The immediate proximity of osseous structures with neurovascular and visceral anatomy establishes a technical challenge with several possible complications to be aware of. But overall, complications tend to be uncommonly observed.

■ Intraoperatively, care should be taken to avoid pleural compromise. This complication is more common when the pleura are thickened in cases involving neoplasm, infection, or previous surgery. If necessary, a chest tube can be placed at the end of surgery.

■ Historically, blood loss has been recognized as a concern for posterolateral approaches but with recent attention to hemostasis, blood loss can be well controlled. Special attention to penetrating arteries is required during dissection and removal of portions of the pedicle and anterior aspect of the vertebral body.

■ The intercostal artery and nerve should be ligated or retracted to avoid significant bleeding during rib resection. Similarly, injury to the intercostal nerve should be avoided to prevent intercostal neuralgia.

■ Other nervous injuries, including nerve root injuries or dural tears are possible. Dural tears should be closed intraoperatively to prevent cerebrospinal fluid leakage.

■ Postoperatively, infectious complications such as pneumonia and urinary tract infection have been noted. Patients who undergo costotransversectomy usually suffer multiple comorbidities, which further complicates postoperative course. Postoperative atelectasis may result secondary to pain and immobility. Wound infections are not common but can be treated with appropriate irrigation and debridement and intravenous antibiotics.

PEARLS AND PITFALLS

Imaging	■ For any lesion requiring costotransversectomy, proper intraoperative imaging is helpful. Use of a radiolucent table will facilitate images. Tucking the arms in will also facilitate fluoroscopy.
Exposure	■ Inadequate rib resection may create a more posterior-directed approach than anticipated, which restrains the view of more anterior structures. This could lead to improper exposure of the lesion necessitating spinal cord manipulation, which should always be avoided. This can be avoided by an adequately lateral rib resection to establish a proper posterolateral approach. ■ Tying off the nerve roots will also allow easier access to the vertebral body and endplates.
Pleural injury	■ In the case of pleural disruption, repair should proceed immediately. Flooding the operative field with irrigation while searching for air leakage during ventilation can check for undiscovered pleural leaks. A chest tube can be placed at the end of the case if need be.
Corpectomy	■ The key to doing an adequate corpectomy is visualization and access. To gain adequate access, tie off the nerve roots and resect the rib as far lateral as necessary to view as much of the vertebra as you need.
Discectomy	■ Obtaining adequate exposure will facilitate the discectomy. Angled instruments will also help. During the discectomy, move the curettes and rasps in a mediolateral direction to avoid injury to the ventral spinal cord.
Hemostasis	■ Hemostasis should be maintained throughout surgery. Take time to obtain good vascular access and to ensure adequate blood products are available. ■ When dealing with tumors, embolization of vascular tumors may decrease blood loss.

REFERENCES

1. Alberstone CD, Benzel, EC. History; Menard's costotransversectomy. In: Benzel, EC. *Spine Surgery: Techniques, Complications, Avoidance, and Management*. 2nd ed. Philadelphia, PA: Elsevier; 2005: 8.

2. Herkowitz HN, Garfin SR, Balderston RA, et al. The Spine. 5th ed. Philadelphia, PA: Elsevier; 2006: 308–319.

3. Bohlman HH, Zdeblick TA. Anterior excision of herniated thoracic discs. J Bone Joint Surg Am 1988;70:1038–1047.

4. Smith JT, Gollogly S, Dunn HK. Simultaneous anterior-posterior approach through a costotransversectomy for the treatment of congenital kyphosis and acquired kyphoscoliotic deformities. J Bone Joint Surg Am 2005;87(10):2281–2289.

5. Garrido E. Modified costotransversectomy: a surgical approach to ventrally placed lesions in the thoracic spinal canal. Surg Neurol 1980;13(2):109–113.

6. Overby MC, Rothman AS. Anterolateral decompression for metastatic epidural spinal cord tumors. Results of a modified costotransversectomy approach. J Neurosurg 1985;62(3):344–348.

7. Fessler RG, Sturgill M. Review: complications of surgery for thoracic disc disease. Surg Neurol 1998;49(6):609–618.

8. Wiggins GC, Mirza S, Bellabarba C, et al. Perioperative complications with costotransversectomy and anterior approaches to thoracic and thoracolumbar tumors. Neurosurg Focus 2001;11(6):e4.

9. Lee DD, Lemma MA, Kostuik JP. Surgical approaches to the thoracic and thoracolumbar spine. In: Frymoyer JW, Wiesel SW, eds. *The Adult & Pediatric Spine*. Philadelphia, PA: Lippincott Williams & Wilkins; 2004: 1011–1041.

10. Papadopoulos SM, Fessler RG. Thoracic spine; Anatomy and surgical approaches and exposures of the vertebral column. In: Benzel EC. *Spine Surgery: Techniques, Complications Avoidance, and Management*. 2nd ed. Philadelphia, PA: Elsevier; 2005: 281–293.

11. Maiman DJ, et al. Lateral extracavitary decompression. In: Benzel EC, ed. *Spine Surgery: Techniques, Complications Avoidance, and Management*. 2nd ed. Philadelphia, PA: Elsevier; 2005: 429–434.

12. Sciubba DM, Gallia GL, McGirt MJ, et al. Thoracic kyphotic deformity reduction with a distractible titanium cage via an entirely posterior approach. Neurosurgery 2007;60(4)(suppl 2):223–230.

13. Cybulski GR, Stone JL, Opesanmi O. Spinal cord decompression via a modified costotransversectomy approach combined with posterior instrumentation for management of metastatic neoplasms of the thoracic spine. Surg Neurol 1991;35(4):280–285.

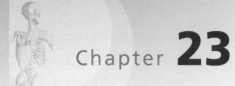

Chapter 23

Primary and Metastatic Tumors of the Spine: Total En Bloc Spondylectomy

Katsuro Tomita, Norio Kawahara, and Hideki Murakami

BACKGROUND

- Conventionally, curettage or piecemeal excision has been the usual approach to vertebral tumors.
- These approaches have clear disadvantages, however, including high risk of tumor cell contamination to the surrounding structures and residual tumor tissue at the site due to difficulty in demarcating tumor from healthy tissue.
- These contribute to incomplete resection of the tumor as well as high local recurrence rates of the spinal malignant tumor.
- To reduce local recurrence and to increase survival, we have developed total en bloc spondylectomy (TES).[10,11,14]
- In this method, the entire vertebra or vertebrae containing the malignant tumor are resected, together with en bloc laminectomy, en bloc corpectomy, and bilateral pediculotomy using a T-saw through the posterior approach.[9]
- Using this technique, we are able to excise the tumor mass together with a wide or marginal margin.

ANATOMY

- The following tissues serve as barriers to spinal tumor progression: the anterior longitudinal ligament (ALL), the posterior longitudinal ligament (PLL), the periosteum abutting the spinal canal, the ligamentum flavum (LF), the periosteum of the lamina and spinous process, the interspinous ligament (ISL), the supraspinous ligament (SSL), the cartilaginous endplate, and the cartilaginous annulus fibrosus. However, both the PLL and the periosteum on the lateral side of the vertebral body are "weak" anatomic barriers. In contrast, the ALL, cartilaginous endplate, and annulus fibrosus are "strong" barriers. In the spine one vertebra could be regarded as a single oncologic compartment and the surrounding tissues as barriers to tumor spread (**FIG 1**).[5]

INDICATIONS

- Surgical indication for primary tumors
  - The surgical strategy for primary spinal tumors used at the authors' institution is based on Enneking's concept of musculoskeletal tumors[3] (Table 1).
- Surgical indication for metastatic tumors
  - Surgical strategy for spinal metastases (Table 2) consists of three prognostic factors: (1) grade of malignancy; (2) visceral metastases; and (3) bone metastases.[12]
  - The extent of the spinal metastases is stratified using the surgical classification of spinal tumors (Table 3), and technically appropriate and feasible surgery is employed, such as en bloc spondylectomy, piecemeal thorough excision, curettage, or palliative surgery.

IMAGING AND OTHER STAGING STUDIES

- Plain radiography
- CT/MRI
- Bone scan
- Angiography and other studies
- Biopsy

SURGICAL MANAGEMENT

- The TES operation was designed to achieve complete tumor resection en bloc, including main and satellite microlesions in a vertebral compartment to avoid local recurrence.
- The primary candidates for TES are primary malignant tumor (stage 1, 2); aggressive benign tumor (stage 3); and isolated metastasis in a patient with long life expectancy (see Tables 1 and 2).
- From the viewpoint of tumor growth (see Surgical classification; Table 3), TES is recommended for types 3, 4, and 5 lesions; and relatively indicated for types 1, 2, and 6 lesions.
- Type 1 or 2 still can be a candidate for radiation therapy, chemotherapy, corpectomy, or hemivertebrectomy.
- TES is not recommended for type 7 lesions. Systemic treatment or hospice care may be the treatment choice for these lesions.[10,11,13] However, the final decision can be made individually based on discussion among the patient and his or her family and doctors.

Preoperative Embolization

- Segmental arteries above and below the feeding artery, as well as the feeding artery itself, should be embolized preoperatively. This embolization technique dramatically reduces intraoperative bleeding without compromising spinal cord function.[4,8,15]

Positioning

- The patient is placed prone over the Relton-Hall four-poster frame for the posterior approach to avoid compression to the vena cava.

Approach

- The surgical approach is decided based on the degree of tumor development or affected spinal level.

Single Posterior Approach

- For TES above L4, a single posterior approach is preferred rather than a postero–anterior combined approach, as long as the tumor does not involve major vessels or segmental arteries.

Anteroposterior Double Approach

- In type 5 or 6 tumors that involve major vessels or segmental arteries, anterior dissection followed by posterior TES is indicated. Currently, a thoracoscopic or mini-open approach is preferred for anterior dissection.

Posteroanterior Double Approach

- Posterior laminectomy and stabilization followed by anterior en bloc corpectomy and placement of a vertebral prosthesis is indicated in spinal tumors at the level of L5 or L4 because of the technical challenge presented by the iliac wing and lumbosacral plexus nerves.

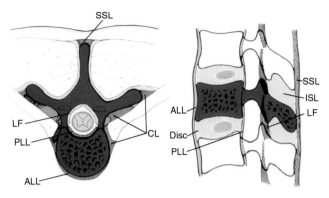

FIG 1 • Compartment and barrier.

Table 1	Surgical Strategy for Primary Spinal Tumors

Surgical Staging	Contamination/ Residual Tumor	Surgical Margin	Spinal Cord Salvage Surgery
Benign tumor			
1. Latent			Don't touch!
2. Active	OK/OK	Intralesional	Debulking (piecemeal)
3. Aggressive	No/no	Intralesional or marginal	Thorough exision (piecemeal/en bloc)
Malignant tumor			
I. Low grade	No/no		
II. High grade	No/no	Marginal or wide	Total en bloc excision
III. With metastases	No/no	(Radical: impractical)	

Table 2	Surgical Strategy for Spinal Metastases

Minimum requirement :
ECOG Performance Status 0 — 3 ---- 5 ◆
or
Karnofsky Performance Scale : 0 — 30 0% ---- ◆

	Prognostic Scoring System		
Factor / Point	Primary tumor	Mets. to vital organ	Bone mets.
1	slow growth	no met : 0	isolated
2	moderate growth	controllable	multiple
3	rapid growth	uncontrollable	

Total P. Score	Life Expentacy	Treatment Aim	Surgery
2			
3	2y <	Long-term local control	En bloc exc.
4			
5	1–2y	Middle-term loca control	Debulking
6			
7	6–12m	Short-term palliation	Palliative decomposition
8			
9	< 3m	Terminal care	No surgical treament
10			

Table 2 Appendix	Points for each primary tumor

1 point = slow growth
- Breast ca.*
- Thyroid ca.*
- Prostatic ca, Testicular ca.

2 points = Moderate growth
- Renal cell ca.*
- Uterus ca. Ovarian ca.
- Colorectal ca

4 points = Rapid growth

ex.
- Lung ca.
- Gastric ca. Esophageal ca.
- Nasopharyngeal ca.
- Hepatocellular ca
- Pancreas ca.etc
- Bladder ca.
- Melanoma
- Sarcoma (osteosarcoma, Ewing sarcoma, Leiomyosarcoma, etc)
- Primary unknown metastasis
- other rare ca.
- ....etc.

*Rare types of the following ca. should be given "4 points" as a rapidly growing cancer: 1 Breast ca., inflammatory type; 2 Thyroid ca., undifferentiated type; 3 Renal cell ca., inflammatory type.

Table 3	Surgical Classification of Spinal Tumors

Intra-Compartmental	**Extra-Compartmental**	**Multiple**
Type 1 vertebral body	**Type 4** spinal canal extension	**Type 7**
Type 2 pedicle extension	**Type 5** paravertebral extension	
Type 3 body - lamina extension	**Type 6** adjacent vertebral extension	

Exposure

- A straight vertical midline incision is made over the spinous processes and is extended three vertebrae above and below the involved segment(s).
- The paraspinal muscles are dissected from the spinous processes and the laminae, and then retracted laterally.
- If the patient underwent a posterior route biopsy, the tracts are carefully resected in a manner similar to that used in limb-salvaging procedures.
- After a careful dissection of the area around the facet joints, a large retractor, the *articulated spinal retractor,* which has a uniaxial joint in each limb and was designed for this surgery, is applied.
- By spreading the retractor and detaching the muscles around the facet joints, a wider exposure is then obtained.
- The operative field must be wide enough on both sides to allow dissection under the surface of the transverse processes.
- In the thoracic spine, the ribs on the affected level are transected 3 to 4 cm lateral to the costotransverse joint, and the pleura is bluntly separated from the vertebra (**TECH FIG 1**).
- To expose the superior articular process of the uppermost vertebra, the spinous and inferior articular processes of the neighboring vertebra are osteotomized and removed with dissection of the attached soft tissues, including the ligamentum flavum.

Introduction of the T-saw Guide

- To make an exit for the T-saw guide through the nerve root canal, the soft tissue attached to the inferior aspect of the pars interarticularis is dissected and removed, using utmost care so as not to damage the corresponding nerve root.

- A C-curved malleable T-saw guide is then introduced through the intervertebral foramen in a cephalocaudal direction.
- In this procedure, the tip of the T-saw guide should be introduced along the medial cortex of the lamina and the pedicle so as not to injure the spinal cord and the nerve root (**TECH FIG 2**).
- After passing the T-saw guide, its tip at the exit of the nerve root canal can be found beneath the inferior border of the pars interarticularis.
- A T-saw is passed through the hole in the wire guide and is clamped with a T-saw holder at each end.
- The T-saw guide is removed, and tension on the T-saw is maintained.

Cutting the Pedicles and En Bloc Laminectomy

- While tension is maintained, the T-saw is placed beneath the superior articular and transverse processes with a specially designed T-saw manipulator. With this procedure, the T-saw placed around the lamina is wrapped around the pedicle.
- With a reciprocating motion of the T-saw, the pedicles are cut, and then the whole posterior element of the spine (the spinous process, the superior and inferior articular processes, the transverse process, and the pedicle) is removed in one piece (**TECH FIG 3**).
- The cut surface of the pedicle is sealed with bone wax to reduce bleeding and to minimize contamination by tumor cells.[1]

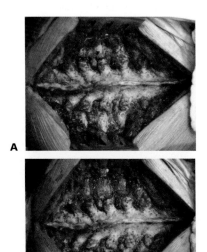

TECH FIG 1 • **A.** Exposure. **B.** Ribs on the affected level are transected 3 to 4 cm lateral to the costotransverse joint.

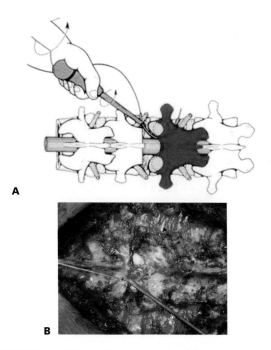

TECH FIG 2 • **A.** Schematic diagram depicting introduction of the the T-saw guide. **B.** A C-curved malleable guidewire is introduced through the right intervertebral foramen in a cephalocaudal direction.

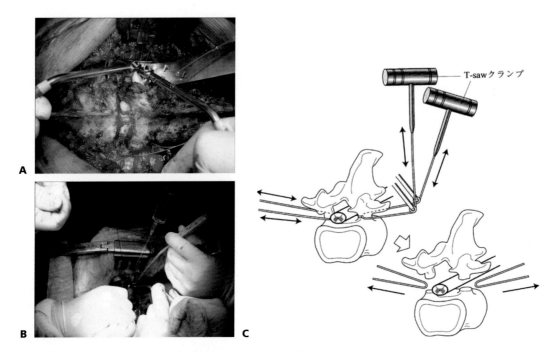

TECH FIG 3 • A,B. Right pedicle is cut with a reciprocating motion of the T-saw. **C.** Schematic drawing of the pediculotomy.

- To maintain stability after segmental resection of the anterior column, a temporary posterior instrumentation ("two above and two below" segmental fixation) is performed.

Blunt Dissection Around the Vertebral Body

- The spinal branch of the segmental artery, which runs along the nerve root, is ligated and divided. In the thoracic spine, the nerve root is cut on the side from which the affected vertebra is removed.
- The blunt dissection is done on both sides through the plane between the pleura (or the iliopsoas muscle) and the vertebral body (**TECH FIG 4**).
- Usually, the lateral aspect of the body is easily dissected with a curved vertebral spatula.
- Then the segmental artery should be dissected from the vertebral body.
- By continuing dissection of both lateral sides of the vertebral body anteriorly, the aorta is carefully dissected posteriorly from the anterior aspect of the vertebral body with a spatula and the surgeon's fingers.
- When the surgeon's fingertips meet with each other anterior to the vertebral body, a series of spatulas, starting from the smallest size, are inserted sequentially to extend the dissection.
- A pair of the largest spatulas is kept in the dissection site to prevent the surrounding tissues and organs from iatrogenic injury and to make the surgical field wide enough for the surgeon to manipulate the anterior column.

Dissection of the Spinal Cord and En Bloc Corpectomy

- Using a cord spatula, the spinal cord (dura mater) is mobilized from the surrounding venous plexus and the ligamentous tissue.

- T-saws are inserted at the proximal and distal cutting levels of the vertebral bodies after confirmation of the disc levels with needles. Recently, a diamond T-saw is now available for corpectomy.
- The teeth-cord protector, which has teeth on both edges to prevent the T-saw from slipping, is then applied.
- The anterior column of the vertebra is cut by the T-saw, together with the anterior and posterior longitudinal ligaments (**TECH FIG 5**).
- The freed anterior column is rotated around the spinal cord and removed carefully to avoid injury to the spinal cord.
- With this procedure, a complete anterior and posterior decompression of the spinal cord (circumspinal decompression) and total en bloc resection of the vertebral tumor are achieved.

Anterior Reconstruction and Posterior Instrumentation

- An anchor hole on the cut end of the remaining vertebra is made on each side to seat the graft. A vertebral spacer such as a titanium mesh cylinder cage with autograft, allograft, or cement (**TECH FIG 6**) is properly inserted to the anchor holes within the remaining healthy vertebrae.
- After checking the appropriate position of the vertebral spacer radiographically, the posterior instrumentation is adjusted to slightly compress the inserted vertebral spacer.
- By this "spinal shortening" procedure, the block cylinder is caught tightly and the anteroposterior 360-degree spinal reconstruction is completed. [2,7]
- If two or three vertebrae are resected, it is recommended that the connector device be applied between the posterior rods and anterior spacer (artificial pedicle).

Anterior Detachment
around the vertebral body

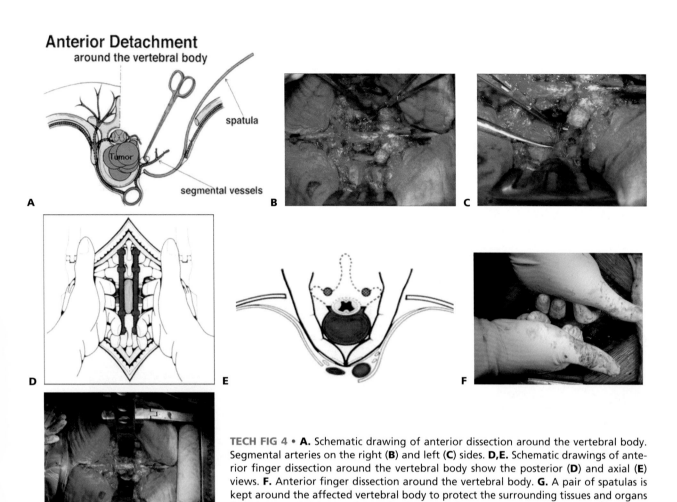

TECH FIG 4 • A. Schematic drawing of anterior dissection around the vertebral body. Segmental arteries on the right (**B**) and left (**C**) sides. **D,E.** Schematic drawings of anterior finger dissection around the vertebral body show the posterior (**D**) and axial (**E**) views. **F.** Anterior finger dissection around the vertebral body. **G.** A pair of spatulas is kept around the affected vertebral body to protect the surrounding tissues and organs from iatrogenic injury and to make the surgical field wide enough for manipulation of the anterior column.

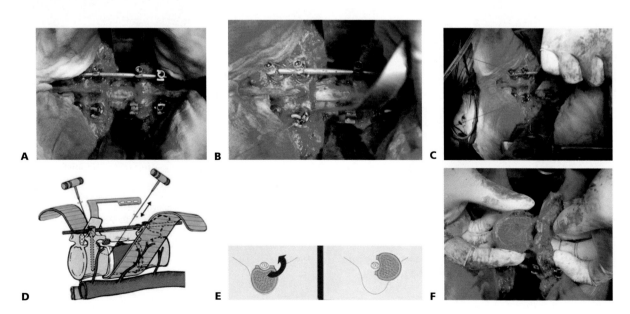

TECH FIG 5 • A. A temporary posterior instrumentation is performed to maintain stability after segmental resection of the anterior column. **B,C.** The anterior column of the vertebra is cut by the T-saw, together with the anterior and posterior longitudinal ligaments. The teeth-cord protector, which has teeth on both edges to prevent the T-saw from slipping, is then applied. **D.** Schematic drawing of cutting the anterior column. **E.** Diagram of en bloc corpectomy. **F.** Intraoperative photograph of specimen from the resected T7 vertebra. *(continued)*

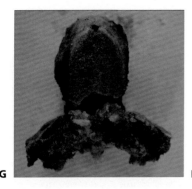 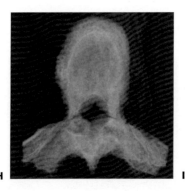 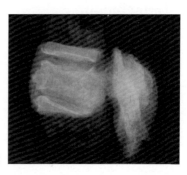

TECH FIG 5 • *(continued)* **G.** Specimens resected along with the compartment and barrier concept. **H,I.** Radiographs of resected specimens from metastatic tumor of T7 showing the complete vertebra in horizontal (**H**) and lateral (**I**) views.

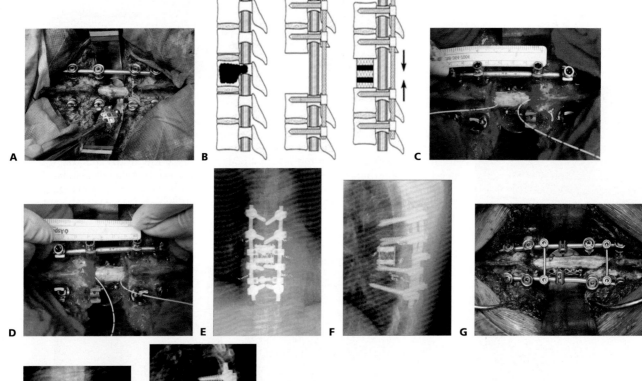

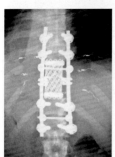 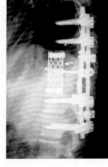

TECH FIG 6 • **A.** A vertebral spacer is properly inserted to the anchor holes within the remaining healthy vertebrae. **B.** Schema of reconstruction (lateral view). **C,D.** After checking the appropriate position of the vertebral spacer radiographically, the posterior instrumentation is adjusted to slightly compress (10 mm in this case) the inserted vertebral spacer. **E,F.** Postoperative radiograph after spinal column shortening shows three pairs of preoperative embolization coils. **G–I.** Resection of two vertebrae. **G.** Bilateral artificial pedicles are placed. **H,I.** Postoperative radiographs of reconstruction with artificial pedicle.

PEARLS AND PITFALLS

Bleeding from the epidural venous plexus[12]	■ 1.5 mL of fibrin glue injected manually into the epidural space in both the cranial and caudal direction of the targeted vertebra after en bloc laminectomy helps reduce oozing from the epidural venous plexus.
Blunt dissection around the vertebral body	■ Careful step-by-step dissection with anatomic consideration is an important fundamental. ■ Preceding TES by a posterior approach, vessels around the vertebral body are managed anteriorly using thoracoscopy or a minimally open approach. This is safer than performing TES by a single posterior approach in a patient in whom the segmental artery(ies) may be involved by the tumor. ■ At lesions of L1 and L2, the diaphragm insertions should be dissected from the vertebral body before the lumbar arteries are dissected, because the segmental arteries run between the vertebral body and diaphragm insertion.[6]
Ligation of the segmental arteries	■ Ligation of the segmental arteries up to three vertebral levels, even including a branch of the artery of Adamkiewicz, may not affect the spinal cord evoked potentials and spinal cord function.[4,8,15]
Spinal cord injury	■ Mechanical damage to the neural structures, especially shifting aside, twisting, and hanging down or upward of the cord, should be avoided. ■ Spinal cord stretching causes irreversible mechanical damage. Excessive nerve root traction also damages the cord due to the root avulsion mechanism.
Risk of tumor cell contamination[13]	■ Double rinsing with distilled water and highly concentrated cisplatinum is recommended to eradicate contaminated cancer cells.
Spinal shortening	■ The posterior instrumentation is adjusted to compress the inserted vertebral prosthesis slightly (5–10 mm) to secure it as a final step of spinal reconstruction using TES. ■ This process of spinal shortening provides two important advantages: (1) increased spinal stability of the anterior and posterior spinal column; and (2) increased spinal cord blood flow, which is desirable to improve spinal cord function.[7]

POSTOPERATIVE CARE

■ Suction drainage is used for 3 to 5 days after surgery.
■ The patient is allowed to start walking within 1 week after surgery.
■ The patient wears a thoracolumbosacral orthosis for 3 to 6 months until bony union is attained.

OUTCOMES

■ From 1989 to 2003, 284 patients with spinal tumors (primary, 86 patients; metastasis, 198 patients) were surgically treated and followed for a minimum of 2 years.
■ Total en bloc spondylectomy was performed in 33 of the 86 patients with a primary tumor; 17 patients with malignant tumors (3 osteosarcoma, 3 Ewing sarcoma, 3 plasmocytoma, 2 chondrosarcoma, and 1 case each of 6 other tumors) and 16 patients with aggressive benign tumors (4 patients with giant cell tumor, 3 patients with osteoblastoma, 3 patients with symptomatic hemangioma, and 1 case each of 6 other tumors).
■ Five-year survival of the 17 patients with primary malignant spinal tumors (stages 1 and 2) who underwent TES was 67%, and that of the 16 patients with aggressive benign tumors (stages 2 and 3) was 100%.
■ In the same periods, TES was performed in 64 of 198 patients with spinal metastases. Of the 64 cases with a metastatic tumor, the primary organs were as follows: kidney, 18 cases; breast, 15 cases; thyroid, 9 cases; lung, 4 cases; liver, 4 cases; and other carcinoma, 14 cases.
■ Forty-three patients with the 2, 3, 4 points out of 64 patients who underwent TES resulted in 2-year survival of 66.6% and 5-year survival of 46.6%.

■ Ninety-two of 97 patients (95%) had no tumor recurrence until death or last follow-up.
■ Five of 97 patients (5%) had local recurrence; the mean length of the recurrence was 22.1 months after operation.
■ In all five patients with local recurrence, the recurrence arose from residual tumor tissue.

COMPLICATIONS

■ Excessive bleeding
■ Injury of the major vessels during blunt dissection of the vertebral body
■ Spinal cord injury
■ Injury of lung or pleura
■ Postoperative hematoma
■ Liquorrhea
■ Pleural effusion
■ Chylothorax
■ Instrumentation failure
■ Infection, especially after preoperative radiation therapy

REFERENCES

1. Abdel-Wanis ME, Tsuchiya H, Kawahara N, et al. Tumor growth potential after tumoral and instrumental contamination: an in-vivo comparative study of T-saw, Gigli saw, and scalpel. J Orthop Sci 2001;6:424–429.
2. Akamaru T, Kawahara N, Sakamoto J, et al. The transmission of stress to grafted bone inside a titanium mesh cage used in anterior column reconstruction after total spondylectomy: a finite-element analysis. Spine 2005;30:2783–2787.
3. Enneking WF, Spanier SS, Goodmann MA. A system for the surgical staging of musculoskeletal sarcoma. Clin Orthop 1980;153:106–120.

4. Fujimaki Y, Kawahara N, Tomita K, et al. How many ligations of bilateral segmental arteries cause ischemic spinal cord dysfunction? An experimental study using a dog model. Spine 2006;31: E781–789.

5. Fujita T, Ueda Y, Kawahara N, et al. Local spread of metastatic vertrebral tumors. A histologic study. Spine 1997;22:1905–1912.

6. Kawahara N, Tomita K, Baba H, et al. Cadereric vascular anatomy for total en bloc spondylectomy in malignant vertebral tumors. Spine 1996;21:1401–1407.

7. Kawahara N, Tomita K, Kobayashi T, et al. Influence of acute shortening on the spinal cord. an experimental study. Spine 2005;30: 613–620.

8. Numbu K, Kawahara N, Murakami H, et al. Interruption of bilateral segmental arteries at several levels. Influence on vertebral blood flow. Spine 2004;29:1530–1534.

9. Tomita K, Kawahara N. The threadwire saw: a new device for cutting bone. J Bone Joint Surg Am 1996;78A:1915–1917.

10. Tomita K, Kawahara N, Baba H, et al. Total en bloc spondylectomy. A new surgical technique for primary malignant vertebral tumors. Spine 1997;22:324–333.

11. Tomita K, Kawahara N, Baba H, et al. Total en bloc spondylectomy for solitary spinal metastasis. Int Orthop 1994;18:291–298.

12. Tomita K, Kawahara K, Kobayashi T, et al. Surgical strategy for spinal metastases. Spine 2001;26:298–306.

13. Tomita K, Kawahara N, Murakami H, et al. Total en bloc spondylectomy for spinal tumors: improvement of the technique and its associated basic background. J Orthop Sci 2006;11:3–12.

14. Tomita K, Toribatake Y, Kawahara N, et al. Total en bloc spondylectomy and circumspinal decompression for solitary spinal metastasis. Paraplegia 1994;32:36–46.

15. Ueda Y, Kawahara N, Tomita K, et al. Influence on spinal cord blood flow and spinal cord function by interruption of bilateral segmental arteries at up to three levels: experimental study in dogs. Spine 2005; 30:2239–2243.

Chapter 24 | Adult Scoliosis

Andrew P. White, James S. Harrop, and Todd J. Albert

DEFINITION

- Adult scoliosis is a coronal deformity of the spine, typically also involving axial and sagittal plane abnormalities.
- Adult scoliosis may be categorized by patient presentation.
  - One group, predominantly defined by lumbar stenosis and neurogenic claudication with degenerative deformity, has surgical management typically achieved by posterior lumbar procedures.
  - A second group, categorized by progressive deformity, with or without back pain, is more frequently treated with combination anterior and posterior procedures that may involve the thoracic spine to achieve surgical goals.
- While the surgical principles and techniques used to address these different categories are similar, important variations exist.

ANATOMY

- Anatomic characterization of adult spinal deformity involves the coronal, sagittal, and axial plane.
  - Lumbar degenerative scoliosis is characterized by loss of lordosis and intervertebral disc height, as well as listhesis in the anteroposterior, lateral, or rotary direction (**FIG 1A,B**).
  - Long curves, typically the result of a preexisting spinal deformity, may involve the entire thoracolumbar spine and may be associated with a significant rotational component (**FIG 1C,D**).

PATHOGENESIS

- Adult scoliosis develops either as the progression of a spinal deformity that was present in adolescence, or as the development of a deformity related to other spinal disorders.
  - The progression of the adolescent spinal deformity is related to increasingly unbalanced forces in the axial skeleton over time.
  - De novo adult deformity is commonly the result of degenerative disease and may also be related to osteoporotic fragility fractures of the vertebrae, resulting in a deformity frequently associated with spinal stenosis and mechanical back pain.

NATURAL HISTORY

- The progression of an adolescent deformity is often seen as a long thoracolumbar curve in the adult.
  - Curves that reach a magnitude of more than 50 degrees are more likely to progress, resulting in symptom exacerbation.
  - As patient age increases, curve flexibility decreases.
- Lumbar degenerative curves typically involve fewer segments and may be limited to the lumbar spine.
  - Degeneration and deformity can cause central, lateral recess, and neural foraminal stenosis as a result of:
    - Loss of intervertebral height
    - Hypertrophy of facet joints
    - Buckling of the ligamentum flavum
    - Compression deformities
  - Neurogenic claudication, as well as radiculopathy and back pain, may result.

PATIENT HISTORY AND PHYSICAL FINDINGS

- Determining the reason for the patient's presentation is the first step in establishing the goals of surgical treatment.
- Patients with extensive thoracolumbar deformity may present with concerns related to curve progression with an impact on:
  - Balance
  - Ambulation
  - Pain
  - Cosmesis
- Patients with lumbar degenerative scoliosis classically present with complaints of neurogenic claudication.
  - Hip and knee flexion contractures, related to the typical forward-flexed ambulation that limits the symptoms of neurogenic claudication, may be found (**FIG 2**).
  - Major focal neurologic abnormalities are unusual in this patient group, although relatively mild degrees of weakness in the tibialis anterior and extensor hallucis longus are not uncommon.
- Physical examination should include the following:
  - Assessment of sagittal balance based on lateral observation of the patient standing with knees extended. A plumb line is dropped from the ear and the deviation (anterior or posterior shift) at the greater trochanter is measured, as is the regional (lumbar) lordosis and (thoracic) kyphosis. An upright posture with head over trunk and trunk over pelvis is a critical treatment goal.
  - Assessment of coronal balance based on posterior observation of the patient standing. A plumb line is dropped from the occiput and the deviation (leftward or rightward shift) at the sacrum is measured. A centered posture reduces gait abnormality.
  - The clinician should observe and palpate the vertical relationship of the right and left acromions with the patient standing. Shoulder asymmetry may indicate coronal postural compensation to maintain upright stance.
  - The clinician should observe and palpate the vertical relationship of the right and left iliac crests with the patient standing on the right, left, and both legs. Pelvic obliquity may be a primary or compensatory mechanism with spinal deformity.
  - Assessment of hip and knee range of motion. Longstanding sagittal plane deformities, as well as neurogenic claudication, may result in hip and knee flexion contractures.
  - Focal findings may be uncommon, but a thorough neurologic examination must be performed.

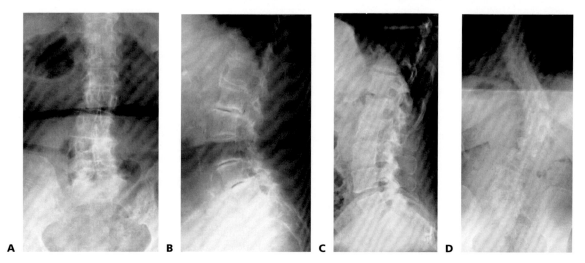

FIG 1 • A,B. Degenerative lumbar scoliosis in PA (**A**) and lateral (**B**) radiographs. Lateral, rotary, and anterolis-theses are seen, with significant loss of disc height, osteophyte formation, and subchondral sclerosis. The coronal deformity is limited to the lumbar region. **C,D.** A long scoliosis involving the lumbar and thoracic regions, associated with rotational deformity, shown in PA (**C**) and lateral (**D**) radiographs.

IMAGING AND OTHER DIAGNOSTIC STUDIES

Radiographs

- Standing posteroanterior (PA) radiographs on 36-inch cassettes characterize the spinal deformity by:
  - The magnitude of primary and compensatory curves, by the Cobb method (**FIG 3**)
  - Coronal balance: the relationship between the C7 plumb line and center of S1 on PA views (**FIG 4**)

- The apical vertebrae (most laterally deviated; **FIG 5A**)
- The stable vertebra (caudal vertebra that is transected by the z axis; **FIG 5B**)
- Rotary and lateral listhesis
- Standing lateral radiographs on 36-inch cassettes characterize the spinal deformity by:
  - Regional lordosis and kyphosis (**FIG 6**)
  - Sagittal balance; the relationship between the C7 plumb line and center of S1 on lateral views (**FIG 7**)
  - Anterolisthesis or retrolisthesis

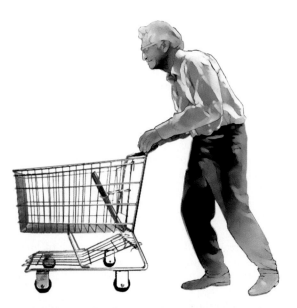

FIG 2 • Neurogenic claudication is frequently associated with this gait abnormality. A forward-flexed posture may provide postural relief of posterior foraminal stenosis but typically alters the sagittal balance, as depicted here. Hip and knee flexion contractures may be associated.

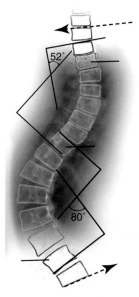

FIG 3 • The Cobb method is used to measure the coronal deformity. Vertebral endplates (or the margins of pedicles) are used to extend lines as depicted for each of the curves involved. Lines orthogonal to these are then compared to determine the scoliosis angle. Vertebrae are typically selected to maximize the Cobb angle on each measurement.

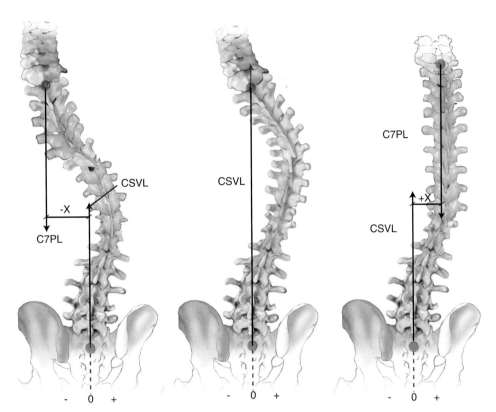

FIG 4 • Coronal balance is evaluated on the standing PA radiograph. A virtual plumb line is dropped from the center of C7. The lateral distance between that plumb line and the center of S1 is then measured. (*Left to right*) Negative coronal decompensation, coronal compensation, and positive coronal decompensation. CSVL, center sacral vertical line.

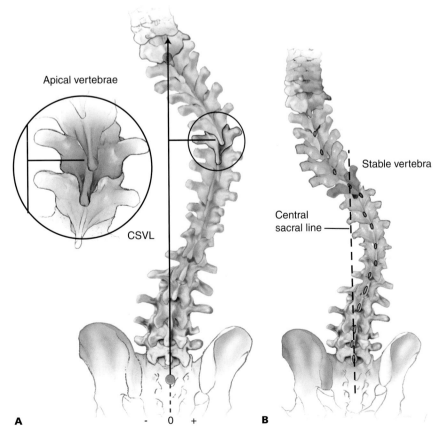

FIG 5 • **A.** The apical vertebra is defined as that which is most deviated laterally on the PA radiograph. **B.** The stable vertebra is defined as the caudal vertebra that is transected by the vertical plumb line extending from the center of S1 on the standing PA radiograph. CSVL, center sacral vertical line.

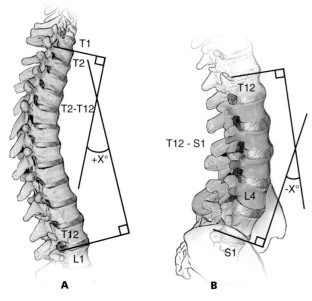

A   **B**

FIG 6 • Regional lordosis and kyphosis are measured on the standing lateral radiograph. Typically the vertebral endplates are used as references for measurement.

- Right- and left-bending PA radiographs (**FIG 8**) are used to:
  - Evaluate spinal flexibility
  - Determine the structural or nonstructural nature of the curve
- Supine traction radiographs may also be used to evaluate curve flexibility.

CT Scans

- Axial CT images, reformatted in the plane of the superior endplates of each vertebra, may be used to measure pedicle dimensions for preoperative planning.
- Plain radiographs and CT images can be used to assess the degree of bone loss and tailor the reconstructive techniques to the bone quality of the patient.

MRI

- MRI is used to assess neurologic compression (**FIG 9**) as well as the status of the disc, ligamentum flavum, and other soft tissues.

Dual-Energy Radiographic Absorptiometry

- Dual-energy radiographic absorptiometry (DEXA) is often performed for patients with identified risk factors[15]:
  - History of fracture as an adult or fracture in a first-degree relative

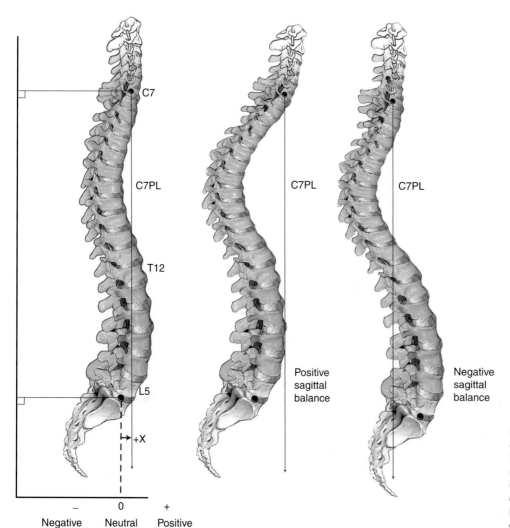

FIG 7 • Sagittal balance is evaluated on the standing lateral radiograph. It is measured as the anterior (positive) or posterior (negative) distance between the C7 plumb line and the center of the L5-S1 disc space.

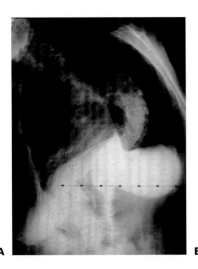
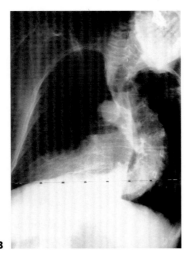

FIG 8 • Bending radiographs aid in determining the flexibility of the spinal curves and are also used to determine the structural or nonstructural nature of the curves.

- White race
- Advanced age
- Smoking
- Low body weight
- Female gender
- Dementia
- Poor health or general fragility

Provocative Tests

- Discography can be useful to assess for painful segments, particularly in the lower lumbar spine.
- Facet blocks have been employed to determine levels that should be included, or need not be included, in the fusion. This may be particularly relevant at the lumbosacral junction.[20]

NONOPERATIVE MANAGEMENT

- A physical therapy regimen may be tried, focusing on:
  - Stretching and core-strengthening exercises
  - Postural training
  - Gait training
  - Resolution of hip and knee flexion contractures
  - General conditioning

- Nonsteroidal anti-inflammatory medications may be used if safely tolerated

SURGICAL MANAGEMENT

- The treatment of adult scoliosis is complex because of the global nature of the spinal deformity and the multiple causes of this disorder.
- Efficiency, safety, and effectiveness in meeting surgical goals are each optimized by a well-designed procedure.

Preoperative Planning

- Preoperative planning is instrumental to a successful treatment algorithm; avoiding both short- and long-term complications is paramount.
- In 1968, the complications associated with surgical correction of adult deformity were estimated to include[31]:
  - 5% risk of death
  - 6% risk of major neurologic deficit
  - 20% risk of correction loss
  - 10% risk of deep infection
  - 40% risk of major medical complication

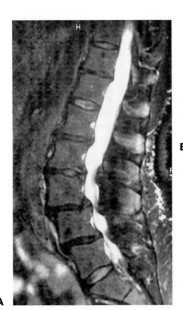
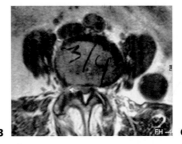
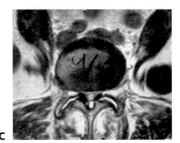

FIG 9 • MRI is particularly useful in evaluating patients with neurologic symptoms such as claudication. It is used to assess neurologic compression as well as the status of the disc, ligamentum flavum, and other soft tissues.

- With advances in surgical and anesthesia techniques, neurophysiologic monitoring, and improvements in perioperative management, these risks have been significantly decreased.[2]
- The patient with adult scoliosis may carry a myriad of comorbidities that may increase the risk of a spinal operation or even contraindicate it. A complete preoperative assessment of those considering surgical treatment provides the opportunity to minimize risks by optimizing health status.
- Modifiable conditions that affect surgical risk include:
  - Tobacco smoking[40]
  - History of asthma or chronic obstructive pulmonary disease[38]
  - Coronary or cerebrovascular disease[1,27]
  - Diabetes[29]
  - Nutritional deficiency[18,30]
  - Osteoporosis[3,23]
  - Depression[34]
  - Current significant life stressors[6]
- Collaboration with consulting medical specialists who are trained in perioperative management is an important technique to optimize outcomes for patients with adult scoliosis.
- Anesthesia colleagues familiar with this surgical course may also reduce risks.
- Certain medical considerations directly affect the selection of surgical techniques for a patient with adult scoliosis.
  - Assessment of bone quality plays a critical role in the design of the operation.
  - Osteoporosis is the rule, not the exception.[22]

Approach

- Posterior surgical approaches are typically used for the treatment of adult deformity correction.
- Anterior surgery may be used alone in isolated cases but is more frequently combined with posterior surgery to augment the deformity correction, reconstruction, or both.
- Anterior exposure allows the soft tissue releases that are often required for adequate deformity correction.

General Procedures

Fixation Strategies for Osteoporotic Bone

- Spinal instrumentation with pedicle screw fixation is less effective in osteoporotic bone.[8,14]
  - Trabecular bone is predominantly affected by osteoporosis.
  - Since pedicle screws have cortical contact limited to the pedicle isthmus, a "windshield wiper" mode of failure typically leads to screw loosening.[24]
- Fixation strategies for osteoporotic bone are targeted toward:
  - Taking advantage of the relatively stronger cortical bone[7]
  - Augmenting the fixation of a pedicle screw within the existing trabecular bone[39]
- Bone-implant interface complications in the osteoporotic spine can be reduced by various methods.
  - Sublaminar wires and pediculolaminar fixation[16] take advantage of the cortical bone composition of the posterior spinal lamina (**FIG 10**).
  - Fixation of pedicle screws within osteoporotic trabecular bone may be improved by polymethylmethacrylate (PMMA) cement augmentation.[36]
    - Fluoroscopy is used to visualize the placement of 2 to 3 cc of PMMA per pedicle to ensure that cement does not migrate to the neural elements.

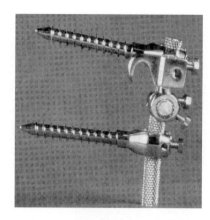

FIG 10 • Fixation strategies for osteoporotic bone may include the use of multiple fixation points in a vertebra. Such instrumentation, as depicted here, incorporates pedicle screw and laminar hook instrumentation at the same vertebral level.

- Calcium sulfate paste may also be used; this has the theoretical advantage of becoming replaced by bone over time.[35]
- Modified pedicle screws may also be used, including conical screws, hydroxyapatite-coated screws, and expandable screws.

PEDICLE SCREW ELECTION AND PLACEMENT

- Screw pullout strength is improved when high insertional torque is achieved[42] by:
  - Undertapping (or not tapping) the screw path
  - Using tapered screws. These are limited by the absolute restriction that they cannot be reversed or backed out; such an action would remove the screw's contact with the bone.
  - Using larger-diameter screws. Increased cortical contact may increase insertional torque but may increase the risk of pedicle fracture as well.
  - Using longer screws: Bicortical purchase can increase screw pullout strength but may pose the possibility of injury to abdominal or vascular structures.

Fusion and Bone Grafting

- Establishment of a solid fusion is critical.
- The pseudarthrosis rate in one large series of adult deformity patients after long fusion procedures was 24%. Statistically significant risk factors for pseudarthrosis in that study included[17]:
  - Thoracolumbar kyphosis
  - Hip osteoarthritis
  - Use of a thoracoabdominal (versus paramedian) approach
  - Positive sagittal balance greater than 5 cm
  - Age greater than 55 years
  - Incomplete sacropelvic fixation
- These risk factors emphasize the importance of surgically establishing the proper mechanical environment, including overall sagittal balance and appropriate fixation.

BONE GRAFT SELECTION

- Appropriate graft selection may reduce pseudarthrosis risk.
- Bone grafts and alternatives may serve multiple roles in the surgical treatment of adult scoliosis; fusion-promotion and deformity-correction techniques both may influence graft selection.

An anterior interbody graft may need to be structural to correct a deformity.

If a structural graft is used anteriorly first, it is with the anticipation that further deformity correction at that segment will be limited by posterior manipulation.

Anterior structural interbody grafts can be instrumental in preventing a kyphosis when the convexity of a deformity is compressed in a reduction maneuver.

Structural grafts can be placed with a bias toward the concavity in order to assist in the deformity correction.

Structural interbody grafts serve a critical role in supplementing the stability of a reconstruction, particularly at the caudal end of a construct, at the lumbar–sacral junction.

Morselized grafts may allow for deformity correction by subsequent posterior manipulation.

Our typical strategy is as follows:

Use structural grafts at the caudal end of the construct (two to four levels).

Overzealous posterior manipulation can cause loosening or displacement of an anterior structural graft.

Use morselized graft rostrally.

Subsequent deformity correction during the posterior procedure will be limited mainly to those levels with morselized (or no) anterior graft.

INTERBODY GRAFT MATERIALS

Graft selection is guided by:

The goal of fusion success

The potential utility of structural roles for the graft

The risk of potential complications and other shortcomings

Costs

Interbody grafts may be composed of:

Bone (autograft or allograft)

Metal

Carbon fiber

PEEK

Other synthetic material

To reduce the risk of graft subsidence, a graft with a modulus of elasticity similar to that of the native bone can be employed.

Iliac crest autograft is typically the best modulus match but is associated with well-established harvest-related morbidity.

In osteoporosis, we have used allograft harvested from the iliac crest of a donor, which offers:

A relatively high proportion of trabecular to cortical bone compared to a long bone allograft, and an improved modulus match

More rapid biologic incorporation of trabecular grafts

Carbon fiber and PEEK interbody cages offer a lower (and more closely matched) modulus compared to metal cages; we typically avoid metal cages in the reconstruction of osteoporotic spinal deformities.

Autograft remains the gold standard material for establishing a solid arthrodesis but has shortcomings:

Morbidity of iliac crest autograft harvest

Chronic donor-site pain

Postoperative hematoma, infection

Nerve or vessel injury

Iliac graft harvest may be undesirable when iliac instrumentation is planned.

Autograft may be insufficient for an extensive thoracolumbar fusion.

Autograft alternatives include allograft products, synthetics, and bone morphogenetic proteins (BMP).

The fusion efficacy of BMP-2 has recently been demonstrated in patients with adult spinal deformity.

Seventy adult patients underwent scoliosis fusion with anterior or posterior BMP-2 application, with either local bone graft only (posterior) or no bone graft (anterior), obviating rib, iliac crest, or other autograft harvest morbidity.

Fusion rates were satisfactory, with 96% anterior fusion success and 93% posterior fusion success.[26]

BONE MORPHOGENETIC PROTEIN

Attention to certain surgical techniques reduces the risk of complications and may also improve efficacy.

The risks associated with the use of BMP in the cervical spine include[41]:

Complications related to soft tissue swelling

Inappropriate bone formation

Accelerated graft resorption

In the lumbar spine, there also have been reports of undesirable effects, including:

Inappropriate bone formation around neural elements[28]

Postoperative radiculitis

Accelerated resorption of interbody grafts, increasing the risk of pseudarthrosis, has also been reported in a study of single-level uninstrumented anterior lumbar interbody fusion.[33]

Structural allograft with appropriate doses of BMP at the lower two to four levels in adult thoracolumbar fusions can, however, be used with minimal risks of complications.

Example: BMP-augmented transforamimal lumbar interbody fusion (TLIF)

Care is taken to reduce the risk of inappropriate bone formation.

These steps may help ensure maintenance of the BMP and limit the BMP from affecting adjacent tissues:

Irrigate before the placement of the BMP packed cage, not afterward.

Pack the BMP sponge entirely within the cage, avoiding "overstuffing."

Place additional sponge only anterior to the cage.

Use a repairable "trapdoor" annulotomy.

A three-sided annular flap is created, hinging medially, such that when the flap is held open with sutures at its corners, it augments the protection of the thecal sac.

After discectomy and placement of BMP, anterior graft, and TLIF cage, the annulotomy is repaired with suture and augmentation of the closure with an adjuvant sealant.

Sagittal Balance

The single most important principle in the surgical treatment of adult scoliosis is achieving and maintaining a proper sagittal balance.

Balanced spinal posture with neutral positioning:

Provides for decreased energy requirements with ambulation

Limits pain and fatigue

Improves cosmesis and patient satisfaction

Limits complications associated with unresolved (or new) deformities

FUSION LEVEL SELECTION

- Sagittal balance must be achieved.
- Junctional problems must be avoided.
- Presenting symptoms can guide level selection.
  - Discography can be useful to assess for painful segments, particularly in the lower lumbar spine, that may be incorporated in the fusion.
  - Facet blocks have been employed to determine levels that should be included or need not be included. This may be particularly relevant at the lumbosacral junction.[20]

RADIOGRAPHS

- 36-inch standing PA and lateral
- PA (left and right) bending views, to determine if the main curves are structural
  - If the Cobb angle is greater than 25 degrees on side-bending radiographs, then it is considered to be a structural curve.[25]
- Curve magnitude and flexibility and the apical vertebral translation of the thoracic and lumbar curves are measured.
- The relationship between the C7 plumb line and the center sacral vertical line is considered.
- Radiographic signs of degenerative disease are categorized.
- Listheses (rotary and lateral) are noted. Degenerative segments often are associated with stenosis; this must be considered in the treatment algorithm.

FUSION TO THE SACRUM

- Extension of the fusion to the sacrum for the adult scoliosis patient is an important and controversial subject. There is no consensus as to the best strategy for all clinical scenarios, but certain guidelines and lessons have been developed.
- There is a relatively high rate of pseudarthrosis (and other complications) after L5–S1 fusion.[11,19] For these reasons, in part, some have advocated avoiding fusion to the sacrum whenever possible.[5]
- Certain scenarios do require lumbosacral fusion:
  - Symptomatic L5–S1 spondylolisthesis
  - Other instability
  - Oblique take-off with over 15 degrees of scoliosis at the L5–S1 segment often requires reduction and fusion for adequate correction of deformity.
  - For correction of lumbar hypolordosis to achieve proper sagittal balance
- The risk of pseudarthrosis at the lumbosacral junction can be limited by:
  - Employing combined approaches to perform a meticulous 360-degree fusion at the L5–S1 segment
  - BMP may be applied to further increase the chances of solid arthrodesis.
  - Anterior instrumentation has been advocated:
    - Fixed-angle plates
    - Vertebral body compression screws
  - Isolated posterior instrumentation may be satisfactory if good bicortical purchase is achieved with sacral screws, with high insertional torque.
- Additional fixation is required, however, in many cases, and iliac screws or Galveston technique fixation satisfies this need.
- Recently, the use of allograft with BMP and posterior pedicle fixation, without iliac fixation, has been used successfully due to the speed of healing, with the caveat that this depends on the length of fusion.

Specific Management Strategies by Diagnosis

Degenerative Lumbar Scoliosis

- The patient with adult lumbar scoliosis typically has some component of back pain and may also present with radiculopathy or claudication.
- For the typical patient presenting with stenosis complaints, decompression of the neural elements is a priority.
- Deformity correction with proper sagittal balance also is a critical goal of surgery.
  - Loss of lumbar lordosis is associated with increased pain.[37]
  - Restoration of proper sagittal balance is the most important factor associated with clinical outcome.[13]
- The typical patient presents with hypolordosis and varying degrees of scoliosis, typically associated with relatively flexible thoracic compensatory curves less than 30 degrees or no thoracic curve (**FIG 11A,B**).
- Common radiographic findings include:
  - Degenerative disease, most commonly at L5–S1
  - Rotary subluxation at L3–L4 (**FIG 11C,D**)
  - Obliquity at L4–L5 (**FIG 11E,F**)
- The choice of surgical approach for the treatment of lumbar adult scoliosis depends on:
  - The levels of the pain-generating segments
  - The flexibility of the curve
  - The coronal obiquity of the distal vertebrae
  - The extent of the curve
- While in situ fusion may be an option for patients with small-magnitude deformity and poor bone quality, typically restoration of lordosis and coronal realignment are desired (**FIG 12**). This can be accomplished with a variety of methods, many of which require restoration of anterior height.

TLIF for Deformity Correction and Reconstruction

- TLIF may achieve these goals with a posterior-only approach.
- To assist in correction of the deformity, the cage may be biased to the concavity of the scoliosis to address the coronal plane.
- After facetectomy and posterior compression, lordosis can be restored.
  - In general, a posterior interbody technique (posterior or thoracic lumbar interbody fusion) is less effective than an anterior interbody approach for restoring lordosis.
  - The use of an operating table that produces extension of the lumbar spine (Jackson) to maximize positional lordosis is critical.
- The decision of the levels to include in the treatment of a degenerative lumbar deformity may be determined by a variety of influences.
  - It can be useful to preoperatively determine which segments contribute to a patient's pain.
  - The apex of the deformity is included (typically L3 or L4).
  - Levels that are severely degenerated may also be included, particularly if they exhibit lateral or rotary listhesis.
- There is no general consensus as to where a lumbar construct should terminate cranially, but it should be at least at a stable end vertebra (ie, the cranial-end level of the fusion construct should be bisected by the center sacral line on a lateral radiograph).
- If the goal is to treat neurogenic claudication, relieve stenosis, and prevent future progression, a short-segment construct (often L2–L5) is sufficient if adequate lordosis is attained and the cranial and caudal vertebrae are well balanced.

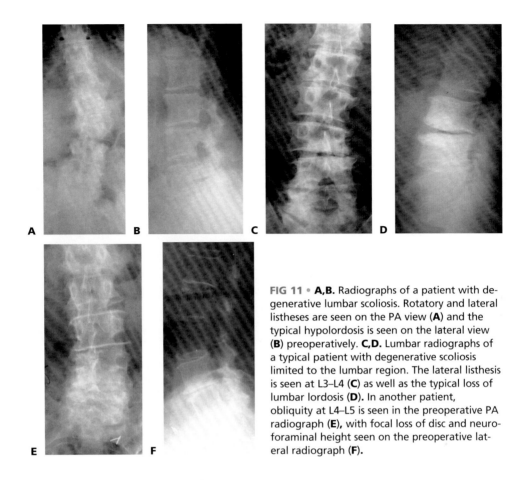

FIG 11 • **A,B.** Radiographs of a patient with degenerative lumbar scoliosis. Rotatory and lateral listheses are seen on the PA view (**A**) and the typical hypolordosis is seen on the lateral view (**B**) preoperatively. **C,D.** Lumbar radiographs of a typical patient with degenerative scoliosis limited to the lumbar region. The lateral listhesis is seen at L3–L4 (**C**) as well as the typical loss of lumbar lordosis (**D**). In another patient, obliquity at L4–L5 is seen in the preoperative PA radiograph (**E**), with focal loss of disc and neuroforaminal height seen on the preoperative lateral radiograph (**F**).

- In many scenarios, however, such as when the Cobb angle is from L1 to L5, it is necessary to continue the fusion cranially past the thoracolumbar junction.
- When this is the case, one should take care not to end the fusion at the thoracolumbar junction or at the apex of the thoracic kyphosis.

- Extending the fusion to the thoracolumbar junction provides fixation into the more stable rib-bearing vertebrae and is more likely to terminate within the sagittal plumb line, reducing the risk of instrumentation failure or junctional kyphosis.
- A frequent decision-making dilemma is where to end the caudal end of the fusion reconstruction.

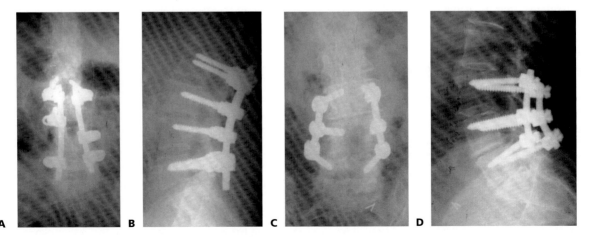

FIG 12 • **A,B.** After decompression of the patient in Figure 11A,B, spinal reconstruction is achieved with recreation of coronal (**A**) and sagittal (**B**) balance. **C,D.** In the patient in Figure 11E,F, postoperative reconstruction after decompression of the neural elements recreates lumbar lordosis to achieve proper sagittal balance.

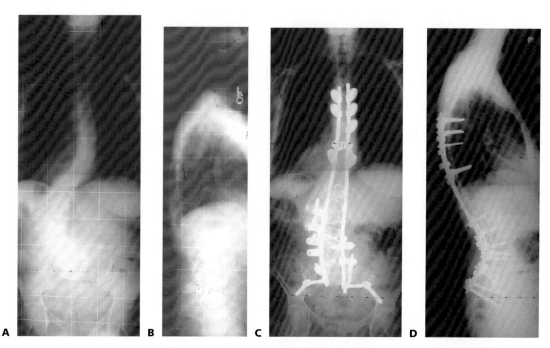

A   B   C   D

FIG 13 • These standing radiographs were performed on 36-inch cassettes before and after scoliosis fusion from T4 to the ileum. **A,B.** Iliac fixation was motivated, in part, by the obliquity at the lumbosacral junction. Concerns related to this patient's osteoporosis led the surgeons to use a combination of fixation techniques, including pedicle screw fixation and sublaminar wiring, to take advantage of the relatively well-preserved cortical bone. There is restoration of coronal (**C**) and sagittal (**D**) balance.

- Accepted indications to fuse to the sacrum include[4]:
  - Spondylolisthesis or previous laminectomy at L5–S1 (**FIG 13A**)
  - Stenosis requiring decompression at L5–S1
  - Severe degeneration
  - An oblique take-off (above 15 degrees) of L5 (**FIG 13B**)
- Fusions to the sacrum in adults with lumbar scoliosis have been found to:
  - Require more additional surgery than those to L5
  - Have more postoperative complications
- On the other hand, fusions to L5 have been associated with:
  - A 61% rate of adjacent segment disease
  - An associated shift in sagittal balance[12]
- When fusion to the sacrum is performed, iliac fixation should be considered, particularly if the fusion includes more than three levels (**FIG 13C,D**).
- Augmentation of the lumbosacral reconstruction with interbody fusion at L5–S1:
  - Improves biomechanical stability[32]
  - Reduces the risk of lumbosacral pseudarthrosis[21]
- A structural graft at L5–S1 can:
  - Recreate lordosis, partially restoring sagittal balance
  - Diminish stenosis by restoring intervertebral height
- Hip and knee flexion contractures can be common in this group, with patients accustomed to ambulating with flexed posture.
  - A flexion contracture at the hip limits the patient's ability to extend the sagittal plumb line posterior to the hips.
  - It may be necessary to address the patient's hip pathologies before planning any surgical correction of a spinal deformity.

Thoracic and Lumbar (Double-Curve) Scoliosis

- Patients with double major adult scoliosis may present with axial skeletal pain.
- Complaints of progressive deformity may be manifested as:
  - Changes in balance
  - Gait abnormalities
  - Alterations in cosmesis
- The surgical treatment of double-curve scoliosis often combines anterior and posterior procedures (**FIG 14**).
  - Long deformities that are relatively inflexible may require anterior releases to accomplish effective reduction and fusion with posterior surgery.
- In part because of the typical degeneration in adult patients, fusions into the caudal lumbar spine are more frequently required.
  - Bending films determine whether the lumbar flexibility is adequate for the scoliosis to "bend out" (see Fig 8).
    - Curve stiffness is related to both patient age and curve magnitude.
    - Flexibility decreases by 10% with every 10-degree increase in coronal deformity beyond 40 degrees.
    - Flexibility decreases by 5% to 10% with each decade of life.[9]
- The correction of a double-curve deformity can be accomplished with a variety of methods. The primary goal of achieving a proper sagittal balance must be emphasized. Reduction of the coronal and rotational deformities follows in priority, with the goal of establishing coronal balance and reduction of rib asymmetry for enhanced cosmesis and patient satisfaction, if possible.

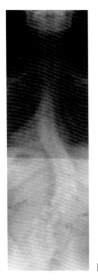
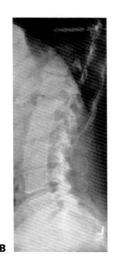
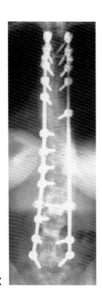
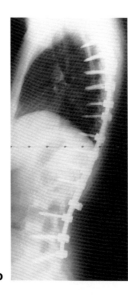

A   B   C   D

FIG 14 • This long thoracolumbar scoliosis was treated with a fusion from the upper thoracic spine to L5. To reduce the risk of pseudarthrosis at the caudal end of the construct and to assist in the recreation of lordosis, structural interbody grafts were placed in the three most caudal disc spaces of the fusion, with morselized graft above, after releases of the anterior interbody soft tissues were performed. Subsequently, a posterior fusion was performed with pedicle screw instrumentation.

- Analogous to the design of the operation for adult lumbar deformities, the decision of whether to extend the fusion to the sacrum may be difficult.
- Lumbosacral fusion is recommended when[5]:
  - Decompression of L5–S1 stenosis is required
  - There is a fixed obliquity over 15 degrees at L5–S1 (see Fig 13B)
- Long fusions to the sacrum increase the risk of pseudarthrosis and reoperation. These may be minimized by anterior augmentation and iliac fixation, as previously discussed (see Fig 14).
- The cranial end of the fusion should include the thoracic curve and should not stop caudal to any structural aspect of it.
- All fixed deformities and subluxations should be included in the fusion.

- Rod cross-links increase the stiffness of long constructs[10] and are recommended (see Fig 14C). They should be avoided at the thoracolumbar junction; however, where they may increase the risk of pseudarthrosis.[17]
- Vertebral derotation
  - Curve stiffness may limit the surgeon's ability to reduce the rotational deformity in the adult population.
  - For relatively flexible rotational deformities, rotational reduction can be achieved with effective improvement in trunk symmetry, which can significantly improve patient satisfaction (**FIG 15**).
  - Additional release maneuvers may be necessary in stiff curves, including thoracoplasty, concave rib osteotomies, and aggressive facetectomies.

PEARLS AND PITFALLS

Reduction of complications associated with BMP	■ The surgeon should minimize the dose of BMP specific to each application. ■ The surgeon should minimize diffusion of the protein from the site of desired action. 　■ Meticulous hemostasis should be achieved before BMP implantation; a postoperative hematoma may provide an avenue for the spread of the protein. 　■ Wound irrigation should be performed before BMP implantation, not afterward. 　■ The BMP should be contained within a rigid structure to limit compression of the implant, to prevent pressure-induced diffusion. 　■ A barrier should be created between the protein implant and sensitive tissues. Thrombin glue has been used to seal the epidural space from the BMP. 　■ Hemostatic sponges and suction drains may permit protein to migrate to adjacent tissues and should not be placed adjacent to the protein implant.
Prevention of adjacent-segment disease	■ The preoperative status (or health) of the segment or disc is the greatest predictor for the development of adjacent segment disease. ■ For the population with adult scoliosis, where some identifiable degenerative disease is nearly ubiquitous, this is particularly relevant. 　■ The surgeon should not end a fusion adjacent to a severely degenerated disc. 　■ The surgeon should not end a fusion adjacent to a segment with fixed obliquity or subluxation. 　■ The surgeon should preserve the supra-adjacent facet. 　■ The surgeon should preserve the intraspinous and the supraspinous ligaments. 　■ The surgeon should not violate the cranial disc space with pedicle screws.

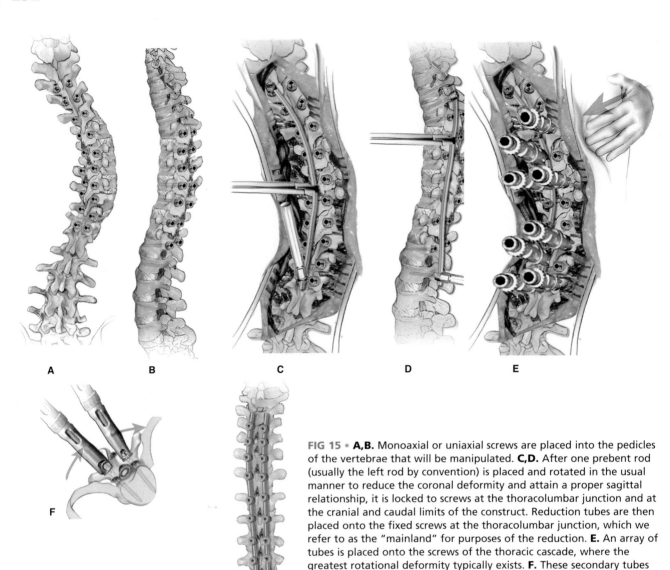

A   B   C   D   E

F

G   H

FIG 15 • A,B. Monoaxial or uniaxial screws are placed into the pedicles of the vertebrae that will be manipulated. **C,D.** After one prebent rod (usually the left rod by convention) is placed and rotated in the usual manner to reduce the coronal deformity and attain a proper sagittal relationship, it is locked to screws at the thoracolumbar junction and at the cranial and caudal limits of the construct. Reduction tubes are then placed onto the fixed screws at the thoracolumbar junction, which we refer to as the "mainland" for purposes of the reduction. **E.** An array of tubes is placed onto the screws of the thoracic cascade, where the greatest rotational deformity typically exists. **F.** These secondary tubes are then aligned toward the mainland vertebrae, effecting the rotational reduction, and locked to the rods. **G.** Rotational reduction is then applied one vertebra at a time in the lumbar region, caudal to the mainland, since the lumbar lordosis often limits the application of more than one set of reduction tubes concurrently. **H.** The prebent contralateral rod is then placed and locked to screws at the thoracolumbar junction as well.

POSTOPERATIVE CARE

- If a brace is used, it must be custom-molded postoperatively, after surgical deformity correction is accomplished.
- Application of a preoperatively molded brace is counterproductive and should be avoided.
- Postoperative physical therapy regimen should focus on:
  - Range-of-motion and flexibility improvement, often in response to chronic hip and knee loss of motion or contractures
  - Gait training, to include balance rehabilitation
  - General conditioning

REFERENCES

1. Auerbach AD, Goldman L. Beta blockers and reduction of cardiac events in noncardiac surgery: clinical applications. JAMA 2002;287: 1445–1447.
2. Baron EM, Albert TJ. Medical complications of surgical treatment of adult spinal deformity and how to avoid them. Spine 2006;31: S106–S118.
3. Berven S, Hu SS. Reconstruction of the osteoporotic spine. In: The Adult and Pediatric Spine, 3rd ed. Philadelphia: Lippincott Williams & Wilkins, 2004:1179–1188.
4. Bridwell KH. Selection of instrumentation and fusion levels for scoliosis: where to start and where to stop. J Neurosurg Spine 2004;1:1–8.
5. Bridwell KH, Edwards CC, Lenke LG. The pros and cons to saving the L5–S1 motion segment in a long scoliosis fusion construct. Spine 2003;28:S234–S242.
6. Clarke DM, Russell PA, Polglase AL. Psychiatric disturbance and acute stress responses in surgical patients. Aust NZ J Surg 1997;67: 812–813.
7. Coe JD, Warden KE, Herzig MA, et al. Influence of bone mineral density on the fixation of thoracolumbar implants: a comparative study of transpedicular screws, laminar hooks, and spinous process wires. Spine 1990;15:902–907.

8. Cook SD, Salkeld SL, Stanley T. Biomechanical study of pedicle screw fixation in severely osteoporotic bone. Spine J 2004;4: 402–408.

9. Deviren V, Berven S, Kleinstueck F, et al. Predictors of flexibility and pain patterns in thoracolumbar and lumbar idiopathic scoliosis. Spine 2002;27:2346–2349.

10. Dick JC, Zdeblick TA, Bartel B, et al. Mechanical evaluation of cross-designs in rigid pedicle screw systems. Spine 1997;22:370–375.

11. Eck KR, Bridwell KH, Ungacta FF. Complications and results of long deformity fusion down to L4, L5, and the sacrum. Spine 2001;26: E182–E192.

12. Edwards CC II, Bridwell KH, Patel A, et al. Thoracolumbar deformity arthrodesis to L5 in adults: the fate of the L5–S1 disc. Spine 2003;28: 2122–2131.

13. Glassman SD, Berven S, Bridwell K, et al. Correlation of radiographic parameters and clinical symptoms in adult scoliosis. Spine 2005;30: 682–688.

14. Halvorson TL, Kelley LA, Thomas KA, et al. Effects of bone mineral density on pedicle screw fixation. Spine 1994;19:2415–2420.

15. Heineman DF. Osteoporosis: an overview of the National Osteoporosis Foundation Clinical Practice Guide. Geriatrics 2000;55:31–36.

16. Hilibrand AS, Moore DC, Graziano GP. The role of pediculolaminar fixation in compromised pedicle bone. Spine 1996;21:445–451.

17. Kim YJ, Bridwell KH, Lenke LG, et al. Pseudarthrosis in long adult spinal deformity instrumentation and fusion to the sacrum: prevalence and risk factor analysis of 144 cases. Spine 2006;31: 2329–2336.

18. Klein JD, Hey LA, Yu CS, et al. Perioperative nutrition and postoperative complications in patients undergoing spine surgery. Spine 1996;21:2676–2682.

19. Kostuik JP, Hall BB. Spinal fusions to the sacrum in adults with scoliosis. Spine 1983;8:489–500.

20. Kostuik JP. Treatment of scoliosis in the adult thoracolumbar spine with special reference of fusion to the sacrum. Orthop Clin North Am 1988;19:371–381.

21. Kuklo TR, Bridwell KH, Lenke LG, et al. Minimum 2-year analysis of sacropelvic fixation and L5–S1 fusion using S1 and iliac screws. Spine 2001;26:1976–1983.

22. Lane JM, Riley EH, Wirganowicz PZ. Osteoporosis: diagnosis and treatment. J Bone Joint Surg Am 1996;78A:618–632.

23. Lane JM, Russell L, Khan SN. Osteoporosis. Clin Orthop Relat Res 2004;425:126–134.

24. Law M, Tencer AF, Anderson PA. Caudo-cephalad loading of pedicle screws: mechanisms of loosening and methods of augmentation. Spine 1993;18:2438–2443.

25. Lenke LG, Betz RR, Harms J, et al. Adolescent idiopathic scoliosis: a new classification to determine extent of spinal arthrodesis. J Bone Joint Surg Am 2001;83A:1169–1181.

26. Luhmann SJ, Bridwell KH, Cheng I, et al. Use of bone morphogenetic protein-2 for adult spinal deformity. Spine 2005;30:S110–S117.

27. Mangano DT, Layug EL, Wallace A. Effect of atenolol on mortality and cardiovascular morbidity after noncardiac surgery. N Engl J Med 1996;335:1713–1720.

28. McKay W, Sandhu HS. RhBMP-2 use in spinal fusions: focus issue on bone morphogenetic proteins in spinal fusion. Spine 2002;27:S66–S85.

29. Moitra VK, Meiler SE. The diabetic surgical patient. Curr Opin Anaesthesiol 2006;19:339–345.

30. Moore FA, Feliciano DV, Andrassy RJ, et al. Early enteral feeding, compared with parenteral, reduces postoperative septic complications. Ann Surg 1992;216:172–183.

31. Nachemson A. A long-term follow-up study of scoliosis. Acta Orthop Scand 1968;39:466–476.

32. Polly DW, Klemme WR, Cunningham BW, et al. The biomechanical significance of anterior column support in a simulated single-level spinal fusion. J Spinal Disord 2000;13:58–62.

33. Pradhan BB, Bae HW, Kropf MA, et al. Graft resorption with rhBMP-2 in anterior cervical discectomy and fusion: a radiographic characterization of the effect of rhBMP-2 on structural allografts. Spine J 2005;5:181S–189S.

34. Rosenberger PH, Jokl P, Ickovics J. Psychosocial factors and surgical outcomes: an evidence-based literature review. J Am Acad Orthop Surg 2006;14:397–405.

35. Rothmiller MT, Schwalm D, Glattes RC, et al. Evaluation of calcium sulfate paste for augmentation of lumbar pedicle screw pullout strength. Spine J 2002;2:255–260.

36. Sarzier JS, Evans AJ, Cahill DW. Increase pedicle screw pullout strength with vertebroplasty augmentation in osteoporotic spines. J Neurosurg 2002;96:309–312.

37. Schwab FJ, Smith V, Biserni M. Adult scoliosis: a quantitative radiographic and clinical analysis. Spine 2002;28:602–606.

38. Smetana GW. Preoperative pulmonary evaluation. N Engl J Med 1999;340:937–943.

39. Tan J, Kwon B, Dvorak MF, et al. Pedicle screw motion in the osteoporotic spine after augmentation with laminar hooks, sublaminar wires, or calcium phosphate cement: a comparative analysis. Spine 2004;29:1723–1730.

40. Warner MA, Offord KP, Warner ME. Role of preoperative cessation of smoking and other factors in postoperative pulmonary complications: a blinded prospective study of CAB patients. Mayo Clin Proc 1989; 64:609.

41. White AP, Brothers J, Albert TJ, et al. Surgical techniques to maximize safety of bone morphogenetic proteins in spinal surgery. Minerv Orthoped Traum 2007. In press.

42. Zindrick MR, Wiltse LL, Widell EH. A biomechanical study of intrapedicular screw fixation in the lumbosacral spine. Clin Orthop Relat Res 1986;203:99–112.

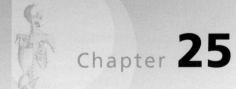
Smith-Petersen Osteotomy and Pedicle Subtraction Osteotomy

Lukas P. Zebala and Keith H. Bridwell

DEFINITION

▪ Smith-Petersen osteotomy (SPO) is a chevron resection of the posterior elements that shorten the posterior column and lengthen the anterior column upon closure (**FIG 1**). The chevron osteotomy is called a SPO if performed through a prior fusion or a Ponté osteotomy if done through a nonfused spinal segment.

▪ Pedicle subtraction osteotomy (PSO) is a posterior based osteotomy that requires resection of the posterior elements, pedicles, and decancellation of the vertebral body in a V-shaped fashion through the transpedicular corridor (**FIG 2**). The osteotomy hinges on the anterior column with closure of the middle and posterior columns creating a large cancellous bone footprint for fusion.

ANATOMY

▪ A thorough understanding of spinal anatomy including spinal cord, nerve root, and vertebral segments is needed to safely perform these procedures. For an SPO, understanding the relationship of the interspinous ligaments, ligamentum flavum, facet joints, nerve roots, and spinal cord is important to resect enough posterior elements to allow osteotomy closure without posterior impingement. In a PSO, it is important to understand these same relationships, but in addition, the relationship of the exiting and traversing nerve roots to the corresponding pedicle is necessary to allow safe osteotomy closure.

▪ SPO involves creating a chevron trough in the posterior elements by resecting the posterior elements through the facet joints and pars intra-articularis and posterior ligaments

(supraspinous, intraspinous, and ligamentum flavum). A mobile disc space allows for closure of the middle and posterior columns and spontaneous opening of the anterior column.

▪ A pedicle subtraction osteotomy requires a wide laminectomy from the pedicle above to pedicle below the osteotomy level, resection of the bilateral pedicles at the PSO level, and vertebral body decancellation to the anterior vertebral body in a wedge shape.

PATHOGENESIS

▪ Sagittal imbalance has been classified into both type I and type II. Type I sagittal imbalance is when there is a region of the spine that is fused in a hypolordotic or kyphotic position, but overall sagittal balance is satisfactory (sagittal C7 plumb falling through the L5 to S1 disc space or slightly behind it on a standing long cassette lateral radiograph), as the patient is able to compensate through nonfused segments. A type II imbalance is one in which the patient cannot compensate due to adjacent level degeneration resulting in a positive sagittal imbalance (patient leans forward in the sagittal plane). Type I patients often maintain their balance by hyperextending through mobile lumbar segments below the kyphotic segment. In type II imbalance, vertebral segments above or below the kyphotic area are substantially degenerated or fused and, therein, the spine is unable to hyperextend and maintain balance (**FIG 3A,B**).

▪ Kyphosis can be smooth and span several segments, such as in Scheuermann kyphosis (**FIG 4A,B**), or sharp and angular, over one or two segments, such as in congenital or posttraumatic kyphosis.

Smith-Petersen Osteotomy

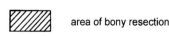

FIG 1 • Drawing depicting area of bone resection for a Smith-Petersen osteotomy.

Three Column Pedicle Subtraction Osteotomy

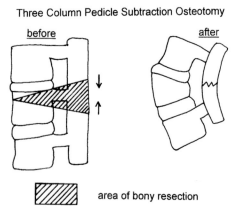

FIG 2 • Drawing depicting area of bone resection for a pedicle subtraction osteotomy.

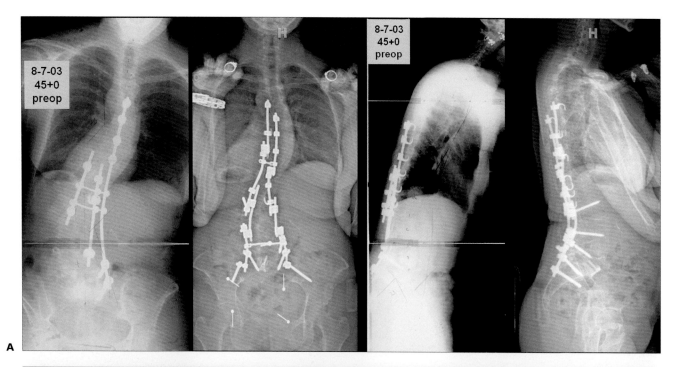

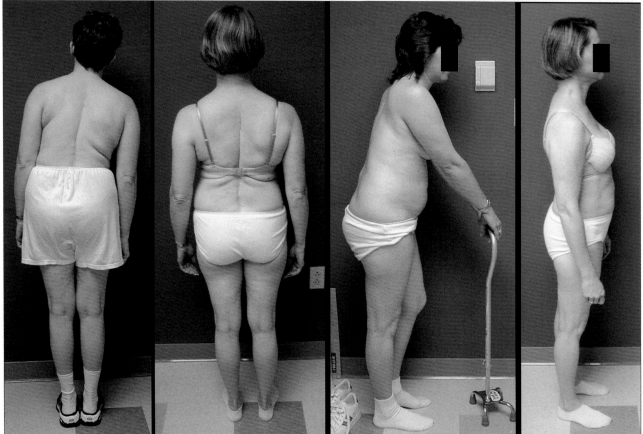

FIG 3 • A and B: Patient (45-year-old woman) with eight prior spinal fusions presenting with fixed sagittal and coronal imbalances. An asymmetric L2 pedicle subtraction osteotomy was performed for spinal realignment. At 6 years follow-up, a solid fusion was achieved with improvement in radiographic and clinical appearance.

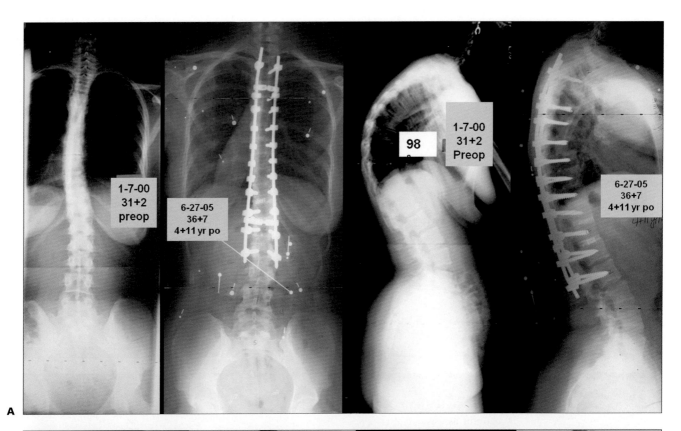

A

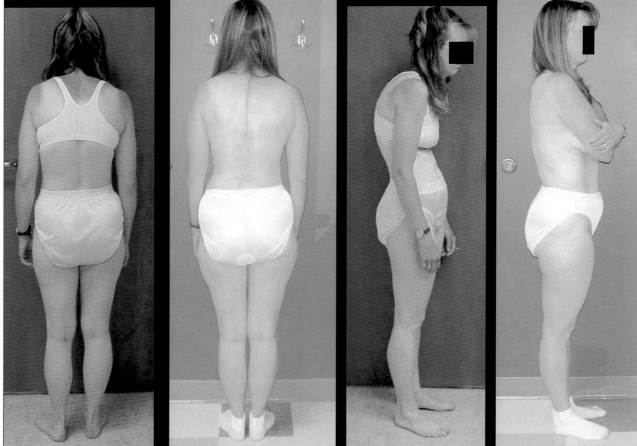

B

FIG 4 • A and B: Patient (31-year-old woman) with three prior posterior spinal fusions at outside institution for treatment of Scheuermann kyphosis presented with worsened thoracic kyphosis, multiple pseudarthrosis, and sagittal imbalance. A revision T3 to L2 posterior spinal fusion with Smith-Petersen osteotomies T5 to T12 and anterior spinal fusion was performed for spinal realignment. At 4+11 year follow-up, a solid anteroposterior fusion was achieved with improvement in radiographic and clinical appearance.

▪ These osteotomies are most often used for the correction of sagittal imbalance or kyphosis. SPOs are most often used to correct sagittal imbalance between 5 and 10 cm or smooth gradual kyphosis, whereas a PSO is used to treat sagittal imbalance >10 cm or sharp, angular kyphosis within the lumbar spine. An asymmetric PSO can be done for a deformity that has both a coronal imbalance and sagittal imbalance together. A vertebral column resection (VCR) may be use to treat sharp, angular kyphosis within the thoracic or thoracolumbar spine.

NATURAL HISTORY

▪ The natural history of the diseases/conditions leading to sagittal imbalance and kyphosis are variable and a complete workup is necessary before recommending an osteotomy as a corrective operation.
▪ Deformities that progress become rigid and, uncompensated, may present with intolerable pain, decreased ability to perform activities of daily living, or myelopathy and nerve root impingement.

PATIENT HISTORY AND PHYSICAL FINDINGS

▪ The thorough history should include an understanding of the patient's main reason(s) for seeking treatment, for example, progressive deformity, pain, loss of function, neurologic deterioration.
▪ The history should include a careful assessment of current pain medication usage, as preoperative narcotic usage may complicate the perioperative care. Additionally, any medications that may confer a risk of increased bleeding (eg, acetylsalicylic acid [ASA]) should be noted, and the patient is cautioned to stop them prior to surgery.
▪ Patients should be questioned on their use of nicotine-containing products, particularly cigarettes as the risk of perioperative complications and pseudarthrosis is increased in these patients and may be a relative contraindication to these procedures.
▪ Those patients with diabetes mellitus must have well controlled blood glucose levels before and after surgery, as uncontrolled blood glucose levels are associated with increased risk of perioperative infection.
▪ A patient's nutritional status should be assessed and optimized prior to surgery. In addition, a bone density test should be performed to assess for osteoporosis and appropriate treatment of these deficiencies or referral for their treatment should be initiated.
▪ Patients with respiratory disease may require consultation with a pulmonologist or assessment of lung function by pulmonary function tests. Cardiac history should be assessed with the assistance of a cardiologist. Often, coordination with the patient's primary care physician is necessary to get the patient ready for these surgeries.
▪ The overall coronal and sagittal plane balance should be observed with the patient standing upright in the clinical exam.
▪ The deformity should be assessed for its flexibility by placing the patient prone and supine on the exam table. Several minutes of supine positioning will allow one to assess the flexibility of a kyphotic deformity.
▪ A detailed neurologic exam assessing sensation, strength, reflexes, and pathologic reflexes is necessary. A complete neurologic examination should assess for signs of myelopathy (gait disturbance such as a wide-based gait, imbalance) or

nerve root palsies (foot drop). In addition, assessment of hip and knee contractures is required as these conditions may make osteotomy correction and postoperative recovery more difficult.

IMAGING AND OTHER DIAGNOSTIC STUDIES

▪ Radiographic assessment includes a series of standing full length 36-inch radiographs in the anteroposterior (AP) and lateral planes, left and right side bending radiographs if coronal deformity is present, and full length supine or prone radiographs to assess spontaneous deformity correction.
▪ Hyperextension radiographs (bolster placed at apex of kyphosis) and hyperflexion radiographs (bolster at apex of lordosis) help assess sagittal plane rigidity.
▪ For sagittal plane deformity, comparison of standing AP and lateral radiographs to prone and/or supine fulcrum hyperextension long-cassette radiographs will help assess deformity flexibility.
▪ CT scan is often obtained to assess prior fusion masses, bone quality, relevant bone anatomy at proposed osteotomy site, and bone anomalies (small pedicles) that may preclude safe fixation point placement. A CT myelogram may help assess areas of stenosis.
▪ MRI is often obtained to evaluate the spinal cord and nerve roots in addition to assessing for neural axis anomalies.
▪ If SPOs are planned, assessment for mobile disc spaces is paramount as this is a requirement for this osteotomy.

DIFFERENTIAL DIAGNOSIS

▪ Smooth global kyphosis (Scheuermann kyphosis)
▪ Sharp angular kyphosis (posttraumatic)
▪ Sagittal imbalance (type I and II) (flat-back syndrome, postlaminectomy kyphosis)

NONOPERATIVE MANAGEMENT

▪ Patients with static deformities and only mild pain or physical impairment should be managed with a trial of nonoperative therapy.
▪ This includes a directed physical therapy program, to include cardiovascular conditioning, postural training, and abdominal strengthening.
▪ For those patients with moderate to severe pain, a referral to a pain specialist, most notably for those patients with complaints of pain not consistent with their presenting pathology, or other signs of nonorganic causes of pain.
▪ Epidural and transforaminal steroid injections offer a less invasive potentially diagnostic and/or therapeutic intervention for patients with nerve root compression.

SURGICAL MANAGEMENT

▪ SPO is often used to treat smooth, gradual kyphotic deformities or positive sagittal imbalance of 5 to 10 cm. Usually, multiple SPOs through the apex of the deformity are performed (**FIGS 5–7**). It is important to perform a wide facetectomy as posterior compression closes down the neural foramina and may cause nerve root impingement. In general, the degree of kyphotic correction with a single SPO is 10 degrees per level or 1 degree per millimeter of bone resected.
▪ A pedicle subtraction osteotomy is most often performed for sharp angular kyphosis, gradual kyphosis that lacks mobile

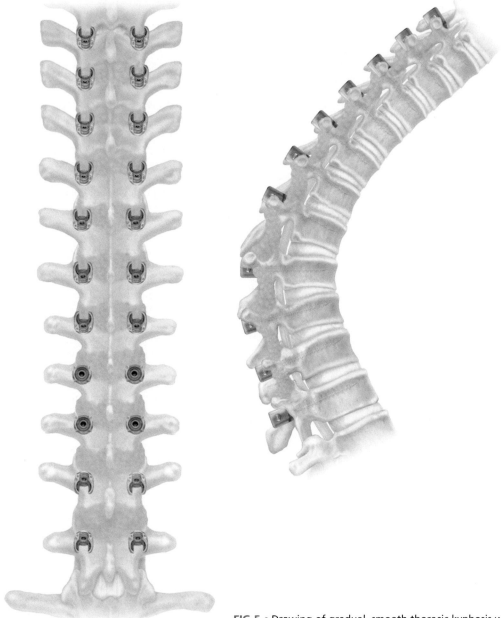

FIG 5 • Drawing of gradual, smooth thoracic kyphosis with multilevel pedicle screw placement.

disc spaces or positive sagittal imbalance greater than 10 cm. In general, the degree of kyphotic correction with a lumbar PSO is approximately 30 to 40 degrees.

Preoperative Planning

■ A multidisciplinary team approach is often necessary in the treatment of patients with complex deformity that require multilevel SPOs or a PSO.

■ Preoperative assessment of the patient's cardiovascular, pulmonary, nutritional, hematologic, and metabolic systems is required to maximize the patient's preoperative reserve. SPOs can be performed within any region of the spine, most often in the thoracic or lumbar spine. PSOs are most often performed in the lumbar spine, usually at L2 or L3. A PSO in the lower lumbar spine, L4 or L5, reduces the number of available distal fixation points.

Positioning

■ An Orthopedic Systems Incorporated (OSI) Jackson frame with six pads is the authors' preferred operative table when performing corrective deformity surgery. The pads are strategically placed to allow the abdomen to rest free, reducing intra-abdominal pressure and intraoperative bleeding. In addition, the axilla should be free to help reduce the risk of brachial plexus injury.

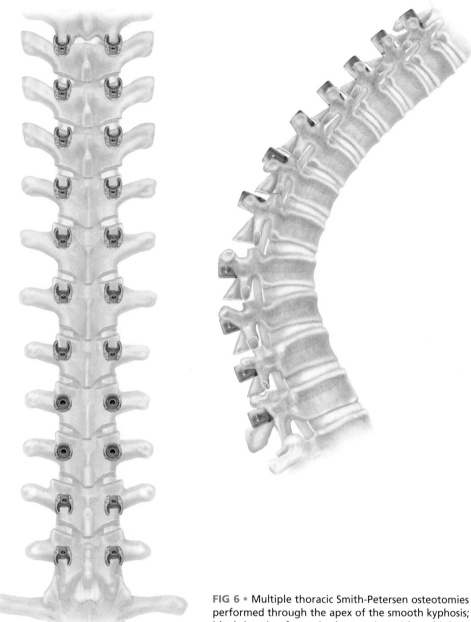

FIG 6 • Multiple thoracic Smith-Petersen osteotomies performed through the apex of the smooth kyphosis; an ideal situation for sagittal correction with multiple Smith-Petersen osteotomies.

■ We prefer to place a halo or Gardner-Wells tongs with 5 to 15 lb of traction that allows for rigid positioning of the skull and allows the face and eyes to remain free during surgery.
■ Arms are placed in a 90/90 position on padded arm boards with no pressure on the axillae and elbow padding to decrease the risk of brachial plexopathy or ulnar nerve neuropathy.
■ The hips are gently extended, and the knees slightly flexed. For PSO correction, the hips can be extended further to help close down the osteotomy.
■ Spinal cord monitoring leads are placed to monitor the sensory and motor function of the lower extremities.

Approach
■ The standard posterior subperiosteal approach is used from the transverse processes of the most superior instrumented level to the most distal vertebra or ilium that are to be fused.
■ The approach can be done in stages, lumbar followed by thoracic or vice versa, to help reduce blood loss if adequate surgical help is not available. In conjunction with the anesthesiologist, hypotensive anesthesia is used to help reduce blood loss.
■ In addition, the use of antifibrinolytic medications can assist in helping reduce blood loss during these procedures.

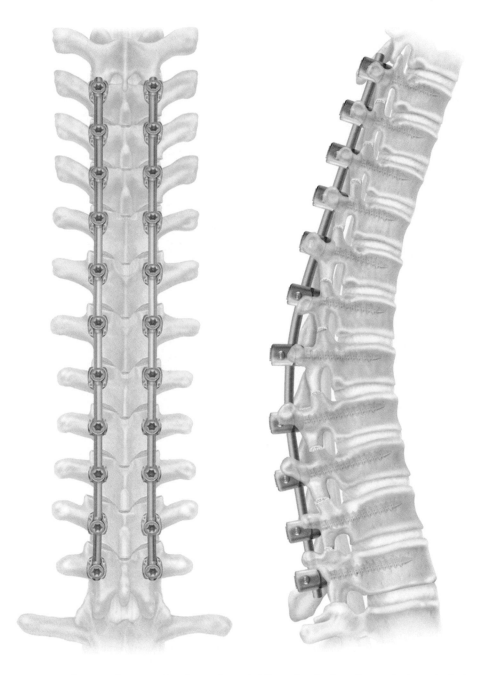

FIG 7 • Cantilever and compression forces through bilateral rods allow for gradual, controlled correction of the smooth kyphosis by closing down of the Smith-Petersen osteotomies.

Smith-Petersen Osteotomy

- Step 1. Identify the pedicles at all levels where SPOs are planned by placing pedicle screws. Alternatively, SPOs can be done prior to placement of pedicle screws. For large deformities or abnormal pedicle anatomy, performing a SPO first can help identify the medial and superior borders of the pedicle to assist in locating of the starting point for pedicle screw placement.
- Step 2. Remove the interspinous ligaments down to level of ligament flavum and identify the median raphe.

Ensure adequate space between ligament flavum and dura with a Woodson elevator and use Kerrison punches to resect a V of bone that starts centrally and works out laterally through the facet joints and pars (**FIG 1**).
- Step 3. Closure of the osteotomy is through a combination of compression and cantilever forces (**FIGS 5–7**). In treatment of a smooth gradual kyphosis, bilateral rods are contoured to the desired sagittal plane profile and secured into the cephalad pedicles. Gradual cantilever

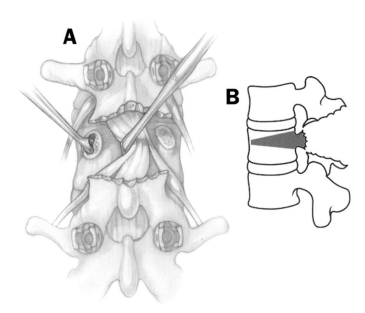

TECH FIG 1 • **A and B:** Resect all the posterior elements around the pedicles

(downward) force is applied and the rods are sequentially captured within the caudally located pedicle screws. Once the rod is captured within the pedicle screws, sequential compression through the pedicle screws towards the deformity apex can be added to close down the SPOs. Compressive forces reduce spinal kyphosis.

Pedicle Subtraction Osteotomy

- Step 1. Resect all the posterior elements around the pedicles with a combination of Leksell rongeurs, high-speed burr, and Kerrison punches. The pedicles are surrounded medially, laterally, superiorly, and inferiorly (**TECH FIG 1**).
- Step 2. Decancellate the pedicles and the vertebral body (**TECH FIG 2**).

- Step 3. Thin the posterior vertebral body wall with a curette until it is wafer thin. Greenstick the posterior vertebral cortex with a Woodson elevator or reverse angled curette (**TECH FIG 3**).
- Step 4. Resect the lateral vertebral cortex with a Leksell rongeur bilaterally (**TECH FIG 4**).
- Step 5. Closure of the osteotomy. Gentle downward pressure on the two segments along with compression through the pedicle screws and rods can be used to approximate the two osteotomy edges. Cantilevering through the rods can also assist in osteotomy closure. Sometimes placing more pillows/pads underneath the patient's hips and legs can extend the pelvis/hips and help with osteotomy closure. A third rod technique can also be used. This relies on establishing midline fixation

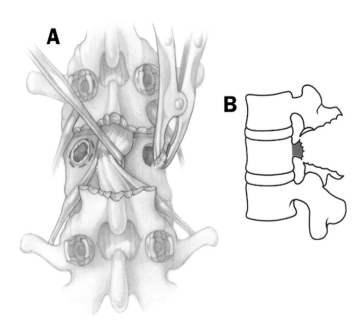

TECH FIG 2 • **A and B:** Decancellate the pedicles and the vertebral body

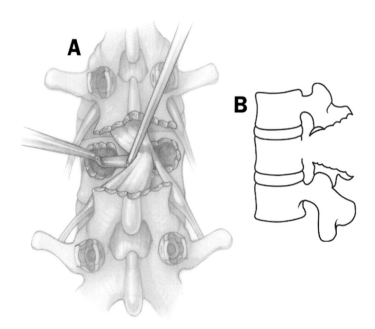

TECH FIG 3 • **A and B:** Greenstick the posterior vertebral cortex with a Woodson elevator or reverse angled curette.

points, often through a prior fusion mass, above and below the PSO site. A rod within these fixation points can then be used to use sequential compression to bring the osteotomy to closure. We do not routinely use special osteotomy tables; however, these do exist that can be used to assist in gradual osteotomy closure. (**TECH FIG 5**).

■ Step 6. Inspect the osteotomy site to make sure that there is adequate decompression without dorsal impingement of the thecal sac or nerve roots after the osteotomy is closed (**TECH FIG 6A,B**). An asymmetrical PSO requires resection of more bone on the convex side

of the deformity when creating the wedge resection so that during closure the convex side is closed more than the concave side allowing rebalancing of the patient in the coronal plane and sagittal plane. Not only is the posterior column resection bigger on the convexity, but the middle and anterior columns have to be resected more generously on the convexity as well. This involves turning the corner on the vertebral body and what amounts to resecting two-thirds of the convexity of the vertebral body both laterally and anteriorly, which otherwise would not be necessary with a standard PSO.

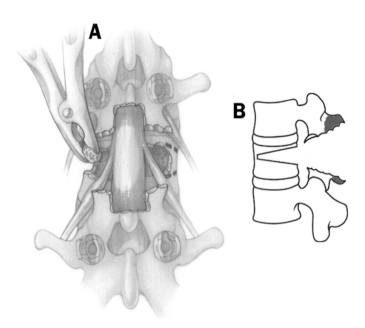

TECH FIG 4 • **A and B:** Resect the lateral vertebral cortex with luxell bilaterally.

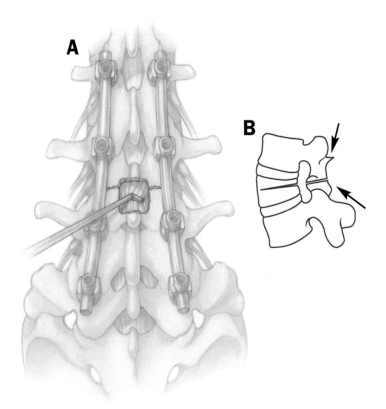

TECH FIG 5 • **A and B:** Close down the osteotomy by compression, cantilever, and extension of chest and lower extremities.

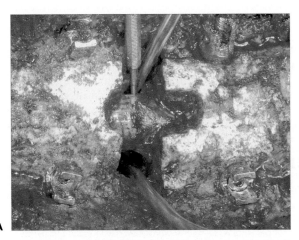
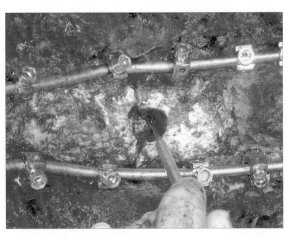

TECH FIG 6 • **A and B:** Intraoperative photograph showing the surgeon assessing for adequate decompression posteriorly at the pedicle subtraction osteotomy (PSO) site prior to and after PSO closure to help prevent iatrogenic impingement of neural elements with PSO closure.

PEARLS AND PITFALLS

Smith-Petersen osteotomy	■ Fixation points can be placed before or after the osteotomies are performed.
	■ For large deformities or abnormal pedicle anatomy, performing an SPO first, prior to pedicle screw placement, can help in identifying the medial and superior borders of the pedicle to assist in locating the starting point.
	■ Undercut the lamina as much as possible to remove all ligamentum flavum.
	■ If possible, limit the amount of forces placed on the pedicle screws and apply forces more through the posterior elements.
Pedicle subtraction osteotomy	■ Resect a symmetrical wedge of bone within the vertebral body to minimize the potential for coronal decompensation with osteotomy closure.
	■ Ensure that the ventral dura is free from the posterior vertebral cortex and that the posterior vertebral cortex is adequately thin to allow for controlled implosion of the bone into the osteotomy site.
	■ Attempting to greenstick the posterior vertebral cortex that is too thick may require too much force and increases the risk of a ventral dural tear.
	■ Remember, as the osteotomy is closed, the contour in the rods will have to change. As more closure is achieved, more lordosis is needed in the rods.
	■ If possible, limit the amount of forces placed on the pedicle screws and apply forces more through the posterior elements.
	■ With pedicle subtraction procedures, there is some risk of dural buckling and the posterior elements impinging on the dura. Our preference is to enlarge the field centrally to observe dural buckling and to "feel" the dorsal canal with nerve hooks/Woodson elevators. Watch carefully for vertebral subluxation at the osteotomy site.
	■ Neuromonitoring is followed for up to 1 hour after final osteotomy compression. A formal wake-up test is often done after the osteotomy closure, as neuromonitoring is at times unable to detect nerve root injury. A formal wake-up test is performed prior to leaving the operating room.

POSTOPERATIVE CARE

■ Patients are often sent to the intensive care unit for close monitoring (for 24 to 48 hours as needed) and then transitioned to the hospital ward.

■ Patients are mobilized on postoperative day 1.

■ Drains are retained until recorded output is less than 30 mL per 8-hour shift.

■ Diet is advanced slowly, with the return of bowel sounds.

■ Deep vein thrombosis prophylaxis is provided with sequential compressive devices and thromboembolic deterrent hose.

■ Avoid flexion and axial loading of the spine for at least 4 months postoperatively.

■ No cast or brace is necessary

OUTCOMES

■ Studies have shown improvement (20% to 30%) in Scoliosis Research Society (SRS)-30 and Oswestry Disability Index scores in most patients at 2- and 5-year follow-up.[1–4]

■ Three SPOs accomplish approximately what is accomplished with one pedicle subtraction procedure. The blood loss is greater with a pedicle subtraction procedure.[1,6]

COMPLICATIONS

■ Substantial complications associated with pedicle subtraction osteotomies include neurologic deficit, substantial blood loss, and adding on to the sagittal deformity if the entire thoracic and lumbar spine is not fused.[2]

■ The neurologic risk with performing a pedicle subtraction procedure in the lumbar spine exceeds the risk associated with three SPOs. The complications associated with the procedure in older patients are more substantial.[5]

■ A review of 108 pedicle subtraction osteotomies revealed an intraoperative and postoperative neurological deficit rate of 11.1 % with 2.8% of deficits being permanent.[5]

■ Multiple SPOs can accomplish substantial correction of major fixed sagittal imbalance. However, there is a risk of pitching the patient to the concavity because of the fact that the osteotomies are often performed through areas of residual scoliosis and the SPO shortens the concavity/posterior elements and lengthens the convexity/anterior disc spaces.[1]

REFERENCES

1. Booth KC, Bridwell KH, Lenke LG, et al. Complications and predictive factors for the successful treatment of flatback deformity (fixed sagittal imbalance). Spine 1999;24(16):1712–1720.
2. Bridwell KH, Lewis S, Edwards C, et al. Complications and outcomes of pedicle subtraction osteotomies for fixed sagittal imbalance. Spine 2003;28(18):2093–2101.
3. Bridwell KH, Lewis SJ, Rinella A, et al. Pedicle subtraction osteotomy for the treatment of fixed sagittal imbalance: Surgical technique. J Bone Joint Surg [Am] 2004;86A(1):44–50.
4. Bridwell KH, Lewis S, Edwards C, et al. Complications and outcomes of pedicle subtraction osteotomies for fixed sagittal imbalance. Spine 2003;28(18):2093–2101.
5. Buchowski JM, Bridwell KH, Lenke LG, et al. Neurological complications of lumbar pedicle subtraction osteotomy: a 10-year assessment. Spine 2007;32(20):2245–2252.
6. Cho K, Bridwell KH, Lenke LG, et al. Comparison of Smith-Petersen versus pedicle subtraction osteotomy for the correction of fixed sagittal imbalance. Spine 2005;30(18):2030–2037.

Chapter 26

Vertebral Column Resection for Severe Rigid Spinal Deformity through an All Posterior Approach

Michael P. Kelly, Lukas P. Zebala, and Lawrence G. Lenke

DEFINITION

■ Posterior vertebral column resection (VCR) entails the removal of the anterior, middle, and posterior columns of the vertebra(e) through a posterior-alone approach. VCR is often performed at the apex of a deformity for severe, rigid scoliotic and kyphotic spinal deformities.

ANATOMY

■ A thorough understanding of the anatomy of the vertebral segment and spinal cord is needed to safely perform this procedure. This includes understanding the peculiarities of rotated vertebral segments in severe scoliotic deformities. The morphologic and iatrogenic changes of the posterior elements must be appreciated, as must the course of the spinal cord and nerve roots.

PATHOGENESIS

■ The origins of these deformities are multiple and varied, including congenital, idiopathic, neoplastic, traumatic, and iatrogenic causes.

NATURAL HISTORY

■ The natural history of the diseases leading to severe scoliotic, kyphotic, or combined deformities are variable.
■ Those that do progress to severe, rigid deformities may present with intolerable deformity, severe pain, decreased ability to perform activities of daily living, myelopathy/spinal cord compression, and pulmonary dysfunction.
■ Those fixed deformities that are asymptomatic (i.e., a well-balanced patient without complaint) may be managed nonoperatively. However, one must obtain careful follow-up to assess for possible deformity progression over time.

PATIENT HISTORY AND PHYSICAL FINDINGS

■ The overall coronal and sagittal plane balance should be observed with the patient standing upright.
■ The deformity should be assessed for any flexibility by placing the patient prone and supine on the exam table. Several minutes of supine positioning will allow one to assess the flexibility of a kyphotic deformity. Often, we will have the patient lie supine on the examining table, turn the lights off, and return in 15 to 20 minutes for repeat evaluation.
■ The history should include a careful assessment of current pain medication usage, as preoperative narcotic usage may complicate the perioperative care. Additionally, any medications that may confer a risk of increased bleeding (e.g., aspirin)

should be noted, and the patient cautioned to stop them prior to surgery.
■ The use of nicotine-containing products, particularly cigarettes, is a relative contraindication to this procedure as the risk of pseudarthrosis is increased as well as perioperative complications.
■ Those patients with diabetes mellitus must have well controlled blood glucose levels before surgery, as uncontrolled blood glucose levels are associated with increased risk of perioperative infection.
■ A patient's nutritional status should be assessed and optimized prior to surgery. In addition, a bone density test should be performed to diagnosis presence of osteoporosis and initiation of preoperative treatment of any deficiencies.
■ The patient's gait should be assessed for evidence of myelopathy (e.g., wide based, shuffling gait).
■ A detailed neurologic examination must be performed and documented including examination for pathologic reflexes, like asymmetric abdominal reflexes, Babinski's response, and sustained clonus. Pathologic reflexes must alert the surgeon to possible intraspinal pathologies (e.g., Chiari II, syrinx, tethered cord) that may need to be addressed prior to the deformity correction.
■ Preoperative examinations by a primary care physician, a cardiologist (including stress testing as indicated), and an anesthesiologist is mandatory to mitigate any risks of perioperative morbidity and mortality.
■ A review of systems should include a review of the respiratory system and any history of respiratory compromise or distress. Preoperative pulmonary function tests should be obtained in all patients with a deformity severe enough to be considered for a VCR procedure.

IMAGING AND OTHER DIAGNOSTIC STUDIES

■ A radiographic spinal deformity series is obtained, which includes standing anteroposterior (AP) and lateral long-cassette radiographs, left and right side bending, full AP, and lateral supine or prone images (**FIGS 1 TO 3** [Case 1]).
■ Flexibility radiographs include push-prone and axial traction X-rays and help assess coronal plane rigidity.
■ Hyperextension radiographs (bolster placed at apex of kyphosis) and hyperflexion radiographs (bolster at apex of lordosis) help assess sagittal plane rigidity.
■ A three-dimensional (3D) CT scan is obtained to evaluate the entire anterior and posterior spinal column. This aids in the identification of important vertebral landmarks (**FIG 4A,B**).
■ Skull to sacrum MRI is necessary to evaluate the entire neural axis (e.g., Chiari malformation, syringomyelia, tethered spinal cord) (**FIGS 5 AND 6** [Case 2]).

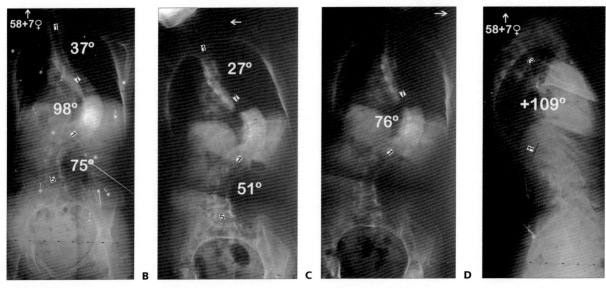

FIG 1 • **A–D.** Case 1. Fifty-eight-year-old woman with adult idiopathic thoracic kyphoscoliosis.

DIFFERENTIAL DIAGNOSIS

- Severe scoliosis
- Global kyphosis
- Angular kyphosis
- Kyphoscoliosis
- Fixed coronal and sagittal imbalance syndrome (e.g., status post-Harrington rod instrumentation)

NONOPERATIVE MANAGEMENT

- Patients with static deformities and only mild pain or physical impairment should be managed with a trial of nonoperative therapy.
- This includes a directed physical therapy program, to include cardiovascular conditioning, postural training, and abdominal strengthening.

- For those patients with moderate-to-severe pain, a referral to a pain specialist, most notably for those patients with complaints of pain not consistent with their presenting pathology, or other signs of nonorganic causes of pain.
- As with nerve root compression, epidural and transforaminal steroid injections offer a less invasive potentially diagnostic and/or therapeutic intervention.

SURGICAL MANAGEMENT

- Classically, rigid deformities were treated with staged anterior and posterior procedures to resect and reconstruct the spine through the rigid segment.[1-3] The posterior vertebral column resection allows a similar correction of deformity, with the benefits of shorter total operative time, and lower blood loss.[4]

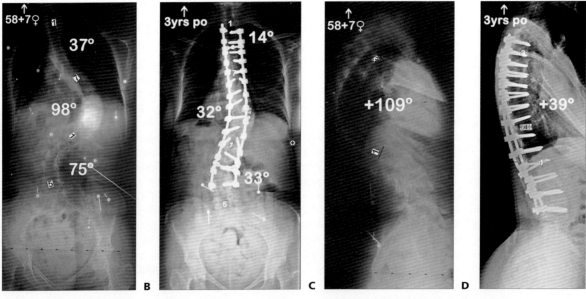

FIG 2 • **A–D.** Case 1. Patient underwent a posterior spinal fusion T2–L4 with a T10 VCR with radiographs demonstrating excellent alignment at 3 years postoperative.

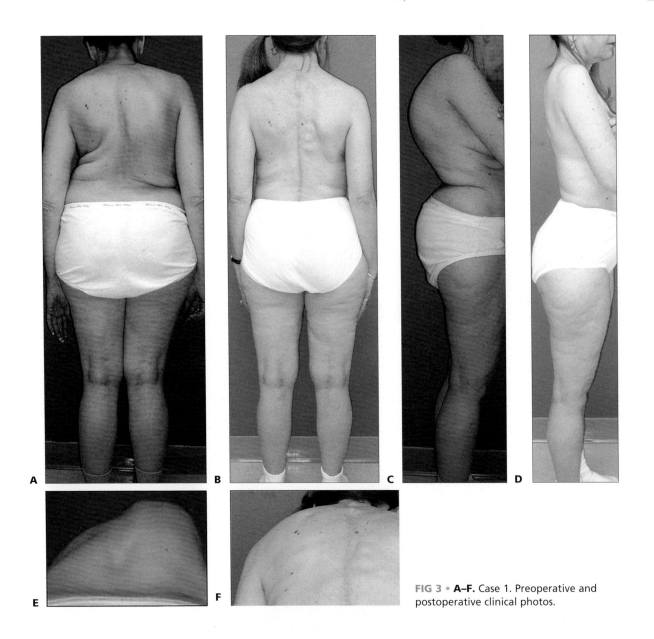

FIG 3 • **A–F.** Case 1. Preoperative and postoperative clinical photos.

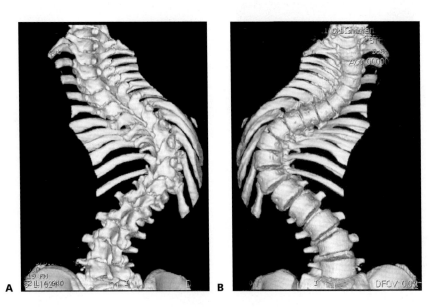

FIG 4 • **A.** Posterior and (**B**) anterior 3D CT scan of a severe idiopathic scoliosis patient.

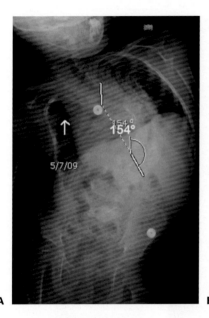
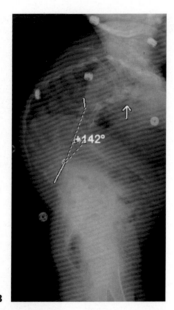

FIG 5 • **A,B.** Case 2. Six-year-old male with severe congenital kyphoscoliosis.

- Location of the deformity often determines whether a VCR (thoracic) or pedicle subtraction osteotomy (lumbar) will assist in correction of sagittal imbalance. For less severe and flexible deformity with mobile disc spaces, multilevel Ponte/Smith-Petersen osteotomies may be adequate for deformity correction.[5]

- Flexibility films will help determine whether a three-column osteotomy is needed versus posterior column osteotomies alone. Posterior column osteotomies may on average correct 10 degrees of kyphosis per level of osteotomy dependent on the spinal level being osteotomized. For large, angular deformities, a three-column osteotomy allows for greater correction in the coronal and sagittal planes.

- We perform VCR in place of anterior and posterior procedures, electing to perform the correction through one single approach.

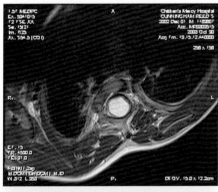
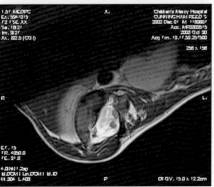
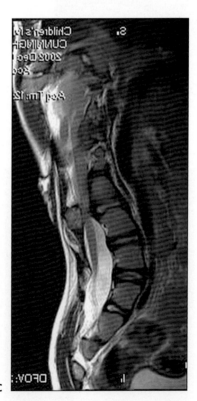

FIG 6 • **A–C.** Case 2. Patient's total spine MRI demonstrated a syringomyelia, diplomyelia, and a tethered spinal cord.

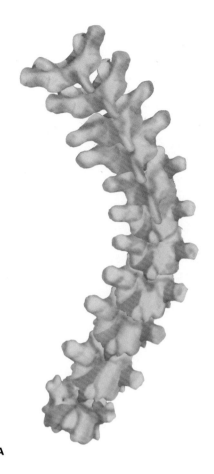

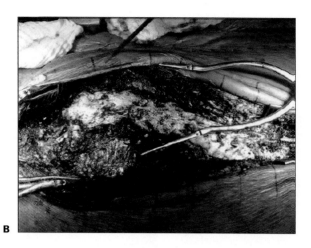

FIG 7 • A. Schematic of posterior exposure. **B.** Intraoperative view of posterior exposure of fusion mass in preparation for VCR.

■ The VCR is almost invariably performed at the apex of the deformity.

Preoperative Planning

■ A multidisciplinary team approach is often necessary in the treatment of patients with complex deformity that requires a VCR.
■ Preoperative assessment of the patient's cardiovascular, pulmonary, nutritional, hematologic, and metabolic systems is required to maximize the patient's preoperative reserve.

Positioning

■ The patient is positioned prone on an OSI Jackson frame with six pads, which are placed strategically to allow the abdomen to rest free, reducing intra-abdominal pressure and intraoperative bleeding.
■ We prefer to place a halo or Gardner-Wells tongs with 5 to 15 lb of traction that allows for rigid positioning of the skull with the face free.
■ The arms are placed in a 90–90 position with care to position the axillae free and elbows well padded to decrease the risk of brachial plexopathy or ulnar nerve neuropathy.

■ Pressure areas are carefully padded as the length of the procedure increases the risk of position-related complications (e.g., skin macerations, plexopathies).
■ The hips are gently extended and the knees slightly flexed with the use of multiple pillows.
■ Spinal cord monitoring leads are placed to monitor the sensory and motor function of the lower extremities.

Approach

■ The standard posterior, subperiosteal approach is used from the transverse processes of the most superior instrumented level to the most distal vertebra or ilium to be instrumented/fused (**FIG 7A,B**). Careful examination of the preoperative CT scan should alert the surgeon to areas of bony deficiency in the posterior elements, to prevent incidental durotomies (**FIGS 8 TO 11** [Case 3]).
■ Thoracoplasties may be necessary at apical vertebrae to obtain adequate exposure of the transverse processes at the apex of a severe scoliosis or kyphoscoliosis deformity.
■ Intraoperative radiographs or fluoroscopy should always be used to confirm vertebral levels.
■ An efficient, meticulous exposure is necessary to minimize blood loss.

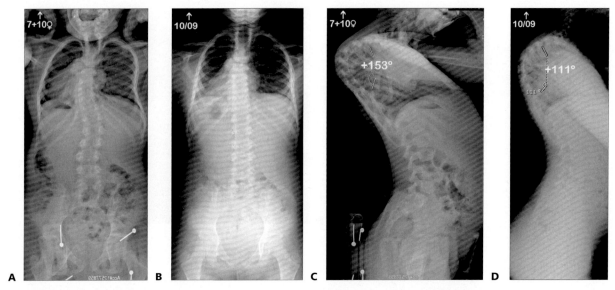

FIG 8 • A–D. Case 3. Seven-year-old girl with a severe 153-degree postlaminectomy kyphosis with myelopathy. She was placed in preoperative halo-gravity traction.

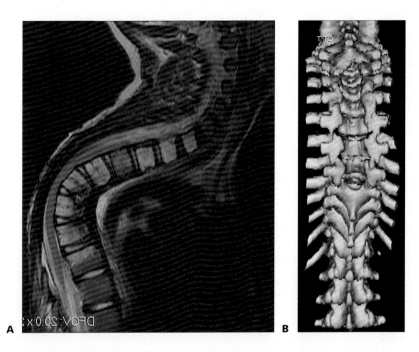

FIG 9 • A,B. Case 3. Patient's preoperative 3D CT scan shows the laminectomy defect.

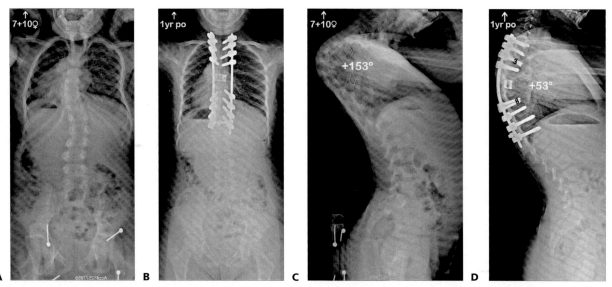

FIG 10 • A–D. Case 3. Patient underwent a two-level posterior vertebral column resection and posterior spinal fusion T1–T11 with complete relief of her myelopathy.

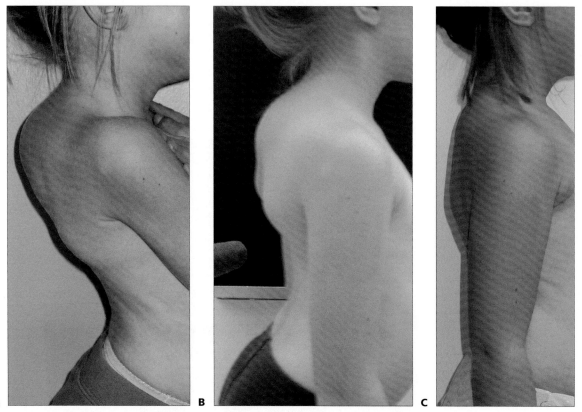

FIG 11 • A–C. Case 3. Preoperative, traction, and 1-year postoperative clinical photos.

FACET OSTEOTOMIES

- Inferior facetectomies are performed at every level where motion exists, resecting approximately 3 to 4 mm of the inferior facet joint.
- Ponte or Smith-Petersen osteotomies are performed around the apex of the deformity, usually from the upper end vertebra to one level below the lower end vertebra. The ligamentum flavum and facet joints are excised.
  - These osteotomies allow for more harmonious correction of the deformity as well as offering access to the medial pedicle to aid in screw placement at the concavity of the deformity.
- In those patients with severe apical kyphosis, we will place pedicle screws prior to any osteotomies. A temporary rod is placed prior to any osteotomy to prevent sagging of the vertebral column, which can put the spinal cord at risk of neurologic impairment.

PEDICLE SCREW PLACEMENT

- We employ a modified anatomic freehand technique with a straight-ahead screw trajectory to increase pedicle pull-out strength.[6] Assessment of preoperative imaging allows for assessment of pedicle screw diameter and length at each vertebra (TECH FIG 1A–D).
- Pedicle screw placement is performed in a sequential fashion from distal to proximal.
- Placement of segmental apical screws is important to ensure rigid stabilization of the VCR site.
- Intraoperative use of fluoroscopy, CT scan, or navigation may be used in assisting the placement of screws, especially through areas of prior fusion with distorted anatomy.
- Multiaxial screws (or multiaxial reduction screws) are most commonly used.
  - Reduction screws are used when cantilever bending is needed for reduction of the rod and deformity. This is often at the distal end of a construct and in areas of hyperlordosis, where rod reduction may be difficult.

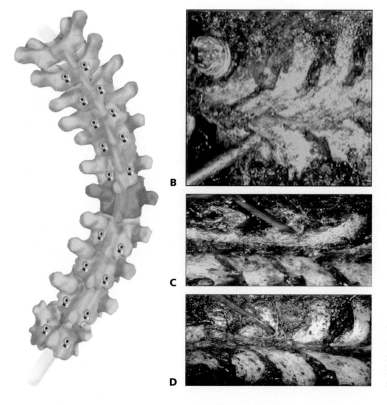

A

B

C

D

TECH FIG 1 • A. Pedicle screws placed segmentally except at shaded apical level where resection is planned. **B–D.** Freehand pedicle screw placement.

TECHNIQUES

VERTEBRAL COLUMN RESECTION

- In the thoracic spine, bilateral costotransversectomies are performed at the level of resection (**TECH FIG 2**).
  - Five to 6 cm of medial rib is resected prior to the laminectomy to minimize the risk of canal intrusion.
  - After subperiosteal dissection, the medial rib fragment is removed, ideally with the rib head attached. Often, however, the rib head remains attached at the vertebral body and can be removed later during the corpectomy.
- The ribs are kept intact, not morselized, which are used as structural grafts to bridge the laminectomy site after osteotomy closure. Next, a wide laminectomy is performed extending from the cranial vertebral pedicles of the level(s) of resection to the caudal vertebra pedicles (**TECH FIG 3A,B**).
- A thorough central decompression is necessary to prevent dorsal dural compression with osteotomy closure. Exiting nerve roots are isolated by removing the facet joints and pedicles bilaterally.
- The nerve roots at the level of the osteotomy are temporarily clamped with a bulldog type vascular clamp for 5 to 10 minutes and attention is turned to any spinal cord monitoring data changes (**TECH FIG 3A,B**).
  - In the thoracic spine, we prefer to ligate the nerve roots medial to the dorsal root ganglion.
    - If spinal cord monitoring data remains stable, then the nerve root is ligated with two 2-0 silk sutures.

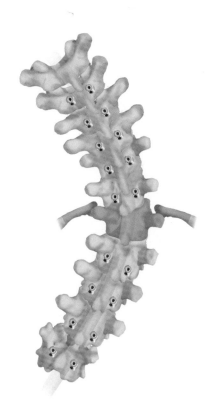

TECH FIG 2 • Shaded area on ribs adjoining to vertebra to be resected via bilateral costotransversectomy.

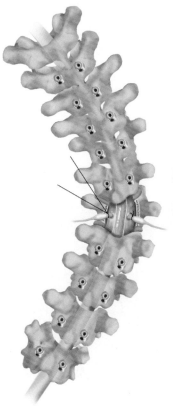

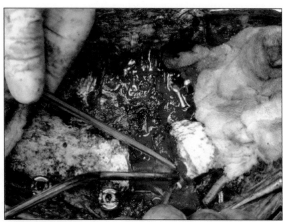

B

A

TECH FIG 3 • A. Laminectomy and nerve root ligation. **B.** Laminectomy and undercutting of ventral aspect of fusion mass.

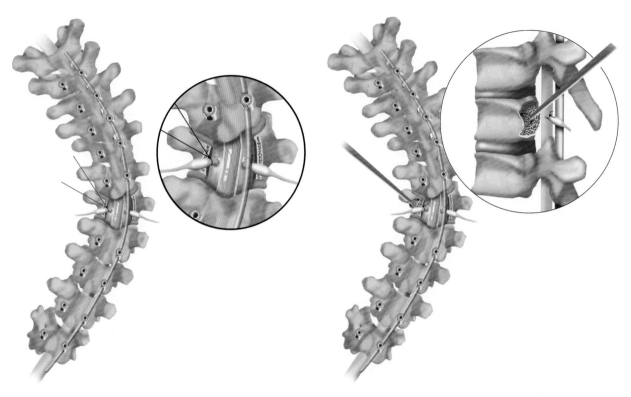

TECH FIG 4 • Stabilizing rod placement.

TECH FIG 5 • Lateral vertebral body access.

- ▪ In our experience, two or three contiguous, unilateral thoracic roots can be sacrificed without neurologic deficits, except for occasional chest wall numbness.
- ▪ In the lumbar spine, the nerve roots are preserved.
- ▪ In preparation for the vertebral body resection, a unilateral stabilizing rod is placed with pedicle screws two or three levels above and below the level of resection (**TECH FIG 4**).
  - ▪ For extreme angular kyphotic or kyphoscoliotic deformities, bilateral rods are used to prevent subluxation of the vertebral column.

- ▪ The cancellous bone of the vertebral body is accessed via a lateral pedicle body window. Subperiosteal dissection on the lateral vertebral body is done with a combination of blunt dissection tools and electrocautery. The paraspinal structures are carefully peeled away until access to the anterior vertebral body is gained. Special retractors may help protect these structures during the corpectomy (**TECH FIG 5**).
  - ▪ The cancellous bone is then curetted and saved for use as local bone graft.
  - ▪ Resecting the concave pedicle poses a challenge, as it is very cortical.

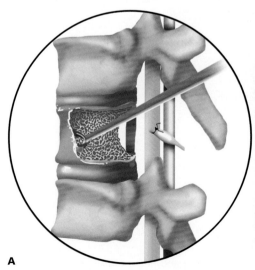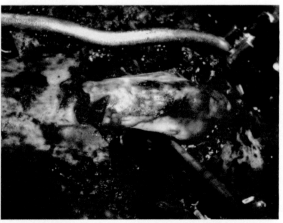

A **B**

TECH FIG 6 • **A.** Vertebral body removal beginning at posterolateral edge of vertebra. **B.** Vertebral body removal continued.

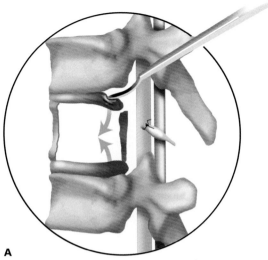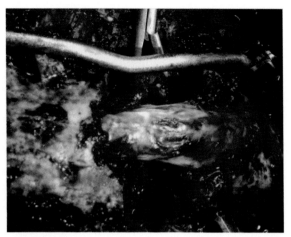

A   B

TECH FIG 7 • A. Discectomy is performed above and below corpectomy level. **B.** Intraoperative view of discectomy.

- In a pure scoliosis deformity, the dural sac and cord rest on the medial pedicle, with no ventral body due to rotation.
- We prefer to use a matchstick burr to remove this cortical bone in these situations.
  - In these deformities, most of the vertebral body will be removed from the convexity.
  - The concave pedicle is removed first, as blood may obscure the field if the convexity is removed first. This also allows the cord to drift medially, away from the majority of the resection.
- The entire vertebral body is removed except for a thin section preserving the anterior longitudinal ligament (ALL) (**TECH FIG 6A,B**).
- Discectomies are performed at the levels above and below the vertebral body resection (**TECH FIG 7A,B**).
  - Care must be taken to preserve the endplates for cage placement.
  - The last section of the vertebral body, which is removed by impaction, is the posterior vertebral body wall or ventral spinal canal (**TECH FIG 8**).
  - The dural sac must be freed from the posterior longitudinal ligament.

- The posterior body wall is removed with reverse-angle curettes, Woodson elevators, or a specialized posterior wall resector (PSO tool set; Medtronic Spinal and Biologics, Memphis, TN).
- Care must be taken to remove any posterior osteophytes to prevent cord impingement during the correction.

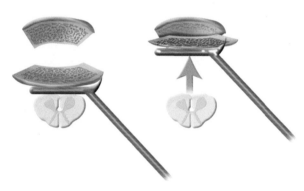

TECH FIG 8 • Posterior vertebral body wall impaction in final aspect of body removal.

CLOSURE OF RESECTION SITE

- Closure of the resected area is now performed with compression (**TECH FIG 9**). Compression of the convexity allows for shortening of the spinal column. Sequential compression on the convexity and distraction of the concavity, performed in an alternating fashion, allows for safe reduction of the deformity through a shortening procedure. Distraction is not an initial technique, as this may put traction on the spinal cord and cause a neurologic deficit.
  - In cases with large degrees of kyphosis, a structural cage is placed anteriorly. This prevents overshorten-

ing and acts as a hinge for greater correction of the kyphotic deformity (**TECH FIG 10**).
- In cases with good pedicular fixation, compression is applied through the screws.
- In cases with less rigid pedicular fixation, a closure is performed, with dominoes at the level of the resection.
  - Care must be taken to watch for subluxation or dural sac impingement during closure.
  - To create a configuration, rods are cut and contoured to fit the deformity above and below the

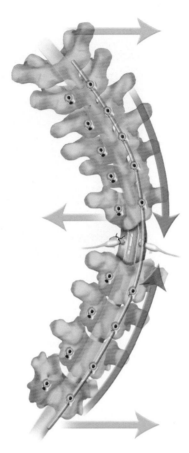

TECH FIG 9 • Posterior shortening is always the initial corrective maneuver.

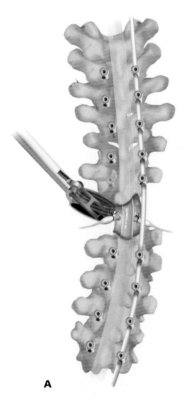

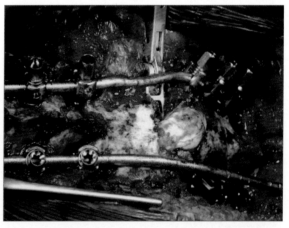

TECH FIG 10 • **A.** Cage placement is performed prior to final closure. **B.** Intraoperative view of cage placement.

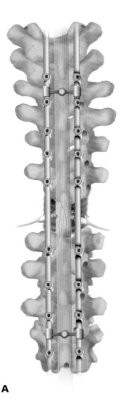

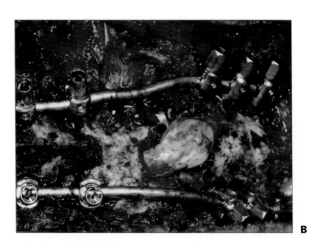

TECH FIG 11 • A,B. Final correction with both rods placed.

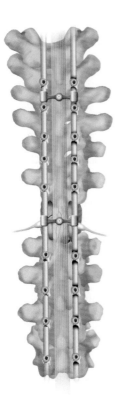

TECH FIG 12 • Note rib grafts placed over laminectomy defect.

level of resection. These rods are then fixed in place with set screws, which are tightened. The rods are connected to each other via domino connectors. Thus, compression and distraction forces are applied to the rods through the domino and a rod gripper, with the forces distributed across the multiple pedicle screws above or below the domino connector.

- After the closure is performed, a contralateral rod is placed. The temporary stabilization rod is removed, and a final rod is placed (TECH FIG 11A,B).
- In situ contouring of the rods is performed, again with care taken to watch for subluxation at the resection, or dural sac impingement.
- Intraoperative radiographs are obtained to check alignment.
- Decortication of dorsal laminae and transverse processes is performed with a matchstick burr.
- The laminectomy defect at the site of resection is covered with the resected rib sections (from the previously performed costotransversectomy) (TECH FIG 12).
  - The ribs are split longitudinally, and placed, cancellous side down, from the lamina above to the lamina below.
  - The ribs may be secured with sutures or a crosslink, if space allows.
  - A final circumferential check of the dura is performed to ensure no dural sac impingement.

WOUND CLOSURE

- Deep drains are placed, and the fascial layer closed using 0 Vicryl (Ethicon, Somerville, NJ). A suprafascial drain is placed and the subcutaneous layer closed using 2-0 Vicryl suture. The skin is closed using absorbable 3-0 Vicryl suture.

- An intraoperative wake-up test is performed. The patient should rehearse the wake-up test at the preoperative visit and in the preoperative holding area.
- Final radiographs are obtained to confirm implant position and overall alignment.

POSTOPERATIVE CARE

- Patients are often sent to the intensive care unit for close monitoring (for 24 to 48 hours as needed), then transitioned to the hospital ward.
- Patients are mobilized on postoperative day 1.
- Drains are retained until recorded output is less than 30 mL per 8-hour shift.
- Diet is advanced slowly with the return of bowel sounds.
- Deep vein thrombosis prophylaxis is provided with sequential compressive devices and thromboembolic deterrent hose.

OUTCOMES

- 107 consecutive posterior VCRs performed by single surgeon (LGL)
  - Pediatric (63) and adult (44)
  - Primary (47) and revision (60)
  - Region of spinal cord (99) and lumbar spine (8)
- 1-level (73), 2-level (28), 3-level (6)
- Diagnoses: severe scoliosis (29), global kyphosis (16), angular kyphosis (25), kyphoscoliosis (37)
- Average correction: severe scoliosis (69%), global kyphosis (54%), angular kyphosis (63%), kyphoscoliosis (56%)
- Mean estimated blood loss: 1,300 mL; mean operative time: 9 hours/37 minutes

COMPLICATIONS

- Twelve spinal cord monitoring changes: All reversed with intraoperative measures to restore spinal cord blood flow (increased mean arterial pressure, wider decompression, larger interbody cage, reduced subluxation). No neurologic deficits upon wake up.
- Two neurologic deficits: spinal cord monitoring not available on either because of preexisting severe myelopathic disease. Both awoke paraplegic with intact sensation. Both have improved and are able to walk.

PEARLS AND PITFALLS

Preoperative planning	■ A multispecialty approach to preoperative surgical clearance and should include cardiac, pulmonary, hematologic, and bone mineral density workups. ■ Use of neuromonitoring of motor and sensory pathways is mandatory.
Vertebral column resection	■ Prior to starting VCR, MAPs should be kept at 80 mm Hg to help with spinal cord perfusion, hemoglobin should be close to 30, and room should be warmed. ■ Subperiosteal dissection of lateral vertebral body wall with careful attention to save segmental vessels will minimize blood loss. ■ Temporary rod placement prior to decompression to prevent subluxation. ■ Wide laminectomy from superior to inferior level pedicles with complete facetectomies. ■ Identification of bilateral nerve roots. In the thoracic spine, often only one nerve root needs to be sacrificed. Tieing off nerve root should be done medial to dorsal root ganglion. ■ Resection of vertebral body should be accomplished as much as possible from one side to minimize the number or exchanges necessary of the temporary rods. ■ The spinal cord should be free from the PLL/dorsal vertebral body prior to removal of the posterior vertebral body wall. ■ Osteotomy closure should be done slowly with constant neuromonitoring. ■ Limit osteotomy closure to approximately 2.0–2.5 cm to prevent overshortening of spinal cord. ■ Use of an anterior intervertebral cage will limit amount of spine shortening and should be placed after initial round of osteotomy closure.
After resection complete	■ Neuromonitoring is followed for up to 1 hour after final osteotomy compression, and a formal neurologic examination is performed prior to leaving the OR. ■ Rib autograft should be used as a bridge over osteotomy site to protect neural elements. ■ Deep and superficial drains may reduce postoperative hematoma/seroma formation.

REFERENCES

1. Dick J, Boachie-Adjei O, Wilson M. One-stage versus two-stage anterior and posterior spinal reconstruction in adults. Comparison of outcomes including nutritional status, complications rates, hospital costs, and other factors. Spine (Phila Pa 1976) 1992;17:S310–S316.
2. Johnson JR, Holt RT. Combined use of anterior and posterior surgery for adult scoliosis. Orthop Clin North Am 1988;19: 361–370.
3. Leatherman KD, Dickson RA. Two-stage corrective surgery for congenital deformities of the spine. J Bone Joint Surg Br 1979;61-B:324–328.
4. Lenke LG, Sides BA, Koester LA, et al. Vertebral column resection for the treatment of severe spinal deformity. Clin Orthop Relat Res 2010;468:687–699.
5. Cho KJ, Bridwell KH, Lenke LG, et al. Comparison of Smith-Petersen versus pedicle subtraction osteotomy for the correction of fixed sagittal imbalance. Spine (Phila Pa 1976) 2005;30: 2030–2037; discussion 8.
6. Lehman RA Jr, Polly DW Jr, Kuklo TR, et al. Straight-forward versus anatomic trajectory technique of thoracic pedicle screw fixation: a biomechanical analysis. Spine (Phila Pa 1976) 2003;28: 2058–2065.

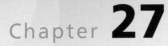

Chapter 27

Smith-Petersen Osteotomy for the Management of Sagittal Plane Spinal Deformity

Selvon St. Clair and William C. Horton III

DEFINITION

▪ A number of osteotomy techniques have been described to treat severe or rigid sagittal plane spinal deformity.

▪ These include multilevel anterior interbody radical discectomy and release, posterior pedicle subtraction osteotomy (PSO), vertebral column resection (VCR), and Smith-Petersen osteotomy (SPO).

▪ This chapter reviews the SPO (also known as "chevron" osteotomy or "Ponte" osteotomy), a mainstay in the treatment of sagittal deformity since it was first described in 1945 by Smith-Petersen and associates.[1]

ANATOMY

▪ The SPO is indicated for correction of a fixed or partially fixed sagittal plane spinal deformity, including hyperkyphosis typified by Scheuermann kyphosis (**FIG 1**).

▪ Although commonly used in the thoracic spine, it has also been used in the lumbar region to correct flatback syndrome or loss of normal lordosis.

PATHOGENESIS

▪ The various causes of flatback syndrome include Harrington distraction instrumentation,[2–4] anterior column degeneration, chronic vertebral compression fractures, adjacent segment degeneration, and iatrogenic causes with pseudarthrosis resulting in loss of sagittal plane correction.[5,6]

▪ Additionally, the concepts behind SPO have been applied at the cervicothoracic junction for kyphosis such as in ankylosing spondylitis.

▪ Regardless of the etiology, the clinical presentation of patients with sagittal plane spinal deformity is quite similar.

PATIENT HISTORY AND PHYSICAL FINDINGS

▪ Patients usually complain of back pain due to muscle fatigue, but can also present with the inability to stand erect without compensating by bending their knees, stumbling while walking, and a feeling of leaning forward (**FIG 2**).[7]

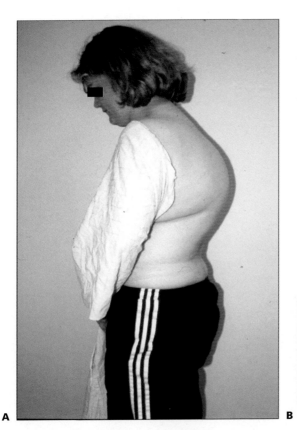
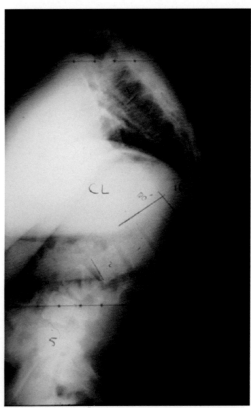

A **B**

FIG 1 • **A.** Preoperative clinical photograph and (**B**) lateral radiograph of 100-degree Scheuermann kyphosis.

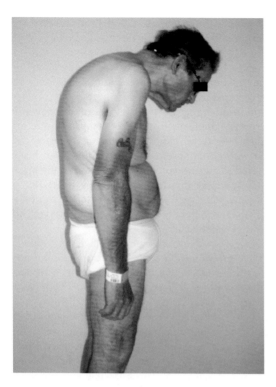

FIG 2 • Clinical photograph of a patient with sagittal plane deformity.

IMAGING AND OTHER DIAGNOSTIC STUDIES

▪ The flexibility of the deformity should be evaluated by both physical examination and preoperative planning radiographic evaluation.

▪ Radiographically, sagittal spinal deformity is evaluated with anterior posterior (AP), posterior anterior (PA), and lateral full-length radiographs with the knees extended and the hands resting on the clavicles (**FIG 3**).[8]

▪ The bolster supine hyperextension lateral radiograph or the push prone radiograph is also helpful to assess the rigidity of the deformity (**FIG 4**). Further detailed analysis of coronal plane and segmental anatomy can be determined by CT scan.

▪ Sagittal imbalance is usually determined by the vertical plumb line technique[9–11] as assessed on 36-inch plain film.

▪ Neutral sagittal balance: vertical plumb line falls at center of dens or middle of C7 vertebral body aligned with the posterior superior aspect of the S1 endplate on standing upright films.

▪ Positive sagittal balance: vertical plumb line falls anterior to the posterior superior aspect of S1 by a minimum of 2 to 3 cm.

▪ Types of sagittal imbalance include (1) compensated abnormalities with neutral sagittal balance and (2) uncompensated abnormalities with positive sagittal balance that can be rigid or fixed. Attention must also be placed on the femurs and on pelvic parameters in evaluating global balance and in preoperative planning.[12]

SURGICAL MANAGEMENT

Procedure Overview

▪ Standard SPO essentially involves complete resection of the facet complex bilaterally as well as any overlapping lamina and spinous process.

▪ The posterior column bone resection must extend from pedicle to pedicle in a cephalocaudal direction. Facetectomies allow for shortening of the posterior column and a component of subsequent lengthening of the anterior column with middle column as fulcrum (**FIG 5**).

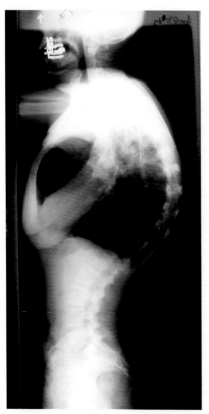

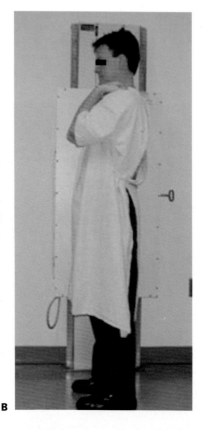

FIG 3 • **A.** Thirty-six-inch film with arms straight out obscuring view of C7–T4 area. **B.** Demonstration of correct position for 36-inch film to allow view of upper T spine and not affect balance.

A   B

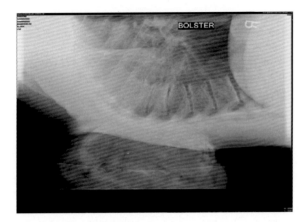

FIG 4 • Supine bolster lateral X-ray.

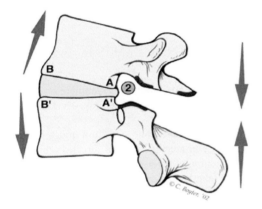

FIG 5 • Schematic illustration of the bony resection required for and the angular correction that is obtainable with Smith-Petersen osteotomy.

■ If done in the thoracic spine, the rib head and costovertebral articulation will also act with the middle column as the fulcrum for extension.

■ The end objective is increased lordosis by shortening the posterior column to restore the sagittal balance such that the head is centered over the sacrum.[11]

■ Modification of the SPO involves placement of an interbody graft or spacer in the disc space after complete discectomy and interbody arthrodesis. This method permits a greater degree of lordosis without compromising neural foraminal height and can be used to address coronal plane deformity by placing the interbody spacer asymmetrically in the disc space.[11]

■ It must be recognized that the degree of correction is governed by the flexibility of the anterior column and the effective preoperative disc height.

■ Ankylosis or bridging anterior osteophytes may significantly block the correction (**FIG 6**). In cases of rigid deformity, true anterior column osteoclasis helps to achieve a correction of up to 40 degrees to 50 degrees, as may be seen with ankylosing spondylitis.[13]

■ Although it is commonly estimated that 1 mm of posterior bone resection results in approximately 1 degree of sagittal correction, this may vary depending on the flexibility through the disc. If a radical anterior release is performed before extension osteotomy, the combined anterior distraction and posterior shortening can increase the segmental correction by a factor of 2.5.[12]

Preoperative Planning

■ The more caudal the level considered for an SPO, the greater the effect will be on overall alignment.

■ More mobile and taller interbody disc spaces allow for greater correction than severely degenerated, less mobile disc spaces.

■ Due to the potential for natural long-term postoperative degeneration of adjacent disc levels that may have a kyphogenic effect, overestimating the required correction by a few degrees is preferred.

■ Disperse SPO over multiple levels.

■ Avoid SPO adjacent to the lowest instrumented vertebra (LIV) or upper instrumented vertebra (UIV) to minimize the risk of end vertebrae fixation pullout.

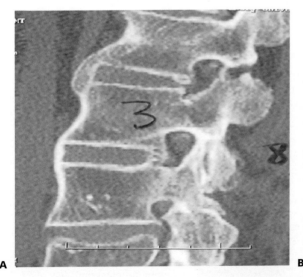
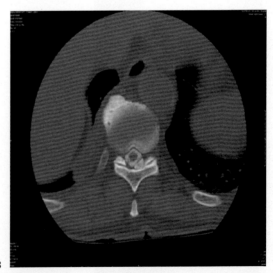

FIG 6 • **A,B.** Showing a patient with ankylosing spondylitis with only one disc that might move with Smith-Petersen osteotomy and another patient with ossification of the ligamentum flavum, which if not resected, might prevent Smith-Petersen osteotomy closure and neurologic compromise.

Indices / Indications[9–11]

- Type I smooth thoracic and/or lumbar kyphosis
- Type I sharp, angular kyphosis in the thoracic spine
- Type II smooth kyphotic deformity of thoracic and/or lumbar spine when associated with minor (6 to 8 cm) positive sagittal balance
- Type II smooth kyphotic deformity of thoracic spine when associated with major sagittal imbalance (>12 cm)
- In scoliosis for three-dimensional deformity correction

Contraindications

- Sharp, fixed angular type II deformity that cannot be corrected by SPO[9–11]
- Anterior fixation, a collapsed or immobile disc space, or an anterior bridging osteophyte at the level of a planned SPO (an open, mobile disc space is prerequisite)
- Posterior wound infection
- Anterior or lateral bridging osteophytes (**FIG 6**), or congenital bars that can not be released

Relative Contraindications

- Calcification of the great vessels is a relative contraindication
- Ossification of the dura
- Inability to achieve appropriate segmental control with fixation

Equipment

- Posterior based segmental instrumentation system
- Open frame that will allow the kyphosis to reduce, radiolucent operating table
- Neurologic intraoperative monitoring is highly recommended
  - Transcranial motor evoked potential (TcMEP): essential in kyphosis correction
  - Somatosensory evoked potentials (SSEP): essential in kyphosis correction
  - Electromyography (EMG): free running of lower extremities and evoked with pedicle screw fixation (optional)
  - D-wave monitoring

Patient Positioning

- The patient is placed in the prone position with the hips flexed initially. For lumbar deformities, the hips can be extended later in the case during correction to help close the osteotomy.

- Posterior extension osteotomies are done at the apex of the deformity. The procedure's objective is (1) to shorten the posterior column by closing down the disc space posteriorly pivoting on the posterior longitudinal ligament (PLL) and (2) to thereby extend the anterior column (see FIG 5).[1]
- The rule of thumb is for every 1 mm of posterior bone resection, 1 degree of correction can be expected.[14]

STEPS

1. First, obtain meticulous clean wide exposure of spinous process, lamina, pars, facets, out to the tips of transverse process (TP) as well as the lateral border of any old fusion. Strive for meticulous hemostasis; use bipolar cautery respecting bilateral segmental perfusion dynamics. Avoid Gelfoam, or if needed it should be removed before osteotomy closure (**TECH FIG 1**).
2. Removal of overlapping spinous processes to cleanly delineate ligamentum flavum and its midline raphe.
3. Removal of inferior facets bilaterally at the desired spinal level, exiting inferior to the base of the TP.
4. Ligamentum flavum resection from pedicle to pedicle to avoid any mass effect from redundant ligament dorsally on the neural structures once the SPO is closed down.
5. Bilateral superior articular facet resection, which ends flush to the top of the TP.
6. Smoothing out cut edges to avoid any obstruction to closure or possible iatrogenic injury to dura or nerves.
7. If there is no coronal deformity to be corrected, the osteotomy should be symmetrical.
8. To address a coronal deformity, an asymmetric SPO can be used with the wider osteotomy on the side of convexity.[11]
9. Removal of laminar bone should be adequate and account for possible desired contact between the superior and inferior lamina after closure that may aid fusion.

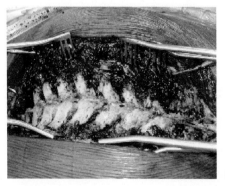 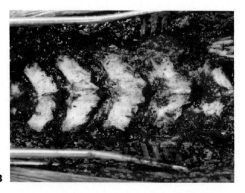

TECH FIG 1 • Intraoperative photographs (**A**) prior to and (**B**) after Smith-Petersen osteotomy.

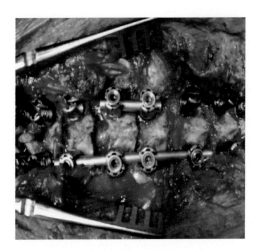
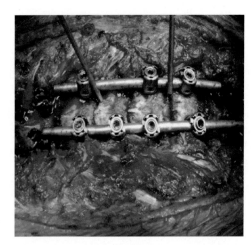

TECH FIG 2 • Sequential temporary apical rod technique for segmental reduction.

Typically, the osteotomy width is between 6 and 10 mm cephalocaudally.

10. The gap created by the osteotomy is compressed, hinging on the posterior aspect of the disc space causing posterior column shortening and anterior column extension.

11. The compression is held in place with posterior spinal instrumentation (**TECH FIGS 2 AND 3**).

12. The lamina and the spinous process of the upper and lower vertebra is decorticated in preparation for arthrodesis.

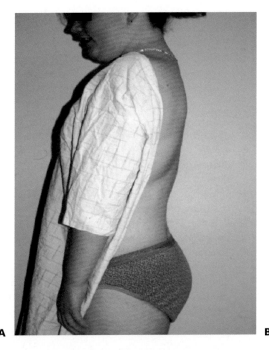
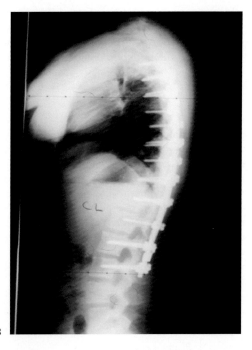

A

B

TECH FIG 3 • **A.** Postoperative clinical photograph and (**B**) lateral radiograph after Smith-Peterson osteotomy correction of 100-degree Scheuermann kyphosis.

PEARLS AND PITFALLS

- Attention to cardiovascular parameters can assist with limiting blood loss.
  - In adults, mild hypotension during exposure can help reduce blood loss; however, during osteotomy and manipulation, the pressure should be elevated; mean arterial pressures (MAPs) greater than 80 mm Hg are ideal.
  - In the pediatric population, MAPs are maintained between 50 and 60 mm Hg during the approach with an increase from 70 to 80 mm Hg before deformity correction.[15]
- Avoid bone wax where it can inhibit fusion.

- Carefully plan for soft tissue coverage. Initial exposure should meticulously preserve full thickness flaps especially at the deformity apex. Flaps may be necessary to get tensionless closure in revision cases. Low profile instrumentation or monoaxial screws may need to be considered in kyphosis with severe gibbus deformity and thin tissue cover.
- Beware of ossification of the ligamentum flavum (OLF), which can best be seen on preop scans (see **FIG 6B**). These areas are frequently stenotic and adhered to dura dorsally. OLF must be fully resected before any closure is attempted.
- During the SPO, the pedicles should remain undisturbed. One must be especially careful with osteotomes, which may propagate a crack into the pedicle if dull or not well directed. Invasion of pedicles may weaken critical fixation points requiring an alternate approach to adequately allow for closure of the osteotomy.
- Avoid the use of large Kerrisons: size 2 or 3 mm is recommended particularly when working on the concavity of deformity with associated scoliosis.
- Look out in rare cases with dorsal displacement of spinal cord or roots, which may have frequent adhesions that need to be resected.
- If multiple SPOs are planned, dorsal compression should be performed in a way that redistributes forces over the largest area possible; either via cantilever or via apical compression techniques (**FIG 7**). If using cantilever methods, manipulate two rods simultaneously to distribute corrective loads, and carefully monitor stress on end vertebrae fixation.
- End segments are most likely to pullout so optimization of screw length and diameter is critical.
- In higher degree thoracic kyphotic patients, cranial traction may be helpful. In severe lumbar deformity, extending the table during correction may facilitate osteotomy closure but beware of pressure on the thighs and tibiae, or the patient shifting under the drapes.
- Before closing any osteotomy, the neural foramina should be probed gently to ensure they are patent. It is common to discover a small superior tip of a resected superior facet retained in the foramen (especially in thoracic spine), or a remaining spike of either facet base.
- In cases where osteotomy fails to close down, check for residual lateral facet bone or bridging osteophytes or anterior column obstruction. You may need to do more SPOs or convert to pedicle subtraction osteotomy if the anterior column will not release.
- During closure, anteriorly directed manual pressure directed near the apex can help provide additional corrective force. Any time instruments are used for pushing down on the apex to assist reduction, be certain that the canal is safe and there is no risk if an instrument inadvertently slips.
- In the lumbar spine where lordosis increases during closure, the dura may buckle slightly. If this is seen, create additional central opening by resecting and beveling the midline laminae to provide extra space.
- Ensure TP decortication laterally, and in the midline use careful decortication technique mindful of fixation points and any exposed neural elements. Carefully pack generous bone around all osteotomy points avoiding any material into the canal.
- Cross-table postreduction lateral imaging should be done to ensure that adequate correction has been obtained.

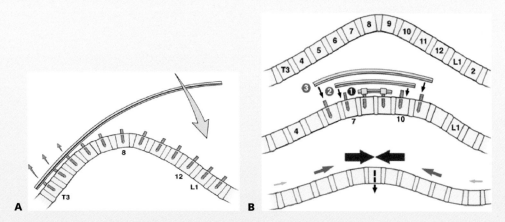

FIG 7 • A. Illustration showing cantilever reduction technique and (**B**) apical-based sequential temporary apical rod technique.

COMPLICATIONS

Intraoperative

- Subluxation
- Dorsal root compression
- Spinal cord traumatic injury
- Dural buckling
- Cerebrospinal leak
- Great vessel injury
- Pedicle fracture

Postoperative

- New neurologic deficits secondary to intraoperative spinal cord or nerve root injury
- Radiculopathy from neural foraminal compression (rare unless there is baseline foraminal stenosis)[4]
- Superior mesenteric artery syndrome, intestinal obstruction,[14,16] and prolonged ileus
- Epidural/intraspinal hematoma
- Deep venous thrombosis and pulmonary embolism
- Pseudarthrosis is another reported complication
- Adjacent segment disease/junctional kyphosis

REFERENCES

1. Smith-Peterson MN, Larson CB, Aufranc OE. Ostetomy of the spine for correction of flexion deformity in rheumatoid arthritis. J Bone Joint Surg Am 1945;27:1–11.

2. Casey MP, Archer MA, Jacobs RR, et al. The effects of Harrington rod contouring on lumbar lordosis. Spine 1987;12:750–753.

3. LaGrone MO. Loss of lumbar lordosis: A complication of spinal fusion for scoliosis. Orthop Clin North Am 1988;19:383–393.

4. Lagrone MO, Bradford DS, Moe JH, et al. Treatment of symptomatic flatback after spinal fusion. J Bone Joint Surg Am 1988;70:569–580.

5. Berven SH, Deviren V, Smith JA, et al. Management of fixed sagittal plane deformity results of the transpedicular wedge resection osteotomy. Spine 2001;26:2036–2043.

6. Bridwell KH, Lenke LG, Lewis SJ. Treatment of spinal stenosis and fixed sagittal imbalance. Clin Orthop 2001;384:35–44.

7. Joseph SA Jr, Moreno AP, Brandoff J, et al. Sagittal plane deformity in the adult patient." J Am Acad Orthop Surg 2009;17(6):378–388.

8. Horton WC, Brown CW, Bridwell KH, et al. Is there an optimal patient stance for obtaining a lateral 36″ radiograph? A critical comparison of three techniques. Spine (Phila Pa 1976) 2005;30(4): 427–433.

9. Bridwell KH. Decision making regarding Smith-Petersen vs. pedicle subtraction osteotomy vs. vertebral column resection for spinal deformity. Spine (Phila Pa 1976) 2006;31(19)(suppl):S171–S178.

10. Booth KC, Bridwell KH, Lenke LG, et al. Complications and predictive factors for the successful treatment of flatback deformity (fixed sagittal imbalance). Spine (Phila Pa 1976) 1999;24(16): 1712–1720.

11. La Marca F, Brumblay H. Smith-Petersen osteotomy in thoracolumbar deformity surgery. Neurosurgery 2008;63(3)(suppl):163–170.

12. Lee MJ, Wiater B, Bransford RJ, et al. Lordosis restoration after Smith-Petersen osteotomies and interbody strut placement: a radiographic study in cadavers. Spine (Phila Pa 1976) 2010;35(25):E1487–E1491.

13. Simmons EH. Kyphotic deformity of the spine in ankylosing spondylitis. Clin Orthop Relat Res 1977;(128):65–77.

14. Gill JB, Levin A, Burd T, et al. Corrective osteotomies in spine surgery. J Bone Joint Surg Am 2008;90(11):2509–2520.

15. Diab MG, Franzone JM, Vitale MG. The role of posterior spinal osteotomies in pediatric spinal deformity surgery: indications and operative technique. J Pediatr Orthop 2011;31(1)(suppl):S88–S98.

16. Dorward IG, Lenke LG. Osteotomies in the posterior-only treatment of complex adult spinal deformity: a comparative review. Neurosurg Focus 2010;28(3):E4.

Chapter 28

Sacropelvic Fixation Techniques

Christopher T. Martin and Khaled M. Kebaish

DEFINITION

▪ Sacropelvic fixation is a term used to describe instrumentation into the sacrum and pelvis.

▪ The most common indication is a long spinal fusion to the sacrum. Other indications include high-grade spondylolisthesis, flat back syndrome requiring corrective osteotomy, and correction of pelvic obliquity.

▪ The purpose is to provide secure distal fixation points that resist the strong flexion moments and cantilever forces present at the lumbosacral junction.

▪ Multiple techniques are used including the Galveston rod, the iliac screws, and the S2 alar iliac (S2AI) technique.

ANATOMY

▪ A clear understanding of the anatomy of the sacrum and pelvis is crucial to the safe and accurate placement of sacral and pelvic instrumentation. Familiarity with the anatomy of the sacrum, ilium, and sacroiliac joint is of particular importance.

The Sacrum

▪ The sacrum lies at the junction between the mobile and fixed portions of the spine and functions as a keystone that unites the two hemipelvises.

▪ The sacral vertebrae are fused and the transverse processes merge into the expanded lateral sacral ala.

▪ The majority of the bone in the sacrum has a cancellous osseous structure.[1] The trabecular density is greatest in the pedicle and body of the vertebrae, and least in the sacral ala.[1] Therefore, sacral pedicle screws are best directed toward the midline.[2]

▪ The sacrum does not contain a true pedicle, but rather a confluence of cancellous bone between the sacral body and the ala. Compared to pedicles in the mobile spine, this area is capacious. The S1 pedicle has a mean length of 46.9 ± 3.3 mm in women and 49.7 ± 3.7 mm in men, and is angled roughly 40 degrees from the midline (**FIG 1**).[3]

▪ Numerous critical structures—including the internal iliac artery and vein, middle sacral artery and vein, sympathetic chain, lumbosacral trunk, and sigmoid colon—lie directly on the sacrum at some point and could potentially be injured by the instrumentation used in sacropelvic fusions (**FIG 2**).[4]

The Ilium

▪ The ilium is the most superior of the three bones that make up the os coxa.

▪ In adolescents, the ilium is connected to the pubis and the ischium through the triradiate cartilage. Fusion of this cartilage completes between 13 and 16 years of age in most patients.

▪ In thin patients, the posterior superior iliac spine (PSIS) is marked by an overlying dimple in the skin. A transverse line drawn between these two dimples crosses the sacrum at the level of S2.

▪ The structures of the greater sciatic foramen are at risk of damage during instrumentation of the pelvis.[5]

The Sacroiliac Joint

▪ The sacroiliac (SI) joint is an L-shaped synovial joint with an irregularly contoured surface that interlocks in order to resist movement. The joint functions to transfer axial load from the torso onto the hemipelvises.

▪ The joint is stabilized by the anterior sacroiliac ligament, interosseous SI ligament, and the posterior SI ligament (**FIG 3**).

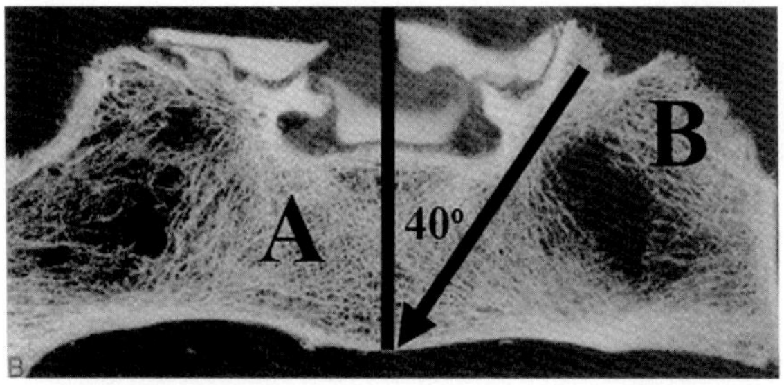

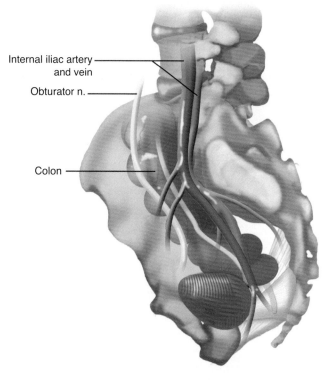

Internal iliac artery and vein

Obturator n.

Colon

FIG 1 • Cross section of sacrum. The bone density is greatest in the pedicle and body of the vertebrae (**A**) and lowest in the ala (**B**). *Arrow* marks the location of S1 pedicle. (Figure modified from Peretz, AM Hipp, JA Heggeness, MH. The internal bony architecture of the sacrum. Spine 1998;23(9):971–974, with permission)

FIG 2 • Important anatomic structures overlying the sacrum. (Adapted from Anatomic consideration for sacral screw placement. Spine 1991;16(6S):S286–294.)

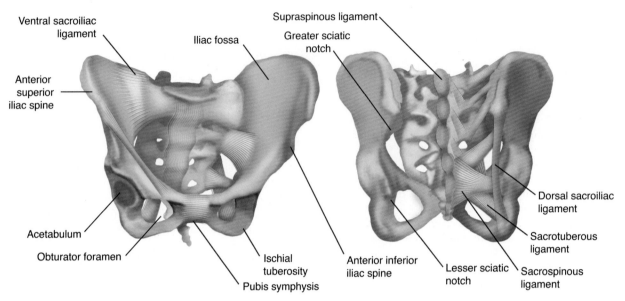

FIG 3 • Ligamentous support and bony anatomy of the pelvis.

BIOMECHANICS

■ Fusions across the lumbosacral junction are a particular challenge for spine surgeons and this location has a high incidence of pseudarthrosis.[5]

■ Substantial biomechanical forces are concentrated at the lumbosacral junction. The fusion mass above the sacrum acts as a long lever arm that transmits flexion, extension, and torsional forces from the spine above. These forces cause motion at the junction that may increase the risk of pseudarthrosis.[6,7]

■ Furthermore, the density of bone in the sacrum is poor, and obtaining adequate fixation is a particular challenge.[8]

■ McCord et al[9] introduced the concept of the lumbosacral pivot point (**FIG 4**), which is defined as the middle of the osteoligamentous column at the junction between L5 and S1.

■ The farther that the pelvic implant progresses anterior to this point, the more stable the construct. Furthermore, instrumentation that crosses the SI joint is not effective unless it passes anterior to this pivot point.[9]

■ O'Brien et al. introduced the concept of three zones of sacropelvic fixation (**FIG 5**).[10] Fixation in zone 3 has the highest biomechanical strength and allows placement of the instrumentation the farthest anterior to the pivot point.

SURGICAL MANAGEMENT

Indications

1. Long spinal fusions

   ■ The most common indication for sacropelvic fixation is a long spinal fusion to the sacrum.[5] The definition of a long spinal fusion is controversial. Most agree that fusions that cross the thoracolumbar junction and progress to the pelvis should be augmented with pelvic anchors. However, we feel that pelvic anchors should also be considered in fusions that extend above L2 and progress to the pelvis.

   ■ Conditions that commonly require a long spinal fusion include lumbar scoliosis in adults, children with a structural lumbosacral scoliotic curve, paralytic kyphoscoliosis,

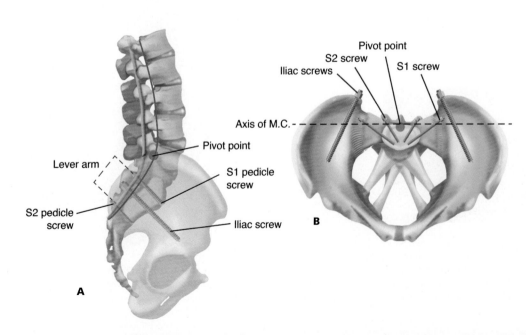

FIG 4 • Lumbosacral pivot point. **A.** Lateral view and (**B**) axial view of the pivot point. (Adapted from McCord DH, Cunningham BW, Shono Y, et al. Biomechanical analysis of lumbosacral fixation. Spine 1992;17:S235–43.)

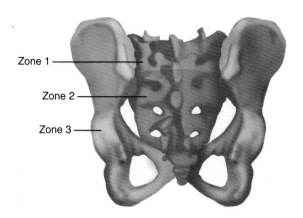

FIG 5 • Zones of pelvic fixation. Biomechanical strength increases as you progress from zone 1 to zone 3. Furthermore, zone 3 allows placement of the instrumentation the farthest anterior to the pivot point. (Modified from O'Brien M.F. Sacropelvic Fixation in Spinal Deformity. In: Dewlad RL, ed. *Spinal Deformities: The Comprehensive Text.* New York: Thieme; 2003:601–614.)

paralytic and neuromuscular kyphoscoliosis, and congenital scoliosis.[2]

2. High-grade spondylolisthesis
   ▪ Correction of grade III or higher spondylolisthesis places excessive force on the posterior implants.[11]
   ▪ Instrumentation into the pelvis serves as an adjunct to the S1 pedicle screws and may reduce the incidence of pseudarthrosis and implant failure.[2]

3. Flat back syndrome requiring corrective osteotomy
   ▪ Flat back syndrome refers to the loss of lumbar lordosis following a posterior spinal fusion.[12] Patients present with pain, loss of sagittal balance, and caudad disc degeneration.
   ▪ Correction of the deformity frequently requires multiple osteotomies and a long fusion to the sacrum.[12] These fusions should be supplemented with pelvic instrumentation to decrease the risk of pseudarthrosis.

4. Correction of pelvic obliquity
   ▪ Pelvic obliquity is common in patients with neuromuscular deformities.
   ▪ Correction of the obliquity frequently requires pelvic fixation.[13]

5. Other disorders
   ▪ Less common indications include sacrectomy performed for sacral tumors, for sacral fracture, and for osteoporosis in the presence of lumbosacral fusion.[2]

Preoperative Planning

▪ A C-arm should be available for intraoperative imaging if necessary.
▪ Planning the extent and type of procedure to be performed requires a thorough understanding of the anatomy of the patient's deformity.
▪ Patients with significant pelvic obliquity may have significant differences between the two sides of the pelvis, and the trajectory of the anchors may need to be modified accordingly.
▪ Patients with significant osteoporosis may require larger size screws, up to 10 mm, in order to obtain adequate purchase.
▪ Patients who have had prior bone taken from the iliac crest may not be candidates for iliac bolts and an alternative technique such as the S2AI method should be considered.

▪ Patients with deficient iliac bone—for example, patients with sacropelvic resection for tumor—may require additional points of fixation on the intact side.

Imaging

▪ Standing 36-inch lateral and posteroanterior (PA) plain radiographs should be the initial diagnostic study in most patients and can be used to evaluate overall alignment of the spine and bony pathology.
▪ Due to the complex and variable anatomy of the sacrum, CT imaging may be helpful for planning of screw placement but is not always necessary.
▪ Identification of anatomic abnormalities such as dural ectasia, Tarlov cyst, or prior harvesting of iliac crest bone which might alter the necessary surgical approach should be completed prior to the surgical procedure.

Positioning

▪ The patient is positioned prone on a radiolucent frame, usually a Jackson table, per routine for posterior spinal procedures.
▪ A transverse pad should run across the chest at the level of the shoulders. A second transverse pad should run across the pelvis at the level of the anterior superior iliac spine (ASIS). The chest wall and abdomen should be free to expand without touching the table to insure adequate space for chest wall movement during ventilation.
▪ The drapes should be placed distally enough to expose the start of the gluteal cleft, taking care not to drape out the PSIS.

Approach

▪ The approach depends on the technique used and specific points for each technique are below.
▪ In general, the approach for the open procedures is an extension of the midline incision (**FIG 6**), centered over the spinous processes of the vertebrae, and with some modification distally based on the technique.
▪ The goal should be to quickly expose the entire area of the spine that is going to be instrumented, with removal of soft tissue out to the transverse processes bilaterally.
▪ The exposure should extend caudally enough to expose the dorsal S1 sacral foramen in order to allow for the placement of sacropelvic fixation.
▪ The iliac screw and Galveston techniques require additional soft tissue dissection laterally out to the iliac crest in order to expose the starting point on the PSIS.

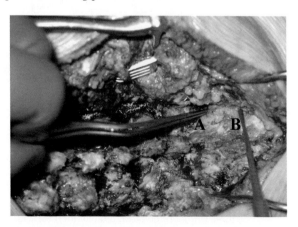

FIG 6 • Standard midline exposure. Probes mark the location of the S1 and S2 dorsal sacral foramina at points *A* and *B*, respectively.

■ Although many techniques exist for sacropelvic fixation, only three are currently in widespread use.[5] Here, we will focus only on those three: the Galveston L-rod technique,[14] the iliac screw technique,[15] and the newer S2AI technique.[16,17]

THE GALVESTON L-ROD TECHNIQUE[14]

■ Placement of the Galveston rods proceeds after a standard midline exposure centered over the spinous processes (**FIG 6**). Here, we will focus only on those steps necessary for placement of pelvic fixation. Specific steps necessary for placement of the sublaminar wires or for correction of the deformity in scoliotic or myelodysplastic spines are beyond the scope of this chapter, but can be found elsewhere.[18]

■ After placement of sublaminar wires at all spinal levels that are to be instrumented, exposure of the ilium is begun by palpating the PSIS, and then dissecting off the subcutaneous tissue from the lumbosacral fascia starting in the midline and proceeding out bilaterally toward the PSIS using cobb elevators and bovine electrocautery.

■ The gluteal musculature should be dissected away from the outer portion of the ilium subperiosteally until the greater sciatic notch is accessible with a finger.

■ A longitudinal or oblique incision is made in the fascia overlying the PSIS.

■ A 3/16-inch stainless steel pelvic pin is then driven into the ilium toward the AIIS to a depth of 6 to 9 cm. The starting point is just posterior to the SI joint at the level of the PSIS. Placement of a finger into the sciatic notch can help guide the pin toward the AIIS.

■ The pin is left in place in order to facilitate correct bending of the L-rod, which is a 3/16-inch diameter stainless steel rod.

■ The first bend in the L-rod creates the short end, which will be placed into the table of the ilium and can be approximated by placing the short end of the rod parallel to the pelvic pin in the table of the ilium. The second bend turns the long end of the rod cephalad (**TECH FIG 1**).

■ Next, the pelvic pin is removed, and the short end of the L-rod is driven into the table of the ilium.

■ The long end of the L-rod is then attached to the mobile spine by using the previously placed sublaminar wires (**TECH FIG 2**).

■ Alternatively, some surgeons choose to attach the Galveston rod to the heads of pedicle screws.

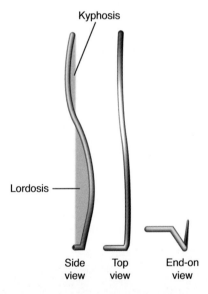

TECH FIG 1 • Appropriate shaping of the L-rod. (Adapted from Allen BL, Jr, Ferguson RL. The Galveston technique for L rod instrumentation of the scoliotic spine. *Spine*. 1982;7:276–284.)

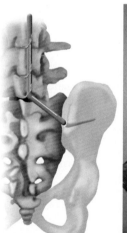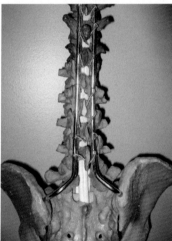

TECH FIG 2 • Line diagram (*left*, adapted from Allen BL, Jr, Ferguson RL. The Galveston technique for L rod instrumentation of the scoliotic spine. *Spine*. 1982;7:276–284.) and model (*right*) showing proper placement of the Galveston rod into the table of the ilium.

SACRAL TRICORTICAL PEDICLE SCREWS[19]

■ The iliac screw and S2AI methods for sacropelvic fixation begin with placement of sacral (S1) screws, which should be completed prior to placement of the pelvic fixation.

■ Sacral pedicle screws can be placed through either two or three (through the sacral prominatory) cortices, but tricortical screws have been shown to have twice the insertional torque of bicortical screws, and this is the preferred technique.[19]

■ An awl is used to breach the dorsal cortex of the sacrum at the starting point 1 cm proximal and immediately lateral to the S1 sacral foramen (**TECH FIG 3A**).

■ A slightly curved large pedicle finder (gearshift-type) is used to sound the cancellous bone. The path should be directed 30 to 40 degrees anteromedially and 15 degrees cephalad toward the anterior tip of the sacral promontory (**TECH FIG 3B**).

Kyphosis

Lordosis

Side view   Top view   End-on view

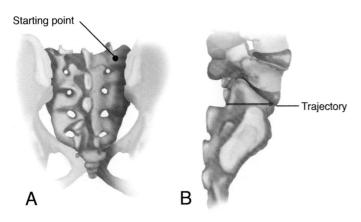

Starting point

Trajectory

A   B

TECH FIG 3 • Starting point (*black dot* in **A**) and trajectory (**B**) for the tricortical S1 screws.

- The direction toward the anterior tip of the promontory can be estimated from preoperative plain radiographs and confirmed intraoperatively with lateral fluoroscopy prior to placement of the screw (**TECH FIG 4**).

- The pilot hole is tapped using a tap size 1mm less than the screw to be inserted, typically a 6 mm tap is used and a 7mm screw is placed (**TECH FIG 5**).
- All five boundaries of the screw hole are sounded using a ballpoint probe in order to verify that the bony cortex has not been breached.
- Screw length is then measured using a ballpoint depth gauge. Screws are typically placed with a bicortical purchase.
- The screws are then placed under direct visualization.

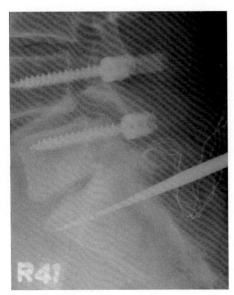

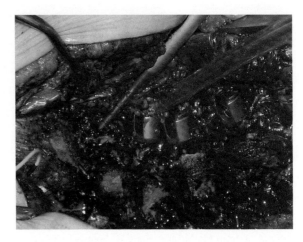

TECH FIG 4 • Intraoperative fluoroscopy showing the trajectory of the pedicle finder, which is 30 to 40 degrees anteromedially and 15 degrees cephalad toward the anterior tip of the sacral promontory.

TECH FIG 5 • Placement of the S1 tricortical screw. The pilot hole is tapped using a tap size 1mm less than the screw to be inserted, the depth is measured using a ball-point depth gauge, and an appropriate length screw is placed along the path obtaining a bicortical purchase.

THE ILIAC SCREW TECHNIQUE[2,15]

- We recommend that the iliac screw be placed only after other points of fixation, including the S1 screws, have already been secured. When placing the iliac screws using the S2AI technique, inserting the proximal screws, especially the S1 PS, helps in guiding the surgeon in fine tuning the lat/medial starting point for the S2AI screws so as to end with a straight inline anchor at the lumbosacral junction facilitating rod placement.
- The PSIS is palpated, and the subcutaneous tissue is dissected off the lumbosacral fascia bilaterally toward the PSIS using cobb elevators and bovine electrocautery (**TECH FIG 6**).

- A longitudinal or oblique incision is made in the fascia overlying the PSIS.
- The incision is extended both caudally and cephalad along the ilium with respect to the PSIS (**TECH FIG 7A**).
- A rongeur or burr is used to breach the cortex overlying the PSIS, approximately 1 cm from the distal ilium. The amount of bone resected depends on the bulkiness of the implant, and the goal should be to minimize implant prominence.
- With a pedicle seeker or curette, the path into the ilium down toward the ASIS is then developed (**TECH FIG 7A**).

TECHNIQUES

- The path averages 25 degrees lateral to mid-sagittal plane and 30 to 35 degrees caudal to the transverse plane toward the ASIS. Fluoroscopy may be used to confirm the path. Alternatively, placement of a finger into the sciatic notch provides an anatomic landmark which can help guide the path (TECH FIG 7B).
- The path is then palpated with a ballpoint probe in order to verify that neither the medial nor lateral iliac crest cortex has been breached.
- Screw lengths are then measured by marking the depth on the ballpoint probe. Common screw sizes are 7 to 8 mm in diameter and 70 to 80 mm in length.
- The screw path is then tapped using a handheld tap, and an appropriate length screw is inserted.
- Lastly, the screw must then be attached to the longitudinal rods of the main spinal construct by using a modular connector system. The connectors are tunneled anterior to the paraspinal muscles (TECH FIG 8).
- Pelvic radiographs or C-arm fluoroscopic images may be taken in order to confirm placement of the instrumentation. The trajectory and starting point of the screw should be assessed. For the iliac screw, the starting point should be over the PSIS, and directed towards the AIIS, proximal to the sciatic notch. For the S2AI screw, the starting point is midway between S1 and S2 sacral foram-

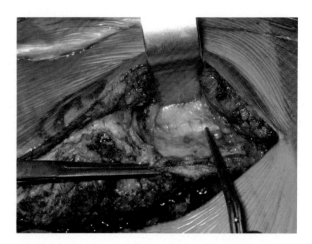

TECH FIG 6 • Extension of the midline incision out to the posterior superior iliac spine (PSIS) for placement of the iliac screws. The paraspinal muscles are held out of the field with a clamp and the PSIS is marked by the forceps.

ina and directed towards the AIIS, using an AP view will ensure the cephalad/caudad position, a tear drop view will ensure no breach to the medial or lateral cortices of the Ilium.

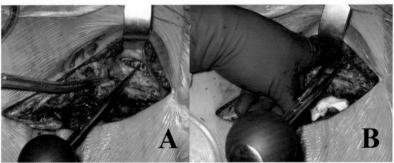

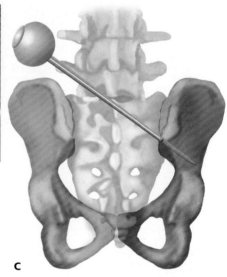

TECH FIG 7 • An oblique incision is made in the fascia overlying the posterior superior iliac spine. Subsequently, the pedicle seeker is driven into the table of the ilium, angled toward the anterior superior iliac spine (A). Placement of a finger into the greater sciatic notch can help guide the pedicle seeker (B). C. Line diagram of trajectory (A, B, from Moshirfar A, Rand FF, Sponseller PD, et al. Pelvic fixation in spine surgery: Historical overview, indications, biomechanical relevance, and current techniques. J Bone Joint Surg Am 2005;87 Suppl 2:89–106 with permission).

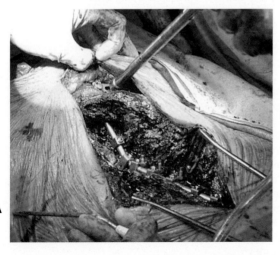

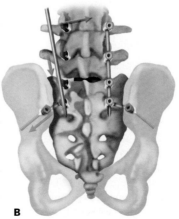

TECH FIG 8 • The iliac screw is attached to the main spinal construct by using a modular connector system, which is tunneled anterior to the paraspinous muscles. A, (from Moshirfar A, Rand FF, Sponseller PD, et al. Pelvic fixation in spine surgery: Historical overview, indications, biomechanical relevance, and current techniques. J Bone Joint Surg Am 2005;87 Suppl 2:89–106.)

OPEN S2AI TECHNIQUE[16,20]

- The placement of the S2AI screw should take place only after the other points of fixation, including the S1 screws, have been secured.
- After placement of the S1 screw, the position of the S1 dorsal sacral foramen is identified using standard antero-posterior (AP) and pelvic inlet fluoroscopic views.
- An awl is used to breach the dorsal cortex over the starting point, located in line with the lateral edge of the S1 foramen and 5 to 10 mm distal to the S1 foramen (**TECH FIG 9A**).
- The ideal S2AI trajectory averages 40 degrees of lateral angulation in the transverse plane and 40 degrees of caudal angulation in the sagittal planes, directed toward the ASIS (**TECH FIG 9B,C**).
- A 2.5-mm pelvic drill bit (extended length) is used to tap drill through the sacral ala, the SI joint, and into the ilium. This distance is roughly 30 to 45 mm in most patients (**TECH FIG 10**).
- At this point, the drill bit is removed and replaced with a 3.2-mm drill bit in order to reduce the risk of breakage in

harder bone and is advanced for a total depth of approximately 80 to 90 mm.
- Once the drill has reached the ilium, the drill itself is removed. A ball-point depth gauge is then inserted into the hole in order to determine the length of the screw.
- Next, a 1.45-mm guidewire mounted on a handheld driver is advanced for an additional 10 to 20 mm in order to seat the guidewire in bone (**TECH FIG 11**). Angulation continues to be directed down toward the ASIS.
- Placement can be confirmed with intraoperative fluoroscopy or a single pelvic radiograph.
- The hole is then manually tapped over the guidewire using a cannulated tap (**TECH FIG 12A**), and an appropriate length screw is placed (**TECH FIG 12B**). Screw sizes of 8 to 10 mm by 80 to 100 mm are common in adults.
- Because the screws are in line with the rest of the spinal construct, no additional cross connectors are required for assembly (**TECH FIG 13**).

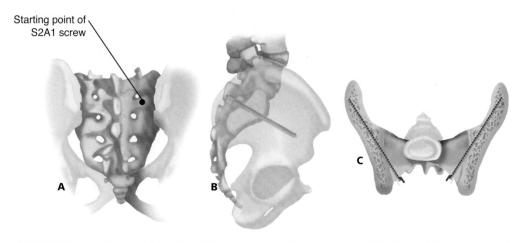

Starting point of S2A1 screw

TECH FIG 9 • Starting point for the S2AI screw marked by a *black dot* (**A**). Sagittal (**B**) and coronal (**C**) views of the final trajectory of the S2AI screw.

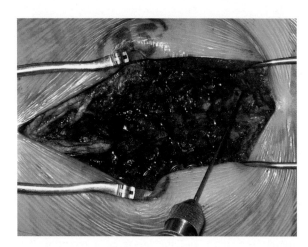

TECH FIG 10 • A drill is used to tap through the sacroiliac articulation.

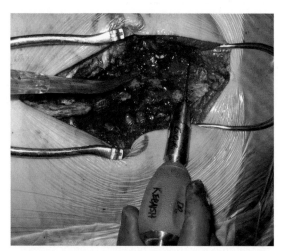

TECH FIG 11 • The drill is removed and a 1.45-mm guidewire mounted on a handheld driver is advanced into the table of the ilium toward the anterior superior iliac spine.

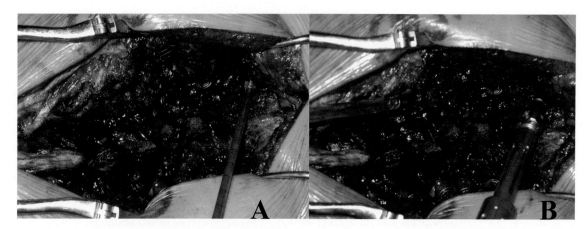

TECH FIG 12 • Tapping the S2AI screw **hole** over the guidewire (**A**) and placement of the S2AI screw (**B**).

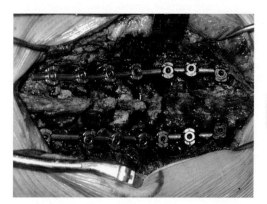
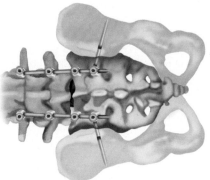

TECH FIG 13 • Final alignment of the S2AI screw and spinal construct above.

PERCUTANEOUS S2AI TECHNIQUE[21,22]

- Because the S2AI screw is in line with the spinal construct attached to the mobile spine, the S2AI technique is amenable to a minimally invasive percutaneous approach.[21]
- The percutaneous sacropelvic fixation is frequently combined with a minimally invasive percutaneous fixation of the lumbar spine, but this may not be required depending on the indication.
- The approach to the sacrum is a 3 cm midline incision at the level of the S1 and S2 dorsal foramen.
- The starting point, located in line with the lateral edge of the S1 foramen and 5 to 10 mm distal to the S1 foramen (TECH FIG 9A), is identified using standard AP and pelvic inlet fluoroscopic views.
- A Jamshidi needle is angled toward the anterior ASIS and advanced 20 mm into the sacral ala. The ideal S2AI trajectory is the same as in the open procedure and averages 40 degrees of lateral angulation in the transverse plane and 40 degrees of caudal angulation in the sagittal planes, but varies with pelvic obliquity (TECH FIG 9B,C).
- A teardrop view is then obtained in order to verify the positioning (TECH FIG 14).
- The teardrop view is a fluoroscopic view obtained by rolling the C-arm roughly 45 degrees over the table, and

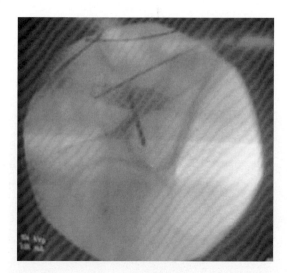

TECH FIG 14 • Representative fluoroscopic teardrop view, obtained by rolling the C-arm roughly 45 degrees over the table and tilting it roughly 45 degrees cephalad, which creates an overlap of the anterior superior iliac spine and the posterior superior iliac spine, and the image of a teardrop. (From Martin CT, Witham T, Kebaish KM. Sacropelvic fixation: two case reports of a new percutaneous technique. Spine 2011; 36(9):e618–21.)

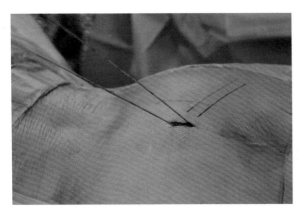

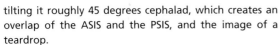

TECH FIG 15 • Percutaneous guidewire placement.

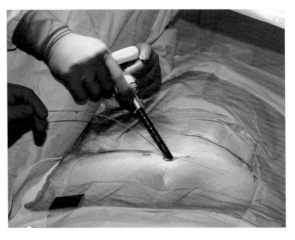

TECH FIG 16 • A cannulated handheld tap is used to tap the screw hole over the guidewire.

tilting it roughly 45 degrees cephalad, which creates an overlap of the ASIS and the PSIS, and the image of a teardrop.
- The needle position is adjusted to be coaxial with the teardrop and then advanced 10 mm past the sacroiliac joint.
- Next, a 1.45-mm guidewire is passed through the Jamshidi needle, again angling toward the ASIS.
- The Jamshidi needle is removed, and the guidewire is advanced into the ilium through the cancellous bone between the cortices of the ilium until the distal cortex is reached (TECH FIG 15).
- Positioning and angulation of the wire can be confirmed with fluoroscopic views as needed.
- Screw lengths are then measured by marking the depth of the guidewire. Screw sizes of 8 to 10 mm by 80 to 100 mm are common in adults.

- The hole is manually tapped over the guidewire using a cannulated tap (TECH FIG 16), and an appropriate length screw is placed (TECH FIG 17A).
- Because the screws are in line with the rest of the spinal construct, no additional cross connectors are required for assembly.
- In cases in which a percutaneous lumbar spinal procedure has also been performed, the S2AI screw can be attached to the main spinal construct by threading a rod under the skin from proximal to distal, and maneuvering the rod with a premade rod-guidance tube (TECH FIG 17B).
- The final trajectory and placement of the screw is identical to that of the open S2AI technique (TECH FIG 9B,C).

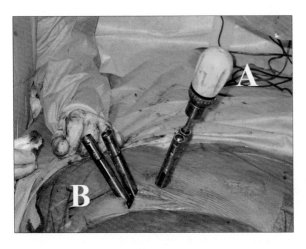

TECH FIG 17 • **A.** The screw is placed with a handheld drill. **B.** In cases in which a minimally invasive lumbar spine procedure has also been done, the rod can be attached to the main spinal construct by passing it underneath the skin with the assistance of premade rod guidance tubes. (From Martin CT, Witham T, Kebaish KM. Sacropelvic fixation: two case reports of a new percutaneous technique. Spine 2011;36(9):e618–21.)

AUTHOR'S PREFERRED TECHNIQUE

- At our institution, the S2AI technique has been adopted as the procedure of choice for sacropelvic fixation in both adult and pediatric cases.

PEARLS AND PITFALLS

Indications	■ Long spinal fusions to the sacrum are the most common indication for sacropelvic fixation.
Teardrop fluoroscopic view	■ The teardrop is created by the overlap of the ASIS and PSIS and represents a bony canal through which the pelvic fixation may be safely placed.
Damage to surrounding soft tissues	■ Structures in the sciatic notch are at risk. ■ Minimized by verifying a bony endpoint with a blunt probe prior to screw placement.
Implant prominence	■ Most common reason for revision. ■ Minimized by creating a notch prior to placement of the iliac screw, by burying the screw beyond the PSIS, by choosing a medial starting point for the screw, or by using the S2AI technique.
Instrumentation loosening	■ Minimize by using largest acceptable diameter screw. ■ Addition of an anterior fusion increases construct stability.

POSTOPERATIVE CARE

■ The patient should be awoken in the operating room and a detailed neurologic examination should be conducted immediately following surgery. If a neurologic deficit is detected, appropriate imaging and surgical intervention may be necessary.
■ The postoperative diet and patient pain control can be managed as per routine postoperative care.
■ No additional external immobilization such as an orthotic or plaster cast is necessary.
■ The patient should be placed in a regular hospital bed and early ambulation should be encouraged.
■ Physical therapy should be started as soon as feasible following the surgical procedure.
■ After discharge, follow-up at regular intervals is important, including appropriate radiographs as indicated depending on the procedure performed.

OUTCOMES

■ Excellent fusion rates have been achieved with all three techniques.[13–15,20]
■ Implant prominence and pain is a common reason for instrumentation removal in both the iliac screw and the S2AI techniques. However, less than 2% of patients with S2AI screws require implant removal after 2 years, as compared to up to 22% of patients with iliac screws.[23,24]
■ The screw in the S2AI technique breaches the synovial cartilage of the SI joint in approximately 60% of cases. However, a recent study showed no adverse effects on the SI joint at 2 years follow-up.[20]

COMPLICATIONS

■ Modern techniques for sacropelvic fixation have helped to minimize the incidence of complications. However, serious complications still can and do occur. A brief discussion of these complications and ways to minimize them is presented here.

Instrumentation Misplacement and Injuries to Adjacent Structures

■ The structures in the greater sciatic foramen and those overlying the anterior surface of the sacrum are at risk during placement of the instrumentation.[5]
■ However, injury to these structures is very uncommon,[5] and the risk can be minimized by using a blunt probe to ensure a proper bony endpoint prior to screw placement.

■ Fluoroscopic imaging can also be useful, particularly in patients with difficult anatomy.

Implant Prominence

■ Implant prominence can lead to significant pain and discomfort and is the most common reason for revision of this procedure.[5]
■ The risk of this complication is highest in thin patients and is higher with the iliac screw and Galveston techniques.[5]
■ The risks can be minimized by creating a notch prior to placement of the iliac screw, by burying the screw beyond the PSIS, by choosing a medial starting point for the iliac screw, or by using the S2AI technique, which on average allows for 15 mm deeper placement of the screw head as compared to the iliac screw technique.[17]

Implant Loosening

■ Loosening is a second common reason for implant removal, but it may remain asymptomatic if fusion can be achieved prior to its onset.[5]
■ Loosening is caused by repeated micromotion of the implants and is visible radiographically as a radiolucency around the screw or rod.
■ In the Galveston L-rod technique, loosening of the short arm of the L-rod is particularly common, and this complication is called the windshield wiper effect.[13,25]
■ In some patients treated with the Galveston technique, the windshield wiper effect may lead to pain and the need for implant removal.[13,25]
■ With the S2AI and iliac screw techniques, choosing the largest diameter screw possible (usually 8 to 10 mm in adults) can help to delay implant loosening and maximize the chances of a successful fusion.

Wound Problems and Infection

■ Few studies have reported definitive infection rates associated with sacropelvic fixation.
■ Furthermore, the infection rate associated with sacropelvic fixation alone is difficult to ascertain because these techniques are often combined with fusions of the mobile spine above which requires additional incisions and soft tissue dissection.
■ Infection rates associated with the Galveston L-rod have been reported to range from 3% to 10%.[13,26]
■ In a study of 81 patients treated with iliac screw fixation, the infection rate was reported as 4%.[15]

- A study of 27 patients treated with the S2AI technique showed an infection rate of 0%.[20]
- Significantly less dissection is required for the S2AI technique, which may account for the lower infection rates reported with that procedure.

Nonunion and Instrumentation Failure

- If bony fusion does not occur, the instrumentation is destined to fail, often through implant failure or breakage.
- Augmentation of sacropelvic fixation with an anterior interbody lumbar fusion at L4–L5 and L5–S1 can optimize fusion stability and increase the chances of a successful fusion.[27-29]

REFERENCES

1. Peretz AM, Hipp JA, Heggeness MH. The internal bony architecture of the sacrum. Spine (Phila Pa 1976) 1998;23:971–974.
2. Moshirfar A, Rand FF, Sponseller PD, et al. Pelvic fixation in spine surgery. Historical overview, indications, biomechanical relevance, and current techniques. J Bone Joint Surg Am 2005;87 Suppl 2:89–106.
3. Xu R, Ebraheim NA, Yeasting RA, et al. Morphometric evaluation of the first sacral vertebra and the projection of its pedicle on the posterior aspect of the sacrum. Spine (Phila Pa 1976) 1995;20:936–940.
4. Mirkovic S, Abitbol JJ, Steinman J, et al. Anatomic consideration for sacral screw placement. Spine (Phila Pa 1976) 1991;16:S289–S294.
5. Kebaish KM. Sacropelvic fixation: techniques and complications. Spine (Phila Pa 1976) 2010;35:2245–2251.
6. Devlin VJ, Boachie-Adjei O, Bradford DS, et al. Treatment of adult spinal deformity with fusion to the sacrum using CD instrumentation. J Spinal Disord 1991;4:1–14.
7. Camp JF, Caudle R, Ashmun RD, et al. Immediate complications of cotrel-dubousset instrumentation to the sacro-pelvis. A clinical and biomechanical study. Spine (Phila Pa 1976) 1990;15:932–941.
8. Jackson RP, McManus AC. The iliac buttress. A computed tomographic study of sacral anatomy. Spine (Phila Pa 1976) 1993;18:1318–1328.
9. McCord DH, Cunningham BW, Shono Y, et al. Biomechanical analysis of lumbosacral fixation. Spine (Phila Pa 1976) 1992;17:S235–S243.
10. O'Brien MF, Sacropelvic fixation in spinal deformity. In: Dewlad RL, ed. Spinal Deformities: The Comprehensive Text. New York, NY: Thieme; 2003:601–614.
11. Cunningham BW, Lewis SJ, Long J, et al. Biomechanical evaluation of lumbosacral reconstruction techniques for spondylolisthesis: an in vitro porcine model. Spine (Phila Pa 1976) 2002;27:2321–2327.
12. Wiggins GC, Ondra SL, Shaffrey CI. Management of iatrogenic flatback syndrome. Neurosurg Focus 2003;15:E8.
13. Gau YL, Lonstein JE, Winter RB, et al. Luque-galveston procedure for correction and stabilization of neuromuscular scoliosis and pelvic obliquity: a review of 68 patients. J Spinal Disord 1991;4:399–410.
14. Allen BL Jr, Ferguson RL. The galveston technique of pelvic fixation with L-rod instrumentation of the spine. Spine (Phila Pa 1976) 1984;9:388–394.
15. Kuklo TR, Bridwell KH, Lewis SJ, et al. Minimum 2-year analysis of sacropelvic fixation and L5-S1 fusion using S1 and iliac screws. Spine (Phila Pa 1976) 2001;26:1976–1983.
16. O'Brien JR, Yu WD, Bhatnagar R, et al. An anatomic study of the S2 iliac technique for lumbopelvic screw placement. Spine (Phila Pa 1976) 2009;34:E439–E442.
17. Chang TL, Sponseller PD, Kebaish KM, et al. Low profile pelvic fixation: anatomic parameters for sacral alar-iliac fixation versus traditional iliac fixation. Spine (Phila Pa 1976) 2009;34:436–440.
18. Allen BL Jr, Ferguson RL. The galveston technique for L rod instrumentation of the scoliotic spine. Spine (Phila Pa 1976) 1982;7:276–284.
19. Lehman RA Jr, Kuklo TR, Belmont PJ Jr, et al. Advantage of pedicle screw fixation directed into the apex of the sacral promontory over bicortical fixation: a biomechanical analysis. Spine (Phila Pa 1976) 2002;27:806–811.
20. Sponseller PD, Zimmerman RM, Ko PS, et al. Low profile pelvic fixation with the sacral alar iliac technique in the pediatric population improves results at two-year minimum follow-up. Spine (Phila Pa 1976) 2010;35:1887–1892.
21. Martin CT, Witham TF, Kebaish KM. Sacropelvic fixation: two case reports of a new percutaneous technique. Spine (Phila Pa 1976) 2011;36(9):E618–E621.
22. O'Brien JR, Matteini L, Yu WD, et al. Feasibility of minimally invasive sacropelvic fixation: percutaneous S2 alar iliac fixation. Spine (Phila Pa 1976) 2010;35:460–464.
23. Kebaish KM, Pull ter Gunne AF, Mohamed AS, et al. A new low profile sacropelvic fixation using S2 alar iliac (S2AI) screws in adult deformity fusion to the sacrum: a prospective study with minimum 2-year follow-up. Presented at: the North American Spine Society Annual Meeting; November 10–14, 2009; San Francisco, CA.
24. Emami A, Deviren V, Berven S, et al. Outcome and complications of long fusions to the sacrum in adult spine deformity: Luque-Galveston, combined iliac and sacral screws, and sacral fixation. Spine (Phila Pa 1976) 2002;27:776–786.
25. Broom MJ, Banta JV, Renshaw TS. Spinal fusion augmented by luque-rod segmental instrumentation for neuromuscular scoliosis. J Bone Joint Surg Am 1989;71:32–44.
26. Nectoux E, Giacomelli MC, Karger C, et al. Complications of the luque-galveston scoliosis correction technique in paediatric cerebral palsy. Orthop Traumatol Surg Res 2010;96:354–361.
27. Kostuik JP, Hall BB. Spinal fusions to the sacrum in adults with scoliosis. Spine (Phila Pa 1976) 1983;8:489–500.
28. Kostuik JP, Errico TJ, Gleason TF. Techniques of internal fixation for degenerative conditions of the lumbar spine. Clin Orthop Relat Res 1986;(203):219–231.
29. Ogilvie JW, Schendel M. Comparison of lumbosacral fixation devices. Clin Orthop Relat Res 1986;(203):120–125.

Chapter 29

Management of Intraoperative Cerebrospinal Fluid Leaks: Techniques of Dural Repair, Dural Patching, and Placement and Management of Subarachnoid Lumbar Drains

Christopher G. Kalhorn and Kevin M. McGrail

INTRODUCTION

Management of intraoperative durotomies and the postoperative management of cerebrospinal leaks can pose serious problems in spinal surgery. This chapter addresses the intraoperative management of durotomies as well as postoperative care. We first discuss risk factors that can predispose patients to the occurrence of an intraoperative durotomy. We review the surgical instruments, biological agents, and drainage catheters that are of assistance with repair of durotomies. A discussion then occurs with respect to the particular challenges at varying locations within the spinal axis when it is approached either anteriorly or posteriorly.

AVOIDANCE OF DUROTOMY DURING EXPOSURE OF THE SPINE

- Careful study of preoperative imaging studies may yield valuable information with respect to potential pitfalls during exposure of the spine.
- Look out for postoperative changes from previous laminectomies or laminotomies.
- Spina bifida occulta is reported in up to 10% to 15% of normal healthy adults and is a potential site for durotomy during exposure.
- Incomplete ossification of the C1 laminar arch should be kept in mind during any posterior approach to the high cervical spine or craniocervical junction.
- The L5 S1 interspace is a widened interspace and is a frequent area for incidental durotomy during exposure of the lumbar spine.
- Ossification of the posterior longitudinal ligament, especially in the cervical and thoracic spine can often be recognized on preoperative imaging studies and carries a high risk of intraoperative cerebrospinal fluid (CSF) leak.

PRINCIPLES OF REPAIR: DUROTOMY DURING EXPOSURE OF THE SPINE

- Often, these durotomies occur in the midline and can be repaired primarily with simple interrupted or running sutures. 4-0 or 5-0 monofilament suture such as Prolene (Ethicon, Somerville, NJ) or nylon are appropriate.
- We prefer a repair with a small tapered needle such as an RB-1 in a simple running fashion.
- A good needle driver such as Castro-Viejo can be helpful to repair a tear in the lateral recess.

GENERAL PRINCIPLES AND PATIENT SAFETY

- When an intraoperative durotomy has occurred, care should be taken to avoid any injury to the underlying neural elements.
- Surgical cautery (Bovie) use should be limited when in proximity to neural elements.
- Minimize the use of high-speed cutting drill bits near the spinal canal. A diamond drill bit is a much safer instrument especially in less experienced hands.
- The use of appropriate sized suction tips is recommended once a durotomy has occurred. The smallest suction tip that can be used to keep the surgical field clear should be employed.
- Suction tips that allow for regulation of the strength of the suction at the handpiece are extremely useful.
- Suction tips that have their apertures on the side and not on the tip (Grossman suction tips) are also very useful in these situations.
- Suction lines that are soft and flexible allow for rapid "clamping off" when a durotomy has occurred. This can prevent a suction tip from inadvertently sucking up nerve roots.
- Make sure that you have a capable and experienced assistant. Sometimes what you really need is an extra pair of experienced hands to maximize your exposure so that you can work on primary repair of the dural defect.
- Once a durotomy has taken place, protect the neural elements with a soft Cottonoid (Codman, Warsaw, IN).
- Focus is then directed toward minimizing and further extension of the durotomy and attaining sufficient bone exposure to allow for primary dural repair when possible.
- Whenever possible, achieve a watertight primary dural repair and reinforce with dural sealant when indicated.
- Decompression of the lumbar cistern through the release of spinal fluid can also alleviate the extramural forces on the epidural venous plexus. This can result in large amounts of bleeding which can normally be controlled with bipolar cautery or thrombin-soaked Gelfoam (Baxter Healthcare Corporation, Hayward, CA).

DURAL SUBSTITUTES

- There are a number of commercially available dural substitute materials.
- Most of these are derivatives of bovine collagen.
- They are available as suturable or onlay dural grafts.
- Bovine pericardium is also commercially available as a suturable dural graft.

▪ There are case reports of aseptic or chemical meningitis associated with bovine pericardial grafts.

▪ Autologous grafting materials include pericranium, fascia lata, and autologous muscle grafts that can be used as a plug to prevent a leak.

DURAL SEALANTS

▪ There are a number of commercially available dural sealants.

▪ Most are derivatives of fibrin glue.

▪ Thin layers of these sealants can be applied with aerosolizers to reinforce a dural repair.

▪ Some of these products have been reported to swell postoperatively. For this reason, a minimum of product should be used to reinforce the repair and avoid postoperative compression of the neural elements.

DUROTOMIES DURING POSTERIOR LUMBAR SURGERY

▪ Lumbar dural tears may occur during exposure of the lumbar spine, during the course of decompression of the neural elements, or during the placement of spinal hardware.

▪ If possible, avoid a leak in the first place. This can be done by avoiding sharp bone edges along the margins of a decompressive laminectomy.

▪ Make good use of your assistant. In the lumbar spine, have your assistant utilize a blunt nerve hook or a no. 4 Penfield to gently displace the dura away from the bone edge while you are doing your decompression.

▪ Most midline durotomies lend themselves to primary dural repair.

▪ Durotomies which occur in the lateral recess or overlying the exiting nerve root sheath are more difficult to repair.

▪ When a CSF leak occurs in the lateral recess, first obtain wider bone exposure. A primary dural repair should then be attempted.

▪ Large dural defects that cannot be repaired primary should be grafted (eg, with bovine pericardial graft or dural substitute). These grafts should be sewn in place in a watertight manner when possible.

▪ For dural tears that cannot be repaired primarily or patched, consider an onlay dural substitute graft reinforced with a dural sealant.

▪ When CSF leaks occur over the nerve root sheath, these are often difficult to repair primarily and can be treated successfully with dural sealant or fibrin glue.

▪ Occasionally, one can face a fairly small lumbar durotomy through which multiple rootlets of the cauda equina can herniate. In this situation, it may be necessary to enlarge the durotomy and even to drain some spinal fluid to allow for safe reduction of the rootlets back into the spinal canal followed by primary repair of the dura.

DUROTOMIES DURING REVISION LUMBAR SURGERY

▪ Patients with a history of CSF leak with previous surgery should be counseled preoperatively that they are likely at a higher risk of recurrent CSF leak.

▪ During exposure of the spine, the use of sharp curettes to define normal facet and bone anatomy is extremely useful.

▪ The use of a diamond drill around the margins of a previous laminectomy may help prevent a leak.

▪ When scar is densely adherent to the underlying dura, it may be prudent to leave areas of adherent scar attached to avoid a CSF leak.

DUROTOMIES DURING POSTERIOR THORACIC SURGERY

▪ Many of the same principles as outlined in repair of CSF leaks during posterior lumbar surgery apply in the posterior thoracic spine.

▪ If a leak occurs over a thoracic nerve root sheath, the root itself can be ligated and sacrificed to prevent further leakage of CSF.

▪ With CSF leak in the setting of posterior lumbar or thoracic surgery we will often recommend a period of flat bedrest for the first 48 hours to allow for short-term healing of the repair.

▪ After 48 hours, we will mobilize the patients ad lib.

DUROTOMIES DURING POSTERIOR CERVICAL SURGERY

▪ Durotomies during posterior spinal surgery normally are midline or paramedian in location and lend themselves to primary dural repair. This can be supplemented with dural sealant.

DUROTOMIES DURING ANTERIOR CERVICAL SPINAL APPROACHES

▪ CSF leaks are not as common in anterior cervical approaches as they are in lumbar spinal procedures.

▪ Most leaks that we have observed during anterior cervical discectomy and fusion (ACDF) have been in association with the use of high-powered drills.

▪ These leaks normally occur at the site of the takeoff of the cervical root sheath. In this location the dura takes a slight superior course as the nerve root exits the foramen, making the dura more likely to be injured in this location.

▪ Durotomies during ACDF can be extremely difficult to repair primarily.

▪ Most of these durotomies can be treated with an onlay dural substitute and a widely fitting bone graft that occupies the width of the discectomy defect.

▪ Consideration should be given to the placement of a lumbar subarachnoid drain.

DUROTOMIES DURING ANTERIOR THORACIC SPINAL APPROACHES

▪ Durotomies that occur during anterior thoracic approaches are of concern because of the large potential space of leak and frequent requirements for postoperative chest tubes.

▪ Attempt should be made to repair the dura primarily if possible.

▪ Often, these leaks can only be repaired with onlay dural substitute and dura sealant together.

▪ Attention should be given to the postoperative chest tube output.

▪ If there is a question about whether chest tube fluid represents normal pleural fluid or CSF, a sample of fluid can be collected and sent for beta 2 transferrin which is positive in CSF.

▪ With a persistent CSF leak occurs in the setting of a chest tube with CSF coming out of the chest tube, we recommend taking the chest tube off of negative pressure suction when feasible and continuing the lumbar drain until the chest tube can be removed.

■ Our experience has been that recurrent CSF leaks in the chest are unusual.

PLACEMENT OF LUMBAR SUBARACHNOID DRAINS

■ We will most often place a lumbar drain in cases of recurrent CSF leak after primary repair or in cases that are deemed to be high risk for postoperative CSF leak.
■ Lumbar subarachnoid drains can either be placed surgically at the time of a lumbar decompressive laminectomy or separately through a 14-gauge Tuohy needle.
■ The purpose of a lumbar drain is to divert spinal fluid and alleviate pressure to allow for the repaired area of CSF leak to heal.
■ Care should be taken at the time of lumbar catheter placement not to attempt to reposition the drain catheter while the spinal needle is in place. This can result in inadvertent shearing of the catheter.
■ Lumbar drains are connected to a sterile drainage system.
■ Most common site of insertion is from L2 to L5.

POSTOPERATIVE MANAGEMENT OF LUMBAR DRAINS

■ Careful postoperative orders must be given regarding the management of lumbar drains.
■ Drainage systems are most commonly placed at the level of the patient's spine and the height of the drainage collection device is adjusted to maintain a CSF output of approximately 80 mL of spinal fluid per 8-hour shift.
■ Patients are frequently maintained on intravenous antibiotics while the spinal drain is in place. We use prophylactic Ancef until the drain is removed.
■ The drain is normally left open for 3 to 7 days to allow time for healing of the durotomy.
■ The lumbar drainage system is the clamped and the patient is observed for signs or recurrent CSF leak.
■ If there is no further evidence of CSF leak after the drain has been clamped for 24 hours, the lumbar subarachnoid drain is removed.
■ Overdrainage of CSF through a lumbar drain can result in tearing of cranial bridging veins and acute subdural hematoma formation.
■ The risk of infection with prolonged indwelling drains can be minimized with good sterile technique. Drains can also be tunneled, which also helps to minimize infection risk. It has been our practice to maintain our patients on intravenous antibiotics while the drain is in place and we make an effort not to extend CSF diversion through a lumbar drain beyond 7 days.

POSTOPERATIVE MANAGEMENT OF WOUND DRAINS

■ We will place wound drains (wound Hemovac) in the setting of a repaired CSF leak.
■ The intention of placing a wound drain is to help prevent the postoperative occurrence of an epidural hematoma.
■ Epidural hematoma is of concern due to a loss of turgor pressure within the thecal sac and decompression of the lumbar epidural venous plexus.
■ These drains can later be removed or taken off of suction if the drain outputs are high or the patient develops a spinal headache.

CLINICAL SIGNS OF ONGOING CSF LEAK

■ These include low-pressure headache (spinal headache). These headaches often will be present when the patient is in the upright position and will resolve or improve when the patient is recumbent.
■ New onset cranial nerve palsies (abducens nerve palsy). As the sixth cranial nerve has the longest intracranial course, this is presumably due to traction on the sixth nerve with excessive CSF drainage.
■ Nausea and vomiting.

WHAT TO DO WHEN YOUR DRAIN DOES NOT WORK (THE RECURRENT LEAK)

■ For cases of recurrent CSF cutaneous fistulas or recurrent symptomatic CSF leaks which have not resolved with CSF diversion, oftentimes the only option is reexploration and attempted repair of the leak if it can be located.

PSEUDOMENINGOCELE

■ Pseudomeningocele should be divided according to small or asymptomatic collections and larger, symptomatic, or cosmetically disfiguring collections.
■ Small, asymptomatic collections can be observed.
■ Large, symptomatic collections will usually require reexploration and repair with possible CSF diversion through a lumbar subarachnoid drain.
■ Patients who have symptomatic pseudomeningocele may complain of pain or swelling at the surgical site or symptoms of low CSF pressure. These symptoms include persistent positional headache, nausea, vomiting, or occasionally photophobia. These symptoms are exacerbated in the upright position (**FIG 1**).

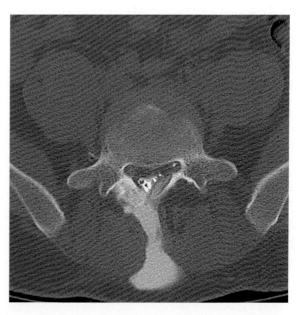

FIG 1 • Axial CT myelogram demonstrating dye extravasation into a pseudomeningocele cavity consistent with cerebrospinal leak.

Chapter 30

Revision Lumbar Surgery: Strategies and Techniques

Todd B. Francis and Gordon R. Bell

DEFINITION

- There are a multitude of different reasons why a patient may need to undergo revision lumbar surgery. Of all patients who have an operation for degenerative lumbar disease, approximately 15% will require a revision surgery.[1]
- The term "failed back syndrome" (FBS) has been used to describe patients that experience poor clinical outcomes following lumbar surgery for degenerative causes, usually involving the intervertebral disc.[2] Although this is a significant diagnosis in patients requiring lumbar revision surgery, it is not all-inclusive in that it typically does not include patients with trauma, tumor, infection, or nondegenerative deformity who require reoperation.

ANATOMY

- It is mandatory to obtain weight-bearing preoperative films to visualize the anatomy and to aid in localization. This is especially true when identifying hardware and intact bony elements as landmarks for the correct level to be operated upon.
- When reoperating on patients having had previous back surgery, spinal anatomy can be considerably distorted. In the majority of cases, the normal bony landmarks and natural anatomic planes are often not present and may be replaced with dense fibrous scar. The dura underlying the scar can be densely adherent to it and the surgeon can easily cause an unintended durotomy if dissection is not carried out with caution.
- In general, the key to exposing a previously operated spine is to identify the normal anatomy and to ultimately identify the lateral wall of the bony canal which is a key landmark in identifying the neural elements. Residual bone lateral to the spinal canal (eg, the facet joints or bony fusion mass) and implanted instrumentation can also serve as valuable and reliable landmarks. When reoperating on the lumbar spine, especially if hardware is in place, dissection is best started laterally by identifying the facets or hardware. From here, the surgeon can work medially to remove scar and identify dura, if necessary.
- In patients without implanted hardware, it is safest to extend the original incision, exposing normal anatomy above and below the previous operative site. This makes it easier to identify the correct level, and dissection can proceed toward the area where the anatomy is uncertain.

PATHOGENESIS

- The risk of developing a recurrent lumbar disc herniation after discectomy is approximately 5% to 18%.[3,4]
- Some common causes for persistent or recurrent symptoms after lumbar surgery include failure to identify or address all of the pathology (eg, lateral recess stenosis, foraminal stenosis, or disc herniation), postoperative instability (eg, spondylolisthesis, scoliosis, kyphosis, and flat back deformity), adjacent level disease, and scar formation.[5]

- Some element of scarring occurs after all surgeries. The presence of peridural fibrosis following decompressive spinal surgery therefore does not necessarily implicate it as a cause of the patient's symptoms. However, patients undergoing lumbar revision surgery tend to have poor outcomes when significant fibrosis is present.[6]
- Pseudoarthrosis in the setting of spinal fusion surgery refers to the radiologic failure of new bone to form across the intended joint space.
- The underlying reason why a patient may require lumbar revision surgery can be suggested by evaluating the duration of symptom relief following the initial surgery. If the patient had no symptom relief following surgery, then either the surgeon did not address the genesis of the pain or perform an inadequate surgical procedure. Transient relief of symptoms (less than 6 months) suggests the development of scar tissue as a cause of recurrence of symptoms. Finally, if the patient experienced a long duration of relief of his or her symptoms (typically longer than 6 to 12 months), this suggests development of new pathology at either the same level or at a new level.

NATURAL HISTORY OF RECURRENT SYMPTOMATIC PATHOLOGY

- The natural history of recurrent pathology following initial surgery is not completely known but is likely similar to that of the original condition. In other words, the natural history of a recurrent disc herniation, for example, is likely similar to that of the original herniation: spontaneous resolution of symptoms in many cases. Therefore, a trial of conservative treatment should be tried prior to surgical intervention.

PATIENT HISTORY AND PHYSICAL FINDINGS

- It is important to determine that the patient has been correctly diagnosed and treated. The three broad questions that need to be determined and asked, based on the history and physical exam, are: was the original diagnosis correct, was the choice of type of surgery appropriate, and was the actual surgical technique appropriate?
- When evaluating a patient with persistent symptoms after lumbar surgery, it is important to carefully review the patient's medical and surgical history. It is useful to categorize the patient's chief complaint into one of three groups: leg pain predominant, back pain predominant, or leg and back pain equal. This will aid the physician in determining the potential source of the patient's continuing symptoms and guide his or her medical decision making appropriately. Predominant leg pain, for example, suggests a neurogenic cause for the pain. Predominant back pain, on the other hand, is likely not due to a neurogenic cause and the genesis of which is much more difficult to identify.

■ A detailed history of present illness and past medical history should be obtained. In particular, it is important to establish a surgical timeline. The onset and characteristics of initial symptoms, a detailed description of all spinal surgical interventions, and the presence or absence of symptom-free periods should be documented. All medications, especially narcotic analgesics and anticoagulants, must be recorded. It is important to review the patient's original presenting symptoms and compare these to the surgical procedure performed to ensure that the correct procedure was chosen. In this regard, it is extremely helpful to review preoperative clinical notes and operative reports. These should be obtained whenever possible. The operative note should be scrutinized for comments about potential intraoperative adverse events, such as durotomy.

■ The presence of additional factors that could affect outcome or recurrence of symptoms should be investigated. These include the presence of a work-related injury, particularly if associated with a pending compensation claim. The likelihood of secondary gain is a potentially significant factor in these patients. In addition, the surgeon must be cognizant of psychosocial issues before planning a revision operation. This includes depression and narcotic addiction. The presence of these psychosocial factors (worker's compensation, depression, anxiety, litigation, etc.) can have a significant negative impact on patient outcome after lumbar surgery.[7] When in doubt about potential significance of such psychosocial factors, a psychological evaluation should be obtained.

■ The quality and pattern of the patient's pain can provide significant information about the nature of the pain. Leg pain that is described as "burning," for example, suggests neuropathic pain, which is generally unresponsive to further surgical intervention. Similarly, leg pain that is present constantly and is unchanged by activity generally suggests the presence of underlying changes in the nerve that are unlikely to be significantly changed by additional surgery. Such nonmechanical pain is not typical of neurogenic pain that is amenable to surgery, which is generally mechanical in nature.

■ In patients with leg pain, careful examination of the lower extremity joints and pulses is important to rule out nonspinal causes of this pain. This is particularly important in older patients, in whom spinal disease frequently coexists with other degenerative conditions such as peripheral vascular disease and joint arthritis.

■ The presence of Waddell signs should also be documented, if present. One of the more significant Waddell signs is overreaction to pain. Other signs include superficial skin tenderness, regional disturbances, distraction phenomena, and simulation. The presence of three or more Waddell signs indicates that the patient's pain is likely nonorganic and portends a poor prognosis, particularly with further surgery.[8] Distraction testing includes the "flip test" in which a patient demonstrates a positive straight leg raise (SLR) test in the supine position but not in the seated position (**FIG 1**). An SLR test in a patient who is exhibiting pain behavior will be easily achieved to 90 degrees, whereas a patient with pain from a true radiculopathy will "flip" back on their hands when attempting a sitting SLR in order to relieve tension in the sciatic nerve.[9] With simulation, anticipatory behavior can be elicited through simulated movement. For example, the patient will report back pain through maneuvers that do not typically move the back, such as mild trunk rotation through hip rotation (Table 1).

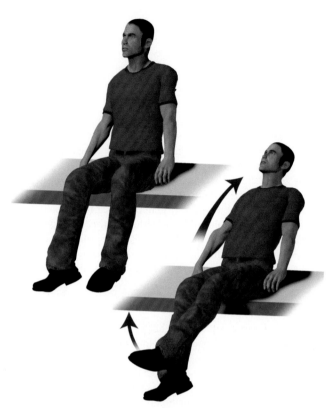

FIG 1 • Flip test. Patient should flip back on hands if straight leg raise test is truly positive.

IMAGING AND OTHER DIAGNOSTIC STUDIES

■ Ideally, all of the patient's preoperative and immediate postoperative films should be reviewed. This assures that surgically correctable pathology was initially present and that it was addressed surgically, both in terms of operating at the correct level and by doing an adequate decompression.

■ All patients being evaluated for revision lumbar surgery should have a current standing anteroposterior (AP) and lateral plain X-ray of their lumbar spine. This should also include a coned-down spot lateral view of the lumbosacral level, especially in patients with prior surgery at L5–S1. This provides valuable information about sagittal and coronal alignment, hardware position and integrity, and bony anatomy. If iatrogenic injury to the pars interarticularis is suspected, oblique views of the lumbar spine can be useful.

■ Flexion-extension lateral views of the lumbar spine can be useful to evaluate for segmental instability.

■ Most patients who have persistent back pain or leg pain after lumbar surgery will have an MRI of their lumbar spine. In patients with a suspected recurrence of a disc herniation, it is important to make the distinction between recurrence and scar since the former is potentially amenable to surgery, whereas the latter is generally not. A precontrast and postcontrast (gadolinium) MRI is helpful to distinguish scar from recurrent disc herniation. Disc material is avascular, and therefore will not enhance following gadolinium administration. Scar, on the other hand, is vascular and will therefore enhance with gadolinium.

Table 1	Vascular versus Neurogenic Claudication	
Examination	**Vascular**	**Neurogenic**
Walking distance	Fixed	Variable
Palliative factors	Standing	Sitting/bending
Provocative factors	Walking	Walking/standing
Walking uphill	Painful	Painless
Bicycle test	Positive (painful)	Negative (painless)
Pulses	Absent	Present
Skin	Loss of hair/shiny	Normal
Back pain	Occasionally	Commonly
Back motion	Normal	Limited
Pain character	Cramping/ distal to proximal	Numbness/aching/ proximal to distal
Atrophy	Uncommon	Occasionally

- In patients with older stainless steel implants, MRI is generally not useful because of significant metal artifact that obscures detail. Under such circumstances, a combined myelogram/CT scan study is very useful. Distortion with titanium implants is less of an issue, but in some cases, distortion from titanium implants can occur, requiring a myelogram/CT scan to identify neural compression. Finally, patients who have an implantable pacemaker or internal defibrillator or who are claustrophobic are not candidates for MRI and should have a myelogram/CT scan to visualize compressive pathology.
- CT without myelography utilizing coronal and sagittal reconstructions is very useful to evaluate hardware placement (especially pedicle screws) and to evaluate an interbody fusion for evidence of pseudoarthrosis.
- Three foot long AP and lateral scoliosis X-rays are sometimes useful and are mandatory to evaluate overall spinal alignment.

DIFFERENTIAL DIAGNOSIS OF PAIN FOLLOWING PREVIOUUS LUMBAR SURGERY

- Wrong diagnosis
  - Pathology not present at time of original surgery
  - Surgery performed for poor indications
- Pathology originally present but not adequately addressed
  - Wrong level surgery
  - Inadequate surgery (pathology incompletely addressed)
- New pathology
  - At same level as prior surgery
    - Recurrent herniated nucleus pulposus (HNP)
    - Recurrent stenosis
    - Arachnoiditis
    - Epidural scar tissue
  - At different level
    - HNP
    - Stenosis
    - Adjacent level disease (including spondylolisthesis)
    - Other pathology (eg, tumor)
- Complications
  - Infection
    - Discitis
    - Osteomyelitis
    - Superficial or deep wound infection
    - Infection associated with hardware
  - Hardware failure
    - Hardware breakage or loosening
    - Hardware misplacement
  - Pseudoarthrosis
  - Durotomy
  - Neural injury
  - Iatrogenic instability or deformity
    - Iatrogenic flat back
    - Pars destabilization and resulting spondylolisthesis
- Others
  - Noncompressive pathology
    - Nonspinal pathology (eg, neuropathy, hip pathology)
  - Psychosocial issues (including chronic pain behavior, depression, worker's compensation, or litigation)
  - Sacroiliac disease or extraspinal joint disease
  - Peripheral nerve syndromes

NONOPERATIVE MANAGEMENT

- It is advisable to try a course of conservative management, similar to that utilized for the index condition, for recurrent disc herniation or stenosis. Many patients will improve with physical therapy, nonsteroidal anti-inflammatory drugs, injection therapy, or other pain management treatments.
- Injections with a local analgesic and steroid may provide relief in patients with sacroiliac disease or other extraspinal joint disease, such as hip arthritis. Spinal epidural injections are unpredictable in the setting of failed back surgery, although they may have a role. Transforaminal injections may be useful as a diagnostic aid in localizing radicular pain to a particular nerve root.
- Patients with multilevel degenerative disease and primary back pain refractory to other treatments may benefit from a multidisciplinary chronic pain management program. These programs typically include pain management specialists, physical therapists, physiatrists, and psychiatrists/psychologists who focus on a physical and cognitive approach to chronic back pain treatment.
- Spinal cord stimulation is an option in patients with persistent and refractory back or leg pain in whom no identifiable cause for the pain can be identified.

SURGICAL MANAGEMENT

Preoperative Planning

- Carefully consider the initial indication for surgery. Operating on the wrong patient or for the wrong indication is a recipe for failure.
- Evaluation of the patient's symptoms, physical exam, and radiographic findings will help the surgeon tailor his or her operative plan most appropriately. It is imperative that the surgeon performs a careful history and physical exam and that imaging findings are correlated with clinical findings. Patients who have predominant back pain and a prior failed fusion surgery may have a pseudoarthrosis or another hardware-related problem that might explain the pain. Patients with leg pain as their primary complaint may have neural compression from stenosis or disc herniation. It is important for the surgeon to correlate preoperative and postoperative clinical and imaging findings.

Positioning

■ It is generally important that the patient's abdomen be free of compression in order to minimize epidural bleeding. There are many options to accomplish this, and the authors prefer a Jackson table (Mizuho OSI, Union City, CA). This table allows the abdomen to hang freely, thereby reducing intra-abdominal pressure and minimizing epidural bleeding. In addition, this table also facilitates achieving lumbar lordosis (**FIG 2**). The kneeling position can also be used for simple revision decompressions and discectomies (**FIG 3**). It is not advised for multilevel revision fusions as it produces pressure on the knees and may result in iatrogenic flat back.

■ Gardner-Wells tongs are recommended for lengthy procedures in order to avoid pressure on the globe and to reduce the likelihood of pressure or abrasions on the patient's face.

■ Elevate the head of the bed to reduce facial edema and reduce intraocular pressure.

■ Padding of all bony prominences is advised to prevent compressive neuropathies. This included the ulnar nerve at the elbow and the lateral femoral cutaneous nerve at the level of the anterior superior iliac spine.

Approach

■ In general, when possible, try to avoid operating through a prior anterior or lateral exposure for revision unless absolutely necessary. The scar tissue from these procedures can make the revision approach difficult and dangerous. If an anterior approach is absolutely required, the approach can be made from the opposite side.

■ The posterior approach is generally preferred, as this is the most familiar surgical approach for most surgeons, and most pathology in patients having had prior surgery can be easily dealt with through this approach. The posterior approach gives the surgeon easy access to the pedicles in case instrumentation is needed, permits exposure of the entire lumbar and thoracolumbar spine if needed, and provides adequate access to the intervertebral discs.

■ Bleeding during revision lumbar surgery is variable. To some extent, the present of avascular scar tissue reduces the amount of bleeding. On the other hand, the amount of dissection is generally considerable, and the extent of the construct is often significant. To a large extent, the amount of bleeding is directly related to the length of the incision and the length (duration) of the surgery. In many, if not most, posterior revision cases both are considerable. Therefore, careful hemostasis is mandatory. This can be facilitated by the use of the Aquamantys (Medtronic, Portsmouth, NH), which is a hemostatic device that utilizes a combination of radiofrequency (RF) and saline to reduce blood loss. Additional blood conservation can be achieved by the use of cell salvage, in which intraoperative blood loss is given back to the patient.

■ Anterior or lateral procedures can be used to augment a posterior procedure in order to increase fusion rates by directly accessing the intervertebral disc. The anterior approach may be useful to treat a pseudoarthrosis following a posterior fusion by providing direct access to the disc through an unoperated tissue plane. In addition, the anterior approach enables a more thorough removal of disc material and facilitates placement of a large graft to increase the likelihood of achieving fusion. This avoids the potential difficulty of trying to achieve a posterior fusion in the presence of a previously operated and scarred posterior fusion site. The anterior or lateral approach may be used in unusual situations such as to address an anteriorly extruded intervertebral graft or cage.

■ The major disadvantage to the lateral and anterior approach is that they generally provide a more limited exposure to the lumbar spine than a posterior approach. They are therefore often reserved for focal revision lumbar surgery when the initial approach was posterior.

■ Minimally invasive techniques can be used for selected patients requiring lumbar revision surgery. These patients may include obese patients with a recurrent disc herniation or a new herniation at a different level. It is generally not advisable to perform a minimally invasive surgery in a patient requiring extensive reconstruction and instrumentation for deformity or pseudoarthrosis, although exceptions do exist.

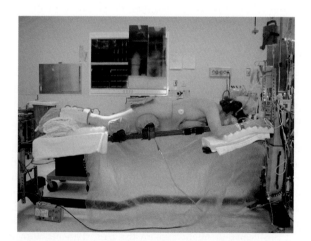

FIG 2 • The Jackson table allows the patient's abdomen to hang freely below the surgical field, minimizing epidural bleeding and enhancing lumbar lordosis. This position is preferred for lumbar fusion cases to preserve lumbar lordosis during instrumentation.

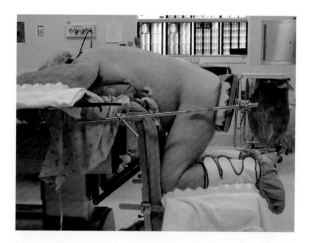

FIG 3 • The abdomen is also allowed to hang freely in the kneeling position. This position is advantageous for revision discectomies or decompressions not requiring instrumentation and fusion, as this position flattens the lumbar spine, distracting the posterior elements and facilitating approach to the disc.

POSTERIOR APPROACH FOR REVISION LUMBAR SURGERY: LAMINECTOMY AND DISCECTOMY

- After induction of anesthesia and intubation, the patient is positioned with the abdomen hanging freely, either prone on a Jackson table or on another frame that eliminates abdominal compression such as a Wilson frame or a four-poster frame. A Wilson frame offers the advantage of reducing lumbar lordosis and distracting the posterior elements, thereby facilitating the approach to the intervertebral discs. Alternatively, the patient may be placed in the kneeling position. For lengthy cases, it is recommended that the patient be placed on a Jackson table with the head placed in Gardner-Wells tongs with 10 lb. of traction. It is imperative that all extremities and bony prominences are carefully padded.

- The preoperative films should be studied to provide optimum exposure. Generally, the surgeon will be going through the same incision as the previous surgery. However, the normal bony landmarks may be significantly distorted or absent. In cases where the posterior bony elements have been completely removed, the surgeon may choose to lengthen the incision proximally or distally to include adjacent normal bony landmarks as a reference. It is generally safer to proceed from normal anatomy to abnormal (previously operated) levels.

- The incision is deepened, identifying any remnants of normal anatomy that may be present such as the spinous processes, laminae, and facet joints. Care must be taken to avoid injury to the dura, which may be unprotected if a prior laminectomy has been performed.

- In many revision surgeries, there will be significant scar tissue present, which may be firm and adherent to surrounding structures (including the dura). In general, dissection should be carried out laterally along the bony wall of the canal rather than diffusely in the midline, since the area of interest is the nerve root. Separation of the lateral edge of the dural sac and nerve root is facilitated by the use of either a Penfield no. 1 or a small curette. Care must be taken not to carry the dissection too far laterally in order to avoid inadvertent injury to the pars. Some surgeons prefer to identify the lateral extent of the pars in order to visualize it, thereby minimizing the risk of injury to it.

- The nerve should be followed along its entire course, including the lateral recess and neural foramen, if necessary. As with nonrevision surgery, the key to proper orientation is identifying the pedicle, since the nerve passes beneath the pedicle. This is more important in revisions since other landmarks are often absent. At the end of the decompression, the nerve should be relatively easily retractable medially and a probe should be able to be passed dorsal and ventral to the nerve root. The pedicles can be palpated with a Woodson.

POSTERIOR APPROACH FOR REVISION LUMBAR SURGERY: FUSION AND INSTRUMENTATION

- The patient is positioned prone on a Jackson table. Pressure points are padded and care is taken to ensure that the chest pad is not compressing breast tissue in female patients. Standard Jackson table attachments (iliac and thigh pads) are used to allow maximum natural lumbar lordosis and allow the abdomen to hang freely.

- The presence of normal anatomy, such as preexisting spinous processes that were not removed during the previous surgery, is an excellent starting point for dissection. The amount, if any, of any such bone remaining may vary depending on the type and extent of the previous surgery. Since implanted hardware provides an excellent known landmark for exposure, it is generally useful to initially identify and expose laterally placed hardware. After the dissection is carried through the deep fascial layer, the dissection should be skived (angled) laterally toward the hardware rather than plunging deeply toward unprotected dura. This will bring the dissection down to the rods and screw heads. Once the screw heads are exposed, the facets are easily identified (**TECH FIG 1**). Care should be taken to avoid inadvertent injury to facet joints proximal and distal to the existing fusion unless they are to be included in an extension of the fusion. Once the hardware is visualized, the lateral edge of the bony canal is easily identified. From here, dissection can be carried out medially. Attention is first turned to separating the scar and pseudomembrane from the lateral bony canal.

There is generally little to be gained by trying to remove scar from the midline dura, and such attempts may lead to inadvertent durotomy.

- Once the hardware is exposed, the next step is to remove the screws and rods. Corresponding screw widths and lengths should be recorded at each level.

- The preexisting posterior fusion mass is then exposed, noting any evidence of pseudoarthrosis. Fibrous tissue within the pseudoarthrosis is removed using curettes in order to preserve the intact fusion mass as much as possible.

- Preexisting holes that contained the pedicle screws are probed to check integrity and length of the hole measured. When possible, it is generally recommended that a slightly longer and wider diameter screw be used for the revision hardware. If larger diameter screws are not available, additional augmentation may be provided by the application of polymethylmethacrylate (PMMA) bone cement, especially in osteoporotic patients.

- If broken screws are encountered, several solutions are possible. If the broken screw is in the middle of a construct, that level can usually be skipped and a cross connector can be added in order to provide additional stability. If the broken screw is at the terminal end of a construct, the instrumentation may be extended at a level below or above the involved level, if feasible. If it is felt that instrumentation at the level of the broken screw is necessary, the screw may be removed using a

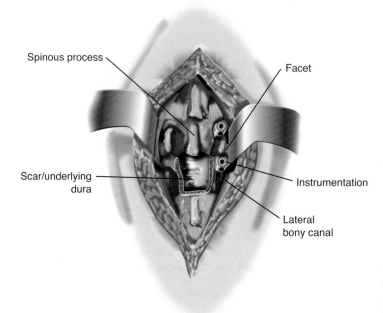

Spinous process
Facet
Scar/underlying dura
Instrumentation
Lateral bony canal

TECH FIG 1 • When performing revision exposure, the safest strategy is to proceed from normal anatomy above/below and from lateral to medial, identifying the edges of the prior laminectomy from know to unknown.

removal kit or by removing additional bone to expose the broken screw. The latter may necessitate additional augmentation with cement (**TECH FIG 2**).

- Fusion mass may be augmented by the use of autologous iliac crest bone graft; local bone from laminectomy, if available, by graft extenders such as demineralized bone matrix (DBM); or by the off-label use of bone morphogenetic protein (BMP).

- Pseudoarthrosis after a posterolateral instrumented fusion is often most optimally treated by the addition of an interbody fusion through nonoperated and therefore unscarred tissue. This provides a healthy focus for fusion. When a posterior approach is being utilized, this is most efficiently achieved through a transforaminal lumbar interbody fusion (TLIF). A TLIF may not be advisable or possible in the presence of significant scar from prior surgery. But if scar is minimal, a TLIF provides a safe and effective way to achieve additional anterior column support to facilitate fusion.
  - This is achieved by a unilateral (or if desired, bilateral) facetectomy with a pedicle-to-pedicle exposure, thereby unroofing the neural foramen entirely, and allowing the root and thecal sac to be gently retracted medially.
  - The intervertebral disc is then sharply incised with a scalpel and the disc is removed piecemeal using curettes and pituitary rongeurs.
  - The cartilaginous endplates are then removed by using a special set of dilators and scrapers.

- Once cartilage has been removed from the bony endplates, spacers are used to estimate proper graft size. An interbody graft or synthetic cage (usually a polyether ether ketone, or PEEK) is then filled with autologous bone, allograft bone, and/or a collagen sponge soaked in BMP used in an off-label manner and placed in the disc space.

- Placement is verified using X-ray and the interbody graft or cage is locked into place by compressing across the previously placed pedicle screws and rods.

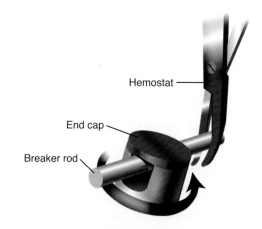

Hemostat
End cap
Breaker rod

TECH FIG 2 • Salvage technique for saw removal.

ANTERIOR APPROACH FOR REVISION LUMBAR SURGERY

- Anterior lumbar interbody fusion (ALIF), when feasible, provides excellent exposure to the intervertebral disc and allows the surgeon maximal access to the disc space. It is a good adjunct to a posterior fusion, especially in the presence of a pseudoarthrosis after posterolateral instrumented fusion.

- The ALIF allows access to disc spaces that may be difficult to access posteriorly because of tenacious scar.

It also allows the placement of larger grafts than can be inserted through a TLIF approach; this maximizes end-plate contact with the graft and increases the chances of fusion, especially when combined with a posterior instrumented fusion.[10]

■ A standard anterior retroperitoneal approach to the lumbar spine is used.

■ Revision anterior procedures in patients with previous anterior lumbar surgery can be difficult and dangerous due to significant scarring. The risk of vascular injury is significant, and exposure by an experienced vascular surgeon is recommended.

ANTEROLATERAL RETROPERITONEAL APPROACH FOR REVISION LUMBAR SURGERY

■ This approach is beneficial to address interbody pathology that is not otherwise accessible from a purely anterior or posterior approach.

■ The patient is placed on a standard operating room (OR) table in a right lateral decubitus position. The hip is positioned behind the table break in order to create separation between the ribcage and the iliac crest.

■ This position can treat pathology from L3 to L5. If L2 exposure is needed, it will likely be necessary to resect the 12th rib.

■ In certain circumstances, it may be advantageous to approach from the right side, but in general avoidance of the inferior vena cava and the liver via the right lateral decubitus position is favorable.

■ The patient is secured to the table with cloth tape. The left arm is suspended in an arm sling and padded and secured to the sling with tape.

■ Fluoroscopy is used to demarcate the level of pathology. This general area is marked on the skin in order to plan the incision.

■ A curvilinear incision is planned beginning in front and superior to the iliac crest, curving under the 12th rib and following this rib to the insertion on the spine.

■ Once the incision is made, the subcutaneous tissue is retracted and the first muscle that is visible will be the latissimus dorsi. This muscle is sharply divided and retracted.

■ The next layer will be the posterior inferior serratus muscle and the internal and external oblique muscles. These muscles are also divided sharply by using Bovie cautery. Care must be taken not to violate the peritoneum directly below these muscles.

■ The peritoneal layer is retracted anteriorly while the ureter and the kidney are retracted to the right, bringing into view the quadratus lumborum. The 12th rib is also identified and may be resected if higher approaches are to be attempted. The neurovascular bundle should be preserved; if this is not possible it can be tied off and divided.

■ The retroperitoneal tissue overlying the lumbar spine is bluntly dissected and brought anteriorly. Care is taken to preserve the ilioinguinal and iliohypogastric nerves that will run between the quadratus lumborum and the psoas muscle.

■ Once this is performed, the lateral surfaces of the lumbar vertebrae are brought into view.

PEARLS AND PITFALLS

Diagnostic pitfalls	■ Account for proper pathology. ■ Double check surgical indications. ■ Take into account other pathology (vascular, joints, etc.). ■ Back pain vs. radiculopathy recurrence: Back pain is much less amenable to reoperation than radiculopathy.
Surgical planning pitfalls	■ Obtain proper imaging studies. Pre- and post-gadolinium MRI should be performed on patients evaluated for recurrent disc pathology or stenosis. If there is a question of global imbalance or deformity, obtain standing 3-foot X-rays. ■ Select correct procedure. ■ Examine all old medical records. ■ Ensure proper OR tools are available (eg, a universal driver set for removing hardware). ■ Prepare the iliac crest in every patient for possible use.
Surgical technique pitfalls	■ Properly position the patient. Elevate the head of the bed and ensure the abdomen hangs free in the prone position to minimize epidural bleeding. Use a head holder with pins if prolonged surgery is planned. ■ Address neural compression. ■ Pay attention to overall alignment. Standing X-rays can help the surgeon evaluate this. ■ Start at the bone and work toward the unknown. ■ No central scar tissue removal, stay lateral where there is bone present and work toward the midline. ■ Ensure adequate lateral gutter decompression.

POSTOPERATIVE CARE

▪ Standard postoperative care of spine surgery patients is indicated in the vast majority of patients undergoing revision surgery. Pain control can be a significant issue in patients undergoing revision lumbar surgery, both because of frequent significant preoperative narcotic requirements making postoperative pain control difficult and because of the sheer magnitude of the surgery. When possible, the use of an epidural pain catheter should be considered. This may not always be possible if there is significant epidural scar tissue present, making the passage of the catheter difficult. Another alternative for pain control is the use of patient controlled analgesia (PCA), whereby the patient controls, within certain predetermined limits, the amount of narcotic analgesic delivered.

▪ If the surgery was significantly long (6 hours or more) and required significant amounts of blood products and fluids, it is usually advantageous to leave the patient intubated overnight and admitted to an intensive care unit (ICU). Oftentimes, the reason for prolonged postoperative intubation is largely related to the amount of facial and airway swelling present. The use of the Jackson table with Gardner-Wells tongs and head of bed elevation results in a significant reduction in facial and airway edema, thereby making it more likely that the patient can be extubated in the OR. Multilevel revision surgery or extensive front–back procedures also usually will require an ICU admit.

▪ Standard neurologic checks in the immediate postop period are performed to assess for neural recovery or new deficits.

▪ Upright X-rays are obtained in patients with hardware placement. These are usually performed within a few days of surgery or as soon as the patient is able to comfortably stand for the X-rays.

OUTCOMES

▪ Patient outcomes depend largely on initial patient diagnosis. There is a wide variety of pathology that a patient can present with after lumbar surgery, and the surgeon must carefully assess all of the information at hand to make the most informed decision.

▪ The patient with recurrent leg pain or leg pain in a different distribution than preoperative has a good chance of benefitting from a second operation.[11] Recurrent leg pain in the same distribution as preoperative suggests reherniation of the same disc, whereas new leg pain may represent a different disc herniation.

▪ The patient with predominant axial back pain (and normal sagittal and coronal alignment), however, will most likely not benefit from another operation. In these patients, it is very difficult for the surgeon to pinpoint the source of the back pain.

COMPLICATIONS

▪ Neural injury is one of the most feared complications of revision surgery. To a large extent, the magnitude of this risk is dictated by the distortion of the normal anatomy and by the presence of scar tissue. Careful adherence to the principles outlined in this chapter will help reduce this risk.

▪ Durotomy is a relatively common occurrence in revision lumbar surgery, as the dura is often adherent to and obscured by the overlying scar and pseudomembrane. When a durotomy is encountered, it should be repaired immediately, if possible. Failure to repair a durotomy promptly can result in the loss of thecal sac turgor and the tamponade effect that a turgid sac produces on the epidural veins. This can result in more blood loss and more difficulty with repair of the durotomy. If the overlying scar is thick enough, it may be included in the suture line. If not, work to expose the free edges of the dura and close primarily. A patch of muscle or fascia may be sewn under the suture line to attempt to tightly appose the defect. An absorbable hemostatic agent such as Surgicel (Ethicon, Menlo Park, CA) and/or fibrin glue may be used to cover the suture line as well.

▪ Infection is always possible after revision surgery. It should be treated in the standard manner that all spine postoperative infections are treated: antibiotics and surgical debridement and washout if the wound is frankly purulent and draining. With an initial infection following an instrumented fusion, it is generally recommended that the instrumentation be kept in place if it is providing stability. This requires a period of parenteral followed by an oftentimes prolonged period of oral antibiotics, with some infectious disease consultants recommending that oral antibiotics be continued indefinitely, as long as the hardware is present. In general, the initial surgical debridement is accompanied by wound closure. If a subsequent episode of infection occur, use of vacuum dressing may be required with delayed wound closure.

▪ Pseudoarthrosis may occur following an initial surgery or revision surgery. Smokers have a higher risk of pseudoarthrosis than nonsmokers do. Consequently, patients should be counseled to stop smoking preoperatively. Our current practice is to mandate that patients stop smoking 3 months prior to surgery and for at least 3 months postoperatively.

REFERENCES

1. Malter AD, McNeney B, Loeser JD, et al. Five-year reoperation rates after different types of lumbar spine surgery. Spine (Phila Pa 1976) 1998;23:814–820.
2. Onesti ST. Failed back syndrome. Neurologist 2004;10:259–264.
3. Cinotti G, Roysam GS, Eisenstein SM, et al. Ipsilateral recurrent lumbar disc herniation. A prospective, controlled study. J Bone Joint Surg Br 1998;80:825–832.
4. Ambrossi GL, McGirt MJ, Sciubba DM, et al. Recurrent lumbar disc herniation after single-level lumbar discectomy: incidence and health care cost analysis. Neurosurgery 2009;65:574–578; discussion 578.
5. Diwan AD, Parvartaneni H, Cammisa F. Failed degenerative lumbar spine surgery. Orthop Clin North Am 2003;34:309–324.
6. Jonsson B, Stromqvist B. Repeat decompression of lumbar nerve roots. A prospective two-year evaluation. J Bone Joint Surg Br 1993; 75:894–897.
7. Trief PM, Grant W, Fredrickson B. A prospective study of psychological predictors of lumbar surgery outcome. Spine (Phila Pa 1976) 2000;25:2616–2621.
8. Waddell G, Kummel EG, Lotto WN, et al. Failed lumbar disc surgery and repeat surgery following industrial injuries. J Bone Joint Surg Am 1979;61:201–207.
9. McCulloch JA, Transfeldt E, Macnab I. Macnab's Backache. Baltimore: Williams & Wilkins; 1997.
10. Lee SH, Kang BU, Jeon SH, et al. Revision surgery of the lumbar spine: anterior lumbar interbody fusion followed by percutaneous pedicle screw fixation. J Neurosurg Spine 2006;5:228–233.
11. Dai LY, Zhou Q, Yao WF, et al. Recurrent lumbar disc herniation after discectomy: outcome of repeat discectomy. Surg Neurol 2005;64:226–231; discussion 231.

Chapter 31

Revision Cervical Surgery: Strategies and Techniques

Casey C. Bachison and Harry N. Herkowitz

DEFINITION

▪ In recent years, the number of patients undergoing cervical spine surgery has risen dramatically. Cervical spine surgery is used to treat a number of common spinal pathologies including the following:

- ▪ Cervical spinal stenosis
- ▪ Deformity
- ▪ Disc herniation
- ▪ Myelopathy
- ▪ Trauma
- ▪ Pathologic conditions such as neoplasia, infection, and metabolic and inflammatory disease

▪ The surgical procedures used to treat these conditions are generally successful but occasionally result in complications that require revision cervical spine surgery. Unexpected life events after spine surgery such as trauma and cancer can cause instability or neurocompression leading to the need for surgical decompression and/or stabilization at the site of previous operative intervention. The more common complications and conditions are defined here.

- ▪ Pseudarthrosis: The term suggests a "false joint." Pseudarthrosis is a failure of bone fusion or nonunion at the site of attempted arthrodesis. Diagnosis is made after 6 months to 1 year following the index surgery. Pseudoarthrosis may occur following anterior or posterior cervical procedures.
- ▪ Adjacent segment degeneration (ASD) occurs when there are degenerative changes at unfused levels adjacent to prior cervical fusion. ASD is believed to result from excessive motion at the level adjacent to an arthrodesis as it compensates for the fused segment. Some controversy exists as to whether the degeneration occurs as a result of prior arthrodesis or as a result of natural progression in an individual already prone to degenerative disc disease.
- ▪ Postlaminectomy kyphosis (PLK) is a kyphotic deformity of the cervical spine that develops as a result of previous surgery in which the posterior elements of the spine, including the spinous process and lamina, were removed. Removal of the posterior tethering structures, including the spinous processes and the associated supraspinous and interspinous ligaments, predisposes individuals to this condition.
- ▪ Hardware/construct failure: Plates, screws, and rods may loosen or break if bone healing is prolonged or inhibited. Allograft and autograft bone used for structural support of the spine are subject to loading forces that can cause the graft to collapse. Poor bone quality in the patient may allow hardware to migrate or bone graft to subside.
- ▪ Same segment disease/residual compression is persistent or recurrent pain present at the level of previous decompression. Same segment disease results from failed stabilization or inadequate decompression at the site of the initial cervical surgical procedure.
- ▪ Pathologic conditions may be the inciting event for the index surgical procedure or may result in the need for revision surgery. Tumor, infection, trauma, and inflammatory conditions such as rheumatoid arthritis and ankylosis spondylitis may lead to instability, deformity, or neurocompression after an index cervical procedure.

ANATOMY

- ▪ Vertebrae
  - ▪ The cervical spine consists of seven specialized vertebrae.
  - ▪ Transverse foramina are present bilaterally for the passage of the vertebral artery.
  - ▪ The vertebral artery generally enters the cervical spine at C6. Occasionally it will enter at C7 or C5. The artery may also enter the spine at different levels on either side of the cervical spine in the same patient. MRI should be obtained prior to surgical intervention to ascertain the site of vertebral artery entry and any anomalies present along its excursion (**FIGS 1 AND 2**).
  - ▪ The spinous processes of C6–2 are bifid. C7 does not possess a bifid spinous process but is more prominent than the other cervical vertebrae. C7 is often referred to as vertebra prominens.
- ▪ Discs
  - ▪ An intervertebral disc is present between each of the cervical vertebrae from C2 through T1.
  - ▪ The occiput to C1 and the C1–2 articulation do not have intervertebral discs and articulate through true synovial joints.
  - ▪ Each disc consists of an outer annulus fibrosis and inner nucleus pulposus.
  - ▪ Between the annulus fibrosis/nucleus pulposus complex and the vertebral body, a cartilaginous endplate is present. The removal of this cartilaginous endplate is pivotal to a successful interbody arthrodesis. Failure to remove the cartilaginous endplate increases the likelihood of pseudarthrosis.
- ▪ Ligaments
  - ▪ A supraspinous ligament runs dorsally over the top of the spinous processes.
  - ▪ Then, an interspinous ligament is present between two spinous processes at each level.
  - ▪ An anterior longitudinal ligament runs along the front of the spine adherent to the ventral aspect of the vertebral body.
  - ▪ A posterior longitudinal ligament (PLL) runs along the dorsal aspect of the vertebral body and intervertebral discs. It forms a barrier between the discs and the dura/spinal cord.
- ▪ Normal lordosis of the cervical spine averages 14.4 degree.[1]
- ▪ Weight bearing axis of the cervical spine passes through the posterior column.[2]
- ▪ Loss of the posterior tension band after resection of the lamina and spinous processes may lead to kyphosis and a shift in the weight bearing axis of the spine to the anterior column.

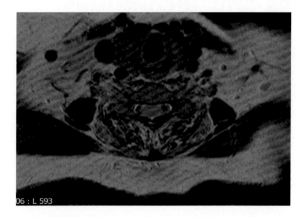

FIG 1 • Axial T2-weighted image through the C6 vertebral body. Note in this patient that the vertebral artery in anomalous and only the right-sided artery enters the spine at this level.

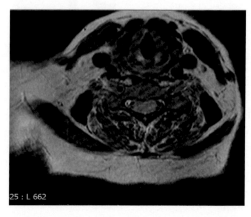

FIG 2 • Axial T2-weighted image through the C5 vertebral body in the same patient as FIG 1. At this level both right and left vertebral arteries have entered the cervical spine.

PATHOGENESIS

- Pseudarthrosis
    - Pseudarthrosis occurs when bone fails to form at the site of attempted arthrodesis. Multiple factors may play a role in the formation of pseudoarthrosis.
    - Risk factors include the following[3]:
        - Multilevel fusions
        - Metabolic abnormalities
        - Smoking
        - Infection
        - Excessive motion
    - Smoking is associated with lower fusion rates in cervical and lumbar fusion. Hilibrand et al. found a higher rate of fusion in nonsmokers (81%) than in smokers (62%).[4] In contrast to the effect of smoking on anterior cervical fusion, Eubanks et al. found smoking did not decrease posterior cervical fusion with lateral mass instrumentation and iliac crest bone grafting.
    - Excessive motion at the site of an anterior cervical discectomy and fusion (ACDF) is associated with increased rates of pseudoarthrosis. Use of anterior cervical plating has been shown in multiple studies to decrease the rate of pseudoarthrosis.[5,6]
    - Corpectomy with the use of autogenous strut grafting should be considered when a multilevel anterior cervical decompression and fusion is performed in patients who are unable or unwilling to stop smoking prior to surgical treatment.[4]
- Adjacent segment degeneration
    - As previously noted, some controversy exists as to whether the degeneration of adjacent segments occurs as a result of prior arthrodesis, which may place increased demands on a level above or below a fusion, or whether the degeneration is a result of natural progression in an individual already prone to degenerative disc disease.
- Deformity, PLK
    - Causes of PLK include the following:
        - Removal of the posterior restraints of the cervical spine, namely posterior bony arch and the supraspinous and interspinous ligaments. Resection of greater than 50% of the facet has been shown to lead to instability.[7]
        - Attenuation or failure of the restraints secondary to radiation
        - Neglect of deformity during index procedure

- Removal of the posterior arch/facets leads to instability, which causes the weight bearing axis of the spine to shift anteriorly.
- Once the axis shifts anteriorly, the posterior cervical musculature fatigues and the kyphosis progresses.[8]
- The load is then transferred to the anterior vertebral bodies and discs.
- Hardware/construct failure[9,10]
    - The likelihood of hardware failure of current cervical instrumentation is small.
    - Anterior cervical hardware or construct failure is an infrequent occurrence; however, complication associated with hardware placement occurs in approximately 22% to 36% of cases.[11]
    - Screw breakage or loosening is often the result of a nonunion or pseudarthrosis, and evaluation of the fusion with flexion/extension views or CT scan is warranted.
    - Infection, osteoporosis, tumor, and trauma can also lead to hardware failure or graft subsidence after cervical fusion with or without instrumentation.
    - The use of multilevel interbody fusion versus corpectomies with strut grafting has been shown to decrease the risk of graft extrusion.
    - Aggressive mobilization and smoking are other potential causes for prolonged healing and hardware failure.
- Same segment disease/residual compression
    - A result of failed or inadequate initial surgical decompression
    - Truumees[12] outlines four general causes for residual compression after cervical surgery. These are the following:
        - Failure to perform a complete decompression at the injured/involved level
        - Failure to decompress adjacent involved levels
        - Migration of graft or fixation materials into the canal or foramen
        - Wrong-level surgery (initial surgery performed at a level that was not responsible for the patient's symptoms; this can occur as a failure to diagnose the offending level correctly or as a result of wrong site surgery)
- Pathologic conditions
    - The pathogenesis of tumor, infection, and inflammatory conditions such as rheumatoid arthritis and ankylosis spondylitis is beyond the scope of the current text. Failure of

the cervical spine as it relates to these conditions is a progressive deterioration of the structural integrity of the bones or erosion of the ligamentous support of the spine. Loss of these structures leads to instability, deformity, or compression of the neural elements.

NATURAL HISTORY

- Pseudarthrosis
  - The most common cause of pain or radiculopathy after ACDF is psuedarthrosis.[13,14]
  - Outcome studies of ACDF show up to 26% pseudarthrosis.[10,13,15,16]
    - Lowery defined pseudoarthrosis as follows[10]:
      - Continued or worsening axial pain 6 months after the initial procedure
      - Complete radiolucency at the host/graft interface
      - Vertebral body motion >2 mm on flexion and extension films
    - Phillips et al.[17] followed 48 patients with radiographic pseudarthrosis:
      - Thirty-two (67%) developed symptoms.
      - Sixteen patients remained asymptomatic for 5.1 years.
      - Nine of the 32 symptomatic patients were pain free for 2 years before trauma caused development of symptoms.
      - Eighty-two percent of patients developed pseudarthrosis at the most caudal level after multilevel fusion.
      - Revision surgery led to good or excellent results in all cases (anterior or posterior).
  - Allograft and multilevel fusion increases the risk of pseudarthrosis.[18]
  - Posterior fusion with lateral mass screws leads to high rate of fusion from 0% to 1.4%; less rigid posterior fixation (wiring) has a less reliable outcome.
- Adjacent segment degeneration
  - Occurs at a rate of 2.9% per year, with 25% of patients developing ASD within 10 years.[19]
  - Patients with degenerative changes at C5–6 or C6–7 at time of initial procedure are at greatest risk for development of ASD.
  - Eck et al. measured disc pressures at C4–5 and C6–7 before and after simulated fusion at C5–6 and found a 73% increase in cranial and 45% in caudal disc pressures during flexion.[20]
- Deformity, PLK
  - Lonstein described PLK as a focal, dramatic angulation of the cervical spine after posterior decompression.[21]
  - Kyphosis is the most common cervical deformity and the most frequent cause is iatrogenic postlaminectomy instability.
  - Patients with PLK generally have a pain-free period following the index surgical procedure followed by the development of persistent pain.
  - Risks of PLK as described by Lonstein[21]:
    - Age less than 30 years
    - Aggressive facetectomy
    - Removal of more than four laminae
    - Preoperative deformity
    - Tumors
    - Removal of C2 posterior elements (major semispinalis insertion)
    - Paraspinal muscle weakness
    - Anterior instability following fracture

- Nowinski et al. studied the effects of progressive facetectomy and recommend posterior fusion when greater than 25% of the facets are sacrificed for decompression.[7] Herkowitz found a 25% incidence of kyphosis in patients with bilateral facet resection.
- Facet capsular resection of greater than 50% increases the risk of progressive deformity.[1]
- Hardware/construct failure
  - Hardware complications following ACDF have been characterized in 22% to 36% of cases.[22]
  - Graft extrusion and malalignment have been described in up to 6% of cases following anterior cervical fusions.[22]
  - When failure occurs, the risk of injury to the tracheoesophageal structures is minimal.[9]
  - Immediate removal of failed hardware is rarely necessary and should only be considered if there is evidence of dysphagia or risk to the spinal cord or nerve roots.
  - Careful and long-term follow-up in patient with loose or broken hardware assures that significant progression of the failure does not occur.
- Same segment disease/residual compression
  - Results from failed or inadequate initial surgical procedure
  - ACDF, posterior cervical fusion, posterior foraminotomy, and micro-ACD ranged from 5% to 36%.[22]
  - Hardware complications following ACDF have been characterized in 22% to 36% of cases.
  - Residual compression after an index spine procedure may result from the following[12]:
    - Failure to perform a complete decompression at the injured/involved level
    - Failure to decompress adjacent involved levels
    - Migration of graft or fixation materials into the canal or foramen
    - Wrong-level surgery
  - Posterior osteophytes may be a significant source of residual compression.[23]
  - Studies have noted limited remodeling or resorption of posterior osteophytes after solid ACDF.[12,24]
  - Kozak et al. has advocated PLL resection to achieve a more complete decompression.[25]
  - Decompression of the neural elements may be needed at the time of surgery for cervical trauma to decrease the potential for compression at the level of the procedure.[26]
- Pathologic conditions: tumor, infection, and inflammatory arthropathies
  - Only 17% of spinal tumors occur in the cervical spine.
  - The most common malignant tumors are chordoma and plasmacytoma, which occur most often in the anterior cervical spine leading to kyphosis.
  - Osteoid osteoma and osteoblastoma are the most common benign tumors of the cervical spine occurring most commonly in the posterior elements.
  - Benign lesion of the spine, and specifically osteoid osteoma, can lead to painful scoliosis, which often improves once the lesion is excised.
  - Three percent to 14% of spinal infections are cervical.
  - Infection of the cervical spine typically begins as a spondylodiscitis causing destruction of the intervertebral disc, which can then spread to the vertebral bodies causing collapse and kyphosis.
  - Metastatic lesions of the cervical spine typically start in the subaxial anterior spine. Progressive destruction of the

vertebral body leads to axial instability first followed by translational and rotational instability.

▪ The natural history of inflammatory arthropathies is a progressive deformity leading to kyphosis.

▪ In the case of rheumatoid arthritis, the cervical spine is affected by one of three potential deforming etiologies: atlantoaxial subluxation, cranial settling, and subaxial subluxation.

PATIENT HISTORY AND PHYSICAL FINDINGS

▪ Patients with prior cervical surgery typically present with complaints of axial pain, radiculopathy, myelopathy, or progressive deformity. They may also have a combination of these symptoms.

▪ It is helpful to know whether the current symptoms are similar or different than the symptoms experienced before the initial surgery.

▪ The evaluation must begin with a complete review of all prior cervical procedures, pain free periods, and trauma.[11,12]

▪ If possible, obtain preoperative imaging and medical records to fully understand the nature and indication for the primary surgery.

▪ Knowing if the original symptoms resolved or persisted after the initial procedure will help ascertain the etiology of the current symptoms.

▪ Ask about any complications following surgery.

▪ Physical exam
  ▪ A complete motor and sensory exam is essential for correct diagnosis of the offending cervical level.

▪ A map of the sensory disturbance can be drawn on the arm with a skin marker.

▪ Evaluate the reflexes, include the biceps (C5), brachioradialis (C6), and triceps (C7). Note that normal reflexes diminish with age and an elderly patient with normal reflexes may be a manifestation of hyperreflexia.

▪ Evaluate for signs of myelopathy, include Hoffman test, dysdiadochokinesia, inverted radial reflex, and the ulnar escape test. In the lower extremities, signs of myelopathy include clonus, an upgoing Babinski reflex, or a wide-based gait.

▪ Note whether the symptoms are unilateral or bilateral and if bowel or bladder dysfunctions are present.

▪ Finally, rule out other potential causes of upper extremity dysfunction, including thoracic outlet syndrome, shoulder impingement/rotator cuff pathology, and/or peripheral nerve compression (cubital tunnel, radial tunnel, carpal tunnel syndromes).

IMAGING AND OTHER DIAGNOSTIC STUDIES

▪ Plain radiographs including anteroposterior, lateral, flexion, and extension views of the cervical spine should be obtained as part of the initial evaluation.

▪ Evaluation of plain radiographs allows for comparison with prior studies to determine if there is deformity, hardware failure, graft subsidence, or spondylosis.

▪ Flexion/extension view allows for evaluation of motion at a level suspected of pseudarthrosis or adjacent segment degeneration.

Methods for Examining the Cervical Spine

Examination	Technique	Illustration	Grading	Significance
Spurling test	Ipsilateral axial rotation, extension, axial compression		Positive test causes radicular symptoms.	Reproduces radicular symptoms when compressive pathology is present. Dermatomal distribution of pain should correlate with level of pathology.
Lhermitte phenomenon	Flexion and/or extension in sagittal plane. The test is generally positive at the extremes of flexion and/or extension.		Positive test causes shock-like sensation running down the spine.	Electric shock-like symptoms in arms and/or legs with extremes of motion. Pain in extension suggests spondylotic myelopathy, whereas symptoms in flexion are more suggestive of posttraumatic or iatrogenic kyphosis.
Hoffman reflex	Elicited by taking the middle finger and flipping the distal phalanx.		Observe for pincer movement between thumb and index finger.	Pincer response has a correlation with cervical spondylotic myelopathy. May be a normal variant. Comparison with contralateral side showing asymmetry may be a better indicator of myelopathy.

(continued)

Methods for Examining the Cervical Spine

Examination	Technique	Illustration	Grading	Significance
Inverted radial reflex	This reflex is demonstrated by tapping the brachioradialis tendon.		A diminished normal reflex is noted along with a reflex contraction of the finger flexors.	Abnormal reflex denotes peripheral compression of the C6 nerve root. Compression at C6 allows pathologic upper motor neuron response.
Finger escape sign (ulnar escape sign)	Performed with eyes closed, fingers adducted. Observe hands while patient is asked to maintain adducted finger position.		Small finger will spontaneously abduct.	Abduction of the small finger indicates intrinsic muscle weakness associated with cervical myelopathy.
Impingement sign	With patient seated and examiner's hand on scapula to prevent rotation, the affected arm is forward flexed causing greater tuberosity to contact the acromion.		Pain at the anterolateral acromion indicates a positive test.	A painful response is indicative of impingement syndrome.
Hawkins modified impingement sign	Forward flexion of the humerus with internal rotation		Pain at anterolateral corner of the acromion.	This test rotates the greater tuberosity under the coracoacromial ligament, and a painful response is indicative of impingement syndrome.
Adson test	Examiner stands behind the patient, radial pulse is palpated with the arm relaxed at the side. The arm is then abducted, extended, and externally rotated. Have patient take a deep breath and turn head to the side being tested. Evaluate pulse again.		Diminution or absence of the radial pulse indicates a positive test.	A positive Adson test indicates compression of the subclavian artery by a cervical rib or tight scalene muscle. This test is used to rule out thoracic outlet syndrome.

- In the case of spinal deformity, flexion/extension views provide information with respect to the reducibility of the cervical deformity to return to normal lordosis.
- Oblique views of the cervical spine allow evaluation of the neuroforamina, uncovertebral joint spurring, facet joints, and fusion mass.
- CT scans
  - CT scans provide the best overall evaluation of the bony architecture of the cervical spine.
  - CT is the modality of choice for the evaluation of a fusion mass and to rule out pseudarthrosis.
  - Myelography of the cervical spine can be used in cases where MRI scan is contraindicated. It is also useful in revision cervical surgery as instrumentation often obscures MRI imaging.
- MRI
  - MRI is the modality of choice for evaluation of the soft tissues and neural elements.
  - The intervertebral disc and spinal cord are best visualized with MRI, which also has the ability to show intramedullary edema of the cord in cases of myelopathy.
  - MRI is noninvasive and does not require intradural contrast medium.
  - In cases of revision surgery, intravenous (IV) contrast medium is used to distinguish between scar tissue, which enhances on gadolinium MRI and recurrent disc herniation which does not enhance with IV contrast medium as it lacks a blood supply.
  - MRI may be contraindicated in patients with pacemakers, spinal cord stimulators, and some cardiac stents.
- Others modalities: nerve conduction studies/electromyography (EMG), bone scans, and pain blocks.
  - Nerve conduction studies and EMG can be used to rule out peripheral nerve compression in cases where a peripheral etiology is suspected. EMG can also assist with determination of the offending cervical level in cases where physical exam findings are confounding.
  - Nuclear tests including bone scans and more specifically a single photon emission computed tomography (SPECT) scan can assist in the diagnosis of pseudarthrosis. Both show increased uptake at the site of stress fracture or pseudarthrosis. The SPECT scan provides a better spatial representation of the cervical spine.
  - Selective nerve root blocks can provide therapeutic relief of pain symptoms and are often incorporated into the nonoperative management for recurrent cervical pain and radiculopathy. In addition, selective root blocks can provide diagnostic data in cases with complex pain or sensory distributions.
- Laboratory workups including blood counts, chemistries, and the inflammatory markers erythrocyte sedimentation rate and C-reactive protein should be obtained prior to revision surgery to rule out infection as a potential cause of pain or dysfunction.

DIFFERENTIAL DIAGNOSIS

- Discogenic, myofasciocutaneous, and cervical facet joint pain
- Adjacent segment degeneration
- Deformity, PLK
- Hardware/construct failure
- Pseudarthrosis

- Recurrent pain from inadequate decompression during initial surgical procedure
- Peripheral neuropathies and pain syndromes that may mimic cervical pathology:
  - Thoracic outlet syndrome
  - Parsonage-Turner syndrome
  - Carpal tunnel syndrome
  - Cubital tunnel syndrome
  - Radial tunnel syndrome
  - Wartenberg's syndrome
  - Ulnar tunnel syndrome
  - Shoulder impingement/rotator cuff disease

NONOPERATIVE MANAGEMENT

- Surgical indications for revision cervical surgery are the same as those for primary surgery: radiculopathy, myelopathy, instability, progressive deformity, and tumor. Surgical outcomes for revision cervical surgery are much less predictable than for primary procedures. Every effort should be made to relieve the patient's symptoms with nonoperative measures prior to consideration of revision cervical surgery. Exceptions to this rule include progressive motor or gait impairment, persistent disabling pain and weakness (3 months), progressive deformity, instability, and neurologic deficits with significant axial or radicular pain.[12]
- Nonoperative modalities
  - Nonsteroidal anti-inflammatory drugs (NSAIDs)
  - Isometric cervical strengthening/physical therapy
  - Selective cervical root injections
  - Epidural steroid injections
  - Pain management clinic
  - Psychological evaluation

SURGICAL MANAGEMENT

- A thorough understanding of the cause of the patient's symptoms is essential for appropriate surgical planning and management.
- Surgical intervention should be considered in patients who have failed a trial of nonoperative intervention and who meet the indication for surgery. These being radiculopathy, myelopathy, instability, progressive deformity, and tumor.
- The goals of surgical intervention are
  - Stabilization of unstable segments
  - Decompression of the spinal cord or nerve roots in cases of myelopathy or radiculopathy
  - Correction of spinal deformity; this can be accomplished through an anterior, posterior, or combined approach and must be tailored specifically for each case.
- Pseudarthrosis
  - In cases of pseudarthrosis, the goal is fusion of the failed segment. This can be accomplished through an anterior or posterior approach.
  - Posterior fusion augments stability, enhances the potential for eventual anterior fusion, avoids the risks of an additional anterior procedure, and is an excellent therapeutic alternative to a second anterior attempt at stabilization.[18]
  - Posterior revision for pseudarthrosis has a 94% to 100% fusion rate.
  - Anterior revision for pseudarthrosis has less blood loss and shorter hospital stays. However, need for second revision is 44% in some series.[27]

- Zdeblick and Coric support use of anterior revision with excellent result and solid fusion obtained by all treated.[5,28]
- Adjacent segment degeneration, residual compression
  - Adjacent segment degeneration is managed with ACDF at the adjacent level.
  - Management of residual compression or recurrent disc herniation is determined by the site of neurologic compromise. A revision ACDF or corpectomy may be required for significant anterior compression. A posterior keyhole foraminotomy can be made to decompress a soft disc herniation.
  - For extension of an anterior fusion to an adjacent level, previous hardware must be removed to allow for extension of the instrumentation. Knowing the manufacturer and required tools for removal is essential. Recently, standalone interbody devices have been introduced on the market that allow instrumentation at an adjacent level without removal of previous hardware.
- Hardware/construct failure
  - Not all hardware failure requires revision surgery. Close follow-up with routine radiographs should be obtained in patients with asymptomatic hardware failure.
  - Surgical intervention is indicated in patients with neurologic compression or soft tissue compromise, instability, or progressive deformity.
  - Anterior failure is approached anteriorly. Posterior failure is approached from the back.
  - Hardware failure is often associated with significant inflammatory reaction and care should be taken as this can obscure the surgical approach.
  - In general, revision instrumentation can be replaced at the site of previous failure. If significant instability is present, a combined anterior/posterior stabilization should be performed.
- Kyphosis
  - The general principles of cervical deformity correction are shortening of the posterior column, lengthening of the anterior column, and use of the PLL as a hinge to facilitate correction.
  - Three general approaches are used to address postlaminectomy kyphosis.
    - Anterior-only approach: This approach corrects kyphosis through corpectomy and strut grafting or multilevel ACDF. The potential for lengthening of the anterior column through placement of interbody biomechanical devices or strut grafting is much greater than the potential of posterior osteotomies to shorten the posterior column. For this reason, an anterior procedure with or without a posterior approach has become the preferred method of deformity correction.[29]
    - Posterior-only approach: This approach uses lateral mass instrumentation with or without posterior osteotomy of the cervical spine to correct the deformity. This approach is limited to deformities that correct passively with flexion/extension views or deformities without significant anterior wedging. Posterior fixation may be limited by poor bone stock following previous laminectomy.
    - Anterior/posterior combined approach: This approach is useful for cases with significant anterior instability and longer fusions over four segments. The combined

approach allows for greater correction of sagittal plane deformity. Although potential for correction is greater with the combined approach, the added risk of a second procedure makes it less appealing to surgeons and patients. Of special note, in some patients with significant deformity with posterior arthrosis or fusions, a three-stage procedure may be required. The first stage performed is a posterior osteotomy of autofusion or levels of arthrosis with placement of instrumentation. The second stage is performed anteriorly with corpectomy and strut grafting or multilevel ACDF. The final stage is performed to secure the posterior fixation.
- Posterior osteotomies for correction of kyphosis
  - Smith-Peterson osteotomy (SPO): This is an osteotomy through the posterior elements only. The lateral masses between two pedicles are resected at the levels of kyphosis, allowing extension of the spine. SPOs can be performed at any level between C3 and C7.
  - Pedicle subtraction osteotomy (PSO): This is a three-column osteotomy involving resection of the posterior elements, pedicles, and a wedge-shaped resection of the vertebral body. A PSO allows for approximately 30 degrees of cervical extension. As the osteotomy passes through all three columns, acceptable levels for PSO are limited to C7 and T1. The vertebral artery passing through the foramen transversarium at C6-1 makes PSO at these levels impossible.

Preoperative Planning

- In most cases, an approach through a previously unexploited plane is the safest.
- If the initial procedure was performed through a right sided approach, then revision should be performed through a left sided approach.
- In cases of anterior surgery, consultation with an otolaryngologist for inspection of the vocal cords confirms that no injury has occurred to the recurrent laryngeal nerve. If vocal fold mobility is abnormal, the approach should be performed through the abnormal side to prevent injury to the healthy fold.
- Consider neuromonitoring
- Identify all implants prior to revision surgery

Positioning

- Modern neuromonitoring has decreased the need for surgeries performed under local anesthetic. This also allows for routine positioning in the prone and supine positions for almost all procedures.
- Supine positioning: anterior cervical procedures (**FIG 3**)
  - Patient is supine on a flat Jackson table or standard operating room (OR) table.
  - A bump or towel role is placed between the scapulae to promote cervical extension.
  - Tape is used to draw the shoulders down allowing for visualization of the cervicothoracic junction.
  - Arms are tucked at the sides with foam around the wrists and elbows to prevent neurapraxia.
  - Padding is places behind the knees and heels.
  - If using a standard OR table, the head rest can be extended to allow further lordosis. Flexion of head rest after placement of interbody grafts provides some compression prior to anterior plating.

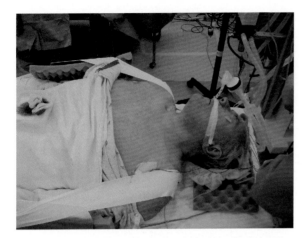

FIG 3 • Patient in the supine position with a bolster between the scapulae, the head slightly extended. The shoulders are taped caudally to allow for visualization of the lower cervical levels. Ask the anesthesiologist to place the tube in the side of the mouth opposite the side anticipated for the approach.

- Baseline neuromonitoring parameters should be established prior to draping.
- Prone positioning: posterior cervical approaches (**FIG 4**)
  - If a Mayfield headholder is to be used, this is placed with the patient in the supine position prior to flipping to the prone position.
  - During placement of the Mayfield tongs, the adjustment arm should be in the forward position directly over the patient's nose. This allows the surgeon to confirm the tongs will not impinge on the nose during intraoperative adjustment of the tongs.
  - For most cases, we use a prone view headholder or a padded face rest.
  - Neuromonitoring is attached prior to prone positioning

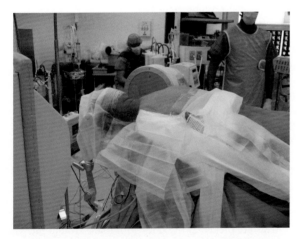

FIG 4 • Patient in the prone position using the Mayfield headrest. The patient may also be placed in a prone view or soft face holder during the procedure. The arms are padded and tucked to the sides. The shoulders are taped caudally to allow for visualization of the lower cervical levels. For upper cervical surgery, the hairline must be trimmed prior to predraping.

- The patient is gently turned to the prone position with the torso on bolsters or a four-point frame.
- If Mayfield tongs are used, attachment to the operating frame is the first priority following the flip.
- All bony prominences are padded to prevent neurapraxia.
- Elbows and hands are padded and the arms tucked to the sides.
- Tape is used to draw the shoulders down allowing for visualization of the cervicothoracic junction.
- Fluoroscopy is be used to confirm cervical alignment.
- Baseline neuromonitoring parameters should be established prior to draping.
- Deep vein thrombosis prophylaxis with thromboembolic deterrent hose and sequential compression devices should be initiated. A warming blanket should be placed prior to draping.

Approach

- Anterior approach
  - A transverse incision is made at the level of pathology.
  - In general, the incision is made on the left side of the neck as the course of the recurrent laryngeal nerve is more predictable on the left side.
  - Superficial landmarks are used to determine the level of the incision. These landmarks are the following:
    - Hard palate: arch of the atlas
    - Lower border of the mandible: C2–3
    - Hyoid bone: C3
    - Thyroid cartilage: C4–5
    - Cricoid cartilage: C6
    - Carotid tubercle: C6
  - For longer exposures, a longitudinal incision is made just medial to the sternocleidomastoid (SCM) muscle.
  - The platysma is split inline with the incision.
  - An interval is then developed between the SCM and carotid sheath laterally and the strap muscles with the tracheoesophageal structures medially.
  - The prevertebral fascia, a loose connective tissue layer, will be encountered over the anterior longitudinal ligament. The fascia is incised and stripped from the spine, exposing the anterior longitudinal ligament and longus colli muscles.
  - The level of pathology is marked with a spinal needle or disc marker and an X-ray obtained to confirm the correct level of pathology.
  - Tips for finding the correct level include palpation of the carotid tubercle and careful evaluation of preoperative X-ray for anterior osteophytes and their relation to the level of interest.
  - Once the level is confirmed, the longus colli are elevated bilaterally and soft tissue retractors are placed below the muscle belly to expose the anterior body and uncinate processes bilaterally.
- Posterior approach
  - The bony prominences of the posterior spine are palpated. C2 has a prominent spinous process as does C7 and T1.
  - A longitudinal incision is made inline with the spinous processes at the levels of pathology.
  - Electrocautery is used to maintain hemostasis throughout the case.
  - The nuchal ligament is followed and divided as it courses down to the spinous processes. The paraspinal muscles in the cervical region often cross midline. The nuchal ligament

appears as a lightly colored pale streak that follows the course of the paraspinal muscles. Following this streak will avoid cutting through muscle fibers and will ultimately lead to the spinous process.

▪ X-rays are obtained with marker on spinous process to confirm correct level surgery.

▪ The deep layer of muscle is stripped from the spinous process and lamina close to the bone with the aid of electrocautery.

▪ Subperiosteal dissection is carried laterally to the border of the lateral masses.

▪ Soft tissue retractors are placed for optimal visualization.

ANTERIOR REVISION FUSION FOR PSEUDOARTHROSIS OR RECURRENT STENOSIS

▪ After anterior approach, previous anterior instrumentation is removed from the spine.

▪ Distraction pins are placed in the levels above and below the pseudarthrosis.

▪ Distraction is placed across the level of pathology and the residual graft and fibrous tissue are removed with a curette or pituitary rongeur.

▪ In cases of severe collapse, the pseudarthrosis may literally be bone on bone. In this case, a high speed burr is used to follow the "scar" or cleft left by the pseudarthrosis. This can be less than 1 mm wide.

▪ Periodically stop and check the scar to confirm you are still in the correct plane. Opening and closing the distraction pins while looking at the pseudarthrosis will show micromotion in the plane of the nonunion.

▪ As the posterior cortex is thinned, a small forward angled curette or micro-Kerrison can be passed through the cortex and the posterior cortex can be removed.

▪ In cases of radiculopathy, the removal of the posterior cortex can be carried out laterally toward the foramen until a nerve hook can be passed out the foramen without impingement.

▪ In primary anterior surgery, resection of the PLL has been advocated for complete decompression. However, this should not be attempted in cases of previous PLL resection as there will be no true plane between the scarred PLL and the dura, increasing the risk of dural injury and cerebrospinal fluid leak. If previous operative notes suggest the PLL was undisturbed, it can be resected at the time of revision.

▪ Following decompression, the interbody space is shaped to accommodate an interbody graft. The graft can be

tricortical autograft or cortical strut allograft. Some controversy exists as to which grafting technique is most appropriate. All techniques mentioned here have found some supported in the literature.

▪ The graft is fashioned using a clamp and high speed burr (**TECH FIG 1**).

▪ Following graft preparation, the block is inserted into the interbody space.

▪ Anterior plating is recommended in all cases of pseudarthrosis.

▪ X-rays are obtained to confirm appropriate placement of the graft and anterior plate.

▪ The incision is closed over a drain.

▪ Cervical collar is placed for immobilization.

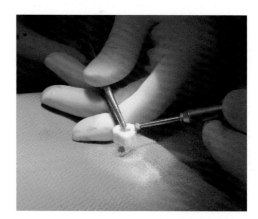

TECH FIG 1 • Graft preparation.

POSTERIOR SPINAL FUSION FOR ANTERIOR PSEUDARTHROSIS

▪ After posterior exposure at the levels of anterior pseudarthrosis, all soft tissue is stripped from the lateral masses bilaterally.

▪ If radiculopathy is present, a laminoforaminotomy is performed. This technique is described in later text.

▪ Several methods of posterior instrumentation exist. At our institution, posterior fixation with lateral mass screws and rods is most frequently performed.

▪ A 2-mm high speed burr is used to make a starting hole 1 mm medial to the center point on the lateral mass.

▪ A 2.4-mm drill bit is used to create a pilot hole for the 3.5-mm lateral mass screw.

▪ The direction of the drill hole is 15 degrees cephalad and 30 degrees lateral.

▪ Drilling begins with a 12-mm depth sleeve and can be increased by 2 mm increments.

▪ After drilling, a depth gauge is used to confirm appropriate screw length.

▪ The hole is tapped with a slightly undersized tap.

▪ The screw is inserted in the same trajectory as the drill and tap.

- These steps are repeated until all lateral mass screws are placed.
- The lateral masses and lamina are then decorticated.
- Appropriate length rods are contoured and then inserted into the heads of the screws bilaterally. Set screws are placed and tightened to appropriate torque.
- Bone graft is then placed over the decorticated lateral masses.
- Closure of the wound in layers.
- Cervical collar is placed for immobilization. (Typically for longer segmental reconstruction.)

ANTERIOR TREATMENT OF POSTLAMINECTOMY KYPHOSIS

- After anterior exposure, scar may be found over the apex of the deformity. Resection of the scar will allow for increased exposure and mobility of the spine.
- At each level of deformity, the intervertebral discs are excised using a pituitary rongeur, curettes, and a micro-Kerrison when needed. The discectomy should be carried down to the level of the PLL.
- Care should be taken to completely remove the cartilaginous endplate to prevent pseudarthrosis.
- In cases of associated radiculopathy, the foramen is decompressed. A nerve hook passed laterally into the foramen confirms the decompression is adequate.
- If multiple interbody grafts are to be used, trial spacers are inserted into the interbody spaces and appropriate grafts are selected for each level.
- The interbody grafts are contoured and inserted into the interbody spaces.
- If strut grafting is desired or required for adequate decompression, a corpectomy is performed by removing the anterior vertebral body with a rongeur.
- A trough is created 16 mm wide in the vertebral body.
- The trough is widened at the lateral uncovertebral joints and deepened to the level of the PLL.
- As the posterior cortex is approached, a high speed burr is used to thin the bone.
- A small angle curette or micro-Kerrison can be introduced below the posterior cortex and this is resected.
- The superior and inferior vertebral endplates are prepared with the high speed burr, creating decorticated bleeding cancellous beds with posterior lips to prevent displacement of the graft.
- A cortical strut is then fashioned from allograft fibula.
- Twenty pounds of traction is placed on the skull with an extension moment to allow for insertion of the contoured graft.
- The graft is inserted and tapped into place with extreme caution to avoid injury to the spinal cord or nerves.
- Anterior cervical plating is recommended in all cases. In multilevel ACDF, there are several sites for screw fixation. For strut grafting, screws are placed above and below the strut. Screws should not be placed through the graft as risk of graft fracture is substantial. If concerned about graft displacement, a nonabsorbable suture can be used to tie the graft to the plate.

POSTERIOR APPROACH FOR POSTLAMINECTOMY KYPHOSIS

- This approach is limited to minor deformities and those that passively correct to normal lordosis on flexion/extension views.
- Prior to the procedure, the Mayfield headholder is positioned on the patient.
- After prone positioning, the Mayfield is secured and the head and neck adjusted until appropriate lordosis is obtained. (Note: Neuromonitoring should be established and ongoing during any manipulation of the cervical spine with the patient under anesthesia.)
- If lordosis is appropriate, lateral mass instrumentation can be placed as outlined previously in the technique for posterior fusion for pseudarthrosis.
- If residual kyphosis is present, posterior osteotomies must be performed prior to lateral mass fixation.
- Once the spine is exposed, the levels of kyphosis undergo posterior osteotomy. This often renders the posterior bone inadequate for isolated posterior fixation and anterior fusion becomes necessary.
- If adequate bone stock is present after osteotomy, then posterior instrumentation with lateral mass screws and fusion is performed as outlined previously.

Combined Anterior Posterior for Postlaminectomy Kyphosis

- Unless significant posterior fusions or arthrosis are present, the combined approach begins with anterior discectomy or corpectomy as outlined under the discussion of isolated anterior treatment of cervical kyphosis.
- Once the anterior instrumentation is complete, the patient is turned to the prone position for lateral mass fixation with or without an osteotomy.
- In general, short anterior procedures of three levels or less do not require posterior stabilization. In cases of four or more levels of reconstruction, posterior instrumentation should be considered.
- Posterior fixation should also be considered in patients with poor bone stock or risks for pseudarthrosis.
- Posterior instrumentation is discussed in detail in the previous section.
- Following combined anterior posterior fusion and instrumentation, the patient should be immobilized in a cervical collar for a minimum of 6 weeks.

Revision for Adjacent Segment Degeneration (Revision ACDF)

- Revision surgery for ASD is similar in many ways to primary ACDF.
- A major difference is the need for approach from a previously unexploited plane. Ear, nose, and throat (ENT) consultation should be obtained and, if vocal cords function normally, the anterior spine is approached from the side opposite that is used during the primary procedure.
- A second difference is the potential need for hardware removal at the site of previous fusion. Every effort should be made to identify the hardware prior to revision surgery.
- With these two exceptions, anterior treatment for ASD is ACDF as outlined under treatment of cervical disc herniation.

Laminoforaminotomy

- Posterior laminoforaminotomy is useful for treatment of nerve root compression in cases of pseudarthrosis, adjacent level degeneration, or recurrent disc herniation at the site of previous anterior fusion.
- After posterior approach at the level of nerve compression, the lamina and lateral mass are identified.
- A burr is used to thin the lateral lamina and medial facet.
- A curved curette is used to create a plane between the medial facet and the ligamentum flavum.
- The anterior facet capsule and additional bone are resected to visualize the exiting nerve root. (Care should be taken to avoid excessive resection of the facet greater than fifty percent of this may cause iatrogenic instability to the cervical spine.)
- The ligamentum is resected and the laminotomy is widened to expose the junction of the thecal sac and nerve root.
- The foramen is probed with a Woodson or nerve hook to confirm decompression, if disc herniation is found, the PLL is incised and the disc fragment removed.
- The spine is closed in layers.
- Soft cervical collar is provided for comfort.

PEARLS AND PITFALLS

Patient selection	Appropriate patient selection is the single most important step to reducing the number of patients requiring revision cervical surgery.
Implants	Identify all previously placed implants prior to revision surgery. Have specific removal equipment available at the time of cervical revision surgery.
Nonoperative management	Nonoperative intervention including NSAIDs, physical therapy, and epidural injections should be attempted prior to surgical intervention.
Imaging	Correlate patient symptoms with positive imaging findings to optimize patient outcomes.

POSTOPERATIVE CARE

- Immediate postoperative care after revision cervical surgery involves immobilization of the spine for 2 to 12 weeks depending on the number of levels addressed during the surgery and the likelihood of instability or nonunion.
- Short fixation over one to two segments is generally immobilized in a cervical collar for 2 weeks. At that time, the patient is allowed to gradually return to activities of daily living. Formal physical therapy evaluation for range of motion (ROM) and strengthening of the cervical spine is typically reserved until fusion mass is seen on plain radiographs.
- Patients with longer fusion and those at risk for poor wound healing and pseudarthrosis are treated in a rigid cervical collar for a minimum of 6 weeks. Formal therapy is started once the fusion is visualized on plain X-rays.
- Physical therapy following revision cervical surgery involves isometric strengthening and ROM prior to returning to unlimited activity.

OUTCOMES

- Overall, revision surgery has less favorable outcomes when compared with primary surgical procedures.
- Outcomes for revision for pseudarthrosis vary with the approach used for revision. Anterior revision surgery is associated with a 57% fusion rate. Several studies reported fusion rates of 94% following posterior revision for pseudarthrosis.
- Zdeblick and Coric reported 100% fusion rates with anterior revision of interbody psuedarthrosis.[5,28] Both autograft and anterior plating were advocated to increase fusion rates.
- The rate of arthrodesis following surgery for adjacent segment degeneration is lower in patients treated with interbody grafting (63%) versus those treated with corpectomy and strut grafting (100%). No statistical significance was found in the clinical outcomes between those treated with interbody fusion and corpectomy with strut grafting.[30]

COMPLICATIONS

- The risk of complications after revision cervical surgery is significantly higher than the risk associated with primary surgery. The overall risk of complication is reported at 27%.[31]
- For each approach, the risk of complication associated with the primary surgery remains with the addition of risks associated with revision circumstances.
- Anterior complications include the following:
  - Esophageal injury: a life-threatening injury; one-third recognized at time of surgery. Early recognition associated with 15% mortality; late recognition associated with 30% mortality.

- Vocal cord paralysis: 15% of cases[31]
- Dysphagia: 10% of cases
- Neurologic injury/monoradiculopathy: 7% of cases
- Durotomy
- Graft site complication

■ Posterior complications include the following:
  - Neurologic injury
  - Durotomy
  - Significant wound complications/infection occurs at a rate of 1.2%

REFERENCES

1. Zdeblick TA, Abitbol JJ, Kunz DN, et al. Cervical stability after sequential capsule resection. Spine 1993;18(14):2005–2008.
2. Panjabi MM, Summers DJ, Pelker RR, et al. Three-dimensional load-displacement curves due to forces on the cervical spine. J Orthop Res 1986;4(2):152–161.
3. Raizman NM, O'Brien JR, Poehling-Monaghan KL, et al. Pseudarthrosis of the spine. J Am Acad Orthop Surg 2009;17(8): 494–503.
4. Hilibrand AS, Fye MA, Emery SE, et al. Impact of smoking on the outcome of anterior cervical arthrodesis with interbody or strut-grafting. J Bone Joint Surg Am 2001;83-A(5):668–673.
5. Coric D, Branch CL Jr, Jenkins JD. Revision of anterior cervical pseudoarthrosis with anterior allograft fusion and plating. J Neurosurg 1997;86(6):969–974.
6. Tribus CB, Corteen DP, Zdeblick TA. The efficacy of anterior cervical plating in the management of symptomatic pseudoarthrosis of the cervical spine. Spine 1999;24(9):860–864.
7. Nowinski GP, Visarius H, Nolte LP, et al. A biomechanical comparison of cervical laminaplasty and cervical laminectomy with progressive facetectomy. Spine 1993;18(14):1995–2004.
8. Albert TJ, Vacarro A. Postlaminectomy kyphosis. Spine 1998;23(24): 2738.
9. Lowery GL, McDonough RF. The significance of hardware failure in anterior cervical plate fixation: patients with 2- to 7-year follow-up. Spine 1998;(23):181–186.
10. Lowery GL, Swank ML, McDonough RF. Surgical revision for failed anterior cervical fusions. Articular pillar plating or anterior revision? Spine 1995;20(22):2436–2441.
11. Boden SD, Bohlman H. *The Failed Spine*. Philadelphia, PA: Lippincott Williams & Wilkins; 2003.
12. Truumees E, McLain R. Failed and revision cervical spine surgery. In: Chapman MW, ed. Chapman's Orthopaedic Surgery. 3rd ed. Philadelphia: Lippincott Williams & Wilkins; 2001: 3846–3860.
13. Simmons EH, Bhalla SK. Anterior cervical discectomy and fusion. A clinical and biomechanical study with eight-year follow-up. J Bone Joint Surg Br 1969;51(2):225–237.
14. Whitecloud TS 3rd, Seago RA. Cervical discogenic syndrome. Results of operative intervention in patients with positive discography. Spine 1987;12(4):313–316.
15. Farey ID, McAfee PC, Davis RF, et al. Pseudarthrosis of the cervical spine after anterior arthrodesis. Treatment by posterior nerve-root decompression, stabilization, and arthrodesis. J Bone Joint Surg Am 1990;72(8):1171–1177.
16. Robinson RA, Walker AE, Ferlic DC, et al. The results of anterior interbody fusion of the cervical spine. J Bone Joint Surg 1962;44(8): 1569–1587.
17. Phillips FM, Carlson G, Emery SE, et al. Anterior cervical pseudarthrosis. Natural history and treatment. Spine 1997;22(14):1585–1589.
18. Lindsey RW, Newhouse KE, Leach J, et al. Nonunion following two-level anterior cervical discectomy and fusion. Clin Orthop Relat Res 1987;(223):155–163.
19. Hilibrand AS, Carlson GD, Palumbo MA, et al. Radiculopathy and myelopathy at segments adjacent to the site of a previous anterior cervical arthrodesis. J Bone Joint Surg Am 1999;81(4):519–528.
20. Eck JC, Humphreys SC, Lim TH, et al. Biomechanical study on the effect of cervical spine fusion on adjacent-level intradiscal pressure and segmental motion. Spine 2002;27(22):2431–2434.
21. Lonstein JE. Post-laminectomy kyphosis. Clin Orthop Relat Res 1977;(128):93–100.
22. Lawrence J, White A, Hilibrand A. Same segment disease after cervical spine surgery. Spine J 2007;7(5):55S.
23. Wu W, Thuomas KA, Hedlund R, et al. Degenerative changes following anterior cervical discectomy and fusion evaluated by fast spin-echo MR imaging. Acta Radiol 1996;37(5):614–617.
24. Stevens JM, Clifton AG, Whitear P. Appearances of posterior osteophytes after sound anterior interbody fusion in the cervical spine: a high-definition computed myelographic study. Neuroradiology 1993;35(3):227–228.
25. Kozak JA, Hanson GW, Rose JR, et al. Anterior discectomy, microscopic decompression, and fusion: a treatment for cervical spondylotic radiculopathy. J Spinal Disord 1989;2(1):43–46.
26. Robertson PA, Ryan MD. Neurological deterioration after reduction of cervical subluxation. Mechanical compression by disc tissue. J Bone Joint Surg Br 1992;74(2):224–227.
27. Carreon L, Glassman SD, Campbell MJ. Treatment of anterior cervical pseudoarthrosis: posterior fusion versus anterior revision. Spine J 2006;6(2):154–156.
28. Zdeblick TA, Hughes SS, Riew KD, Bohlman HH. Failed anterior cervical discectomy and arthrodesis. Analysis and treatment of thirty-five patients. J Bone Joint Surg Am 1997;79(4):523–532.
29. Zdeblick TA, Ducker TB. The use of freeze-dried allograft bone for anterior cervical fusions. Spine 1991;16(7):726–729.
30. Hilibrand AS, Yoo JU, Carlson GD, et al. The success of anterior cervical arthrodesis adjacent to a previous fusion. Spine 1997;22(14): 1574–1579.
31. Gok B, Sciubba DM, McLoughlin GS, et al. Revision surgery for cervical spondylotic myelopathy. Neurosurgery 2008;63(2): 292–298.

Chapter 32

Surgical Excision of Intradural Spinal Tumors

Gerald E. Rodts, Jr. and Daniel Refai

INTRODUCTION

▪ Intradural tumors of the spine are less common than primary or metastatic tumors of the bone or epidural space, and surgical removal of intradural tumors requires delicate technique and maximal avoidance of injury to the spinal cord and nerve roots.

▪ Intradural tumors are rarely the result of metastatic spread of malignant cells. The main categories of intradural tumors are intradural/extramedullary and intradural/intramedullary. Some tumors will exhibit characteristics of both intra- and extramedullary or exophytic growth.

▪ Here we review the primary indications for surgery of intradural tumors as well as the step-by-step techniques used to position the patient, expose the spine, decompression for access to the thecal sac, opening of the dura, intradural resection of tumor tissue, techniques for rotation of the spinal cord for ventral pathology, and dural and wound closure.

PATHOGENESIS

▪ The most common types of tumor that are found in the intradural, extramedullary space are benign meningioma, schwannoma, and neurofibroma.

▪ Teratoma is a more rare intradural tumor that often is both intramedullary and extramedullary.

▪ The most common intramedullary tumors are spinal cord ependymoma, hemangioblastoma, lipoma, astrocytoma, and glioblastoma. They are rarely exophytic except for ependymomas that occur at the conus medullaris.

▪ Nerve sheath tumors (schwannoma, neurofibroma) usually present with radicular symptoms, and myelopathic symptoms develop once the tumor has enlarged to the point where it is causing compression of the spinal cord.

▪ In the lumbar spine (below the conus medullaris), intradural extramedullary tumors commonly cause radicular symptoms (pain, paresthesias, weakness), and low back pain can develop and rapidly progress to an excruciating level when the tumors grow to occupy the majority of the spinal canal.

▪ Intradural, intramedullary tumors can cause axial or radicular pain, but the most common presentation is myelopathy. The progression is typically very slow over many months, unless the pathology is the malignant glioblastoma of the spinal cord. A careful preoperative evaluation must eliminate other pathology of the spinal cord parenchyma such as sarcoidosis, transverse myelitis, multiple sclerosis, etc.

▪ The indications to proceed with surgical resection of intradural tumors of the spine include severe, progressive axial or radicular pain; progressive weakness due to nerve root compression or involvement; and myelopathic symptoms of an upper motor neuron bladder, spastic gait disturbance, incoordination of the upper extremities, generalized weakness, and sensory loss or disturbance. Asymptomatic patients with minimal

or no upper motor neuron signs can be watched closely with serial neurological and MRI examination. Patients with lumbar intradural tumors that are asymptomatic can similarly be watched carefully, but one needs to make sure than even subtle signs of lower motor neuron bladder dysfunction are in fact not present.

PATIENT HISTORY AND PHYSICAL FINDINGS

▪ Presenting symptoms of both intra- and extramedullary spinal cord tumors include axial or appendicular/radicular pain. The pain is usually persistent when either active or at rest. Myelopathic symptoms present as numbness, tingling (paresthesias), gait instability, small motor/hand incoordination (cervical), increasing urinary voiding frequency, difficulty voiding, and general motor weakness. Upper motor neuron signs such as hyperreflexia, Hoffman sign, spreading of reflexes, myoclonus, and Babinski signs are typical.

IMAGING AND OTHER DIAGNOSTIC STUDIES

▪ MRI is the imaging technology of choice for intramedullary and extramedullary spinal cord tumors. Contrast enhancement is necessary. Intramedullary tumors have fairly characteristic appearances on MRI. Astrocytomas will demonstrate variable contrast enhancement and almost never have a solid, homogenous area of enhancement. Ependymomas consistently have a homogenously enhancing mass within the parenchyma of the spinal cord (see **FIG. 1**). T1-weighted images will show low intensity within the tumor mass that enhances brightly upon contrast administration. Often, T2-weighted images will demonstrate surrounding edema within the spinal cord. Hemangioblastomas typically have a cystic area of low-signal intensity on T1-weighted images with a smaller contrast-enhancing nodule on the inside wall of the cyst. Intramedullary lipomas will be nonenhancing and exhibit the typical high signal on T1- and T2-weighted images as seen in bodily adipose tissue.

▪ Extramedullary tumors such as meningiomas will usually enhance positively with contrast in a very homogenous pattern, and often, a "tail" of enhancement will be seen in the location of attachment to the dura (**FIG 2**). Schwannomas and neurofibromas can have homogeneous or heterogeneous enhancement patterns. Some schwannomas will exhibit little to no enhancement, but this is less common.

▪ For patients that cannot undergo an MRI (eg, those with pacemakers, defibrillators, spinal cord stimulators, etc.), CT myelography can be used and can delineate an area of spinal cord swelling or even myelographic block that would indicate the location of an intramedullary tumors. Extramedullary tumors are usually very well outlined by CT-myelography.

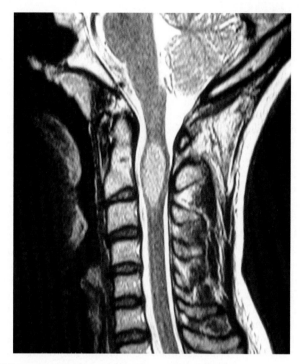

FIG 1 • Ependymoma on contrast-enhanced MRI.

SURGICAL MANAGEMENT FOR INTRADURAL, EXTRAMEDULLARY TUMORS

Preoperative Planning

▪ Surgery for intradural, extramedullary tumors is usually done via a posterior approach. Preoperative intravenous antibiotics with good central nervous system (CNS) penetration such as Nafcillin or Ancef are administered within 1 hour of the skin incision.

Positioning

▪ Patients with tumors located between the skull base and the upper thoracic spine (approximately T4–5) are positioned on chest rolls with the head in the table-mounted, three-pin headholder.
▪ A slightly flexed position is used for most cervical tumors.
▪ If posterior fusion with instrumentation is planned, a more neutral sagittal position is preferred. A urethral catheter is placed in most cases.

Approach

▪ After the skin preparation, a midline incision is made and a subperiosteal exposure of the spine is accomplished.
▪ The dural opening for most intradural, extramedullary tumors will usually need to include a lamina above and below the pathology, so the number of laminae to be removed is usually clear from the sagittal and axial MRI or CT-myelogram images.
▪ The dural opening is usually midline, but the opening can be paramedian in patients with tumors eccentric to one side.
▪ Large schwannomas and neurofibromas will often be visible upon exposure as a dura-covered mass extending out and expanding the neural foramen. In these cases, the dural opening is often laterally with a T-shape extension of the midline opening.
▪ As with all tumors located in or extending out laterally to the neural foramen, the location of the vertebral artery must be clearly known from preoperative imaging studies. This artery is most commonly displaced anteriorly and can remain patent.
▪ In such cases, the vertebral artery can almost always be spared following resection.
▪ In tumors where the vertebral artery is encased within the mass of the tumor, consideration can be given to preoperative endovascular test occlusion and subsequent obliteration via coiling/embolization.

T1 Sag with and without Contrast

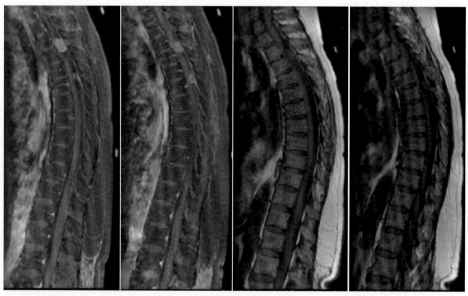

FIG 2 • Intradural, extramedullary contrast-enhancing (left two images) meningioma. Note dural "tail" sign (*arrow*).

MICROSURGICAL TECHNIQUE

▪ For extramedullary tumors such as schwannoma, neurofibroma, and meningioma, the essential techniques of tumor removal consist of internal debulking of the tumor, delicate dissection of the tumor capsule from the pial surface of the spinal cord, and meticulous sparing and protection of surrounding nerve rootlets.

▪ An ultrasonic aspirator is most useful for internal debulking of these tumors.

▪ The surgeon must be careful to avoid going through the capsule of the tumor.

▪ It is helpful to pause from resection every few minutes and three-dimensionally reassess the extent of tumor mass remaining by careful palpation and manipulation of the tumor capsule and remaining tumor mass using microinstruments.

▪ All three of these tumor types typically allow for successful peeling of the final capsule off of the pial surface of the spinal cord.

▪ In cases where the tumor capsule is very adherent to the pial surface or to the surface of posterior or ventral nerve rootlets, the surgeon may elect to leave behind that material and coagulate it with bipolar cautery.

▪ With large, ventral dural-based (meningioma) or nerve root sleeve tumors, it is usually necessary to cut the denticulate ligaments at the equator of the spinal cord. This should be done at several levels, so that manipulation of tumor does not result in excessive torquing of the spinal cord tissue in a small area.

▪ Microscopic monofilament suture (eg, 6-0, 8-0 Prolene [Ethicon, Somerville, NJ]) can be placed through the base of the denticulate ligaments to provide a means of gently rotating the spinal cord.

▪ If rotation is necessary to gain access to large ventral tumors, then the denticulate ligament should be released over several levels (not just in the vicinity of the tumor).

▪ Blood pressure should be maintained at normal levels and consideration can be given to using motor-evoked potential and somatosensory-evoked potentials.

▪ Changes in potential readings during rotation of the spinal cord can allow the surgeon to release the traction to help prevent injury.

▪ In removal of a meningioma, the surgeon should assess the location of the dural attachment and decide whether dural resection and patching is possible, or whether coagulation (alone) of the area is best.

▪ Ideally, resection of the area of dura from which the tumor arose provides the best protection against recurrence. Local fascia or lyophilized bovine pericardium or synthetic materials can be used for sewing in a patch.

▪ With final removal of a schwannoma, all nerve fibers that are not the source of the tumor are carefully dissected off the capsule and preserved. Those that clearly enter the bulk of the tumor are cut and removed with the tumor.

▪ Prior to final closure, meticulous inspection for bleeding is performed. One should limit the amount of bipolar coagulation of pial blood vessels. Often, holding thrombin-soaked collagen sponge with gentle pressure over a small bleeding venule or arteriole is sufficient to stop microscopic hemorrhage.

▪ The dural is then closed with a running (locking or unlocked) monofilament or braided nylon or proline suture. Interrupted dural closure is also acceptable. Fibrin glue or other synthetic glue products are often used to reinforce the suture closure.

▪ The adjuvant use of external lumbar cerebrospinal fluid draining is up to the judgment of the surgeon and may be helpful particularly in cases where weeping of cerebrospinal fluid is seen despite a good suture closure of the dura.

INTRADURAL, INTRAMEDULLARY SPINAL CORD TUMORS

Preoperative Planning

▪ The most common tumor type encountered within the parenchyma of the spinal cord is ependymoma, astrocytoma, hemangioblastoma, and lipoma.

▪ The presenting symptoms of intramedullary tumors are less radicular and mostly myelopathic.

▪ Deep axial or radicular pain is uncommon. Numbness, spasticity, disturbance of bladder function, and quadriparesis are most commonly the presenting symptoms.

▪ Needle biopsy is not recommended due to the risk of spinal cord injury and hemorrhage. Therefore, open biopsy and resection is the standard practice for primary intramedullary tumors.

▪ Patients should be counseled extensively regarding the much higher risk and expectation of new postoperative deficits compared with extramedullary tumors.

▪ Almost all patients will experience some degree of new or increased sensory or motor disturbance as a result of removal of an intramedullary spinal cord tumor.

▪ In the early postoperative state, it is difficult to ascertain what new deficits will be transient and which changes may be permanent. Most patients, however, experience improvement of new neurological findings over time. Some patients will have new permanent deficits, and in some patients there will be progressive neurological deficits as seen in patients with a malignant, incompletely resected astrocytoma of the spinal cord. Often these tumors respond poorly to radiation therapy and chemotherapy.

Positioning

▪ Positioning and laminar bone removal is essentially identical to that performed for extramedullary tumors.

▪ The dural opening is usually made in the midline regardless of the eccentricity of the tumor within the spinal cord.

▪ Although the techniques of internal debulking and tumor capsule dissection are fairly consistent with all solid extramedullary tumors, the strategies of resection for intramedullary tumors varies with tumor type.

▪ MRI characteristics of the tumor preoperatively usually allow the surgeon to anticipate whether there is going to be a demarcation between tumor capsule and spinal cord tissue (as with ependymoma), or whether there is going to be a diffuse blending of tumor tissue with the spinal cord tissue at the periphery of the tumor (astrocytoma, lipoma), or whether there is a large cystic area containing a smaller mural nodule of tumor (hemangioblastoma).

Approach

▪ One important decision involves where to enter the spinal cord. For tumors that come to the pial surface, it is obviously safest to enter there.

■ Many tumors, however, have normal spinal cord tissue between the tumor and the pial surface. They may be eccentric to one side.

■ For centrally located tumors, a midline myelotomy should be considered (**FIG 3**).

■ For eccentric tumors that do not come to the surface, the dorsal root entry zone should be considered.

■ Ultrasound can be helpful in assessing the location and outline of the tumor. The pia is coagulated using micro bipolars at low settings, and a no. 11 blade-scalpel or microscissors are used to open the pial layer.

■ Microinstruments are then used to gently tease open the tissue from inside out, working up and down along the extent of the tumor and respecting the cephalocaudal orientation of the long tracts.

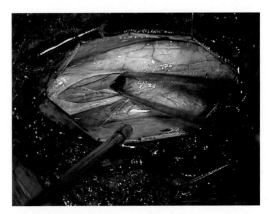

FIG 3 • Initial dissection of the arachnoid, preparing for midline myelotomy. Note dural tack-up sutures.

MICROSCOPIC RESECTION OF INTRAMEDULLARY TUMORS

■ With an ependymoma, the tumor capsule will be a distinctly different color (gray-red) than the surrounding white spinal cord parenchyma (**TECH FIG 1**).

■ When a portion of the tumor capsule has been exposed, the capsule is coagulated and incised with a no. 11 blade scalpel.

■ The ultrasonic aspirator and hand instruments such as cupped forceps or micropituitary rongeur are used to internally debulk the tumor tissue.

■ A portion can be sent for frozen section analysis.

■ The important step in internal debulking of an ependymoma is making sure that one does not penetrate the capsule since there is often normal tissue ventral and lateral to the capsule (**TECH FIG 2**). Also, with this tumor type, there is almost always a ventrally located artery supplying the tumor that one will encounter and need to coagulate as the final, ventral portions of the capsule are resected (**TECH FIG 3**).

■ Small cottonoid patties (Codman, Warsaw, IN) are very useful in "claiming territory" as the capsule becomes soft

and floppy. Multiple cottonoids placed between the capsule and the tumor tissue serve as further protection against instrument damage. Gross total removal of an ependymoma is often feasible.

■ With a spinal cord astrocytoma, the demarcation between tumor tissue and spinal cord parenchyma is often difficult.

■ The goals of surgery are different from an ependymoma removal where gross total resection can be achieved.

■ With an astrocytoma, the surgeon must carefully judge the appearance of the tumor tissue under the microscope. Clearly abnormal tissue that is more yellow or gray can usually be safely removed without devastating consequences.

■ Once the demarcation is no longer clear, one should consider avoiding further tumor removal.

■ In cases where the frozen section results show a high grade (malignant) astrocytoma or glioblastoma, then the prognosis is very poor and the risk of creating devastating neurological loss may not be of value to the patient.

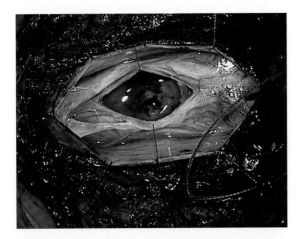

TECH FIG 1 • Myelotomy complete, exposing tumor mass within parenchyma of the spinal cord. Small pia-arachnoid sutures can be seen superiorly and inferiorly holding open myelotomy.

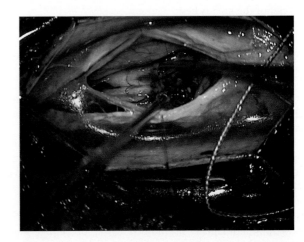

TECH FIG 2 • Final portions of tumor being removed with normal spinal cord tissue at base of cavity within spinal cord.

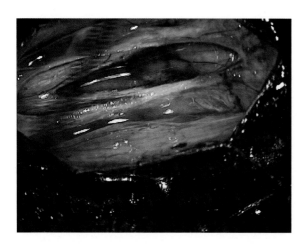

TECH FIG 3 • Tumor removed, pial sutures released.

- Spinal cord lipomas are usually solid, bright yellow tissue and easily distinguished from normal spinal cord parenchyma.
- In rare cases, the tumor mass may be discovered to be in liquid, oily form rather than solid tissue. These tumors usually are visible on the pial surface and can even be exophytic, but ventrally and laterally, the fatty tissue can blend in with the normal parenchyma. Thus, gross total resections may not be possible without the increased risk of neurological injury. Often, a small rim of lipomatous tissue is left behind.
- With cystic hemangioblastomas, the surrounding spinal cord tissue does not necessarily have to be opened along the entire extent of the cystic cavity.
- Attention is paid to where the mural nodule of tumor is located.
- The myelotomy should be performed closest to the level where the nodule is located, and often only a portion of the cystic cavity is exposed that allows adequate visualization of the tumor.
- Vessels identified under magnification that are feeding and draining the tumor are coagulated and cut, and the tumor can often be dissected off of the wall of the cystic cavity.
- The fluid of the cavity typically drains out spontaneously after working and irrigating during tumor removal. Meticulous hemostasis (as always) is confirmed prior to dural closure.

PEARLS AND PITFALLS

▪ Always dissect during the initial myelotomy with the idea of the cephalocaudal orientation of the long tracts.	▪ Frequently zoom out and take in the larger picture of how far along the tumor resection has progressed.
▪ Try and avoid using coagulation on normal pial vessels (gently apply Gelfoam sponge [Baxter Healthcare Corporation, Hayward, CA] and microcottonoid and most bleeding will stop in tiny vessels).	▪ The "backside" or "side walls" of the tumor or tumor capsule will come up faster than you think; avoid breaching that final layer of tumor tissue and injuring normal tissue on the blind side of the tumor.
▪ When dissecting or manipulating normal or tumor tissue, use fine, slow movements to minimize tissue trauma.	

POSTOPERATIVE CARE

▪ Intensive care unit (ICU) observation of immediate postoperative patients is recommended following resection of an intradural, intramedullary, or extramedullary spinal cord tumor so that blood pressure can be monitored, and frequent neurological examinations can be performed to identify those rare patients with a complication such as a postoperative epidural or intramedullary hemorrhage.

▪ The use of corticosteroids is at the discretion of the surgeon.

▪ External cerebrospinal fluid diversion via a lumbar intrathecal drain may be used.

  ▪ Patients with cervical or upper thoracic tumors can be nursed in a partially upright or sitting position as this will decrease the cerebrospinal fluid pressure in the area of the dural closure.

  ▪ Lower thoracic (and lumbar) tumor patients are often kept at flat bed rest, although no guidelines exist for this issue, and the decision is at the discretion of the surgeon.

  ▪ Progressive mobilization and ambulation can begin very soon after surgery or a period of bed rest.

CONCLUSION

▪ The essence of surgery for removal of intradural, extramedullary tumors is internal debulking of the tumor and careful dissection of tumor capsule from the pial surface of the spinal cord.

▪ With ventral tumors, multiple levels of release of the denticulate ligaments is helpful.

▪ In removing intradural, intramedullary tumors of the spinal cord, preoperative knowledge of the anatomical characteristics such as the presence of a cyst, the sharpness of demarcation on imaging of the tumor, the presence of a mural nodule, etc. all help guide the surgeon in deciding the location of the initial myelotomy and the approach to the tumor.

▪ Constant identification and protection of normal spinal cord tissue is obviously essential. In tumors such as astrocytomas, there will often not be any clear margin of tumor and aggressive resection if often best avoided to prevent severe neurological injury.

COMPLICATIONS

▪ The most concerning complication is quadriplegia, and this may occur even when very delicate handling of spinal cord and tumor tissue has been performed. This complication can sometimes not be avoided, but short amplitude, delicate movements of the microinstruments; maintenance of normal blood pressure and oxygenation; and preservation of normal arteries, arterioles, veins, and venules are of great importance.

▪ Postoperative intramedullary hemorrhage is rare and meticulous confirmation of hemostasis while under the microscope is essential.

▪ Cerebrospinal fluid leak is a more common complication. Attention to watertight closure suturing technique is important, and many surgeons use various forms of fibrin glue or synthetic materials to help seal the suture closure.

▪ In patients with thin or easily torn dura and/or leaking of cerebrospinal fluid through the suture holes, postoperative external cerebrospinal fluid drainage via a lumbar intrathecal catheter may be very helpful. Three to five days of drainage in those patients is commonly practiced.

SUGGESTED READING

Angevine PD, Kellner C, Hague RM, et al. Surgical management of ventral intradural spinal lesions. J Neurosurg Spine 2011;15(1):28–37.

Boström A, von Lehe M, Hartmann W, et al. Surgery for spinal cord ependymomas: outcome and prognostic factors. Neurosurgery 2011;68(2):302–308; discussion 309.

Kucia EJ, Bambakidis NC, Chang SW, et al. Surgical technique and outcomes in the treatment of spinal cord ependymomas, part 1: intramedullary ependymomas. Neurosurgery 2011;68(1 Suppl Operative):57–63; discussion 63.

Kucia EJ, Maughan PH, Kakarla UK, et al. Surgical technique and outcomes in the treatment of spinal cord ependymomas: part II: myxopapillary ependymoma. Neurosurgery 2011;68(1 Suppl Operative):90–94; discussion 94.

Chapter 33

Release of the Sternocleidomastoid Muscle

Gokce Mik and Denis S. Drummond

DEFINITION

■ The sternocleidomastoid (SCM) muscle is a major muscle of the neck that laterally flexes and rotates the head.

■ The term *torticollis* comes from the Latin words *tortus* (twisted) and *collum* (neck). It refers to a clinical deformity where the head tilts in one direction and the neck rotates to the opposite side involuntarily.

■ Congenital muscular torticollis (CMT) associated with a contracture of the SCM muscle is the most common etiology of torticollis in infants.

■ CMT is the third most common congenital deformity, next to developmental dysplasia of the hip and congenital clubfoot. The incidence of CMT ranges from 0.4% to 1.3%.[3,6,10]

■ Shortening and contracture of the SCM muscle results in tightness that gives the typical clinical appearance, which is detected at birth or shortly thereafter.

■ Cheng et al[3] subdivided the CMT patients into three groups:
  ■ Clinically palpable sternomastoid "tumor" or pseudotumor
  ■ Muscular torticollis group without palpable or visible tumor but with clinical thickening or tightness of the SCM on the affected side
    ■ All the clinical features of torticollis with neither a palpable mass nor tightness of the SCM muscle

ANATOMY

■ On each side, the SCM muscle passes obliquely across the side of the neck and divides the neck into anterior and posterior triangles.

■ It originates from two heads:
  ■ Sternal head: superior and anterior surface of manubrium sterni.
  ■ Clavicular head: superior surface of medial third of clavicle. With the two heads combining, the muscle ascends laterally and posteriorly to insert in the mastoid process of the temporal bone.

■ The functions of sternocleidomastoid are multiple:
  ■ With unilateral contraction, it:
    ■ Flexes the head and cervical spine ipsilaterally
    ■ Laterally rotates the head to the contralateral side
  ■ With bilateral contraction, it:
    ■ Protracts the head
    ■ Extends the incompletely extended cervical spine

■ The SCM is innervated by the:
  ■ Spinal accessory nerve (XI)
  ■ Ventral ramus of second cervical nerve (C2)

■ The spinal accessory nerve penetrates the deep surface of the SCM muscle, giving off a branch that supplies it. It passes to the posterior aspect of the SCM deep to Erb's point.

■ Erb's point is located roughly in the middle of the posterior border of the SCM muscle. At this point, the anterior branch of the greater auricular nerve crosses the SCM.

■ The external jugular vein is located anterior to the SCM muscle at the proximal part. It crosses the SCM muscle

obliquely at its midpoint and ends at the subclavian vein posteroinferior to the SCM muscle.

■ The SCM protects the carotid artery and internal jugular vein, both of which lie deep to it.

■ The clavicular origin of the SCM muscle can vary in size. In some cases, the width of the clavicular attachment may extend to the midpoint of the clavicle.

■ The anatomy of the SCM muscle and important surrounding structures is shown in **FIGURE 1**.

PATHOGENESIS

■ The most common etiology of CMT in infants is contracture or shortening of the SCM muscle.

■ Infants with CMT most often have a history of difficult or traumatic delivery.

■ Davids et al[7] reported that the position of the head and neck in utero or during labor or delivery can lead to local trauma to the SCM muscle. This is the only muscle in the SCM muscle compartment demonstrated by cadaver studies.

■ Progressive fibrosis and contracture of the SCM muscle may be the sequelae of an intrauterine or perinatal compartment syndrome.[7]

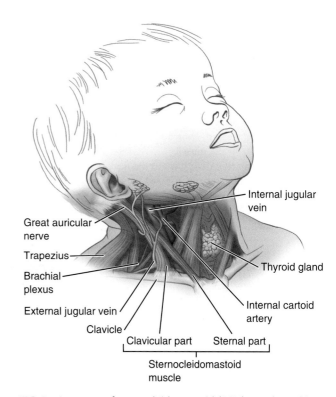

FIG 1 ■ Anatomy of sternocleidomastoid (SCM) muscle and important surrounding structures. Note the course of the external jugular vein and greater auricular nerve; the carotid artery and internal jugular vein lie deep to the SCM muscle.

- CMT may occur in association with oligohydramnios, multiple births, first-born children, and developmental dysplasia of the hip (DDH).
  - These data support the theory of intrauterine restricted fetal motion and malpositioning of the head and neck. These conditions may be associated with more difficult and traumatic deliveries.
  - However, CMT found in the infants who are delivered by cesarean section is not consistent with the theory of birth trauma.
  - The data that show 20% coexistence of developmental dysplasia of the hip support the theory of intrauterine malposition and crowding.[9]
- About 50% of patients with CMT are born with a clinically palpable SCM tumor.[1,5] This tumor or pseudotumor is believed to be a developing hematoma that undergoes subsequent fibrosis. This could result from either birth trauma or intrauterine malposition.
- Electron microscopy studies revealed that the existence of myoblasts in the interstitium of the mass at different stages of differentiation and degeneration might have a significant bearing on the pathogenesis of torticollis.[13]
  - Tang et al[13] explained the success of conservative management (stretching exercises) with the presence of myoblast cells besides fibroblast cells.
  - In vitro, myoblasts could be mechanically stimulated to undergo both hypertrophy and hyperplasia by intermittent stretching and relaxation.
- The pathogenesis of the torticollis resulting from pathologies other than CMT is affiliated with other conditions or syndromes.

NATURAL HISTORY

- Diagnosis of CMT is usually made at or near birth. Other causes of torticollis generally present later (4 months to 1 year).
- A mass (SCM tumor) or fullness in the SCM muscle usually exists within a few weeks or months after delivery.
- Typically, the mass decreases in size and disappears between 6 and 12 months of age.
- If it remains untreated, contraction and sometimes a fibrous bundle can occur in the muscle.
- Flexion and rotation deformity of the neck begins in infancy.
  - Typically the head turns toward the involved side and the chin points to the opposite shoulder.
  - Plagiocephaly and facial asymmetry may be present early on; they increase with time.

- In persistent cases, deformity progresses and becomes inflexible.
- Flattening of the skull and facial bones can develop on the affected or normal side depending on the sleeping position of the child.
- If the child remains untreated until 5 to 7 years of age, contraction of the neck with limited motion becomes resistant to correction. The deformity of the cranium and facial bones also becomes less amenable to spontaneous correction.
  - Formation of a lateral band is mostly responsible for limited neck mobility.
- In older children with persistent deformity, radiographic abnormalities can also occur; they include asymmetry of the articular facets of the axis, tilt of the odontoid process to the side of the torticollis, and possibly cervicothoracic scoliosis.[2,12]

PATIENT HISTORY AND PHYSICAL FINDINGS

- A complete history and physical examination should be done in newborns with torticollis.
  - The incidence of the breech presentation and birth trauma in children with CMT is higher than the general population.
- There is known coexistence of DDH with torticollis.
  - The reported incidence of DDH with CMT varies from 8% to 20%.[9,15]
  - A clinical examination of the hip and ultrasonography screening are thus required for children with CMT.
  - A previous belief that CMT was associated with metatarsus adductus and clubfoot is not supported by the literature.
- Typically, children with CMT hold their head laterally flexed to the affected side and rotate their face to the opposite side.
- Range of neck movement can initially be normal in infants with CMT. Later, the typical deformity can usually be observed. This gradually progresses as the muscle contracture becomes tighter.
  - Any degree of restriction should be noted during the examination.
- The facial bones and cranium are observed for asymmetry. Any flattening of the skull bones is also noted.
- With palpation, a nontender, soft mass of 1 to 2 cm is occasionally found in the lower or middle third of the SCM muscle. With time, the mass changes to a fibrous bundle, and the SCM tendon can then be identified as a tight band that resists correction (**FIG 2**).

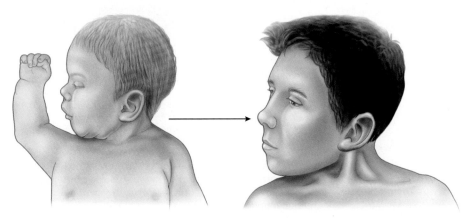

FIG 2 • A nontender, soft mass of 1 to 2 cm can be found in the lower or middle third of the sternocleidomastoid (SCM) muscle within weeks or a few months after delivery. At later ages (usually after 6 to 12 months of age), the mass changes to a fibrous bundle and the SCM tendon then can be identified as a tight band.

■ The flexible deformity seen in the early stage can be corrected by gentle stretching.

IMAGING AND OTHER DIAGNOSTIC STUDIES

■ Radiographs
  ■ Standard cervical spine anteroposterior and lateral views and open-mouth odontoid views are obtained to rule out bony abnormalities such as atlantoaxial instability or fixation, cervical fusion, cervical scoliosis, and odontoid anomalies.
  ■ At the later phases of the developing deformity, radiographic abnormalities such as asymmetry of the articular facets of the axis, tilt of the odontoid process to the side of the torticollis, and sometimes cervicothoracic scoliosis may be observed.[2,12]
■ Ultrasound examination should be performed in children with a palpable SCM mass to demonstrate the fibrotic lesion within the SCM muscle and to differentiate the mass from other pathologies in the neck such as neoplasms, cysts, and vascular malformations.
  ■ In a recent study Tang et al[14] presented their observations with the use of ultrasound for the long-term follow-up of CMT. They noticed that CMT is a polymorphic and dynamic condition rather than a fixed presentation. The alterations of the fibrosis in muscle can affect the type of treatment.
■ Hip ultrasonography should be routinely done in patients born with CMT.
  ■ There is a relatively high incidence of coexistence between CMT and DDH.
■ Some investigators have advised MRI to evaluate the muscle for thickening and fibrosis; however, it does not provide additional information. Further, for infants, MRI requires a general anesthetic, with its associated risks.
  ■ If a posterior fossa tumor is suspected, MRI is indicated.

DIFFERENTIAL DIAGNOSIS

■ Ophthalmologic torticollis occurs with oculomotor imbalance, which is usually observed after the development of focusing skills (3 months). Ophthalmologic torticollis is caused by a weakness of one of the oculomotor muscles of the eye (typically the superior oblique). This causes a strabismus that can be observed if the head tilt is manually corrected. (This maneuver is useful in providing a diagnosis.) Other causes are strabismus and nystagmus.
■ Neurologic causes such as the postural head tilt seen with posterior fossa tumors must be ruled out.
  ■ Nucci et al,[11] in a multidisciplinary study, reported 25 ocular and 4 neurologic causes in 65 children with abnormal head posture.
  ■ About 10% of posterior fossa tumors initially present with torticollis.
■ The other orthopaedic causes of torticollis include congenital cervical vertebral anomalies (scoliosis, Klippel-Feil syndrome) and atlantoaxial rotational instability.
■ Grissel syndrome: torticollis associated with retropharyngeal abscess or post-tonsillectomy status.
■ Neck abscess or inflammatory disorders
■ Sandifer syndrome (reflux)
■ Neurologic
  ■ Posterior fossa tumors
  ■ Dystonia

NONOPERATIVE MANAGEMENT

■ The initial treatment of CMT is nonoperative and is successful in the vast majority of infants by 1 year of age.
■ A program of gentle stretching exercises should include flexion–extension, lateral bending away from the involved side and rotation toward it.
■ Stretching exercises can be done by a physical therapist or by the parents with a home program.
  ■ In our experience, a supervised home program monitored by a physical therapist is the most successful method.
■ Manual stretching should be continued until full neck rotation is achieved.
■ In children 1 year of age or less, the plagiocephaly and facial asymmetry usually remodel spontaneously after the child regains full range of motion of the neck.
■ Cervical orthoses may be an adjunct and support for children whose lateral head tilt does not resolve with exercises, or for older children who no longer tolerate stretching.
■ The duration of the conservative treatment could be longer in children who have SCM tumor at initial presentation.
  ■ The success rate of manual stretching in these patients is lower than those without a SCM tumor.[4]
■ Surgery is recommended for recalcitrant deformity when adequate correction is not achieved by 1 year of age.
■ Children who present after 1 year of age with or without previous treatment are candidates for surgery if they have:
  ■ Significant head tilt with tight band or contracture of the SCM muscle
  ■ Limitation of passive head rotation and lateral flexion by more than 10 to 15 degrees

SURGICAL MANAGEMENT

■ Surgical intervention is indicated for children who have not responded to nonoperative treatment applied for a minimum of 6 months and for children who present with a significant deformity after 1 year of age.
■ The hypothesis is that the sooner correction of the torticollis is achieved, the better the chance for spontaneous correction of the plagiocephaly and facial asymmetry.
■ If there is doubt about the diagnosis of CMT, surgery is contraindicated until a workup has been completed because there could be an underlying disorder causing torticollis, such as ocular or neurogenic pathologies.
■ The operative techniques described for CMT are based on release or lengthening of the tight and shortened SCM muscle.
■ Most commonly preferred procedures include unipolar release, bipolar release with or without Z-plasty lengthening of the sternal head, and the extended procedure for older children and resistant cases.
  ■ Open, percutaneous, and endoscopic techniques have been described for these procedures. We have no experience with endoscopic technique, and we prefer the open approach.

Authors' Preferred Treatment

■ For infants, a home stretching program is taught and supervised by a physical therapist for 6 months.
■ In children with appropriate surgical indications, bipolar release (with or without Z-plasty lengthening) is carried out.
■ In older children with significant deformity, a bipolar release is the first step. Z-plasty may be appropriate in the older children to provide a symmetric appearance postoperatively.

- If satisfactory correction is not demonstrated at intraoperative examination, the distal dissection is extended to permit release of the clavicular head and remaining bands.

Preoperative Planning

- Cervical spine radiographs should be reviewed before surgery to look for bony anomalies or cervical scoliosis.
- In fixed deformities, positioning of the head can be difficult for the anesthesiologist. Flexible fiberoptic intubation should then be considered.
- The ear is taped anteriorly and hair around the mastoid process is shaved.

Positioning

- The procedure is performed under general anesthesia in the supine position. A sandbag is placed to elevate the shoulder on the affected side.

- The endotracheal tube should be kept at the unaffected side so as not to interfere with the operative field.
- Draping should allow the correction to be evaluated by bending the neck. This determines the adequacy of the release intraoperatively.
  - The shoulder draping should permit the anesthesiologist to hold the shoulder, which can maximize tension during this test.
- The neck is bent toward the unaffected side and the head is rotated to the affected side so that the SCM muscle is kept under tension and the origin and insertion can be clearly identified.

INCISION AND DISSECTION

- For the release of the distal pole of the SCM muscle, a transverse, 3- to 4-cm-long incision is made 1 cm superior to the clavicle and between the two heads of the SCM muscle (**TECH FIG 1**).
- The subcutaneous tissue and platysma muscle are divided in the line of incision and the tendon sheaths of the clavicular and sternal heads are exposed.
- For the proximal pole exposure, a 2- to 3-cm horizontal incision is made just distal to the tip of the mastoid process.
- The dissection is carried deeper until the periosteum of the mastoid process is exposed. The insertion of the muscle is then exposed subperiosteally.

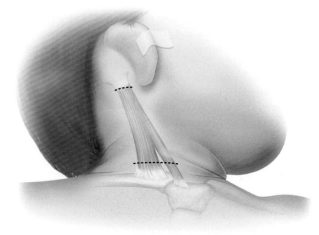

TECH FIG 1 • Proximal and distal incisions (*dotted lines*).

DISTAL UNIPOLAR RELEASE

- Distal unipolar release includes the release of the sternal and sometimes the clavicular heads of the SCM muscle. It may be enough for mild deformities.
- A transverse incision is placed parallel and 1 cm proximal to the clavicle between the clavicular and sternal heads of the SCM.
- An incision that overlies over the clavicle may result in a hypertrophic scar. A higher incision may jeopardize the external jugular vein and may also lead to an unsightly scar.
- Two heads of the SCM muscle are identified as described.
- Surrounding fascia is cleared and the sternal head or both heads are undermined with a curved clamp.
- The muscles are elevated with the help of a clamp and divided using electrocautery (**TECH FIG 2**).
- Alternatively, the sternal head can be lengthened by Z-plasty.

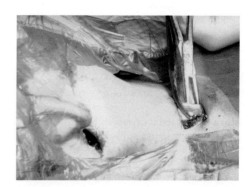

TECH FIG 2 • The origin of the muscle is elevated with the help of a clamp and divided using electrocautery. About 5 to 10 mm of muscle–tendon segment is divided to prevent further contracture and fibrous adhesions.

- About 5 to 10 mm of the muscle–tendon segment is excised to prevent further contracture and fibrous adhesions.
- The adequacy of the release is checked by bending the neck to the contralateral side and rotating it to the ipsi- lateral side while palpating the area with a fingertip to identify any remaining tight bands. They are completely released.
- The incision is closed with subcuticular suture after careful hemostasis.

BIPOLAR RELEASE (AUTHORS' PREFERENCE)

- Bipolar release includes the release of the mastoid insertion of the SCM muscle along with the distal release just described.
- The procedure starts with a distal incision.
- The two heads of the SCM muscle are identified. After undermining the tendons, the curved clamp is left underneath them.
- The curved clamp is left lying superficial to the wound but deep to the tendon. While applying enough tension, ease the proximal exposure and identification of the insertion. The wound is then covered with a moist sponge.
  - With the tension applied by the clamp under the tendon at the distal exposure, a safe identification of the origin has been simplified. Further, the limited exposure avoids the important anatomy (TECH FIG 3A).
- Attention is directed to the proximal insertion and the incision is placed as described before.
- The insertion of the muscle is identified anteriorly and posteriorly. Dissection starts subperiosteally from the mastoid process to avoid the facial nerve anteriorly and the anterior branch of the great auricular nerve inferiorly.

- A curved clamp is passed just deep to the tendon to elevate it so it can be sectioned completely (TECH FIG 3B).
  - There is no need to resect a segment of muscle at the proximal part.
- After the proximal release is performed, attention is then directed back to the distal incision and distal release is completed as described before.
  - Release of the clavicular head with the lengthening of the sternal head by Z-plasty may be appropriate in older children to provide a symmetrical appearance postoperatively (TECH FIG 3C).[8]
- The neck is rotated and bent with the help of the anesthesia team while checking the area with a fingertip to identify any remaining tight bands; they are completely released.
- Both surgical areas are checked to identify if any remaining tight bands or fascial structures are impeding full correction. They are divided carefully.
- Subcutaneous and subcuticular skin closure is then performed after hemostasis.

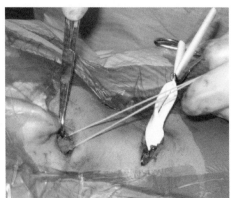
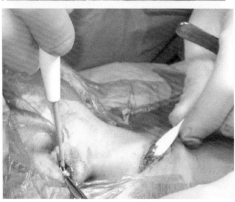
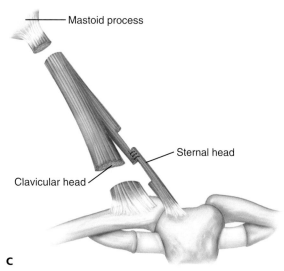

TECH FIG 3 • **A.** With tension applied to the tendon at the distal exposure, a safe identification of the origin has been simplified. Further, the limited exposure avoids the important anatomy. **B.** A curved clamp is passed just deep to the tendon to elevate it for complete sectioning. **C.** Bipolar release with the lengthening of the sternal head by Z-plasty. (**C:** Modified from Ferkel RD, Westin GW, Dawson EG, et al. Muscular torticollis: a modified approach. J Bone Joint Surg Am 1983;65:894–890.)

PEARLS AND PITFALLS

Approach	▪ The distal pole incision is made about 1 cm superior and parallel to the clavicle.
	▪ Superficial scars just over the clavicle may result in hypertrophic scar and unacceptable cosmesis.
	▪ Incisions close to the midpoint of SCM may compromise the external jugular vein and neurologic structures and may lead to an unacceptable scar.
	▪ To avoid complications, the proximal horizontal incision is placed just distal to the tip of the mastoid process. Applying tension under the tendon distally simplifies safe identification of the insertion.
Unipolar release	▪ Unipolar release is used only in younger patients with mild deformities. Generally, a bipolar approach is better.
Bipolar release	▪ A bipolar release is more likely to avoid residual and recurrent deformity. The surgeon should not hesitate to perform this procedure before 1 year of age in resistant cases (9 to 12 months).
	▪ The SCM tendon is first exposed at the origin in the distal wound. The tendon or tendons are elevated to provide tension; the proximal release is then performed; and finally the distal release is completed.

POSTOPERATIVE CARE

▪ Postoperative management includes immobilization of the head and neck in a slightly overcorrected position with a thermoplastic custom-made brace or pinless halo for 3 weeks (**FIG 3**).

▪ The purpose of the brace immobilization is to avoid a habitual posture followed by postoperative scarring. It might also help to reprogram the corrected posture as a norm for the child.

▪ The brace is removed in 3 weeks and passive stretching is recommended as well as active strengthening exercises.

▪ Exercises are continued at home for 3 to 6 months.

OUTCOMES

▪ Early conservative management is successful in over 90% of children with CMT who are younger than 1 year.[3,4,6]

▪ In resistant cases there is still controversy between unipolar and bipolar release.

▪ Cheng et al[3–5] reported excellent results in children operated on at age 6 months to 2 years with unipolar release.

▪ Canale et al[1] found better results after bipolar release, although the difference was not statistically significant.

▪ Wirth et al[16] reported satisfactory results in 48 of 55 patients who had undergone bipolar release, with low recurrence rates (1.8%).

▪ Ferkel et al[8] described a modified bipolar release technique that includes release of the mastoid and clavicular attachments of the SCM muscle and Z-plasty lengthening on the sternal origin to maintain a V contour of the neck distally for cosmesis. They reported 92% satisfactory results with this technique.

▪ We have had one case of recurrence with unipolar release and none with bipolar release in about 50 cases. There have been no wound problems, hypertrophic scarring, or neurovascular complications.

COMPLICATIONS

▪ Wound breakdown
▪ Hematoma
▪ Residual lateral band
▪ Neurovascular damage
  ▪ Spinal accessory nerve
  ▪ Anterior branch of the great auricular nerve
  ▪ External jugular vein
  ▪ Carotid artery
▪ Hypertrophic scar

REFERENCES

1. Canale ST, Griffin DW, Hubbard CN. Congenital muscular torticollis: a long-term follow-up. J Bone Joint Surg Am 1982;64:810–816.
2. Chen CE, Ko JY. Surgical treatment of muscular torticollis for patients above 6 years of age. Arch Orthop Trauma Surg 2000;120:149–151.
3. Cheng JCY, Tang SP, Chen TMK, et al. The clinical presentation and outcomes of treatment of congenital muscular torticollis in infants: a study of 1086 cases. J Pediatr Surg 2000;35:1091–1095.
4. Cheng JCY, Wong MWN, Tang SP, et al. Clinical determinants of the outcome of manual stretching in the treatment of congenital muscular torticollis in infants. J Bone Joint Surg Am 2001;83:679–687.
5. Cheng JCY, Tang SP, Chen TMK. Sternocleidomastoid pseudotumor and congenital muscular torticollis in infants: a prospective study of 510 cases. J Pediatr 1999;134:712–716.
6. Coventry MB, Harris LE. Congenital muscular torticollis in infancy: some observations regarding treatment. J Bone Joint Surg Am 1959;41:815–822.
7. Davids JR, Wenger DR, Mubarak SJ. Congenital muscular torticollis: sequela of intrauterine or perinatal compartment syndrome. J Pediatr Orthop 1993;13:141–147.
8. Ferkel RD, Westin GW, Dawson EG, et al. Muscular torticollis: a modified approach. J Bone Joint Surg Am 1983;65:894–900.
9. Hummer CD, Macewen GD. The coexistence of torticollis and congenital dysplasia of the hip. J Bone Joint Surg Am 1972;54:1255–1256.
10. Ling CM, Low YS. Sternocleidomastoid tumor and muscular torticollis. Clin Orthop Relat Res 1972;86:144–150.

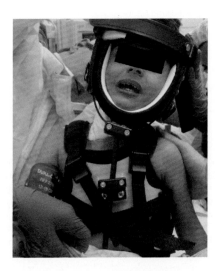

FIG 3 ▪ Pinless halo device for postoperative management.

11. Nucci P, Kushner BJ, Serafino M, et al. A multi-disciplinary study of the ocular, orthopaedic, and neurologic causes of abnormal head postures in children. Am J Opthalmol 2005;140:65–68.

12. Oh I, Nowacek CJ. Surgical release of congenital torticollis in adults. Clin Othop Relat Res 1978;131:141–145.

13. Tang S, Liu Z, Quan X, et al. Sternocleidomastoid pseudotumor of infants and congenital muscular torticollis: fine-structure research. J Pediatr Orthop 1998;18:214–218.

14. Tang SF, Hsu KH, Wong AM, et al. Longitudinal follow-up study of ultrasonography in congenital muscular torticollis. Clin Orthop Relat Res 2002;403:179–185.

15. Walsh JJ, Morrissy RT. Torticollis and hip dislocation. J Pediatr Orthop 1998;18:219–221.

16. Wirth CJ, Hagena FW, Wuelker N, et al. Biterminal tenotomy for the treatment of the muscular torticollis. J Bone Joint Surg Am 1992;74:427–434.

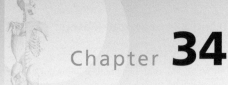

Chapter 34

Segmental Hook and Pedicle Screw Instrumentation for Scoliosis

James T. Guille and Reginald S. Fayssoux

DEFINITION

- Reduction of scoliotic spinal deformity via posterior spinal fusion with instrumentation allows for improvement of the cosmetic appearance of the child or adolescent with scoliosis and prevents curve progression. The goal is to balance these advantages with the inherent risks of instrumentation and reduction maneuvers.
- Instrumentation provides an internal construct holding the spine in its corrected position until spinal fusion is achieved (about 6 months) and obviates the need for postoperative immobilization. A Cobb angle measurement greater than 10 degrees distinguishes minor spine asymmetry from true scoliosis.
- Segmental instrumentation with hooks and pedicle screws provides multiple fixation points, allowing for three-dimensional correction of the scoliotic spine.
- Instrumentation is introduced after posterior exposure of the thoracic or lumbar spine.

ANATOMY

- A thorough knowledge of scoliotic spinal anatomy is critical for the safe placement of instrumentation.
- In the scoliotic spine there is rotation of the vertebral bodies in the transverse plane, with the spinous processes rotating toward the concavity of the curve.
- Anatomy of the posterior elements
  - In the scoliotic spine, the pedicles on the concave side are narrower than those on the convexity, especially at the apex of the curve (**FIG 1A**).[12]
  - The intervertebral foramina in the thoracic spine are larger and deeper than in any other region of the spine, with the exiting nerve root occupying less than 25% of the foramen and coursing through its midportion.
  - Lumbar nerve roots pass adjacent to the inferomedial aspect of the pedicle and lie superior within the foramina.
- Scoliotic deformity affects not only the bony anatomy but also the relationship of the spine to the adjacent soft tissue elements.
  - The aorta is posterolateral to its normal position, putting it at risk for injury with left-sided lateral pedicular breaches (**FIG 1B**).
  - The spinal cord hugs the concavity of the curve such that the width of the epidural space is less than 1 mm at the thoracic apical vertebral levels on the concave side; it is 3 to 5 mm on the convex side.[8]

Thoracic Spine Anatomy

- The thoracic facets are more coronally oriented in comparison to the more sagittally oriented lumbar facets.
- Pedicle anatomy for placement of pedicle screws

- Dimensions
  - In scoliotic spines, average thoracic pedicle length (distance from the posterior cortical starting point to the posterior longitudinal ligament in line with the axis of the pedicle) is 16 to 22 mm.
  - Average thoracic cord length (distance from the posterior cortical starting point to the anterior vertebral cortex in line with the axis of the pedicle) is 34 to 52 mm; it is typically greater on the concavity.
- Coronal anatomy
  - In the scoliotic spine, the medial wall is two to three times thicker than the lateral wall at all thoracic levels. This may be why most screw-related pedicle fractures occur laterally.

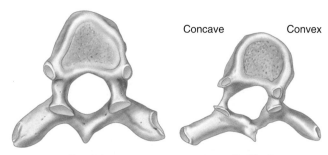

FIG 1 • **A.** Comparison of a normal thoracic vertebra on the left and a scoliotic thoracic vertebra on the right. Note the narrowed concave pedicle on the scoliotic vertebra. **B.** Thoracic-level axial magnetic resonance imaging in a patient with a right thoracic scoliotic curve. Note the posterolateral position of the aorta. (**B:** From Sucato DJ, Duchene C. The position of the aorta relative to the spine: a comparison of patients with and without idiopathic scoliosis. J Bone Joint Surg Am 2003;85A:1461–1469. Reprinted with permission from The Journal of Bone and Joint Surgery, Inc.)

- The coronal anatomy of the thoracic pedicle varies, moving from anterior to posterior. The likelihood of pedicle wall breach is greatest midway between the lamina and body with placement of screws.
- Pedicle width decreases from T1 to T4 and then gradually increases to T12, while pedicle height and length tend to increase from T1 to T12.
  - Main pedicle diameter is 4 to 6 mm in thoracic scoliosis.
  - Endosteal pedicle width in the apical region of the thoracic spine measures 2.5 to 4.2 mm on the concavity of the curve and 4.1 to 5.0 mm on the convexity of the curve.
- In the thoracic spine, transverse processes do not align with the pedicle in the axial plane: they are rostral to the pedicle in the upper thoracic spine and caudal to the pedicle in the lower thoracic spine (crossover occurs at T6–7).
- Transverse orientation
  - T12 pedicles are perpendicular to the floor in the transverse plane.
  - T1 pedicles subtend an angle of about 25 to 30 degrees with the midline in the transverse plane.
  - Thoracic pedicles progressively angle outward in the transverse plane, proceeding superiorly from T12 to T1.
- Thoracic pedicle screw starting points
  - As one proceeds proximally from T12 there is a trend toward a more medial and cephalad pedicle starting point as one proceeds to the apex of the thoracic spine (**FIG 2** and Table 1).
  - This then transitions to a trend toward a more lateral and caudal pedicle starting point as one proceeds proximally from the apex.

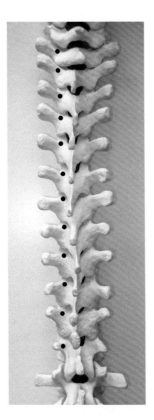

FIG 2 • Thoracic vertebrae starting points (see Table 1).

Table 1	Thoracic Pedicle Screw Starting Points	
Level	**Cephalad–Caudad Starting Points**	**Medial–Lateral Starting Points**
T1	Midpoint TP	Junction TP and lamina
T2	Midpoint TP	Junction TP and lamina
T3	Midpoint TP	Junction TP and lamina
T4	Junction between proximal third and midpoint TP	Junction TP and lamina
T5	Proximal third TP	Junction TP and lamina
T6	Junction of proximal edge and proximal third TP	Junction TP and lamina and facet
T7	Proximal TP	Midpoint facet
T8	Proximal TP	Midpoint facet
T9	Proximal TP	Midpoint facet
T10	Junction of proximal edge and proximal third TP	Junction TP and lamina and facet
T11	Proximal third TP	Just medial to pars
T12	Midpoint TP	At level of lateral pars

TP, thoracic pedicle.

Lumbar Spine Anatomy

- The lumbar vertebral facets are more sagittally oriented in comparison to thoracic vertebral facets.
- Pedicles
  - Dimensions
    - In scoliotic spines, average lumbar pedicle length is 20 to 22 mm.
    - Average lumbar cord length is 45 to 48 mm.
  - Coronal anatomy
    - Average lumbar endosteal pedicle width is 4.8 to 9.5 mm.
    - The larger size of the lumbar pedicles increases the likelihood of optimal placement of pedicle screws.
  - Transverse orientation
    - L1 pedicles are perpendicular to the floor in the transverse plane.
    - L5 pedicles subtend an angle of about 25 to 30 degrees with the midline in the transverse plane.
    - Lumbar pedicles progressively angle outward in the transverse plane, proceeding inferiorly from L1 to L5.
  - Lumbar pedicle screw starting points
    - The long axis of the pedicle pierces the lamina at the intersection of two lines: a vertical line tangential to the lateral border of the superior articular process, and a horizontal line bisecting the transverse process (**FIG 3**).
    - The point of intersection for these two lines lies in the angle between the superior articular process and the base of the transverse process.
- Dangers
  - Medial pedicular breaches endanger the dural sac, especially on the concavity of the curve.
  - Inferior pedicular breaches endanger the nerve root, especially in the lumbar spine.
  - Advancement of pedicle screws following a lateral pedicular breach on the left can endanger the lung, segmental vessels, and sympathetic chain (T4–T12) and the aorta (T5–T10).

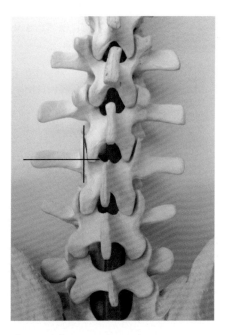

FIG 3 • Lumbar vertebrae starting points.

- Advancement of pedicle screws following a lateral pedicular breach on the right can endanger the lung, segmental vessels, sympathetic chain, and azygous vein (T5–T11).
- Advancement of pedicle screws following a breach of the anterior cortex on the right can endanger the superior intercostal vessels (T4–T5), the esophagus (T4–T9), the azygous vein (T5–T11), the inferior vena cava (T11–T12), and the thoracic duct (T4–T12).
- Advancement of pedicle screws following a breach of the anterior cortex on the left can endanger the esophagus (T4–T9) and the aorta (T5–T12).

PATHOGENESIS

- Idiopathic
- Congenital
  - Failure of formation or segmentation of vertebral precursors leading to asymmetric vertebral growth with subsequent abnormal curvature
- Neuromuscular
  - Variety of etiologies, such as cerebral palsy, muscular dystrophy, polio, spinal muscular atrophy, and myelomeningocele
  - Related to an inability to provide muscular support to the spinal column

NATURAL HISTORY

Idiopathic

- Infantile (0 to 3 years of age)
  - Less than 1% of all cases of idiopathic scoliosis
  - More common in boys
  - Left thoracic curves predominate
  - Most resolve spontaneously
- Juvenile (3 to 10 years of age)
  - 8% to 16% of all cases of idiopathic scoliosis
  - More even female:male ratio
  - Bracing may correct some curves
  - Curves of more than 30 degrees usually progress to surgery

- Adolescent (10 to 18 years of age)
  - Most common form of idiopathic scoliosis
  - Etiology and pathogenesis are not well understood
- Family history is positive in 30% of cases but does not predict curve magnitude or progression.
- More common in girls. The female:male ratio is 1.4:1 for curves 11 to 20 degrees and increases to 5:1 for curves greater than 20 degrees.
- Curves have the greatest chance of progression in the period of peak growth velocity leading up to skeletal maturity (prior to menses in females), after which the potential decreases significantly.[15]
- Scoliotic curves measuring less than 20 degrees are at lower risk for progression.
- Scoliotic curves measuring greater than 50 degrees are at higher risk for further progression during adult life (with a percentage of these progressing at a rate of about one degree per year).[19]
- There are no significant differences in the prevalence of back pain between adults with scoliotic spines and the general population.[17,20]
- Scoliotic curves measuring greater than 100 degrees have an increased prevalence of cardiopulmonary compromise (eg, cor pulmonale, restrictive lung disease).[17]

Congenital

- Severity of deformity related to type and location of anomaly
- Highest chance of curve progression with unilateral unsegmented bar with contralateral hemivertebrae (nearly 100%), followed by a lone unilateral unsegmented bar, double convex hemivertebrae, single convex hemivertebrae, and finally the block vertebrae[16]

Neuromuscular

- Most curves are progressive and are more difficult to manage nonoperatively.
- Curves can cause pelvic obliquity and sitting problems in nonambulatory individuals.

PATIENT HISTORY AND PHYSICAL FINDINGS

- Complete history, including age at onset, timing of growth spurts, menses, presence of pain, family history of scoliosis, nerve, or muscle diseases
- A complete examination is important to obtain a diagnosis because certain etiologies can predispose the patient to increased operative risk (eg, cardiac abnormalities in patients with Marfan syndrome).
- The skin is inspected for café-au-lait spots, the axilla for freckling, and the lumbosacral area for sinus tracts, hairy patches, or dimples. Axillary freckling and multiple café-au-lait spots are associated with neurofibromatosis. Sinus tracts, hairy patches, or dimples in the lumbosacral area are associated with intraspinal anomaly.
- The Adams forward bending test detects curvatures by physical examination. Abnormalities in vertebral rotation become apparent as an asymmetrical rib hump, prominence, or fullness, leading to possible identification of patients at risk for having scoliosis.
- Any shoulder or scapular asymmetry is noted. It is important to point out to parents that this is not always corrected by surgery.

- Pelvic obliquity can indicate a possible leg-length discrepancy that can mimic a lumbar scoliosis.
- Trunk shift and sagittal profile are noted; these indicate coronal balance and sagittal balance, respectively.

IMAGING AND OTHER DIAGNOSTIC STUDIES

- Placement of a pedicle screw at the thoracolumbar junction followed by intraoperative fluoroscopic imaging accurately identifies vertebral level.
- With use of intraoperative fluoroscopic imaging guidance, knowledge of anatomy remains critical in order to orient the intensifier to obtain the best coronal images of the pedicles.
- Radiographic criteria used to evaluate accurate screw placement
  - Harmonious segmental change of the tips of the pedicle screws on the posteroanterior (PA) radiograph
  - No crossing of the medial pedicle wall by the tip of the pedicle screw with reference to vertebral rotation on the PA radiograph
  - No violation of the imaginary midline of the vertebral body by the tip of the pedicle screw on the PA radiograph
  - No breach of the anterior cortex of the vertebral body on the lateral radiograph

DIFFERENTIAL DIAGNOSIS

- Scoliosis
  - Idiopathic
  - Congenital
  - Neuromuscular
- Limb-length discrepancy
- Osteoid osteoma
- Sprengel deformity

NONOPERATIVE MANAGEMENT

- Observation for progression for curves of 0 to 20 degrees. Patients are followed with serial clinical and radiographic examinations.
- Bracing for progressive curves of 20 to 40 degrees if the patient is skeletally immature. Braces are unable to correct curves; their purpose is to prevent curve progression.

SURGICAL MANAGEMENT

Preoperative Planning

- PA and lateral radiographic views of the entire spine.
- Supine bending radiographs may show pedicles not visible on the PA view.
- Convex apical pedicles greater than 5 mm in diameter on the PA radiographs are large enough to accommodate pedicle screw placement.
- Computed tomographic (CT) imaging can be used to evaluate pedicle morphology, with images oriented perpendicular to the plane of the vertebrae.
- Fusion levels are chosen based on the Lenke criteria.

Hook Placement

- Advantages
  - Technically easier, especially at levels with small pedicles (apical concave pedicles)
  - Less operative time

- Disadvantages
  - Increased canal intrusion in comparison to pedicular fixation
  - Lack of three-column fixation
  - Decreased ability to perform correctional derotational maneuvers
- Types of hooks
  - Laminar hooks: should be used with caution in the neurologically intact patient
    - Thoracic laminar hooks: downgoing sloped hooks
    - Lumbar laminar hooks: upgoing or downgoing C-shaped hooks
  - Thoracic transverse process hooks: downgoing C-shaped hooks
  - Thoracic pedicle hooks: upgoing claw-tip hooks placed under the lamina
  - Offset hooks: offset laterally to lie in line with pedicle screws for use in hybrid constructs
- Hook patterns for an isolated thoracic curve
  - Concave side
    - Upgoing pedicle hook on upper end and upper intermediate vertebrae
    - Downgoing laminar hook on lower end and lower intermediate vertebra
  - Convex side
    - Claw construct at upper end vertebrae.
    - Downgoing transverse process hook with upgoing pedicle hook at the same level or next-distal level. Splitting the claw over two levels (split claw) better resists rotational forces.

Pedicle Screw Placement

- Advantages
  - Pedicle screws have significantly higher axial pullout strengths than supralaminar hooks and pedicle hooks.
  - Better correction in the coronal and axial planes.
  - Less decrease in pulmonary function than anterior surgery.
  - No implants in the canal during the correction phase.
  - Correction not gained by pure distraction.
  - Fewer fusion levels.
  - No crankshaft.
  - Larger area for bone graft.
  - Allows earlier postoperative activity.
- Disadvantages
  - Steep learning curve.
  - Caudal or medial penetration can result in dural or neural injury.
  - Lateral penetration can cause vascular injury.
  - Increased operative time.
  - Costly procedures.
- Complications
  - Suboptimal screw position
    - More common in cases of severe deformity
    - Perforation not uncommon (up to 40% of screws in some series)
    - Lateral perforation more common than medial perforation
    - Lowest containment rates in midthoracic spine (T5 to T8)
  - Dural, neural, or vascular injuries occur infrequently.

- Types of pedicle screws
  - Monoaxial
    - No motion between the screw and the screw head
    - Can obtain axial correction of deformity
  - Uniaxial
    - Motion between the screw and the screw head constrained to one plane
    - Can accommodate sagittal contours while retaining ability to obtain axial correction (derotation)
  - Polyaxial
    - Multiaxial motion allowed between screw and screw head
    - For accommodation of sagittal contours
    - Can accommodate malalignment of the starting points in the coronal plane
  - Reduction screw
    - Pedicle screw with breakaway extended tabs
    - Useful for seating rod into pedicle screw for difficult reduction maneuvers
- Freehand placement of thoracic pedicle screws
  - The straightforward trajectory allows for fixed-head screws and true direct vertebral derotation.
  - Anatomic trajectory has a longer bone channel and allows a longer screw to be placed, but mandates the use of a multiaxial screw to connect it to the rod.
  - A straightforward trajectory paralleling the superior endplate has significantly higher pullout strength versus an anatomic trajectory that angles about 22 degrees in the cephalocaudal direction perpendicular to the superior facet.[7]
  - Extrapedicular thoracic pedicle screws
    - Screw inserted at the junction of the cephalad tip of the transverse process and the rib with advancement caudad so that the screw is contained in the pedicle rib unit, defined as the space between the lateral pedicle cortex and medial rib cortex.
    - Similar biomechanical fixation strength of transpedicular screws.
- Confirmation of screw placement
  - Radiographic confirmation
- Neuromonitoring
  - Electromyography to confirm intraosseous screw placement
  - Somatosensory evoked potentials and motor evoked potentials
- Postoperative CT scan routinely performed before patient leaves the hospital to confirm accurate screw placement

Positioning

- Patient is intubated in the supine position on the stretcher.
- Neurologic monitoring leads are placed cranially, on the intercostal and abdominal musculature, and on all four extremities.
- Multiple large-bore intravenous access is obtained for fluid management and an arterial line is placed for intraoperative blood pressure monitoring.
- The patient is transferred to the prone position on a well-padded operating room table such as a Jackson frame (Orthopaedic Systems, Union City, CA).
- Care should be given to the degree of hip flexion–extension, as this can affect the amount of lordosis in the lumbar spine.
- Bolsters underneath the chest and anterior superior iliac spines prevent abdominal compression and allow epidural venous return, thus decreasing epidural bleeding.
- All bony prominences are well padded, including medial elbows, knees, pretibial areas, and ankles.
- Care is taken to avoid abduction and forward flexion past 90 degrees at the shoulder and flexion past 90 degrees at the elbow.
- Skin is shaved if excessively hairy.
- Clear adhesive surgical drapes (3M Steri-Drape Towel Drapes) are placed around the perimeter of the surgical site, extending from the hairline to the top of the gluteal crease (regardless of levels to be fused, the entire spine should be draped).
- If a wake-up test is going to be used by the surgical team, a clear plastic C-arm cover or equivalent clear drape is laid over the exposed feet for visualization during the test.
- A disposable plastic ruler used for measuring the pedicle probe for pedicle depth is placed caudal to the field on the buttocks and covered with a clear Tegaderm dressing.

HOOK PLACEMENT

- Proper hook-site preparation is critical to obtain a stable construct and minimize the chance of hardware failure.
- Ideally, hooks should be placed flush with the bony surfaces to evenly distribute forces and minimize the chance of hook pullout. This is accomplished by meticulous removal of the soft tissues and judicious contouring of the bony surfaces: removing too much bone can weaken hook purchase, whereas removing too little bone can result in improper seating of the hook.

Pedicle Hooks

- Initial pedicle hook-site preparation requires removal of a small portion of the inferior facet with an osteotome (**TECH FIG 1A,B**). The inferior facet of the superior vertebra is osteotomized using an osteotome. A vertical cut is made at the medial edge of the facet, near the base of the spinous process. A horizontal cut in the inferior facet, allowing removal of 3 to 4 mm of bone, follows for insertion of the pedicle hook.
- The exposed hyaline cartilage from the facet joint is removed. A pedicle finder is introduced into the facet joint and gently impacted into place with a mallet (**TECH FIG 1C,D**). Care is taken to avoid canal penetration.
- The permanent pedicle hook is subsequently inserted (**TECH FIG 1E,F**). The surgeon must carefully visualize the facet joint and avoid inserting the pedicle hook into the laminae. If the lamina is split by the hook, fixation will be compromised.

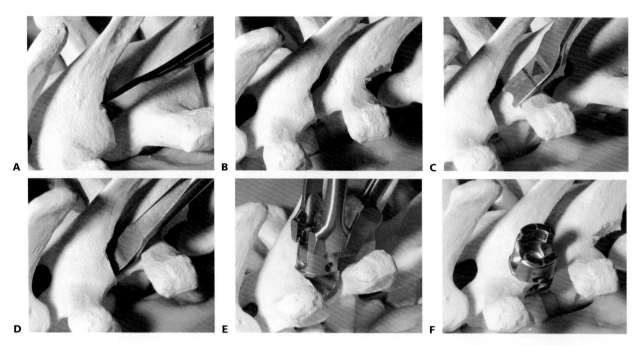

TECH FIG 1 • Placement of pedicle hook. **A,B.** A small portion of the inferior facet is osteotomized. **C,D.** Introduction of pedicle finder into facet joint, taking care to avoid canal penetration. **E,F.** Insertion of pedicle hook.

Laminar Hooks

- Laminar hooks are placed in a similar fashion but require great care because they are positioned in the spinal canal (**TECH FIG 2A,B**).
- To obtain entrance into the canal, the ligamentum flavum is carefully dissected from the laminae and completely removed with curettes and rongeurs until the dura can be visualized. Small laminotomies are performed to allow room for hook insertion (**TECH FIG 2C,D**).
- A hook starter is then used to create a path for the hook (**TECH FIG 2E**). The hook is then placed into the path created (**TECH FIG 2F**).

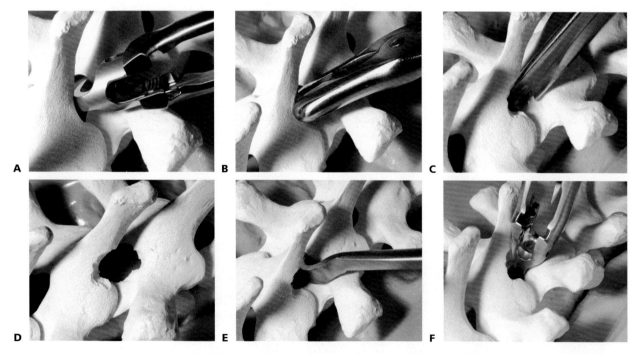

TECH FIG 2 • Placement of supralaminar hook. **A,B.** Placement of a supralaminar hook is difficult without bone removal to allow room for hook insertion. **C,D.** Placement of supralaminar hook. Laminotomies allow room for hook insertion. **E.** Path for hook created with hook starter. **F.** Insertion of supralaminar hook.

Transverse Process Hooks

- Transverse process hooks do not require extensive bone removal but may require minimal contouring to optimize fit (**TECH FIG 3A,B**).

- The costotransverse ligaments on the superior side of the transverse process are divided with a periosteal elevator. The transverse process hook is seated around the transverse process (**TECH FIG 3C,D**).

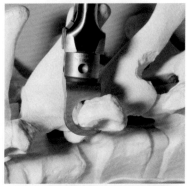
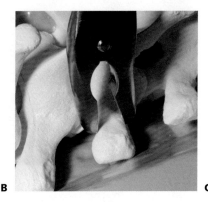
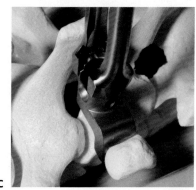
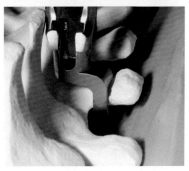

TECH FIG 3 • A,B. Placement of transverse process hook. Contouring of the transverse process is required to optimize fit. **C,D.** Placement of transverse process hook. After contouring the transverse process, the transverse process hook is seated.

EXPOSURE FOR THORACIC PEDICLE SCREW PLACEMENT

- Full exposure of the facet joint, the pars interarticularis, and the entire transverse process aids in identification of the ideal starting point.
- Once the entire spine is exposed, each level is considered independently. The surgeon needs to visualize the local topical anatomy and the effects of the scoliosis on the anatomy (rotation).
- Bovie cautery is used to outline the osseous anatomy at each level. This first entails finding the medial and lateral

border of the facet and the superior and inferior borders of the transverse process (**TECH FIG 4A**).
- The inferior facet of the superior vertebrae is osteotomized using an osteotome at the medial edge of the facet (**TECH FIG 4B**) and at the inferior border of the superior transverse process (**TECH FIG 4C**).
- At this point, the facet joint should be fully exposed (**TECH FIG 4D**), thus facilitating identification of the starting point.

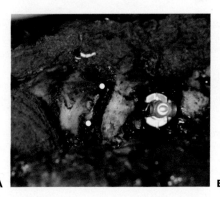
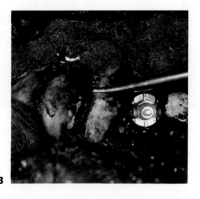

TECH FIG 4 • A. The medial and lateral borders of the facet joint are identified. **B.** The inferior facet of the superior vertebrae is osteotomized at its medial edge. *(continued)*

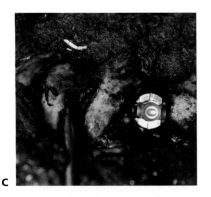

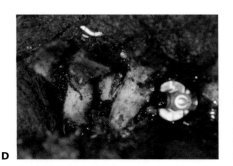

TECH FIG 4 • *(continued)* **C.** The facet is osteotomized at the inferior border of the superior transverse process. **D.** Full exposure of the facet joint facilitates identification of the starting point.

THORACIC PEDICLE SCREW PLACEMENT

- A 3.5-mm acorn-tipped burr is then used to create a hole at the desired starting point (**TECH FIG 5A**). A cancellous blush often heralds entry into the pedicle but can be a false positive found on entry into the transverse process.
- A specialized thoracic probe with a 2-mm blunt tip and a 35-mm curved segment with a rectangular cross section (Lenke probe) is used to create the tract for the pedicle screw.
- The probe is introduced into the starting point with the curvature oriented so the tip is pointed laterally to avoid medial pedicle cortical violation (**TECH FIG 5B**).
- The cancellous soft spot signifies entry into the pedicle.
- The probe is advanced using ventral pressure and axial rotation to a depth of about 15 to 20 mm (the length of the pedicle), using the appropriate orientation for the particular vertebral level and taking care to account for the scoliotic deformity.

- The probe is then removed and reintroduced into the previously developed tract with the tip turned medial to avoid lateral vertebral body cortical violation (**TECH FIG 5C**).
- The probe is advanced to a depth appropriate for the particular vertebral level, taking care to avoid anterior and lateral cortical violation.
- Typical cord lengths (distance from posterior cortical starting point to anterior vertebral cortex in line with the axis of the pedicle):
  - Lower thoracic 40 to 45 mm
  - Midthoracic 35 to 40 mm
  - Upper thoracic 30 to 35 mm
- The tract is probed using a flexible sound and five distinct bony borders are palpated: superior, inferior, medial, and lateral walls and the floor.
- The first 15 to 20 mm of the tract corresponds to the pedicle; its integrity should be critically assessed.

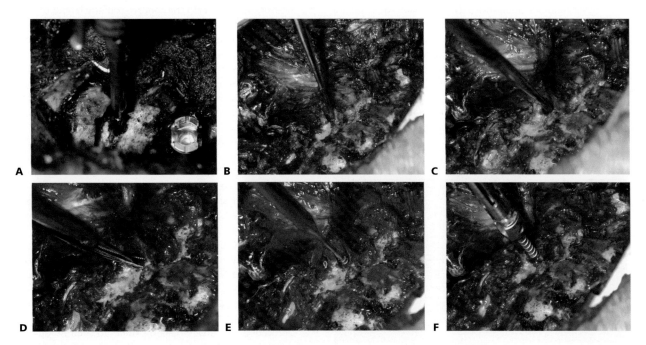

TECH FIG 5 • **A.** A burr is placed at the correct starting point. **B.** After the cortex is breached, a curved probe is placed into the pedicle with the tip pointing laterally to minimize risk of medial pedicle breach and potential cord injury. **C.** After probing past the pedicle, its tip is then turned to point medially to minimize risk of vertebral body cortical breach. **D.** After probing the tract, the depth is measured. **E.** The tract is tapped. **F.** The pedicle screw is inserted.

■ The depth is measured with the flexible sound in the base of the tract using a hemostat (**TECH FIG 5D**).

■ The tract is tapped (**TECH FIG 5E**). Undertapping by 1.0 mm creates a 93% increase in maximal screw insertion torque.[5]

■ The tract is again probed for a breach with the aid of the feel of the tapped threads.

■ Screw diameter is based on radiographic evaluation of pedicles.

■ The screw is placed slowly to allow for viscoelastic expansion of the pedicle (**TECH FIG 5F**).

LUMBAR PEDICLE SCREW PLACEMENT

■ Full exposure of the facet joint, the pars interarticularis, and a portion of the transverse process aids in identification of the ideal starting point.

■ The facet joint is removed to obtain a flat surface before placing the pedicle screw.

■ A 3.5-mm acorn-tipped burr is then used to create a cortical breach at the desired starting point.

■ A specialized probe with a blunt spatula tip and a 35-mm curved segment with a rectangular cross section (lumbar probe) is used to create the tract for the pedicle screw.

■ The probe is introduced into the starting point with the curvature oriented so the tip is pointed laterally to avoid medial pedicle cortical violation.

■ The cancellous soft spot signifies entry into the pedicle.

■ The probe is advanced using ventral pressure and axial rotation to a depth of about 15 to 20 mm (the length of the pedicle), using the appropriate orientation for the particular vertebral level and taking care to account for the scoliotic deformity.

■ The probe is then removed and reintroduced into the previously developed tract with the tip turned medial to avoid lateral vertebral body cortical violation.

■ The probe is advanced to a depth appropriate for the particular vertebral level, taking care to avoid anterior and lateral cortical violation.

■ The tract is probed using a flexible sound and five distinct bony borders are palpated: superior, inferior, medial, and lateral walls and the floor.

■ The first 15 to 20 mm of the tract corresponds to the pedicle; its integrity should be critically assessed.

■ The depth is measured with the flexible sound in the base of the tract using a hemostat.

■ The tract is tapped. Undertapping by 1.0 mm creates a 93% increase in maximal screw insertion torque.[5] The tract is again probed for a breach with the aid of the feel of the tapped threads.

■ Screw diameter is based on radiographic evaluation of pedicles.

■ The screw is placed slowly to allow for viscoelastic expansion of the pedicle.

ROD PLACEMENT

■ Stainless steel is preferred over titanium in patients in whom a derotation maneuver is planned because of the higher modulus of elasticity. The disadvantage is failure occurring at the screw–bone interface instead of via plastic deformation of the rod.

■ Titanium instrumentation allows for magnetic resonance imaging with less metallic artifact and is indicated in patients with nickel allergies or if there are plans to follow the patient with serial MRIs.

■ We use the Bovie cord to measure the length of rod required, although any flexible measuring template may be used (**TECH FIG 6**).

■ Typically, 1 cm is added to the measurement of the concave side to allow for distraction. As most corrective maneuvers are done with the concave rod, the length of the convex rod typically mimics the length of the Bovie cord.

■ The rod is prebent to the appropriate sagittal contour using French benders.

■ The concave-side rod is placed first.

■ There are various methods for rod placement based on the corrective measures that are to be used. We prefer to secure the rod to the hook–screw proximally and work distally.

■ A 90-degree rod derotation maneuver is performed with vise grips. All set screws are then secured to hold correction.

■ The prebent convex-side rod is placed in situ.

■ Compression and distraction maneuvers are performed where needed. In general, care should be taken to "horizontalize" the end vertebrae.

  ■ For selective fusion of Lenke 1A curves, we prefer to horizontalize the lowest instrumented vertebrae (LIV).

  ■ For Lenke 1B curves we prefer to leave a slight obliquity to the LIV.

  ■ For Lenke 1C curves it may be preferable to leave the LIV oblique to prevent coronal decompensation.

■ Derotation maneuvers can be done to address apical rotation.

■ Set screws are tightened to appropriate torque using torque wrench.

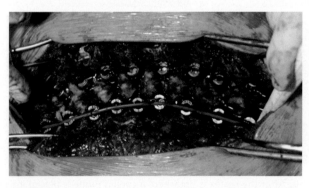

TECH FIG 6 • The length of rod required is determined using the Bovie cord.

PEARLS AND PITFALLS

Violation of the medial wall	▪ Mini-laminotomy ▪ If pedicle feels large enough, the screw is directed more laterally. ▪ Hooks or cables can be used.
Neural injury from medial penetration is rare but does occur	▪ Lateral penetration is more common than medial. ▪ Intraoperative somatosensory evoked potentials, motor evoked potentials, and electromyography can be used to monitor for neurologic compromise and pedicle wall breach. ▪ The surgeon should have a low threshold for a mini-laminotomy and palpation of the pedicle with a Woodson elevator.
Pedicles at the ends of a construct need to be competent	▪ If there is a structural breach, the surgeon can skip a level as long as it is not at the end of the construct. ▪ Hooks can be used in the thoracic level if pedicles are too small.
Screws do not line up well to accept rod	▪ The surgeon should check for aberrant screw placement. ▪ Transverse process can push the screw head medially and the tip laterally. This can be prevented by removing a sufficient amount of transverse process to allow appropriate placement of pedicle screw without impingement by transverse process. ▪ Polyaxial screws can be used.
Unable to locate pedicle entrance	▪ The surgeon should perform a mini-laminotomy. ▪ The surgeon can skip a level and then return if adjacent levels provide additional information. ▪ Hooks or cables can be used.

POSTOPERATIVE CARE

▪ No postoperative immobilization is required with multisegmental constructs.

▪ Postoperative restrictions include limitations with lifting, bending, and twisting.

▪ It is important to maintain mean arterial blood pressure above 70 mm Hg overnight and hemoglobin above 10 g/dL to maintain spinal cord perfusion.

▪ Intravenous antibiotics are maintained for 48 hours postoperatively.

▪ Neurovascular checks are made every 2 hours for the first 8 hours and then every 8 hours.

▪ Patients are out of bed on postoperative day 1.

▪ Foley catheter is removed on postoperative day 2.

▪ Diet is advanced as tolerated.

▪ Patient-controlled analgesia is used for appropriate patients. Continuous narcotic infusion with demand for the first 24 hours is followed by demand only for the next 24 hours, followed by oral pain medications when tolerating diet.

▪ A 4-day hospital course is typical.

▪ Routine follow-up is done at 1, 3, and 6 months and at 1, 2, and 5 years.

▪ Activity is increased based on the degree of fusion.

OUTCOMES

▪ With meticulous attention to detail with regard to instrumentation and fusion techniques, excellent outcomes in terms of straightening and fusion of the scoliotic spine can be expected.

▪ Long-term outcomes are variable and depend on the underlying diagnosis and the extent of retained spinal mobility.

COMPLICATIONS

▪ Wrong-level surgery
▪ Failure of fusion
▪ Hardware malfunction
▪ Neurologic injury
▪ Dural tear
▪ Pneumothorax
▪ Crankshaft
▪ Superior mesenteric artery syndrome
▪ Loss of lumbar lordosis

REFERENCES

1. Karim A, Mukherjee D, Gonzalez-Cruz J, et al. Accuracy and safety of thoracic pedicle screw placement in spinal deformities. J Spinal Disord Tech 2005;18:522–526.
2. Kim YJ, Lenke LG, Bridwell KH, et al. Free hand pedicle screw placement in the thoracic spine: is it safe? Spine 2004;29:333–342.
3. Kim YJ, Lenke LG, Bridwell KH. Comparative analysis of pedicle screw versus hook instrumentation in posterior spinal fusion of AIS. Presented at SRS, Quebec City, September 2003.
4. Kim YJ, Lenke LG, Cheh G, et al. Evaluation of pedicle screw placement in the deformed spine using intraoperative plain radiographs: a comparison with computerized tomography. Spine 2005;30:2084–2088.
5. Kuklo TR, Lehman RA Jr. Effect of various tapping diameters on insertion of thoracic pedicle screws: a biomechanical analysis. Spine 2003;28:2066–2077.
6. Kuklo TR, Lenke LG, O'Brien MF, et al. Accuracy and efficacy of thoracic pedicle screws in curves more than 90 degrees. Spine 2005;30:222–226.
7. Lehman RA, Polly DW Jr, Kuklo TR, et al. Straight-forward versus anatomic trajectory technique of thoracic pedicle screw fixation: a biomechanical analysis. Spine 2003;28:2058–2065.
8. Liljenqvist UR, Allkemper T, Hackenberg L, et al. Analysis of vertebral morphology in idiopathic scoliosis with use of magnetic resonance imaging and multiplanar reconstruction. J Bone Joint Surg Am 2002;84A:359–368.
9. Liljenqvist UR, Link TM, Halm HF. Morphometric analysis of thoracic and lumbar vertebrae in idiopathic scoliosis. Spine 2000;25:1247–1253.
10. O'Brien MF, Lenke LG, Mardjetko S, et al. Pedicle morphology in thoracic adolescent idiopathic scoliosis: is pedicle fixation an anatomically viable technique? Spine 2000;25:2285–2293.
11. Parent S, Labelle H, Skalli W, et al. Thoracic pedicle morphometry in vertebrae from scoliotic spines. Spine 2004;29:239–248.
12. Parent S, Labelle H, Skalli W, et al. Morphometric analysis of anatomic scoliotic specimens. Spine 2002;27:2305–2311.

13. Sucato DJ, Duchene C. The position of the aorta relative to the spine: a comparison of patients with and without idiopathic scoliosis. J Bone Joint Surg Am 2003;85A:1461–1469.

14. Vaccaro AR, Rizzolo SJ, Allardyce TJ, et al. Placement of pedicle screws in the thoracic spine. Part I: Morphometric analysis of the thoracic vertebrae. J Bone Joint Surg Am 1995;77A:1193–1199.

15. Dimeglio A. Growth in pediatric orthopaedics. J Pediatr Orthop 2001;21:549–555.

16. McMaster MJ, Ohtsuka K. The natural history of congenital scoliosis: a study of two hundred and fifty-one patients. J Bone Joint Surg Am 1982;64:1128–1147.

17. Pehrsson K, Bake B, Larsson S, et al. Lung function in adult idiopathic scoliosis. Thorax 1991;46:474–478.

18. Ramirez N, Johnston CE, Browne RH. The prevalence of back pain in children who have idiopathic scoliosis. J Bone Joint Surg Am 1997;79A:364–368.

19. Weinstein SL, Ponseti IV. Curve progression in idiopathic scoliosis. J Bone Joint Surg Am 1981;65A:447–455.

20. Weinstein SL, Zavala DC, Ponseti IV. Idiopathic scoliosis: long-term follow-up and prognosis in untreated patients. J Bone Joint Surg Am 1981;63A:702–712.

Chapter 35 Kyphectomy in Spina Bifida

Richard E. McCarthy

DEFINITION

- Kyphosis in the patient with myelomeningocele can occur at the thoracolumbar junction, the midlumbar spine, or the lumbosacral junction.
- The different types of kyphosis have some bearing on the treatment needed for the repair, but whether the origin is congenital, developmental, or paralytic, the consequences can be devastating for the child with this condition.
- Skin breakdown over the apex of the kyphosis can develop deep wound infections and lead to central nervous system infections.
- Secondary changes in other organ systems can create compromise in the gastrointestinal or genitourinary systems or even potentially disastrous kinking of the great vessels due to compromise in the abdominal height. Diminished absorption frequently occurs in the gastrointestinal tract, and renal calculi may develop from poor urinary drainage.
- Secondary effects on the pulmonary capacity produce thoracic insufficiency syndrome because the abdominal contents are pushed into the thoracic cage. Added to this is a secondary thoracic lordosis cephalad to the kyphosis.
- Bracing generally leads to problems from skin pressure and ultimately does not solve the problem.

ANATOMY

- The kyphotic angle can be gradual or acute.
- The paraspinal musculature is partially innervated in a flexion position lateral to the bony ridges owing to lack of posterior migration from an embryologic origin. In this position, they contribute to forward flexion of the spinal column.
  - The bony ridges laterally in the area of the diastasis leave little bone for fusion mass on the posterior side of the vertebral column.
- The midline defect from the original myelomeningocele characteristically is covered by a fragile dura separated from the overlying skin by a thin layer of subcutaneous tissue.
  - The soft tissue coverage is made worse by poor nutrition.
- One of the most reliably formed vertebral structures is the sacral ala.
- The great vessels generally do not follow the kyphotic contours into the kyphotic apex.

PATHOGENESIS

- Embryologically the notochord is covered dorsally by closure of the ectoderm over top of it, progressing in a cephalic to a caudal direction. In myelomeningocele, the closure is incomplete, usually at the caudal end.
- Less common types of myelomeningocele occur in the thoracic and cervical area. Thoracolumbar, lumbar, and lumbosacral kyphosis is the most commonly seen type and occurs because of lack of posterior migration of the ectoderm surrounding the notochord, leaving the neural placode in a vulnerable position, exposed at birth.
  - Congenital bony defects occurring in this area lead to an early-onset kyphosis that can pose significant problems for the neurosurgeon's closure at birth. This has led some experts to encourage neonatal correction of the kyphosis.
- With further growth and an upright sitting posture, the paraspinal musculature, which has formed in a lateral and anterior position, pulls the upper torso into a more kyphotic position, both actively through muscle contracture and secondarily from gravity.
  - This can lead to further skin compromise and pressure in the soft tissues overlying the kyphosis.
  - Skin breakdown can be a serious problem over the kyphosis.
- The C7 lateral plumb line shows the upper torso to be far out of balance in a forward-flexed posture, leading to thoracic insufficiency from the abdominal contents pressing under the diaphragm.
  - This can render the child a "functional quadriplegic" since he or she uses the upper extremities for balance and to unweight the diaphragm by pivoting on the extended arms for breathing purposes (marionette maneuver; **FIG 1**).
  - From a developmental standpoint, this can further limit the young child's upper extremity interaction with his or her environment, which is essential for the development of normal intelligence.

NATURAL HISTORY

- The natural history of unpublished cases of severe kyphosis is one of thoracic compromise from insufficiency syndrome, progressive decline in pulmonary capacity, and death.

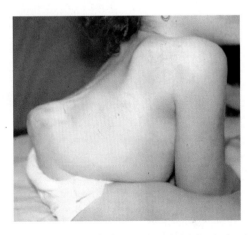

FIG 1 • "Functional quadriplegia" in myelokyphosis; lumbar kyphosis with thoracic lordosis.

PATIENT HISTORY AND PHYSICAL FINDINGS

- A careful history and physical examination should elicit possible signs and symptoms of associated anomalies, including:
  - Chiari malformation
  - Tethered cord
  - Respiratory compromise
  - Gastrointestinal malabsorption
  - Urinary hydrostasis and lithiasis
- Physical examination of the child should include flexibility tests of the curve by physically supporting the child under the armpits to suspend him or her against gravity. Bending back supine on the examining table can also indicate the extent of lumbar flexibility.

IMAGING AND OTHER DIAGNOSTIC STUDIES

- Standard radiographs, anteroposterior (AP) and lateral views of the full spine, in the upright sitting posture assess the effects of gravity upon the curve (**FIG 2A,B**).
  - Supine radiographs are helpful for visualization of bony definition.
  - Flexibility films with traction, manual push, or back bending over a bolster with a shoot-through lateral film, are helpful adjuncts.
- CT scans, especially three-dimensional CT scans, offer the best delineation of the anatomy.
- MRI is critical for assessment of the intrathecal structures and assessing for Chiari malformation, syringomyelias, and tethering (**FIG 2C**).

DIFFERENTIAL DIAGNOSIS

- Congenital versus developmental kyphosis
- Sacral agenesis
- Charcot joints secondary to vertebral column breakdown across the apex of the kyphosis

NONOPERATIVE MANAGEMENT

- Bracing has no place in the treatment of this disorder.
- Occasionally traction is helpful to stretch the kyphosis, especially in a developmental type to aid in correction at the time of surgery.
- This can be done with cervical traction or halo traction, and some authors have promoted the use of this traction during the time of surgery to aid in the correction.

SURGICAL MANAGEMENT

Preoperative Planning

- Vascular monitoring devices are an important adjunct during surgery, and either arterial lines or pulse oximeters on both feet are important to monitor blood supply to the lower extremities at the time of correction.
- A great deal of tension can be placed on the aorta at the time of kyphosis realignment. Thus, arterial and central venous lines are necessary to monitor central pressure and allow for rapid medication administration.
- Areas of skin breakdown should be addressed and healed prior to kyphectomy.
  - Preoperative planning may include assessment by a plastic surgeon and possible need for placement of tissue expanders in the posterolateral axillary margins to aid in skin closure at surgery (**FIG 3**).
- As a part of the preoperative planning, all imaging studies are carefully reviewed to assess flexibility, the adequacy of the vertebral bodies to tolerate pedicle screws, and planning for which levels will need to be decancellized or removed.
  - It is recommended that these plans be recorded on a "blueprint" that can be placed on the operating room wall outlining the location of implants, osteotomies, and order of progression for the surgical plan.
- Assessment by neurosurgery is necessary preoperatively regarding shunt functioning and review of the MRIs.
- Preoperative antibiotics are essential, including gramnegative coverage for urinary pathogens. These are continued postoperatively for 6 to 12 weeks.

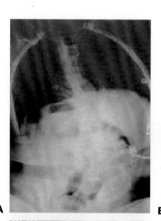
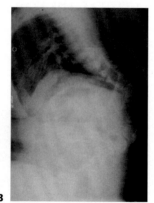
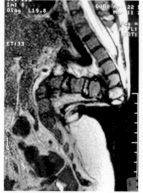

FIG 2 • **A,B.** A 13-year-old with myelokyphosis with diastasis beginning at T6 with 127 degrees of kyphosis. **C.** Preoperative MRI in a 9-year-old with myelomeningocele before undergoing kyphectomy with growing construct.

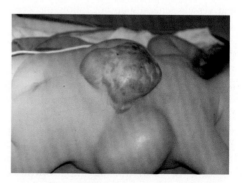

FIG 3 • Myelomeningocele in an 11-month-old with tissue expanders placed bilaterally before delayed closure and kyphectomy.

Nutritional status is maximized and may require hyperalimentation via a gastrostomy tube button months ahead of surgery to maximize postoperative healing.

Positioning

- During positioning, careful padding with extra foam is essential to protect delicate skin during a prolonged operation.
- Eye protection to guard against intraoperative ocular compromise and a spinal frame that allows for suspension of the abdominal structures will diminish the epidural vascular pressure.
- Preoperative assessment of the hips is important to anticipate the intraoperative positioning, and if the flexion contractures about the hips are too severe, a preliminary release of contractures done a few weeks ahead of time may be necessary to allow for proper positioning of the legs at the time of the kyphectomy.

Approach

- The surgical incision may involve excision of compromised skin lesions or scars, although this is best addressed before surgery.

- The previous incisions on a myelomeningocele back may not be midline or ideally placed.
  - The best skin incision for kyphectomy should follow the previous skin incisions to maximize blood supply to the skin edges at closure. Maximum skin and subcutaneous tissue coverage is important for good skin closure.
- If a compromise in the quality of soft tissues is anticipated, then previously placed tissue expanders may be removed from the midline at closure and the expanded tissue brought to the midline.
- There may be times when the poorly healed, convoluted scars from previous neurosurgical interventions may be harbingers of bacteria that will not promote adequate healing or may contribute toward postoperative infection. Preliminary excision of the scars by plastic surgery may afford the best defense against outside-in infections.

INCISION AND LUMBAR DISSECTION

- The incision—either straight or curvilinear—follows the previous scars. It is extended deep to the spinous processes in those sections where they exist.
  - The caudal portion of the incision is made to the level of the dura, with care taken to avoid laceration of the fragile dura.
- The surgical plane is then deviated to the right and left side superficial to the dura while palpating for the lateral bony elements. The deep portion of the incision is directed toward the bone.
  - It is desirable to maintain as much subcutaneous thickness as possible.
- If there are lacerations of the dura, it is best to stop and sew them as one proceeds since the thinned dura may

require a flap of adjacent tissue for a watertight closure. Sometimes it is necessary to sew in a piece of Duragen sealant to ensure a watertight closure.
  - Four-O Neurolon on a small needle in a running fashion works quite well for an incidental durotomy repair.
- As one proceeds from distal to proximal in the lumbar spine, the lateral elements are palpated and with the use of electrocautery, the soft tissues are incised to bone.
- The muscle and soft tissue attachments to the laterally positioned lumbar bones are released to reveal the underlying bony elements that embryologically would have progressed posteriorly to become the lamina and facets (**TECH FIG 1A–C**).

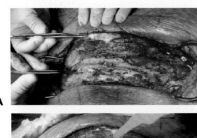

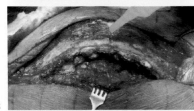

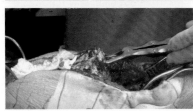

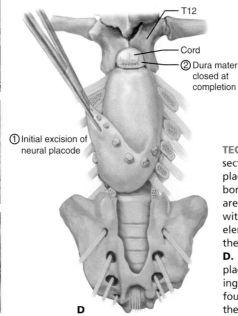

TECH FIG 1 • A. Intraoperative dissection with neuroplacode left in place and forceps placed on bilateral bony ridges. **B.** Paraspinal muscles are dissected away from the kyphosis, with frequent irrigation of neural elements. **C.** In a different patient, the kyphosis has been dissected out. **D.** The neuroplacode can be left in place, mobilized to one side by releasing nonfunctioning nerve roots over four levels, or resecting to the level of the diastasis and oversewing.

- The rudiments of these bones can be visualized along with a transverse process at each level in the bony ridge of the diastasis.
- The medial neural placode is left intact since it acts as third-space filler and padding for the implants.

- There may be instances in which the neuroplacode has to be mobilized, and this is done by releasing nonfunctioning roots on one side and reflecting the dura laterally to gain access to the disc space and underlying vertebrae (**TECH FIG 1D**).

THORACIC DISSECTION

- Once the lumbar spine is dissected, the thoracic area is approached.
  - If one is contemplating a fusion of the thoracic spine, such as in a child over 8 years of age, full dissection out to the tips of the transverse processes should be accomplished.
- If a growing rod construct is being used, such as in a child under age 8 years, this is done with minimal dissection so as to promote growth.
  - If the growing construct is desired, the muscle and soft tissue attachments are cleaned from the sides of the spinous processes as far as the facet joints.

- One needs to be able to visualize the ligamentum flavum sufficiently to pass sublaminar wires for the Luque trolley portion of the "growing" construct.
  - Generally, four thoracic levels for wires are all that is necessary.
- In the lumbar spine, soft tissues should be cleaned from bone sufficiently to allow for fusion between the lateral elements and to the sacrum.

PEDICLE SCREW PLACEMENT

- At this point in the operation, radiographic C-arm guidance is helpful for placement of pedicle screws.
- The entrance point for the lumbar dysplastic pedicles is in a lateral position, with the pedicles directed obliquely toward the vertebral body (**TECH FIG 2**).
  - Bilateral screws can be obliquely placed for fixation.
- Fixation to the pelvis can be done with multiple types of fixation devices, including S-rods, S-hooks, and iliac threaded bolts.
  - Fusion to the sacrum is essential to firmly plant the rod on the pelvis and allow for growth off the top of the rods in the thoracic spine.
- The C-arm is used in both AP and lateral positions to confirm satisfactory placement of the screws in bone. Bicortical fixation is generally not necessary because of the strong fixation supplied by the triangulation of the screws.
- Polyaxial screws are desirable through the lumbar segments.

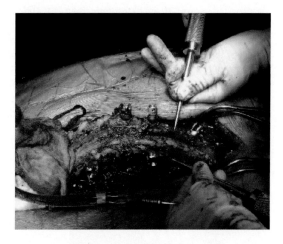

TECH FIG 2 • Screws in place and bilateral curettes in pedicles to decancellize at L3 before doing the same at T12.

DECANCELLIZATION

- Decancellization can be accomplished at multiple levels, leaving adequate vertebral levels for fixation and correction. Ideally, it is accomplished at one or two levels in a location that will leave sufficient midlumbar fixation points to push the vertebrae forward to create lordosis.
  - The levels chosen for decancellization are approached after screw placement, based on the preoperative planning.
- The decancellization begins with a burr at the entrance to the pedicle. It continues with enlarging sizes of curettes, saving the bone for the fusion.
- The inside of the vertebral body is completely cored out, and when bleeding points are encountered, the pedicle can be filled with FloSeal and if necessary further packed with some rolled Gelfoam to stop the bleeding.

- Care is taken to avoid violating the posterior cortex of the vertebral body until the very end, since this is where the epidural vessels are most prolific.
  - The lateral margins of these vertebral bodies are removed, including the transverse process and posterolateral bone.
- The decancellization should be thorough, leaving only the cortex. This is carried out bilaterally followed by implosion of the posterior cortex with an Epstein curette, pushing the bone fragments into the cavity of the vertebral body (**TECH FIG 3**).
  - Bleeding points are stabilized.
- In most instances, decancellization alone at select levels is all that is necessary to gain the mobility for correction.

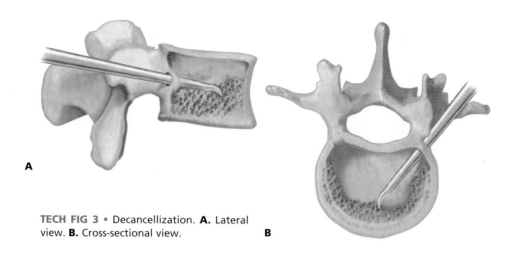

TECH FIG 3 • Decancellization. **A.** Lateral view. **B.** Cross-sectional view.

HORIZONTAL RESECTION

- Occasionally, removal of a vertebral segment may be indicated. If so, it can be accomplished while maintaining the neuroplacode.
- The vertebral section for removal in that instance would be taken from that section of the curve that is horizontal and cephalad to the apex of the kyphosis (**TECH FIG 4**).

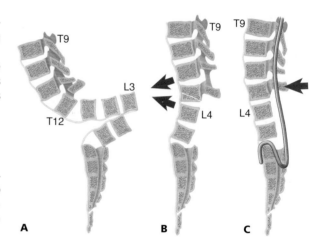

TECH FIG 4 • **A.** If bone is to be resected (due to extreme stiffness), this should be done in the horizontal section at the top of the kyphosis, not at the apex. **B.** After horizontal resection, the bone is pushed forward to realign. **C.** After resection, realignment and fixation are accomplished.

ROD PLACEMENT

- Once these corrective maneuvers have been completed, rods linked to the sacrum can then be placed bilaterally to push the vertebral bodies anteriorly into a straight or preferably a lordotic position (**TECH FIG 5A**).

- Through gradual approximation of the rod forward toward the thoracic fixation points, the lumbar segments are brought into alignment and the rods gradually tightened to the wires of the thoracic spine (**TECH FIG 5B,C**).

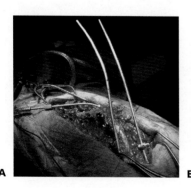
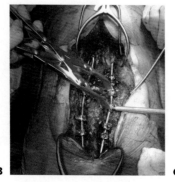
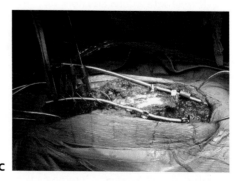

TECH FIG 5 • **A.** Bilateral rods are anchored to L4 and S-hooks in preparation for reduction. **B.** Decancellized levels are crushed by compressing adjacent screw heads. **C.** In a different patient, gradual reduction with wires and provisional tightening are accomplished using a growing construct. *(continued)*

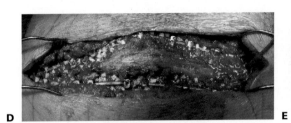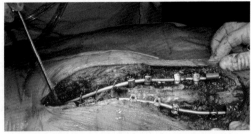

TECH FIG 5 • *(continued)* **D.** Completed reduction in patient in **A** and **B**. Allograft and autograft have been applied to decorticated bone for fusion. **E.** Completed reduction in patient with growing construct in **C**.

- Physiologic kyphosis can be contoured into the thoracic component of the rods to correct the thoracic lordosis.
- Generally, the rods are left one level long at the top to allow for growth in the thoracic spine.

- The final tightening should produce some distraction between the lowest lumbar segment fixation point and the S-hooks pushed against the sacral ala (**TECH FIG 5D,E**). This will set the S-hooks in place securely.
- Final contouring with the in situ benders can allow for further lordosis of the lumbar spine if desired.

ASSESSING AND MANAGING LOWER EXTREMITY HYPOPERFUSION

- Frequently, the initial maneuvers for correction across the kyphosis are accompanied by a decrease in blood flow to the lower extremities. Therefore, it is important to do this corrective maneuver gradually in small increments.
- The baroreceptors in the aorta can accommodate to the change in alignment and stretch. If the blood flow to the

feet is unable to accommodate to the new position of the spine, further decancellization or vertebral body removal will be necessary.
  - This decision is based on the flow to the lower extremities reflected in the pulse oximeter or arterial catheters in the feet.

CLOSURE

- As part of the closure, it is important to grasp the paraspinal musculature with clamps to pull the muscles toward the midline by elevating and mobilizing the muscle layer with a Cobb elevator.
  - Sometimes release of the fascia on the posterior side of the musculature is necessary, and this is best done in the posterior axillary line with a vertical cut in the fascia.
- The paraspinal musculature should be brought as close as possible toward the midline on both sides and sewn down (**TECH FIG 6**).
- At least one and more likely two Hemovac drains should be left, one in the deep and one in the superficial layers, for drainage over 1 week to 10 days postoperatively.
- Subcuticular closures can be used, but they should be reinforced with external suture of some kind, either clips or interrupted nylon sutures on a temporary basis.

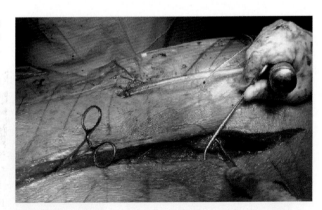

TECH FIG 6 • The paraspinal muscle flaps are brought to midline for final closure.

PEARLS AND PITFALLS

Evaluation	▪ The surgeon can assess flexibility of the curve by physically supporting the child under the armpits to suspend him or her against gravity. Bending back supine on the examining table can also indicate the extent of lumbar flexibility.
Preoperative preparation	▪ Areas of skin breakdown should be addressed and healed before kyphectomy.
Intraoperative monitoring	▪ Vascular monitoring of the lower extremities is a critical part of the intraoperative monitoring.
Preoperative preparation	▪ Preoperative antibiotics are essential, including gram-negative coverage for urinary pathogens. These are continued postoperatively for 6 to 12 weeks.
Managing incidental dural tears	▪ Four-O Neurolon on a small taper needle in a running fashion works quite well for an incidental durotomy repair. Duragen can be sewn over the repair, and occasionally the use of a sealant (Tusseal) is necessary.
Preventing epidural bleeding	▪ Care is taken to avoid violating the posterior cortex of the vertebral body until the very end, since this is where the epidural vessels are most prolific.
Setting the S-hook	▪ The final tightening should produce some distraction between the lowest lumbar segment fixation point and the S-hooks pushed against the sacral ala. This will set the S-hooks in place securely.
Postoperative care	▪ All reasonable measures must be taken to avoid any pressure on the wound or extremities in the postoperative period. All areas of insensate skin must be protected from excessive pressure with frequent change in position on a soft surface. The dressings should be covered with a waterproof covering to protect against secondary contamination from stool.

POSTOPERATIVE CARE

▪ For recovery, patients are placed on their back with an extra-thick foam on top of the mattress to avoid excessive skin pressure.

▪ Logrolling is instituted 6 hours postoperatively and repeated every 2 hours.

▪ Recovery occurs in the intensive care unit until the patient is sufficiently stable.

▪ Although postoperative immobilization is not necessary, if desired it can be accomplished with careful molding of a bi-valved jacket with a Plastizote soft lining.

OUTCOMES

▪ Improved sitting
▪ Improved respiratory function
▪ Better blood supply to skin

COMPLICATIONS

▪ Skin breakdown
▪ Infection, superficial or deep
▪ Vascular compromise to feet with stretch on aorta
▪ Loosening of spinal implants
▪ Pseudarthrosis

REFERENCE

1. McCarthy RE. Myelokyphosis. Shriners Hospitals for Crippled Children, Symposium on Caring for the Child with Myelomeningocele, American Academy of Orthopaedic Surgeons, 2002.

Chapter 36

Anterior Interbody Arthrodesis With Instrumentation for Scoliosis

Daniel J. Sucato

DEFINITION

■ Thoracic scoliosis and thoracolumbar–lumbar scoliosis are typically curves seen in idiopathic scoliosis and can be treated anteriorly.

■ Anterior arthrodesis refers to the fusion of the anterior part of the vertebral bodies, usually with instrumentation for these curve patterns.

ANATOMY

■ Thoracic idiopathic scoliosis usually has an apex at T8 or T9. It is the most common right convex curve pattern and has axial-plane rotational deformity as well as hypokyphosis.

■ The vertebral bodies are nearly normal in their shape, although some distortion of the vertebral body and pedicles is seen, with thin long pedicles on the concavity and shorter, wider pedicles on the convexity.

■ Thoracolumbar–lumbar scoliosis has an apex of the curve at T12 or below and is most commonly a left-sided curve, with or without a compensatory thoracic curve.

PATHOGENESIS

■ The cause of idiopathic scoliosis is not yet known.

NATURAL HISTORY

■ Idiopathic scoliosis progresses with continued growth of the spine, especially during the peak growth periods and when the curve magnitudes are "large" at the completion of growth.

■ Thoracic curves tend to progress at skeletal maturity when the curve is greater than 45 to 50 degrees.

■ Thoracolumbar–lumbar curves tend to progress when the curve is greater than 35 to 40 degrees at the time of skeletal maturity.

PATIENT HISTORY AND PHYSICAL FINDINGS

■ Patients with thoracic scoliosis and thoracolumbar scoliosis should be evaluated for their perception of spine and body deformity to include asymmetric shoulder elevation, trunk shift, waistline asymmetry, and rib or flank prominence.

■ Pain in the axial spine and pain radiating into the lower extremities should be ascertained with a good history; such symptoms warrant an MRI.

■ Neurologic symptoms such as paresthesias, hyperesthesia, or bowel or bladder symptoms are relevant and require further imaging with an MRI.

■ Physical examination should assess the trunk imbalance in the coronal plane, which can be seen with isolated thoracic or thoracolumbar–lumbar curves.

■ The Adams forward bend test characterizes the axial-plane deformity seen in scoliosis and is used to assess rotational deformity of the thoracic rib prominence or the flank prominence. The rotational deformity of the thoracic and lumbar spine is graded using a scoliometer with the patient bending

forward. The rotational deformity seen in scoliosis can be very prominent and the most obvious deformity seen by patient and families.

■ Cutaneous manifestations of dysraphism should also be analyzed.

IMAGING AND OTHER DIAGNOSTIC STUDIES

■ Anteroposterior (AP) and lateral radiographs of the spine should be obtained to review the coronal and sagittal plane deformities, respectively (**FIG 1**).

■ On the AP radiograph, the coronal plane deformity is measured using the Cobb method. Truncal imbalance can be measured using the Floman method (bisecting the distance between the lateral rib margins and comparing this point to the center sacral vertical line [CSVL]).

■ The decompensation of the head relative to the pelvis is measured by the distance between the C7 plumb line and the CSVL.

■ The Risser sign should be evaluated by assessing the ossification of the iliac apophysis, giving it a grade between 0 and 5.

■ The triradiate cartilage status should be assessed as either open or closed.

■ The lateral radiograph is used to measure thoracic kyphosis (measured from T5 to T12) and lumbar lordosis (from L1 to S1) as well as the sagittal balance (comparing a C7 plumb bob line to the front edge of S1).

■ Supine best-bend radiographs can be used to determine the flexibility of the spine and are especially useful to determine

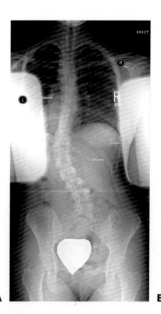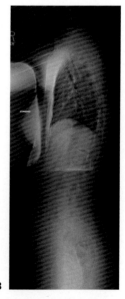

FIG 1 • AP and lateral radiographs of a 51-degree left lumbar curve.

whether the thoracolumbar–lumbar curve is flexible when a primary thoracic curve is present or if the thoracic curve is flexible and compensatory when the primary thoracolumbar–lumbar curve is present.

DIFFERENTIAL DIAGNOSIS

■ Idiopathic scoliosis should be differentiated from other types of scoliosis in which congenital abnormalities are not seen in ambulatory patients. This list includes neurofibromatosis, Marfan syndrome, type 3 spinal muscular atrophy, scoliosis associated with syringomyelia, or tethered cord.

NONOPERATIVE MANAGEMENT

■ Adolescent thoracic and thoracolumbar scoliosis can be treated with bracing when curve magnitudes are between 25 and 45 degrees during peak growth periods.
■ Bracing is used for these curve magnitudes to prevent curve progression and is indicated in Risser grade 0 to 2 patients.
■ Nonoperative management is primarily indicated when the cosmetic appearance of the patient is acceptable to him or her.

SURGICAL MANAGEMENT

■ Surgical indications for thoracic idiopathic scoliosis are curves exceeding 45 to 50 degrees with unacceptable cosmetic deformity.
■ Indications for surgical treatment of thoracolumbar–lumbar curves are curves exceeding 40 to 45 degrees with unacceptable cosmetic deformity.

Preoperative Planning

■ A careful physical examination as noted above is necessary to ensure that there are no neurologic signs or symptoms,

which would indicate neural axis abnormalities. If these are present, MRI of the neural axis is indicated.
■ Radiographic imaging should be used to ensure the curve is characteristic of an idiopathic curve. For thoracic curve magnitudes, this should demonstrate apical lordosis. The atypical curves, such as left-sided thoracic curves or those with significant decompensation despite minimal rotational deformity, or patients who have excessive thoracic kyphosis should be further evaluated with an MRI.
■ The AP radiograph, the lateral standing radiograph, and the supine best-bend radiograph should be used to determine the Lenke classification.
■ Specific detailed analysis of the compensatory curves should be performed to fine-tune a surgical plan to ensure that postoperative decompensation does not occur. This is especially important to determine the flexibility of the lumbar curve and the lumbar modifier for primary thoracic curves, as well as the flexibility of the compensatory thoracic curve for primary thoracolumbar–lumbar curves.
■ Anterior fusion levels for thoracic scoliosis are, in general, proximal-end vertebra to distal-end vertebra. Occasionally a parallel disc is noted at the distal segment. It is controversial whether this disc should be included in the fusion levels. When the curve is relatively small (50 to 60 degrees) and flexible (greater than 50% flexibility index) and the patient is skeletally mature (triradiate cartilage is closed and Risser grade 1 or higher), inclusion of the parallel disc is not often necessary (**FIG 2A,B**).
■ Anterior fusion levels for thoracolumbar–lumbar curves in general are proximal-end vertebra to distal-end vertebra. When the disc below the planned lowest instrumented vertebra is reversing and opening into the fractional lumbosacral curve, then disc wedging is not seen postoperatively. However, a disc below the lowest instrumented vertebra that is parallel preoperatively will often be wedged postoperatively (**FIG 2C,D**).

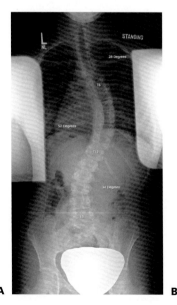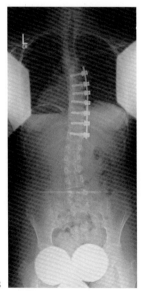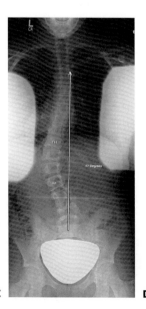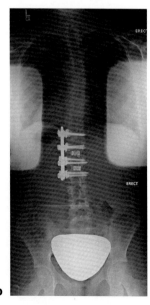

FIG 2 • A. Preoperative radiograph of a 13-year-old girl with a right thoracic curve measuring 52 degrees from T6 to T12. The disc at T11–12 is open into the right thoracic curve while the disc at T12-L1 is parallel. **B.** Thoracoscopic anterior spinal fusion and instrumentation from T6 to T12 demonstrating excellent correction of the main thoracic curve with excellent response of the proximal thoracic and lumbar curves. **C.** A left thoracolumbar curve measured between T11 and L2 with a trunk shift to the left. **D.** Two-year postoperative radiographs following an open anterior fusion and instrumentation from T11 to L2 with dual rod-dual screw system and anterior cages placed at the T12-L1 and L1-L2 levels with excellent coronal plane correction.

Positioning

▪ Positioning for anterior surgery for either the thoracic or thoracolumbar curves is fairly similar.

▪ Patients are placed in the lateral decubitus position with the convex side of the curve up.

▪ An axillary roll is used for safe upper extremity neurologic function (**FIG 3**).

▪ An inflatable bean bag is used to position the patient, and body positioners can be added for further patient stabilization.

▪ For thoracolumbar–lumbar curves, a table that can be flexed allows for greater access to the abdomen and spine. It should be centered over the apex of the curve.

▪ For thoracic scoliosis surgery, the patient can be placed on a flat radiolucent table.

Approach

▪ The anterior approach is used for thoracic scoliosis.

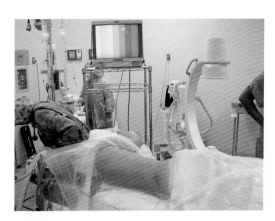

FIG 3 • Positioning for access for a thoracoscopic anterior spinal fusion and instrumentation in the left lateral decubitus position. The arms are positioned at 90 degrees, axillary rolls are placed on the left axilla, and the patient is secured with a bean bag.

TECHNIQUES

OPEN THORACIC ANTERIOR INSTRUMENTATION AND ARTHRODESIS

▪ A curved incision is made over the proximal rib corresponding to the proximal fusion level (ie, commonly T5 with the fifth rib). The incision is carried through the thoracic and abdominal musculature to the periosteum of the rib.

▪ Subperiosteal dissection of the rib is performed circumferentially, and the rib is cut posteriorly and anteriorly.

▪ The parietal pleura is incised in a longitudinal fashion over the vertebral bodies across the intended levels of instrumentation and fusion.

▪ The segmental vessels can be temporarily ligated and spinal cord monitoring should be observed during temporary ligation.

▪ Permanent ligation can be performed after 20 minutes of normal spinal cord monitoring.

▪ Discectomy is performed (see below in the section on the thoracoscopic technique).

▪ Instrumentation is placed (see below).

▪ For the remaining procedures, see details under the thoracoscopic approach.

THORACOSCOPIC ANTERIOR INSTRUMENTATION AND ARTHRODESIS

Positioning, Preparation, and Draping

▪ After true lateral positioning is confirmed, fluoroscopy is used to mark the skin for the proximal-end vertebra and distal-end vertebra on the AP view. The skin markings are made to identify the angle of the proximal-end vertebra on the AP view (**TECH FIG 1**).

▪ The anterior and posterior edges of the vertebral bodies are then marked using the lateral fluoroscopy view.

▪ The chest and flank are prepared and draped in the normal sterile fashion.

Thoracoscopic Portal and Guidewire Placement

▪ An anterior portal is placed, bisecting the distance between the proximal and the distal intended instrumented vertebra, in the anterior axillary line. This portal is used for placement of the camera (**TECH FIG 2A**).

▪ A guidewire is then placed directly over the vertebral bodies over the intended second-most-proximal portal and is visualized with the thoracoscope placed in the anterior portal (**TECH FIG 2B**).

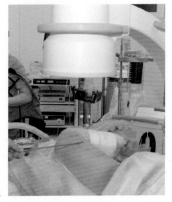

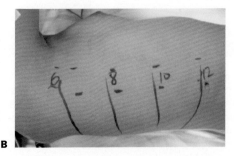

TECH FIG 1 • Fluoroscopic imaging of the spine prior to surgery. **A.** The lateral radiograph is used to identify the anterior and posterior edges of the vertebral body. **B.** The AP radiograph is used to mark the skin over the intended fusion levels to direct portal placement. This example demonstrates a T6–T12 fusion.

A   **B**

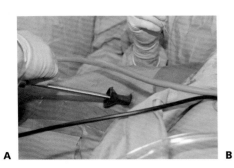

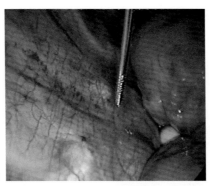

TECH FIG 2 • **A.** The anterior portal is placed in the anterior axillary line with the camera inserted in the portal. The patient is in the left lateral decubitus position: proximal to the right and distal to the left. **B.** A guidewire is placed before placing the posterior lateral portals. The guidewire is directed just anterior to the rib heads and marks a good position for the posterolateral portal.

- After good placement of the guidewire (directly over the rib head), the portal is placed with a transverse incision centered over the rib. This portal can be used for visualization with a thoracoscope to place the remaining portals.
- The most proximal posterolateral portal is placed after the intended second posterolateral portal to ensure exact location of the proximal portal. The proximal portal position is most important, since the most proximal two screws are often placed in small vertebral bodies and have significant coronal angulation, and retraction of the scapula makes this portal difficult.
- The remaining portals are placed in the posterolateral line.
- The portals will house the camera, a fan retractor to retract the lung, a suction device, a working portal, and then a free portal.

Discectomy Technique

- The pleura is incised in the midvertebral line in a longitudinal fashion, keeping the segmental vessels intact (TECH FIG 3A).
- The segmental vessels are then ligated two or three at a time (normotensive anesthesia is used for anterior surgery).
- The parietal pleura is retracted anteriorly, all the way to the opposite side, and access to the anterior longitudinal ligament and the contralateral annulus is allowed (TECH FIG 3B).
- Posterior retraction allows for identification of the rib heads (TECH FIG 3C).
- The disc is incised from the convex rib head to the opposite annulus (TECH FIG 3D).

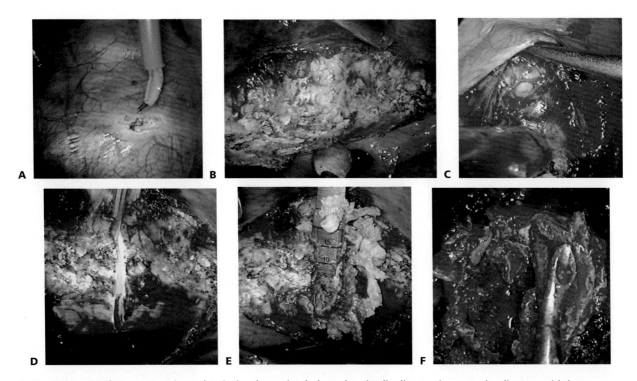

TECH FIG 3 • **A.** Electrocautery is used to incise the parietal pleura longitudinally, starting over the disc to avoid the segmental vessels. The segmental vessels are left intact on the first pass. **B,C.** After ligation of the segmental vessels, the pleura is bluntly retracted. **B.** Anterior dissection circumferentially to the opposite side of the pleura. **C.** Posterior retraction of the parietal pleura beyond the rib head. **D.** A scalpel blade is used to incise the annulus from rib head posteriorly all the way to the opposite annulus. Shown here is the incision up against the rib head after incising the annulus and the anterior longitudinal ligament. **E.** Disc shavers are used to break up the disc material. **F.** An angled curette is used to take down the endplate and tease the periosteum around the corner to get full access to the bone. *(continued)*

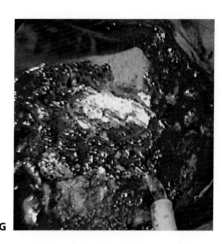

G

TECH FIG 3 • *(continued)* **G.** The most anterior aspect of the rib head is being removed. Electrocautery is used to loosen the soft tissues attaching the rib head to the vertebral body. Part of the rib head has been removed in this photo.

- The periosteum for the proximal and distal vertebra is incised to allow for subperiosteal dissection when the discectomy is performed.
- Disc shavers are used to break up the disc material, using shavers of increasing width (**TECH FIG 3E**).
- A rongeur is used to remove the annulus and nucleus pulposus.
- An angled curette is used to take down the endplate circumferentially (**TECH FIG 3F**).

- The rib head is removed at the T4–T7 levels. Since it is positioned relatively anterior on the vertebral bodies, it allows for good discectomy and good placement of the screws at these levels (**TECH FIG 3G**).
- After discectomy, Gelfoam or Surgicel is placed in the disc space to prevent endplate bleeding.

Implant Placement and Grafting

- Screw placement is performed beginning at the apex of the curve.
- The proper screw position starts just anterior to the rib head and is angled in line with the midaxial plane of the vertebral body (angled anteriorly at the apex especially, with less angulation at the proximal distal levels) (**TECH FIG 4A**).
- Screw position should be parallel to the endplate, and the proximal and distal levels should be angled toward the apex of the curve so that during correction, any screw plow will not loosen screws. Visualization of adjacent screws should confirm good alignment (**TECH FIG 4B**).
- After screw placement, the screw height should be visualized to ensure that rod seating will occur without difficulty (**TECH FIG 4C**).
- Autologous bone is packed into the disc space after removal of Gelfoam or Surgicel.
- Rod placement is performed; rods can be seated either proximally or distally. Depending on rod flexibility and size, a straight rod is placed on the end and the set screws are engaged to secure the rod (**TECH FIG 4D**).

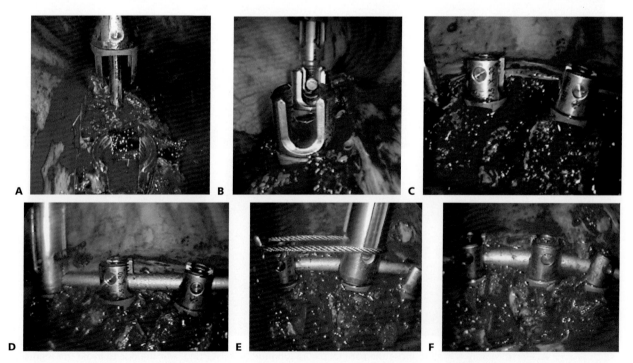

TECH FIG 4 • A. The screw-awl device is placed while visualizing a previously placed screw. The starting point is just anterior to the rib head in this photo. **B.** Final placement of a distal screw while visualizing the more proximal screws. The diaphragm is seen in the background. **C.** After screw placement, the height of the screws should be consistent to allow easy seating of the rod. **D.** The rod is inserted into the most distal screws. **E.** Compression across the most distal segment is first performed using the cable compressor. **F.** After distal compression, the rod is cantilevered to the remaining screw heads. *(continued)*

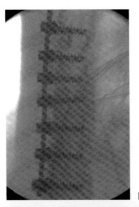
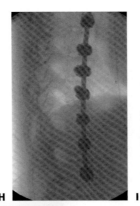
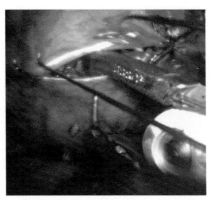
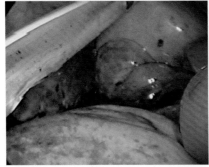

TECH FIG 4 • *(continued)* **G.** AP intraoperative fluoroscopic image confirms good correction of the spine with maintenance of screw position. **H.** Lateral fluoroscopic image demonstrates good position of the screws with restoration of thoracic kyphosis. Rotational correction is also seen with rib margins symmetric. **I.** Closure of the parietal pleura over the instrumentation. **J.** Placement of chest tube under direct visualization while the lung is still deflated.

- Compression across the initial levels is then performed to improve the coronal- and sagittal-plane deformity (**TECH FIG 4E**).
- The rod is then cantilevered down to the remaining screws, and compression is sequentially performed over those levels. Often the rod cannot be cantilevered down to all of the screws, so sequential cantilever and compression are performed (**TECH FIG 4F**).
- Radiographs are obtained at this point and the desired correction is compared with the radiographs. Further compression is performed as needed. Care should be taken to ensure that screw plow or loosening is not occurring radiographically or visually (**TECH FIG 4G,H**).
- Set screws are completely torqued down.
- The pleura is closed over the instrumentation to ensure correct bone graft positioning, decreased chest tube drainage, and improved long-term pulmonary function (**TECH FIG 4I**).
- The lung is inflated under direct visualization.
- A chest tube is placed through the distal portal incision and tunneled to the proximal portal (**TECH FIG 4J**).
- The incisions are closed in the normal fashion.

OPEN INSTRUMENTATION AND ARTHRODESIS OF THE THORACOLUMBAR–LUMBAR SPINE

Preparation and Exposure

- The patient is placed in the lateral decubitus position with the convex side of the spine up.
- An axillary roll is placed.
- The bed can be flexed to allow for easier access to the flank (**TECH FIG 5A**).
- A curved linear incision is made in line with the rib just proximal to the planned upper instrumented vertebra (**TECH FIG 5B**).
- The incision is carried down through the subcutaneous layer through the various muscle layers down over the rib. The incision can be carried out distally lateral to the umbilicus.
- Subperiosteal dissection is carried out around the rib. The rib is transected posteriorly near its insertion to the spine (**TECH FIG 5C**).
- The costochondral junction is then incised. A marking suture is placed at the costochondral junction for later reapproximation (**TECH FIG 5D**).
- Usually at the costochondral level at the 10th rib, access into the retroperitoneal space is quite easy, with retroperitoneal fat evident. The peritoneal contents are then bluntly dissected off the abdominal wall and the undersurface of the diaphragm (**TECH FIG 5E**).
- The diaphragm is then incised just proximal to its insertion, and marking sutures are placed to ensure proper reapproximation (**TECH FIG 5F**).
- A pleural incision is made longitudinally in line with the spine, leaving the segmental vessels intact (**TECH FIG 5G**).
- Segmental vessel ligation is then carried out, maintaining good blood pressure to ensure good spinal cord perfusion (**TECH FIG 5H**).

TECHNIQUES

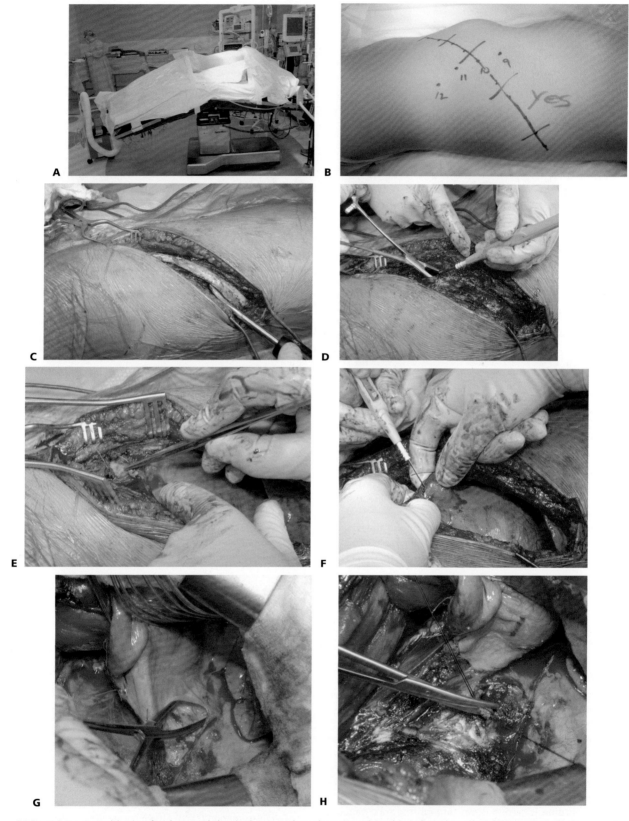

TECH FIG 5 • A. Positioning for thoracoabdominal approach to the spine. The table is flexed to allow full access to the thoracoab-dominal region. **B.** Skin incision is marked. This example is centered over the 10th rib for a T11–L3 fusion. **C.** The incision is made over the rib and subperiosteal dissection is carried out circumferentially around the rib after sequential dissection through the musculature. **D.** The posterior aspect of the periosteum is then incised and the chest is entered. **E.** After incision of the costochon-dral junction, the retroperitoneal fat is visualized and the retroperitoneal cavity is entered. **F.** The diaphragm is incised a finger-breadth proximal to its insertion. **G.** The parietal pleura is incised proximally. **H.** Ligation of segmental vessels after suture tying.

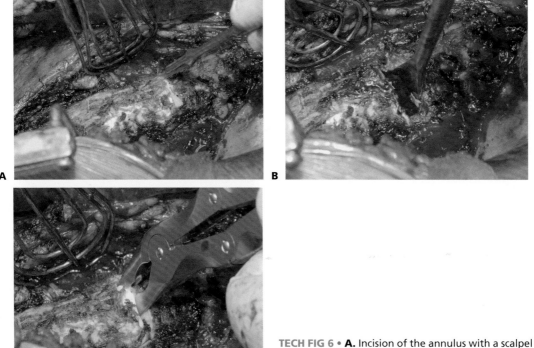

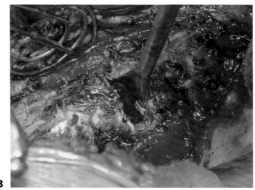

TECH FIG 6 • A. Incision of the annulus with a scalpel blade. **B.** Endplate dissection off the bone using a Cobb elevator. **C.** Lexcel rongeur removal of the disc material.

Discectomy

- Discectomies are performed with incision of the annulus fibrosis (**TECH FIG 6A**).
- Endplate dissection is carried out, using a Cobb elevator to remove the entire endplate disc material back to the posterior aspect of the annulus and to the posterior longitudinal ligament if necessary (for severe curves; **TECH FIG 6B**).
- The disc material is removed completely using rongeurs and curettes (**TECH FIG 6C**).
- The disc space is packed with Surgicel.

Implant Placement, Correction, and Fusion

- The instrumentation is then placed using single large screws with a quarter-inch single-rod implant system, or a dual rod with a 5.5-mm rod (shown here).

- Screws are initially placed at the apex in the middle to posterior third of the vertebral body in the midaxial plane (**TECH FIG 7A**).
- When using a dual-rod system, the posterior screws are initially placed angled in the midaxial plane, while the anterior screws are directed slightly posteriorly. A staple is often used when both the single- and dual-rod screws are used (**TECH FIG 7B**).
- Once screws are placed, the bone graft material is placed as far back toward the posterior longitudinal ligament as possible, or the posterior rim of the annulus fibrosis.
- The operating table should now be leveled to allow for correction of the spine.
- The posterior rod is initially placed with the dual-rod system, and a 90-degree rod rotation removal can be performed (**TECH FIG 7C**).

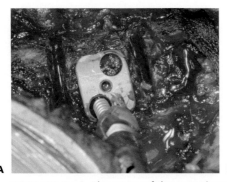

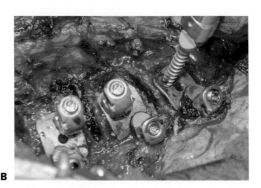

TECH FIG 7 • A. Placement of the posterior screw directed slightly anteriorly with direct visualization of the endplates after complete disc removal. **B.** Anterior screw placement after placement of the posterior screws. The anterior screws are directed slightly posteriorly. *(continued)*

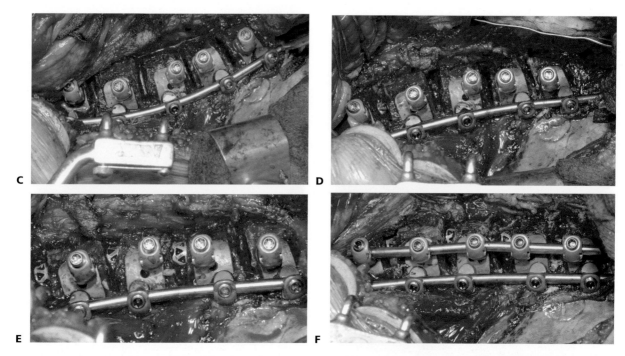

TECH FIG 7 • *(continued)* **C.** Insertion of the posterior rod with lumbar lordosis built into the rod. **D.** After 90 degrees of rod rotation, scoliosis correction is achieved while restoring lumbar lordosis, as shown here. **E.** After rod rotation, the anterior structural support is placed anteriorly and toward the concavity of the deformity. **F.** The anterior rod is seated into the anterior screws.

- Alternatively, directed force on the anterior screws to correct the coronal and axial plane is achieved, and then the posterior rod is inserted (**TECH FIG 7D**).
- After rod rotation with a dual-rod system or single-rod system, or correction with pressure on the anterior screws and fixation with the posterior rod, the anterior structural support is placed. This is most commonly at levels distal to T12 or alternatively at all instrumented levels (**TECH FIG 7E**).
- Compression can then be performed to further correct coronal-plane deformity.
- The anterior structural support should be placed anteriorly and onto the concavity to ensure maintenance of the lordosis and improvement of coronal-plane correction.
- The second anterior rod should be then placed with a dual-rod system and all set screws completely tightened (**TECH FIG 7F**).

- The remaining bone graft material is then placed in the remaining disc space.

Closure

- The pleura is closed as far distally as possible (**TECH FIG 8A**).
- The diaphragm is reapproximated with interrupted Neurolon sutures (**TECH FIG 8B**).
- The costochondral junction is reapproximated, and the periosteum of the rib is reapproximated (**TECH FIG 8C**).
- A chest tube of fairly large diameter is then placed.
- The abdominal wall is reapproximated in layers (**TECH FIG 8D**).
- The remaining muscle layers are closed, as well as the skin and subcutaneous layers (**TECH FIG 8E**).
- The postoperative radiographs are shown in **TECHNIQUES FIGURE 8F AND 8G**.

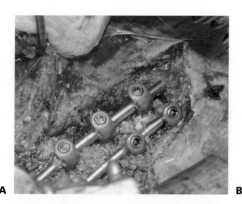

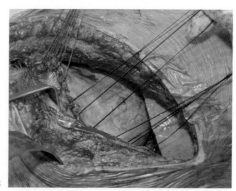

TECH FIG 8 • A. The parietal pleura is closed beginning proximal to the implants. **B.** Interrupted Neurolon sutures are used to close the diaphragm in an anatomic fashion. *(continued)*

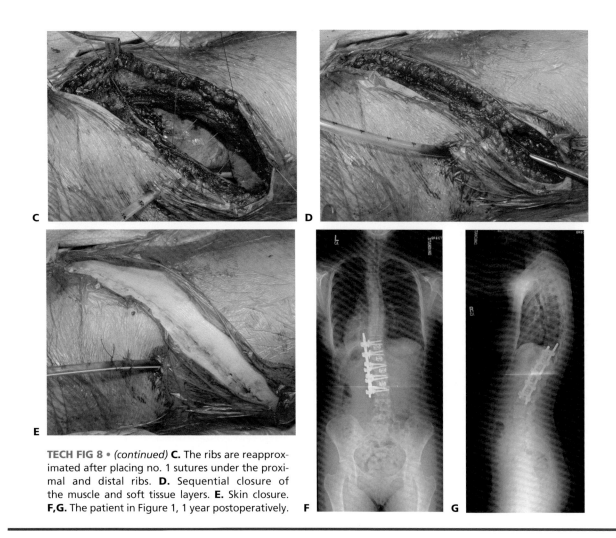

TECH FIG 8 • *(continued)* **C.** The ribs are reapproximated after placing no. 1 sutures under the proximal and distal ribs. **D.** Sequential closure of the muscle and soft tissue layers. **E.** Skin closure. **F,G.** The patient in Figure 1, 1 year postoperatively.

PEARLS AND PITFALLS

Anesthesia	▪ During anterior surgery, normotensive anesthesia should be performed to maintain spinal cord perfusion, especially when segmental vessel ligation is performed. ▪ Complete discectomy is necessary to achieve fusion since pseudarthrosis rates continue to be higher with anterior surgery than with posterior surgery.
Camera performance	▪ Thoracoscopy requires outstanding visualization and camera performance to ensure safe and effective discectomy, as well as instrumentation.
Rib head removal	▪ Rib head removal during thoracic instrumentation from T4 to T7 is necessary to ensure screws are placed posteriorly enough to achieve good purchase.
Discectomy	▪ This is the most important aspect of the procedure to mobilize the spine for correction and to achieve a solid arthrodesis.
Screw placement	▪ Screw placement is always challenging at the proximal and distal levels. Screw trajectories should always be parallel to the endplate, or if anything angled toward the apex of the curve, so that during correction plowing does not result in loosening of the screw.
Deformity correction	▪ Thoracic curve: Compression at sequential levels, followed by cantilever of an undercontoured rod, followed by further compression ▪ Thoracolumbar–lumbar curve: Rod rotation followed by compression

POSTOPERATIVE CARE

- The chest tube should be placed to wall suction and can usually be removed between 48 and 72 hours, when the drainage decreases below 80 cc per shift and when it turns more straw-colored.
- Serial hemoglobin and hematocrit levels should be obtained in the first 48 hours.
- Advancing activities: Sitting in a chair the first postoperative day and walking on the second postoperative day ensures good postoperative pulmonary status and normal bowel function.
- Postoperative bracing is used for 3 months for single-rod anterior thoracoscopic thoracic arthrodesis and instrumentation. No bracing is necessary with single quarter-inch rod instrumentation or dual-rod instrumentation when anterior structural support is used.
- Normal activities are resumed when arthrodesis is visualized (best seen on the lateral radiograph).

OUTCOMES

- Thoracoscopic anterior instrumentation and fusion achieves a good radiographic and functional outcome.
- Thoracoscopic anterior instrumentation and fusion continues to have a fairly high pseudarthrosis rate of 5% to 6%.
- Pulmonary function is somewhat decreased early in the postoperative period with anterior surgery, but then it can return to baseline at 1 to 2 years.
- Thoracolumbar–lumbar anterior instrumentation and fusion results in excellent coronal-, axial-, and sagittal-plane realignment, especially when dual-rod and large single-rod instrumentation systems with anterior structural support are used.

COMPLICATIONS

- Acute complications
  - Infection is rare in anterior spine deformity surgery.
  - Atelectasis and mucous plugs can be seen, especially with single-lung ventilation with anterior instrumentation. Aggressive pulmonary toilet and resuming activities minimize this risk.
- Late complications
  - Pseudarthrosis: The incidence is 4% to 10% for thoracic scoliosis (usually occurs at the apex of the curve) and 4% to 12% for thoracolumbar scoliosis (usually occurs at the distal fusion level).
  - Loss of correction with kyphosis is seen for thoracolumbar–lumbar curves treated anteriorly when anterior structural support is not used.

REFERENCES

1. Bernstein RM, Hall JE. Solid rod short segment anterior fusion in thoracolumbar scoliosis. J Pediatr Orthop B 1998;7:124–131.
2. Betz RR, Shufflebarger H. Anterior versus posterior instrumentation for the correction of thoracic idiopathic scoliosis. Spine 2001;26: 1095–1100.
3. Bitan FD, Neuwirth MG, Kuflik PL, et al. The use of short and rigid anterior instrumentation in the treatment of idiopathic thoracolumbar scoliosis: a retrospective review of 24 cases. Spine 2002;27:1553–1557.
4. Bullmann V, Halm HF, Niemeyer T, et al. Dual-rod correction and instrumentation of idiopathic scoliosis with the Halm-Zielke instrumentation. Spine 2003;28:1306–1313.
5. Kaneda K, Shono Y, Satoh S, et al. New anterior instrumentation for the management of thoracolumbar and lumbar scoliosis: application of the Kaneda two-rod system. Spine 1996;21:1250–1262.
6. Lenke LG, Newton PO, Marks MC, et al. Prospective pulmonary function comparison of open versus endoscopic anterior fusion combined with posterior fusion in adolescent idiopathic scoliosis. Spine 2004;29:2055–2060.
7. Lonner BS, Kondrachov D, Siddiqi F, et al. Thoracoscopic spinal fusion compared with posterior spinal fusion for the treatment of thoracic adolescent idiopathic scoliosis. J Bone Joint Surg Am 2006;88A:1022–1034.
8. Lowe TG, Alongi PR, Smith DAB, et al. Anterior single rod instrumentation for thoracolumbar adolescent idiopathic scoliosis with and without the use of structural interbody support. Spine 2003;28:2232–2242.
9. Newton PO, Parent S, Marks M, et al. Prospective evaluation of 50 consecutive scoliosis patients surgically treated with thoracoscopic anterior instrumentation. Spine 2005;30:S100–109.
10. Ouellet JA, Johnston CE II. Effect of grafting technique on the maintenance of coronal and sagittal correction in anterior treatment of scoliosis. Spine 2002;27:2129–2136.
11. Picetti GD III, Pang D, Bueff HU. Thoracoscopic techniques for the treatment of scoliosis: early results in procedure development. Neurosurgery 2002;51:978–984.
12. Sanders AE, Baumann R, Brown H, et al. Selective anterior fusion of thoracolumbar/lumbar curves in adolescents: when can the associated thoracic curve be left unfused? Spine 2003;28:706–714.
13. Saraph VJ, Krismer M, Wimmer C. Operative treatment of scoliosis with the Kaneda anterior spine system. Spine 2005;30:1616–1620.
14. Satake K, Lenke LG, Kim YJ, et al. Analysis of the lowest instrumented vertebra following anterior spinal fusion of thoracolumbar/lumbar adolescent idiopathic scoliosis: can we predict postoperative disc wedging? Spine 2005;30:418–426.
15. Sucato D, Kassab F, Dempsey M. Thoracoscopic anterior spinal instrumentation and fusion for idiopathic scoliosis: a CT analysis of screw placement and completeness of discectomy. Scoliosis Research Society, Cleveland, Ohio, 2001.
16. Sweet FA, Lenke LG, Bridwell KH, et al. Prospective radiographic and clinical outcomes and complications of single solid rod instrumented anterior spinal fusion in adolescent idiopathic scoliosis. Spine 2001;26:1956–1965.
17. Wong H-K, Hee H-T, Yu Z, et al. Results of thoracoscopic instrumented fusion versus conventional posterior instrumented fusion in adolescent idiopathic scoliosis undergoing selective thoracic fusion. Spine 2004;29:2031–2039.

Chapter 37

Thoracoscopic Release and Fusion for Scoliosis

Daniel J. Sucato

DEFINITION

▪ Thoracoscopy provides the ability to gain access to the thoracic spine via small incisions (portals).

▪ *Anterior release* includes removal of the annulus fibrosis, anterior longitudinal ligament, nucleus pulposus, and, if necessary, the rib head.

▪ *Scoliosis* is a lateral curvature of the spine with axial plane rotation.

▪ *Fusion* is the healing of two vertebral bodies together, usually fused by bone graft or bone graft substitute.

ANATOMY

▪ The thoracic spine spans from the first thoracic vertebra (T1) to the twelfth thoracic vertebra (T12).

▪ The rib head attachment to the vertebral body is more anterior in the proximal thoracic spine than the distal thoracic spine.

▪ The *annulus fibrosis* is the circumferential fibrous tissue that surrounds the nucleus pulposus, which is in the center of the disc.

▪ The anterior longitudinal ligament, which runs on the anterior aspect of the vertebral body, is a strong fibrous tissue that is contiguous throughout the spine. The segmental arteries and veins originate from the aorta and vena cava, respectively, and traverse the vertebral body. The parietal pleura of the chest surrounds the thoracic spine, covering the segmental vessels and the disc and vertebral bodies. The anterior, middle, and posterior axillary lines run (in reference to the axilla) in the anterior, middle, and posterior aspects of the axilla. Scoliotic deformity in the thoracic spine is lateral curvature with axial plane rotation, as well as hypokyphosis (idiopathic scoliosis).

▪ The arch of the aorta and the arch of the azygous vein typically are located at the T4–T5 levels.

PATHOGENESIS

▪ Scoliosis can be grouped into many categories based on pathogenesis.

▪ The most common type of scoliosis seen is idiopathic, in which the etiology and pathogenesis are unknown.

▪ Theories of pathogenesis include hormonal influences, growth disturbance, genetic factors, muscle imbalance, and proprioception and balance abnormalities.

▪ Other types of scoliosis include:

▪ Congenital: abnormal vertebra due to failure of formation or segmentation

▪ Neuromuscular: eg, cerebral palsy, Duchenne muscular dystrophy, spinal muscular atrophy

▪ Neurogenic: eg, neurofibromatosis, spinal cord injury

NATURAL HISTORY

▪ An idiopathic scoliosis curve may progress in two ways:

▪ With continued spine growth

▪ When curve magnitude is greater than 50 degrees at skeletal maturity

▪ Curve progression can be rapid during spine growth, or slow following skeletal maturity (approximately 1 degree per year).

▪ Curve magnitudes above 80 to 90 degrees in the thoracic spine may result in symptomatic pulmonary issues.

▪ Large curves in adulthood can result in pain.[1]

PATIENT HISTORY AND PHYSICAL FINDINGS

▪ The examination for spine deformity should include standing visualization of the spine to look for shoulder height differences, waist asymmetry, overall trunk balance, or coronal head imbalance (**FIG 1**).

▪ Further information is obtained as to the character of the pain (eg, sharp, dull, aching), when the pain occurs (eg, during activity, while attempting to sleep, pain waking from sleep), and the location of the pain (eg, upper, middle, lower back), as well as whether it radiates into the lower extremities.

▪ Other history should include any information on other neurologic symptoms such as bowel or bladder incontinence.

▪ Sensory symptoms should be elicited, especially with hyperesthesias along the chest wall, or upper or lower extremities.

▪ Cutaneous manifestations of dysraphism should be analyzed.

▪ The neurologic examination should include motor strength and a sensory examination of the upper and lower extremities.

▪ The abdominal reflexes are the most important neurologic assessment. They are assessed by stroking the skin adjacent to the umbilicus on the left and right and upper and lower quadrants, and should be symmetrically absent or present. When asymmetric, MRI is necessary to evaluate for neural axis abnormalities.

▪ The lower extremities should be carefully examined for asymmetry with respect to size and strength of the legs, as

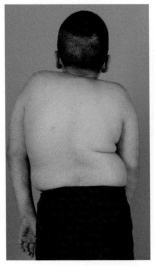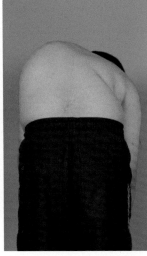

FIG 1 • This 9-year-old boy had a left-sided large thoracic scoliosis but no evidence of neural axis abnormalities on preoperative MRI.

well as foot deformities (eg, cavovarus foot deformities) as an indication for the presence of neural axis abnormalities.

■ Deep tendon reflexes and the Babinski reflex should be investigated.

IMAGING AND OTHER DIAGNOSTIC STUDIES

■ Plain radiography should include a standing posteroanterior (PA) and lateral radiograph of the spine to include the cervical spine to the pelvis and hips.

■ The PA radiograph (**FIG 2A**) should be evaluated for:
  ■ Coronal plane deformities using the Cobb method
  ■ The C7–center sacral vertebral line (CSVL) placement
  ■ A trunk shift using Floman's method (the distance between the CSVL and the mid-distance between the lateral rib margins)
  ■ Evaluation for any congenital abnormalities (eg, hemivertebra, congenital bar)
  ■ The Risser stage (0 through 5)
  ■ The status of the triradiate cartilage (open or closed)

■ The lateral radiographs (**FIG 2B**) should be analyzed to determine:
  ■ Thoracic kyphosis and lumbar lordosis
  ■ Presence of associated spondylolisthesis or spondylolysis
  ■ Sagittal balance (distance between C7 plumb line and the posterior edge of the first sacral vertebral body)
  ■ The Stagnara view is an oblique view to the patient, but an orthogonal view to the coronal curve that is used in severe spinal deformities to better visualize the spine.

■ Indications for MRI include neurologic abnormalities, significant back pain associated with scoliosis, atypical curve patterns such as a left thoracic curve, very young age, congenital scoliosis, neurofibromatosis, Marfan disease.

■ CT scanning may be useful to fully define the osseous anatomy, especially for extremely large curves and congenital curves.

DIFFERENTIAL DIAGNOSIS

■ Idiopathic scoliosis
■ Congenital scoliosis
■ Neurofibromatosis
■ Scoliosis associated with Marfan disease

NONOPERATIVE MANAGEMENT

■ Nonoperative management has little or no role for severe deformity.

■ Patients who are very young with moderate deformity may be treated with a brace to buy time to allow the patient to grow.
  ■ Bracing can be effective to prevent curve progression for small idiopathic curves (ie, 25 to 40 degrees).

SURGICAL MANAGEMENT

■ Anterior thoracoscopic release for spinal deformity has many technical considerations, which are discussed later in this chapter.

■ Indications for an anterior release/fusion
  ■ Severe spinal deformity: scoliosis greater than 80 to 90 degrees with significant rotational deformity or kyphosis greater than 100 degrees with flexibility index less than 50%
  ■ Skeletal immaturity, to avoid the crankshaft phenomenon. Usually performed for children younger than 10 years of age with open triradiate cartilage and Risser grade 0.
  ■ Deficient posterior elements, so that a posterior fusion may be difficult. Such deficiencies occur secondary to previous surgery with laminectomies for tumors or the treatment of neural axis abnormalities.

Preoperative Planning

■ Each patient should be carefully analyzed with respect to those curves that will undergo an anterior release.

■ The radiograph should be viewed to determine preoperatively which levels should be released. Release always includes the apical levels, and usually includes all of the levels within the Cobb measurement.

■ For severe curves, traction in the operating room may be helpful in assisting curve correction.

Positioning and Approach

Lateral Position

■ Advantages
  ■ More familiar and traditional approach
  ■ Conversion to open procedure is easy.
  ■ All thoracic levels can be accessed.
  ■ One can effectively obtain access to the T1 to T5 levels, which are not accessible when the patient is in the prone position.

■ Disadvantages
  ■ Repositioning is necessary for the posterior approach.
  ■ Single-lung ventilation is required.

■ Approach
  ■ Single-lung ventilation is achieved with a double-lumen endotracheal tube or a univent tube.
  ■ Position the patient in the lateral decubitus position.
  ■ Check the endotracheal tube position and the single-lung ventilation status.
  ■ Prepare and drape the chest and side (**FIG 3**).
  ■ Place four portals in the anterior axillary line.

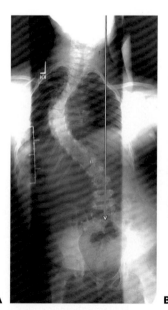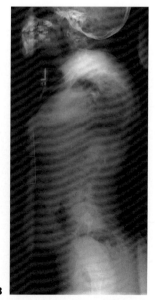

FIG 2 • Preoperative AP and lateral radiographs demonstrate a 93-degree left thoracic scoliosis with a large trunk shift and open triradiate cartilage in the patient shown in Fig 1.

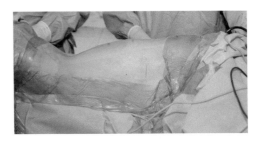

FIG 3 • Lateral positioning. The patient is positioned in the lateral decubitus position with the surgical side up (left in this case). An axillary roll was placed and the patient is in the direct lateral position to assist in surgeon orientation. Proximal is to the right and distal is to the left. A single anterior portal and four posterolateral portals are planned.

Prone Position
- Advantages
  - Not necessary to reposition patient for the posterior procedure
  - No need for single-lung ventilation
  - Significantly decreased respiratory complications. Single double lung ventilation is used.
- Disadvantages
  - Difficult to obtain an anterior release proximal to T5.
  - Conversion to open procedure is difficult.
- Approach
  - Placement of regular endotracheal tube
  - Double-lung ventilation with decreased tidal volumes (about 50% to 60% of normal) and increased ventilatory rate
  - Placement prone on a spine frame (**FIG 4A,B**)
  - Ensure access to the flank and chest.
  - Prepare and drape the back and the chest and flank (**FIG 4C,D**).

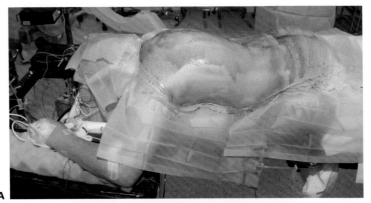

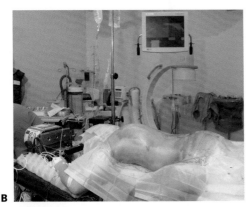

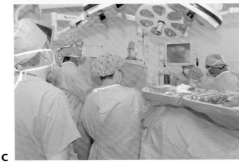

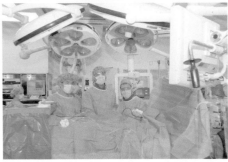

FIG 4 • Prone positioning. **A.** Close-up view of the patient, who has a left thoracic scoliosis. The left flank and spine have been prepared. **B.** The position of the monitor on the opposite side of the patient is shown. **C,D.** Surgical setup for a prone endoscopic release. **C.** View from behind the surgeons. The surgical assistant is on the opposite side of the operating table along with the monitor. The surgeon and first assistant are on the convex side of the patient—in this case, the left side. **D.** View from the opposite side: the surgeons are viewing the monitor. The primary surgeon and two assistants are operating.

THORACOSCOPIC RELEASE AND FUSION FOR SCOLIOSIS

Placement of Portals and Visualization

- Place portals as anteriorly as possible, usually in the midaxillary line (**TECH FIG 1A,B**).
- Insert the camera into the initial portal with the lens directed posteriorly (**TECH FIG 1C**).
- Find a clear space between the posterior chest wall and the lung and advance the thoracoscope.

- Place a small, blunt-tipped cottonoid to retract the lung, to identify the spine and other anatomic structures.
- Place a fan retractor to fully retract the lung, if necessary (**TECH FIG 1D**).
- Place suction into the chest.
- Place working portal.
- Visualize the spine in the horizontal plane with the segmental vessels intact (**TECH FIG 1E**).

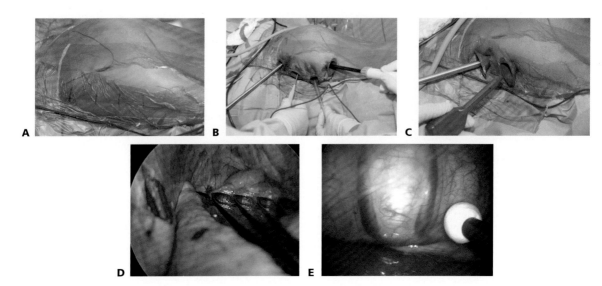

TECH FIG 1 • Prone anterior release. **A.** Skin markings are made to identify the left scapula and the four lateral portals. To the left is proximal. The most proximal portal usually gains access to the T5-6 disc when it is in the mid-scapular region, as shown. **B.** Following placement of the four portals, the thoracoscope is placed in the most proximal working portal with an electrocautery in the second portal, suction is in the third portal, and the fan retractor in the fourth portal. **C.** The first portal is placed first, as shown; in this illustration, it is the most proximal portal, to the left. The secondary portal is then placed approximately two fingerbreadths distally and in line with the first. **D.** A fan retractor is placed to gently push down on the atelectatic lung. Visualized here is the superior-most aspect of the chest. **E.** The spine is visualized in the horizontal plane. The segmental vessels are easily seen.

Exposure and Disc Removal

- Incise the pleura along the mid-vertebral body line (**TECH FIG 2A**).
- Spare the segmental blood vessels to preserve perfusion to the spinal cord.
- Bluntly retract the pleura anteriorly and posteriorly (**TECH FIG 2B**).
- Incise the annulus fibrosis with the scalpel blade circumferentially from lateral rib head to near-opposite rib head (**TECH FIG 2C**).
- Break up the disc with disc shavers (**TECH FIG 2D**).
- Remove the disc material with a rongeur (**TECH FIG 2E**).
- Take down the endplate with a curved curette (**TECH FIG 2F**).
- Place Surgicel (Ethicon, Inc., Somerville, NJ) or other thrombotic agent.
- Remove the disc from all levels planned.
- Place bone graft if desired (**TECH FIG 2G**).
- Close the pleura using the Endostitch device (US Surgical, Warsaw, IN), running one suture from proximal and one from distal (**TECH FIG 2H–J**).
- Place a chest tube (**TECH FIG 2K**).
- Close the portal incisions.

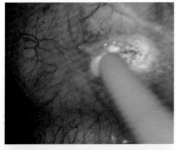

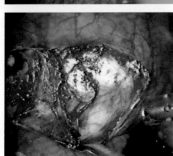

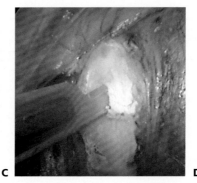

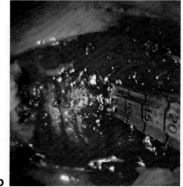

TECH FIG 2 • **A.** Using a curved electrocautery blade, the pleura is incised in the longitudinal fashion, sparing the segmental vessels. **B.** The parietal pleura is retracted anteriorly, as shown, to allow for complete access to the anterior longitudinal ligament, as well as the opposite annulus. The posterior pleura is also retracted. **C.** The annulus is incised parallel to the disc. **D.** Disc shavers are used to break up the disc material. *(continued)*

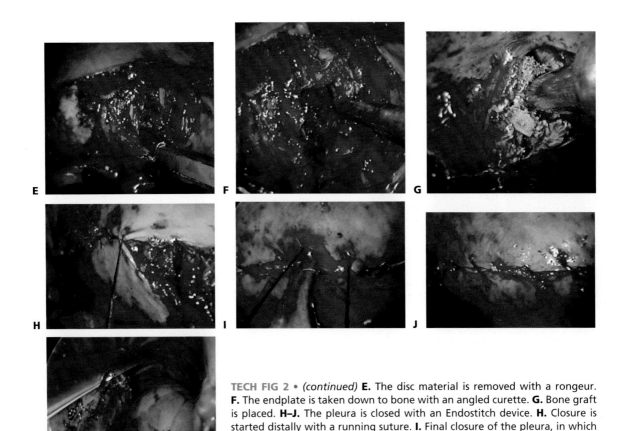

TECH FIG 2 • *(continued)* **E.** The disc material is removed with a rongeur. **F.** The endplate is taken down to bone with an angled curette. **G.** Bone graft is placed. **H–J.** The pleura is closed with an Endostitch device. **H.** Closure is started distally with a running suture. **I.** Final closure of the pleura, in which the proximal suture is brought to the distal suture. **J.** The pleura is closed nicely with a running suture. **K.** Placement of the chest tube at the completion of the procedure, from distal to proximal. The lung is still deflated. The pleura, seen in the background, has been closed previously.

PEARLS AND PITFALLS

Portal placement	▪ Placement of portals is key for visualization and achieving good discectomy. ▪ Place the skin incision for the portal over a rib to allow the portal to be placed above and below the rib (two portals per skin incision). ▪ Ensure that portals are neither too posterior nor too anterior.
Preservation of segmental blood vessels	▪ Incise the pleura in a longitudinal fashion, staying superficial to the segmental vessels. ▪ Use a curved harmonic scalpel or electrocautery. ▪ Incise any adventitial tissue adherent to the pleura over the disc to free up the parietal pleura. ▪ Bluntly retract the pleura to gain access to the disc.

Complete removal of the disc	▪ Develop the same sequence for disc removal:
	  1. Incise the disc with a scalpel blade.
	  2. Break up disc material with shavers.
	  3. Remove loosened disc material.
	  4. Take down the endplates of the vertebral bodies with a curved curette.
	  5. Remove excess endplate material.

Pleural closure	▪ Use the Endostitch device with 2-0 Vicryl suture. ▪ Use two sutures: the first begins in the proximal aspect and is run distally, and the second is started distally and is run proximally.

POSTOPERATIVE CARE

▪ Chest tube management
  ▪ Connect chest tube to wall suction.
  ▪ Obtain daily chest radiographs.
  ▪ The chest tube may be removed when drainage is less than 80 mL over 12 hours and serous color returns (with good pleural closure, removal usually is done on the first day).

▪ Mobilize the patient to chair on postoperative day 1.
▪ Mobilize the patient to ambulation when the chest tube is removed (usually postoperative day 2).
▪ Serial hemoglobin and hematocrit on postoperative days 1 and 2
▪ Advanced activities as tolerated to daily activities in the initial 6 weeks

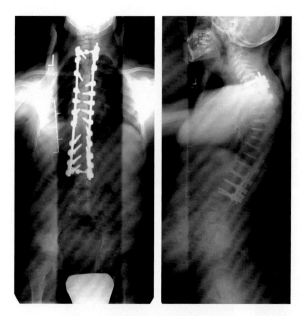

FIG 5 • The 2-year postoperative AP and lateral radiographs of the patient shown in Figures 1 and 2 demonstrated outstanding coronal and sagittal plane correction after prone thoracoscopic anterior release and fusion followed by a posterior spinal fusion and instrumentation from T2 to L2.

■ For the following 6 weeks, physical activities are advanced, depending on posterior constructs.

OUTCOMES

■ The addition of a thoracoscopic anterior release and fusion results in a decrease in pulmonary function in the first 6 weeks; however, at 1 year it is 30% above baseline.
■ Anterior release increases the flexibility of the spine and allows for great coronal, axial plane, and sagittal plane correction.
■ With good surgical technique, an outstanding anterior release can be achieved and will allow for exceptional three-dimensional correction of the spine with posterior instrumentation and fusion (**FIG 5**).

COMPLICATIONS

■ Single-lung ventilation
   ■ Intraoperative complications: inability to ventilate adequately secondary to ventilation-perfusion mismatches, high airway pressures and barotrauma, and underlying pulmonary issues
   ■ Postoperative complications: atelectasis secondary to barotrauma or mucous plugs
   ■ Continuous chest tube drainage, especially when the parietal pleura has not been closed
■ Pneumothorax following chest tube removal
■ Intraoperative injury to the segmental blood vessels or the great vessels
■ Intraoperative injury to the thoracic duct, which usually occurs on the right side at the T11–12 area. This can be avoided by dissection deep to the parietal pleura.
■ Chylothorax is treated with total parenteral nutrition and avoidance of a fatty diet.
■ Intraoperative excessive bleeding secondary to inadvertent segmental vessel injury. Strategies to coagulate the vessel are used.
■ Long-term complications secondary to a thoracoscopic anterior release and fusion are limited.

REFERENCES

1. Al-Sayyad MJ, Crawford AH, Wolf RK. Video-assisted thoracoscopic surgery: The Cincinnati experience. Clin Orthop Relat Res 2005;434:61–70.
2. Crawford AH. Anterior surgery in the thoracic and lumbar spine: Endoscopic techniques in children. Instr Course Lect 2005;54:567–576.
3. Cunningham BW, et al. Video-assisted thoracoscopic surgery versus open thoracotomy for anterior thoracic spinal fusion: a comparative radiographic, biomechanical, and histologic analysis in a sheep model. Spine 1998;23:1333–1340.
4. Newton P, Shea K, Granlund K. Defining the pediatric spinal thoracoscopy learning curve: Sixty-five consecutive cases. Spine 2000;25: 1028–1035.
5. Niemeyer T, et al., Anterior thoracoscopic surgery followed by posterior instrumentation and fusion in spinal deformity. Eur Spine J 2000;9:499–504.
6. Picetti GD III, Pang D, Bueff HU. Thoracoscopic techniques for the treatment of scoliosis: early results in procedure development. Neurosurgery 2002;51:978.
7. Sucato DJ, Elerson E. A comparison between the prone and lateral position for performing a thoracoscopic anterior release and fusion for pediatric spinal deformity. Spine 2003;28:2176–2180.
8. Sucato DJ, et al. Thoracoscopic discectomy and fusion in an animal model: safe and effective when segmental blood vessels are spared. Spine 2002;27:880–886.
9. Huang EY, et al. Thoracoscopic anterior spinal release and fusion: Evolution of a faster, improved approach. J Pediatr Surg 2002;37: 1732–1735.
10. Newton PO, et al. A biomechanical comparison of open and thoracoscopic anterior spinal release in a goat model. Spine 1998;23:530–535.

Chapter 38

Unit Rod Instrumentation for Neuromuscular Scoliosis

Kirk W. Dabney and Freeman Miller

DEFINITION

- Neuromuscular spinal deformity is a result of an abnormal neuromuscular system in childhood, as in cerebral palsy, muscular dystrophy, spinal muscular atrophy, and so forth. It may be related to a pathologic abnormality in muscle tone, motor control, or weakness or a combination.
- While neuromuscular scoliosis (coronal deformity) is the most common neuromuscular spinal deformity, sagittal plane deformity (hyperlordosis and hyperkyphosis) may also occur.

ANATOMY

- The curve patterns of neuromuscular scoliosis are most commonly lumbar or thoracolumbar with associated pelvic obliquity (**FIG 1**).
- Since many children are nonambulatory, associated pelvic obliquity affects sitting balance.
- Ambulatory neuromuscular patients often have decompensation, with the inability to center their head over the center sacral line.

PATHOGENESIS AND NATURAL HISTORY

- The biologic basis of scoliosis or sagittal plane spinal deformity in neuromuscular disorders differs depending on the cause of the specific neuromuscular disease. In general, however, most neuromuscular spinal deformities are largely due to muscle imbalance (low tone or high tone) and abnormal postural reflexes.
- The natural history of neuromuscular scoliosis is usually that of slow progression, beginning with the development of a flexible scoliosis in middle childhood and the more rapid development of a more fixed scoliosis during the adolescent growth spurt. Some neuromuscular conditions are associated with a more progressive scoliosis than others.
- The clinician must weigh the progressive characteristics of scoliosis within each neuromuscular disease with the natural history of the disease itself when deciding on treatment.
- The pathogenesis and natural history of some of the more common disorders associated with neuromuscular spinal deformity and spinal deformity within the disease follow.

Cerebral Palsy

- Cerebral palsy is a heterogeneous disorder that is characterized by a static lesion (eg, injury, congenital defect) to the immature motor cortex of the brain. In modern society, it has become the most common cause of neuromuscular spinal deformity.
- The natural history of neuromuscular scoliosis in cerebral palsy is frequently that of progression. The rate of progression can be very severe in adolescent years (2 to 4 degrees per month).
- Progression also occurs after skeletal maturity, and in curves greater than 40 degrees it may occur at a rate of 2 to 4 degrees per year.[16]

- Curves in the 60- to 90-degree range begin to affect sitting, arm control, and head control. Further progression may prevent the child from sitting in an upright position.
- Conservative treatment with chair modifications and bracing is only a temporary treatment and does not stop curve progression. Conservative treatment is especially helpful in the younger child with a flexible scoliosis to temporarily maintain upright sitting posture. This will allow the spine to grow to its maximum size so that the resulting fusion can correct the spinal deformity without limiting growth.

Muscular Dystrophy

- Duchenne muscular dystrophy is a sex-linked recessive disorder involving a defect on the Xp21.2 locus of the X chromosome resulting in a marked decrease or absence of the protein dystrophin.[5]
- Affected children become progressively weaker with age, eventually becoming nonambulatory.
- Death typically occurs in the second or third decade secondary to pulmonary or cardiac failure.
- Scoliosis is almost universal when the child becomes nonambulatory, and curve progression correlates strongly with a decline in respiratory function.
- The prevalence of scoliosis approaches 100%.[14] For this reason, surgery is done soon after the child becomes nonambulatory, before an irreversible decline in forced vital capacity occurs.

Myelomeningocele

- Myelomeningocele, a congenital malformation of the nervous system, is due to a neural tube defect and results in a spectrum of sensory and motor deficits.

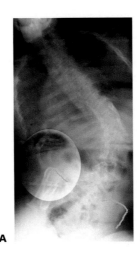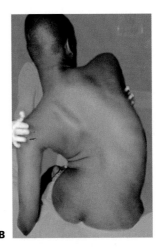

A   **B**

FIG 1 • Typical neuromuscular curve pattern in a child with quadriplegic-pattern cerebral palsy. **A.** Radiograph of long thoracolumbar curve with pelvic obliquity. **B.** Clinical picture of this child with poor sitting balance.

349

- While the level of the spinal cord defect influences the clinical presentation of the disease, neurologic deterioration may occur at any age owing to hydrocephaly, hydrosyringomyelia, Arnold–Chiari deformity, and tethered cord syndrome.
- In general, the higher the level of the defect, the higher the prevalence of scoliosis. Almost 100% of thoracic-level paraplegic patients will develop scoliosis.[17]
- A long C-shaped curve is associated with a high level of paralysis and usually occurs at a young age.
- Hydromyelia and tethered cord syndrome may also be associated with scoliosis and should be suspected if the scoliosis onset is more sudden and associated with other symptoms of acute neurologic deterioration.
- Bracing in younger children can be attempted to slow progression, but it does not stop eventual progression.

Spinal Muscular Atrophy

- This condition is an autosomal recessive disorder resulting in spinal cord anterior horn cell degeneration. Two genes on the chromosome 5q locus have been found to be associated with this disorder: survival motor neuron gene (SMN) and neuronal apoptosis inhibitory gene (NAIP).[15]
- Clinically, progressive muscular weakness occurs, and eventual pulmonary compromise is common.
- Three forms of this disease exist:
  - Type 1 (early, acute Werdnig–Hoffmann)
  - Type 2 (intermediate, chronic Werdnig–Hoffmann)
  - Type 3 (late, Kugelberg–Welander type)
- Most children with the early form of the disease die at an early age and therefore do not require treatment.
- Most children with the intermediate and late type who survive into adolescence develop a progressive spinal deformity. The curvature typically starts in the first decade. Thoracolumbar and single thoracic patterns are most common.
- One third of patients have an associated kyphosis in the sagittal plane. Bracing is ineffective at preventing curve progression but may delay progression in the very young patient to allow further growth of the spine.[1]

Friedreich Ataxia

- This autosomal recessive disorder results in a slowly progressive spinocerebellar degeneration. A defect on chromosome 9 has been identified.
- The incidence of scoliosis is 100%, and progression is related to the age of disease onset. When disease onset is prior to age 10 years and scoliosis onset is before 15 years, scoliosis progression is usually greater than 60 degrees.
- Progressive scoliosis requiring surgery is present in about 50% of patients.[7]
  - Curve patterns are similar to idiopathic scoliosis: double major, single thoracic, and thoracolumbar.
- Orthotic treatment may slow, but usually does not prevent, progression.

Rett Syndrome

- This is an X-linked disorder that affects females almost exclusively. Some children have a mutation on the MECP2 gene.[13] The child's development is normal until 6 to 18 months of age, followed by a rapid deterioration in cognitive and motor function.
- After the initial deterioration in function, the neurologic picture may become relatively static for years. The clinical spectrum is variable, with some children remaining ambulatory and others becoming wheelchair-bound.
- Rett syndrome may be mistaken for cerebral palsy.
- Scoliosis has been reported in up to 80% of patients.[6]
- A long C-shaped thoracolumbar pattern is common. Bracing is typically ineffective and curve progression is common. Surgical stabilization allows maintenance of sitting balance.

Spinal Cord Injury

- Spinal cord injury in the skeletally immature child is associated with a nearly 100% incidence of scoliosis.[3]
- The predominant curve type is a long C-shaped curve. The younger the child, the higher the progression.
- Prophylactic bracing may be effective in smaller curves (under 20 degrees). There are no data to support that bracing is effective in preventing progression in established curves greater than 20 degrees.

PATIENT HISTORY AND PHYSICAL FINDINGS

- The medical history is critical for this group of patients.
  - In patients with cerebral palsy, the medical history correlates very strongly with postoperative complications. This appears to be true also in patients with Duchenne muscular dystrophy and spinal muscular atrophy.
- Important historical information includes respiratory status, cardiac status, gastrointestinal status (eg, gastroesophageal reflux, nutritional intake), and the presence of a seizure disorder.
- Physical examination should assess sitting or standing balance, the pelvic obliquity, and curve magnitude and stiffness (including the curve's coronal, sagittal, and rotational components).
  - Coronal plane stiffness is best assessed by performing the side-bending test (**FIG 2**).
- The physician should also assess for the possible coexistence of hip subluxation or dislocation, which is common in many neuromuscular diseases.
- A complete neurologic examination should also be performed.

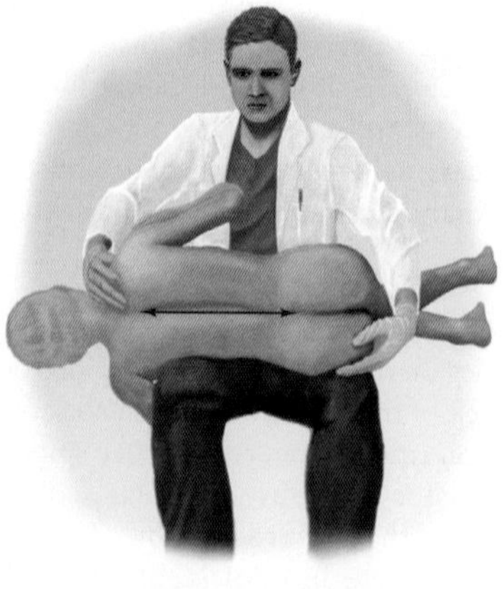

FIG 2 • Side-bending test. Patient is being bent over the examiner's thigh at the apex of the curve. If the patient's curve reverses and the pelvis levels to perpendicular to the trunk, the curve is still flexible enough to correct through posterior fusion and instrumentation alone. If not, an anterior release is performed.

IMAGING AND OTHER DIAGNOSTIC STUDIES

▪ Anteroposterior (AP) and lateral radiographic views should be obtained to assess the Cobb angle and pelvic obliquity in the coronal plane, and lumbar lordosis and thoracic kyphosis in the sagittal plane.
▪ If intraspinal pathology is suspected, especially in the ambulatory patient, a preoperative magnetic resonance imaging (MRI) scan should be obtained.

DIFFERENTIAL DIAGNOSIS

▪ Some neurologic diseases can look similar.
▪ It is important to diagnose progressive neurodegenerative disorders in which mortality from the disease is more rapid than the progression of the spinal deformity.

NONOPERATIVE MANAGEMENT

▪ While there was initially some historical enthusiasm for the treatment of neuromuscular scoliosis with casting or bracing, orthotic management has been found to have little or no impact on neuromuscular deformity.
▪ Flexible curves in younger children may require seating modifications (hip guides and offset lateral seat supports) or a soft thoracolumbar orthosis to maintain balanced seating until the child is at optimal sitting height.
▪ Orthotic treatment does not affect the rate and eventual progression of neuromuscular scoliosis.

SURGICAL MANAGEMENT

Indications

▪ The indications for spinal fusion in neuromuscular scoliosis depend largely on the natural history of the specific neuromuscular disease and the natural history of the scoliosis within the specific disorder.
▪ Examples of two neuromuscular diseases with different indications are Duchenne muscular dystrophy and cerebral palsy.

Duchenne Muscular Dystrophy

▪ The major comorbidity in Duchenne muscular dystrophy is a restrictive type of pulmonary involvement, with forced vital capacity dropping dramatically with scoliosis progression.
▪ Due to the natural history, the indication for fusion is a scoliosis curvature greater than 25 degrees and forced vital capacity greater than 35%.

Cerebral Palsy

▪ The indications for spinal fusion in children with cerebral palsy are a scoliosis curve magnitude approaching 60 degrees in the older child, especially if the curve is becoming stiff by physical examination.
▪ Surgical correction is indicated when the child is not tolerating seating with a combination of either seating adjustments or a soft orthosis.
▪ Less commonly, sagittal plane spinal deformity, hyperlordosis, and kyphosis will cause seating problems or back pain. Cerebral palsy patients with sagittal plane spinal deformity of 70 degrees or more causing seating difficulties or back pain can also benefit from surgical correction.[8]
▪ Typically during the middle part of adolescent growth, the scoliosis becomes much larger and begins to progress and stiffen. Surgical instrumentation and fusion is recommended at this time.

Preoperative Planning

Technical Considerations

▪ Two main technical preoperative questions require careful consideration:
  ▪ Is fusion to the pelvis necessary?
  ▪ Is an anterior release (discectomies around the stiff portion of the curve) necessary?
▪ The only treatment that has made a definitive impact on neuromuscular spinal deformity is instrumentation and fusion.
▪ The standard surgical procedure for neuromuscular scoliosis is a posterior spinal fusion with segmental instrumentation from T1 or T2 down to the sacrum if there is pelvic obliquity.
▪ Even if the pelvis is not involved in a severely involved nonambulatory patient or an ambulatory patient with a poor "righting reflex," the surgeon should still consider fusion to the pelvis to prevent the development of late pelvic obliquity.
▪ Some children with Duchenne muscular dystrophy who have no pelvic obliquity are an exception and can be treated with fusion ending at L5.
▪ The gold standard for neuromuscular scoliosis is Luque rod instrumentation (with Galveston extension for the pelvis), crosslinkage to prevent rod shift and rotation, and sublaminar wires.
▪ The unit rod incorporates these concepts into one instrumentation system[2,4,10,13] (**FIG 3A,B**).
▪ The unit rod has a prebent sagittal contour and comes in sizes of 250 mm to 450 mm. Both quarter-inch and 3/16-inch-diameter rods are available. The quarter-inch rod should be used whenever possible, reserving the 3/16-inch rod for patients with a very thin gracile pelvis.
▪ Some surgeons are using pedicle screws for segmental fixation, especially if there is a severe rotational component to the curvature. Caution should be taken when the bone is severely osteopenic, as the pedicle screws may pull out of the bone.

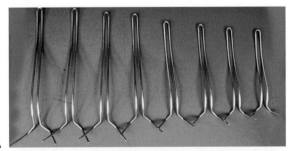

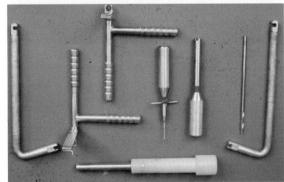

FIG 3 • A. The unit rod is available commercially in a range of sizes. **B.** Drill guides are provided for placement of the pelvic limbs as well as the impactor and pusher for the rod. *(continued)*

C

D

E

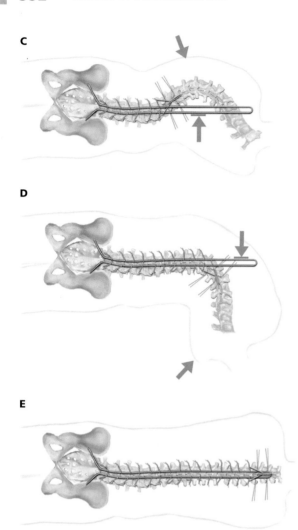

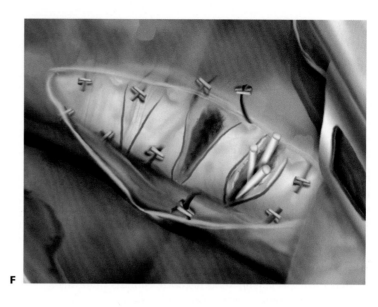

F

FIG 3 • *(continued)* **C–E.** Cantilever effect of the rod correcting pelvic obliquity and scoliosis. The rod is gradually pushed to each vertebra and each wire is tightened, gradually correcting the deformity using transverse forces. **F.** Anterior release: wedge resections of the discs are performed around the apical vertebrae if the spinal deformity is stiff.

- The unit rod is especially powerful as a cantilever to correct pelvic obliquity (**FIG 3C–E**).
- Anterior release for scoliosis is required for larger stiff curves that do not bend out on the bending test (generally greater than 90 degrees) (**FIG 3F**).
  - Anterior release is also recommended for severe hyperlordotic and hyperkyphotic spinal deformities.[8]

Other Preoperative Considerations

- The general medical condition of the child should always be considered first. Many children with neuromuscular conditions will have comorbidities such as pulmonary disease, cardiac disease, seizure disorder, poor nutrition, and so forth.
  - All patients with complex preoperative medical conditions should have the appropriate preoperative workup.
- The surgeon and anesthesiologist should plan for the possibility of large intraoperative blood loss.
  - Type- and cross-matched blood (up to twice the patient's blood volume), fresh-frozen plasma, and platelets should be available.
  - Good vascular access is required, often through central venous access.
- Another consideration is the use of spinal cord monitoring, the role of which is unclear in many patients with neuromus-

cular scoliosis. On the one hand, most children with neuropathies and myopathies can be monitored, while most severely retarded quadriplegic cerebral palsy patients with poor motor function cannot be reliably monitored. In addition, it is hard to justify removing implant hardware if there are signal changes in the child with minimal motor function since the risk of a repeat operation to reimplant hardware is quite high in this population.
  - As a general rule, any child with ambulatory or functional standing (able to assist with standing transfers) should have somatosensory and motor evoked potential monitoring attempted. There may also be some efficacy in monitoring neuromuscular patients with intact sensation and bowel and bladder control.
- A final preoperative consideration is the bone density of the child undergoing spinal fusion. The child who is nonambulatory, poorly nourished, and on seizure medication is at highest risk. Children with low bone density may be difficult to instrument owing to the possibility of sublaminar wires pulling through or screws pulling out of osteopenic bone.
  - Any nonambulatory child with a history of low-impact long-bone fracture should be checked for low bone density using dual-energy x-ray absorptiometry (DEXA scan).
  - Children on seizure medication should have calcium, phosphorus, and vitamin D levels measured.

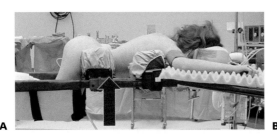 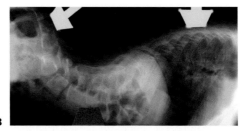

FIG 4 • Positioning the patient should leave the abdomen free and minimize lumbar lordosis by allowing the knees to hang low to optimize pelvic limb placement. If necessary, an unscrubbed assistant can push up on the abdomen (*arrow* in **A**) to aid in the pelvic limb insertion with severe lordosis.

- Patients with bone density two or more z-scores below the mean should be considered for treatment using intravenous pamidronate.

Positioning

- The patient is positioned prone on a Jackson table (a Relton–Hall frame can also be used) with the abdominal area free (**FIG 4**).

- We have adapted special radiolucent posts for the table that can be spaced at a narrower distance compared to the standard posts.
- The hips and knees are bent to minimize lumbar lordosis and to optimize insertion of the limbs of the rod into the pelvis. All bony prominences should be well padded with eggcrate foam.
- Many children with cerebral palsy have significant contractures, making their extremities hard to position. They should be positioned with minimal tension on the joints.

EXPOSURE

- A posterior approach to the spine is performed from T1 to the sacrum.
- A complete subperiosteal exposure of each vertebra is performed, followed by exposure of the outer wing of

each iliac crest down to the sciatic notch and the bottom tips of the posterior superior iliac spines.

PELVIS PREPARATION

- A drill hole is made between the outer and inner cortex of the ilium with a drill bit. Before drilling, the drill bit is marked 10 mm past the drill guide's hook for the sciatic notch in children less than 45 kg and 15 mm past the hook in children greater than 45 kg.
- The right or left drill guide is next inserted into the right or left sciatic notch, respectively.

- The lateral handle of the drill guide is placed parallel to the pelvis (iliac crests) while the axial handle is held parallel to the body axis.
- The pelvis is drilled from the inferior tip of the posterior superior iliac spine in a line just superior and anterior to the sciatic notch, where the bone is densest (**TECH FIG 1**).[11]
- The hole is probed to make certain that the pelvic cortex or the sciatic notch is not penetrated.
- The drill hole can be temporarily packed with Gelfoam to control bleeding.

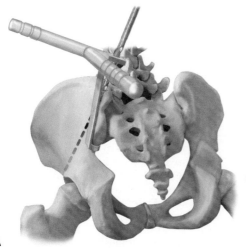

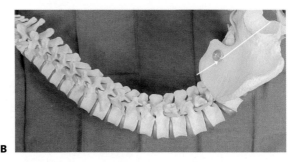

TECH FIG 1 • **A.** Optimal drill hole placement anterior and superior to the sciatic notch. **B.** With severe lordosis, the drill hole starting point is more anterior and aims more posterior.

LUQUE WIRE PASSAGE

- After the spine is completely exposed and pelvis is prepared, the spinous processes are completely removed and the ligamentum flavum is carefully removed to expose the sublaminar spaces.
- Double Luque wires are bent (prebent wires are also available) and passed under the lamina from the lamina of L5 up to and including the T1 lamina.
  - The radius of curvature for the wire bend must approximate the width of the laminae to allow safe passage of the wire.

- Two double wires are passed at the L5 and the T1 lamina only, while a single wire is passed at each of the other levels (**TECH FIG 2A–E**).
- Wires are pulled to equal length and next bent, with the midline bent flat down onto the spinous process beds and the beaded end flat down onto the paraspinous muscles (**TECH FIG 2F**).
  - This helps the wires from getting inadvertently pushed into the spinal canal and allows for easier wire organization.

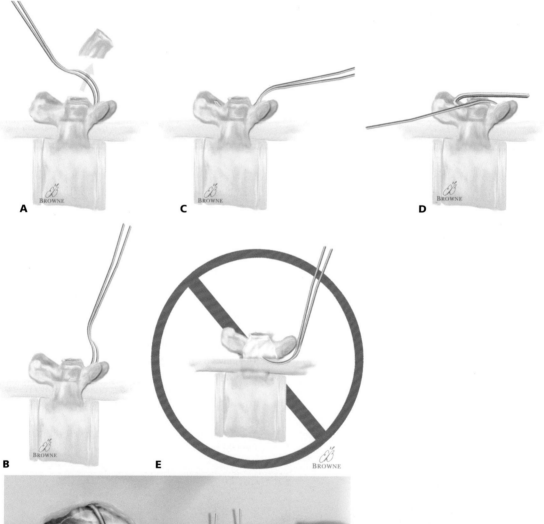

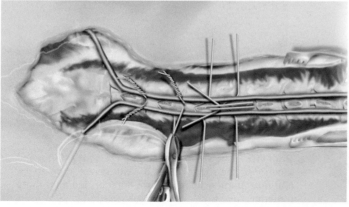

TECH FIG 2 • When passing wires, it is important to roll the wires under the lamina (**A–D**), being careful not to catch the tip under the lamina (**E**), which will lever the wire into the canal and place pressure on the spinal cord. **F.** Wires are bent down to the midline in the middle and the ends are bent down flat against the paraspinous muscles.

ROD SELECTION AND INSERTION

- After the wires are passed, the length of the unit rod is selected.
- This is done by placing the rod upside down with the corner of the rod placed at the drill hole on the elevated side of the pelvis (**TECH FIG 3A**).
  - The proper-length rod should reach T1 (**TECH FIG 3B**).
  - A rod one length shorter should be chosen if there is severe kyphosis because the spine shortens with correction.
  - With severe lordosis, a rod one length longer should be chosen because the spine lengthens with correction.
- It is best to err on the side of the rod being too short because the wires can be brought down to the rod several levels if necessary.
- If the rod is more than 2 cm long, it may be too prominent under the skin.
  - In such cases, cutting the rod and cross-linking the rod may be advisable.
- Facetectomy and decortication of the transverse processes are performed. Corticocancellous allograft (crushed) bone is added (about 180 to 240 mL).

- Insertion of the rod involves crossing the pelvic limbs of the rod to insert them into the previously drilled pelvic holes (**TECH FIG 3C**).
- In patients with pelvic obliquity, the pelvic limb of the rod is placed into the drill hole on the low side of the pelvic obliquity first, with this side crossed underneath the other limb.
- With the rod impactor, the surgeon inserts half to three quarters of this pelvic limb of the rod first and then inserts the opposite pelvic limb, using a rod holder to direct it into the correct direction of the previously drilled hole.
- The rod impactor is next used to drive limbs into the pelvis, alternatively impacting each pelvic leg and making certain to direct each of the legs in the direction of the previously drilled holes.
- At this point, intraoperative fluoroscopy should be used to confirm the correct placement of the rod limbs within the pelvis.
- *Caution:* The surgeon should not try to see if the rod fits by pushing it down into the wound completely in one

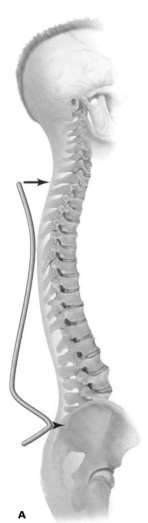

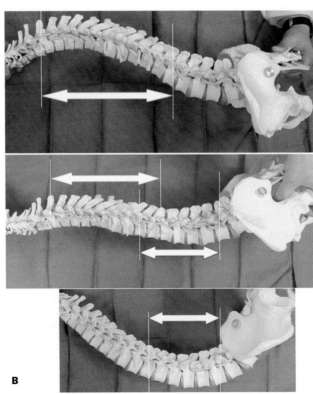

B

TECH FIG 3 • A. Measuring for the proper rod length is one of the most difficult aspects of the surgery and is done by turning the rod upside down and placing the top of the rod at T1 and the bottom corner of the rod at the drill hole in the pelvis. **B.** The spine shortens (*top*) as kyphosis is corrected and lengthens (*bottom*) as excessive lordosis is corrected to normal (*center*). *(continued)*

A

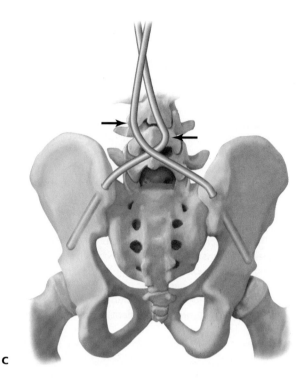

C

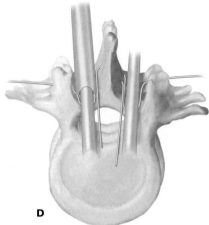

D

TECH FIG 3 • *(continued)* **C.** The pelvic limbs of the unit rod are crossed to insert them into the drill holes into the pelvis. They are gradually impacted 1 cm at a time, alternating between the right and left limbs, until each is completely within the pelvis. **D.** The rod is manually pushed down at each level with a rod pusher before tightening the wires. This is important to prevent wire breakage or cutout through the lamina. It is important to keep the center of the unit rod at the spinous process.

move, as this may cause either the pelvic limbs of the rod to pull out of the pelvis or fracture of the ilium.

- The surgeon should push the rod to line up with the L5 lamina only and then twist the wires (we suggest a jet wire twister). The wires are cut 10 to 15 mm long.

- Now the rod is pushed to L4 and the wires are twisted and cut.
- Next the rod is pushed to L3 and the wires are twisted and cut.
- This process continues one level at a time until the surgeon reaches T1 (**TECH FIG 3D**).

COMPLETION AND WOUND CLOSURE

- All wires are bent down into the midline of the rod and directly caudally. This allows easier exposure of the rod and wires if reoperation should ever become necessary.
- The remaining bone graft is applied (**TECH FIG 4A**).
  - We mix the last 60 cc of allograft with four 80-mg vials of gentamicin. This has lessened the postoperative infection rate.
- If the child is thin and the sacrum is prominent, the sacral spinous processes and lateral processes are trimmed.

- The sacral lamina and lateral processes can be completely removed if they are severely prominent.
- The fascia is closed tightly.
  - No drain is used.
- The subcutaneous tissue and skin are meticulously closed.
- Final radiographs are taken to confirm coronal and sagittal alignment (**TECH FIG 4B–D**).
- In patients with hyperlordosis, pedicle screws with reduction posts are useful in the apex of the sagittal plane deformity to aid in the correction (**TECH FIG 4E,F**).

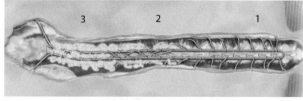

A

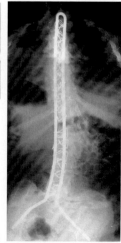

B

TECH FIG 4 • A. Wires are passed and then twisted in a clockwise direction (*1*). Wires are cut about 1 cm and then bent to the midline (*2*). Allograft bone (*yellow*) is placed out laterally along the transverse processes and is impacted into the facet joints after facetectomy (*3*). **B.** AP radiograph of the patient in Figure 1 shows postoperative correction of coronal plane deformity. *(continued)*

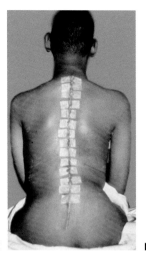
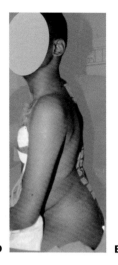
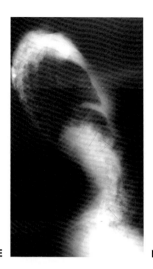
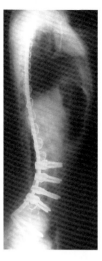

TECH FIG 4 • *(continued)* Clinical photographs show correction of pelvic obliquity (**C**) and good sagittal plane alignment (**D**). Preoperative (**E**) and postoperative (**F**) lateral radiographs of patient with severe hyperlordosis corrected with unit instrumentation and pedicle screws used to correct lordosis in the apex of the deformity.

PEARLS AND PITFALLS

Severe intraoperative hypotension may suddenly occur, especially after decortication.	▪ Constant communication between the surgeon and the anesthesiologist is critical. Type and cross-matched packed red blood cells (1.5 to 2 times blood volume), fresh-frozen plasma, and platelets should be available.
Hypothermia	▪ Hypothermia can be avoided by keeping the room temperature high and using a heated ventilator, a warmer for intravenous fluids and blood, and an airflow heating device.
Excessively stiff scoliosis or accompanying sagittal plane deformity (hyperkyphosis or hyperlordosis)	▪ The surgeon should recognize stiffness preoperatively on the physical examination or bending radiographs to plan for anterior release.
Rod insertion	▪ Using the wires to pull the rod down to the lamina may cause the wires to cut through the lamina. ▪ Relaxing the push on the rod between levels while correcting the major curve may cause an "unzipper" effect, with several wires tearing through laminae or breaking from too much force on the end vertebrae. ▪ The surgeon should use a rod holder to prevent the pusher from slipping off the rod as the top of the rod is approached. ▪ The force from pushing may become large, preventing the patient from being ventilated or causing a drop in blood pressure. If this occurs, the surgeon should relax the push on the rod just enough to allow ventilation and return of pressure.
Pelvic insertion of rod limb in severe lordosis	▪ Difficulty occurs as the surgeon attempts to insert the pelvic limb of the rod and cannot get the rod anterior enough to steer the rod into the drill holes. This may allow the rod to perforate into the sciatic notch or through the inner pelvic table. ▪ Intraoperative fluoroscopy should be used to check proper placement of the pelvic limbs. If pelvic penetration of the rod occurs, the penetrated rod limb should be cut, reinserted into the pelvis, and reconnected with an end-to-end or side-to-side connector.
Misjudgment of rod length	▪ If the rod is too long and prominent, both rods can be cross-linked together and then cut at the T1 vertebrae. If the rod length is misjudged too short by more than two levels, the top of another unit rod can be connected with end-to-end connectors. This is important when there is excessive kyphosis to prevent drop-off of the spine over the top of the rod.
Wires cut through lamina	▪ Only enough bone should be removed to allow wires to pass through the sublaminar space. Wires should not be used to pull the rod to the laminae. This may also be due to inadequate anterior release in a stiff deformity.

POSTOPERATIVE CARE

- Neuromuscular patients are managed in the intensive care unit postoperatively.
  - Most children remain intubated and are ventilated over a 2- to 5-day period. This allows for easier respiratory management and pain management.
- Core body temperature should be increased to 37°C and maintained. Blood clotting is impaired by low body temperature below 33°C, which can easily develop in this patient population.
- Hypertensive episodes are avoided by maintaining increased fluid intake and pressor support as needed. Urine output should be maintained at a minimum of 0.5 cc/kg/hour.
- Most children require aggressive postoperative nutritional support with central hyperalimentation.
  - Typically, a tunneled central venous catheter (Hickman) is placed at the time of surgery.
  - Gastrostomy tube feedings can be started as soon as bowel sounds are present.
  - Gastrojejunostomy or nasojejunostomy tubes may be started as an alternative to hyperalimentation.
- Pancreatic enzyme levels are monitored carefully postoperatively, as elevated amylase and lipase levels are common and indicative of subclinical pancreatitis.
  - Oral or gastrostomy feedings should be delayed if these values are increasing above normal.
  - Adequate nutritional intake for optimal wound healing usually requires about 1.5 times the child's normal preoperative requirements and is continued up to 1 month postoperatively.
- Proper wheelchair assessment postoperatively is also important.

OUTCOMES

- Unit rod instrumentation achieves a scoliosis correction of 70% to 80% of the preoperative curve magnitude and an 80% to 90% correction of pelvic obliquity.[4]
- In a subset of 24 ambulatory cerebral palsy patients who underwent posterior spinal fusion with unit rod instrumentation, all patients had preservation of their ambulatory status.[20]
- Sagittal plane spinal deformity is also well corrected with unit rod instrumentation. Lipton et al[8] showed relief of symptoms and correction of sagittal plane spinal deformity in 24 cerebral palsy patients with hyperlordosis and kyphosis after unit rod instrumentation.
- In one survey of 190 parents and caretakers assessing functional improvement of children with cerebral palsy after posterior spinal fusion, 95.8% of parents and 84.3% of caretakers would recommend spinal surgery again.[18] Positive responses included improved appearance, overall function, quality of life, and ease of care.
- Overall life expectancy of the cerebral palsy child after posterior spinal fusion is also critically important. A survival analysis showed that the presence of severe preoperative thoracic hyperkyphosis and the number of postoperative days in the intensive care unit correlated with decreased life expectancy after evaluating a number of variables.[19]

COMPLICATIONS

- Complications are common but are usually not life-threatening and range from minor to major. They include excessive intraoperative bleeding, neurologic complications, atelectasis, pneumonia, prolonged postoperative ileus, pancreatitis, wound infection, and so forth.
- Mechanical or technical complications also occur and include rod or wire prominence, pseudarthrosis, rod penetration through the pelvis, curve progression after fusion due to crankshafting, and so forth.
- In one study, the curve magnitude, preoperative pulmonary status, and degree of neurologic involvement had the highest correlation with postoperative complications.[9]

REFERENCES

1. Aprin H, Bowen JR, MacEwen GD, et al. Spine fusion in patients with spinal muscular atrophy. J Bone Joint Surg Am 1982;64A:1179–1187.
2. Bell DF, Moseley CF, Koreska J. Unit rod segmental spinal instrumentation in the management of patients with progressive neuromuscular spinal deformity. Spine 1989;14:1301–1307.
3. Dearolf WW III, Betz RR, Vogel LC, et al. Scoliosis in pediatric spinal cord-injured patients. J Pediatr Orthop 1990;10:214–218.
4. Dias RC, Miller F, Dabney K, et al. Surgical correction of spinal deformity using a unit rod in children with cerebral palsy. J Pediatr Orthop 1996;16:734–740.
5. Karol LA. Scoliosis in patients with Duchenne muscular dystrophy. J Bone Joint Surg Am 2007;89A:155–162.
6. Keret D, Bassett GS, Bunnell WP, et al. Scoliosis in Rett syndrome. J Pediatr Orthop 1988;8:138–142.
7. Labelle H, Tohme S, Duhaime M, et al. Natural history of scoliosis in Friedreich's ataxia. J Bone Joint Surg Am 1986;68A:564–572.
8. Lipton GE, Letonoff EJ, Dabney KW, et al. Correction of sagittal plane spinal deformities with unit rod instrumentation in children with cerebral palsy. J Bone Joint Surg Am 2003;85A:2349–2357.
9. Lipton GE, Miller F, Dabney KW, et al. Factors predicting postoperative complications following spinal fusions in children with cerebral palsy. J Spinal Disord 1999;12:197–205.
10. Maloney WJ, Rinsky LA, Gamble JG. Simultaneous correction of pelvic obliquity, frontal plane, and sagittal plane deformities in neuromuscular scoliosis using a unit rod and sublaminar wires: a preliminary report. J Pediatr Orthop 1990;10:742–749.
11. Miller F, Mosely C, Koreska J. Pelvic anatomy relative to lumbosacral instrumentation. J Spinal Disord 1990;3:169–173.
12. Rinsky LA. Surgery of spinal deformity in cerebral palsy: twelve years in the evolution of scoliosis management. Clin Orthop Relat Res 1990;253:100–112.
13. Smeets E, Schollen E, Moog U, et al. Rett syndrome in adolescent and adult females: clinical and molecular genetic findings. Am J Med Genet A 2003;122:227–233.
14. Smith AD, Koreska J, Mosely CF. Progression of scoliosis in Duchenne muscular dystrophy. J Bone Joint Surg Am 1989;71A:1066–1074.
15. Sucato DJ. Spine deformity in spinal muscular atrophy. J Bone Joint Surg Am 2007;89A:148–154.
16. Thometz JG, Simon SR. Progression of scoliosis after skeletal maturity in institutionalized adults who have cerebral palsy. J Bone Joint Surg Am 1988;70A:1290–1296.
17. Trivedi J, Thompson JD, Slakey JB, et al. Clinical and radiographic predictors of scoliosis in patients with myelomeningocele. J Bone Joint Surg Am 2002;84A:1389–1394.
18. Tsirikos AI, Chang WN, Dabney KW, et al. Comparison of parents' and caregivers' satisfaction after spinal fusion in children with cerebral palsy. J Pediatr Orthop 2004;24:54–58.
19. Tsirikos AI, Chang WN, Dabney KW, et al. Life expectancy in pediatric patients with cerebral palsy and neuromuscular scoliosis who underwent spinal fusion. Dev Med Child Neurol 2003;45:677–682.
20. Tsirikos AI, Chang WN, Shah SA, et al. Preserving ambulatory potential in pediatric patients with cerebral palsy who undergo spinal fusion using unit rod instrumentation. Spine 2003;28:480–483.

Chapter 39

Growing Rod Instrumentation for Early-Onset Scoliosis

Victor Hsu and Behrooz Akbarnia

DEFINITION

- Early-onset scoliosis (EOS) is defined by the diagnosis of scoliosis at or before the age of 5 years.
- The many etiologies of EOS include:
  - Congenital vertebral or spinal anomalies: eg, vertebral bars, hemivertebrae, syrinx, tethered cord
  - Neuromuscular diseases: eg, cerebral palsy, spinal dysraphism, muscular dystrophy
  - Syndromes associated with scoliosis: eg, neurofibromatosis
  - Idiopathic causes
- Age of onset is an important aspect of pathology, because progressive curves can be associated with growth disturbances as well as cardiopulmonary compromise, including restrictive lung disease and pulmonary hypertension.

ANATOMY

- Two periods of increased growth velocity are associated with increased incidence of curve progression. The first occurs from birth to 5 years of age; the second includes the adolescent growth spurt occurring after age 10 until just before skeletal maturity.
- The growth velocity from T1 to L5 is greatest from birth until the age of 5. Increases in height during this period average 2 cm per year, and by the age of 5, two thirds of the final sitting height is achieved. The years between 5 and 10 years of age exhibit much less growth. Finally, the adolescent growth spurt causes another increase in growth velocity, at a slower rate than the first growth spurt.
- The increased spinal growth during the first years of life is paralleled by an increase in thorax and lung dimension. Thoracic volume at birth is about 5% of the adult volume; by 5 years of age, it equals 30% of adult volume. A slower rate of thoracic growth occurs from 5 to 10 years of age, by which time it has reached 50% of the adult volume. The final 50% of adult volume is achieved during the adolescent growth spurt from 10 to 15 years of age.
- Lung development also occurs rapidly during the first year of life, and by age 8, most alveolar growth and respiratory branching has occurred.

PATHOGENESIS

- The pathogenesis of EOS depends on its etiology. Vertebral anomalies cause scoliosis by an imbalance in bone growth, whether an increase on a side associated with a hemivertebrae, or retardation on the side associated with a vertebral bar. In neuromuscular and central nervous disorders, an imbalance in muscular forces is the pathogenesis, likely following the Heuter-Volkmann principle.
- The etiology and pathogenesis of infantile idiopathic scoliosis (IIS) (0–3 years of age) is, by definition, unknown. There probably is a genetic component that provides a susceptibility to develop scoliosis. The external factors needed to produce the scoliosis are not yet clearly delineated but may include intrauterine molding as well as infant positioning. The etiology of IIS most likely differs from that of adolescent idiopathic scoliosis (AIS).

NATURAL HISTORY

- The natural history also depends on the etiology. The natural history of EOS due to IIS is favorable when compared with late-onset scoliosis (LOS). Spontaneous resolution occurs in a large number of patients. Progression of congenital curves depends on the type of anomaly and growth potential. EOS due to neuromuscular etiologies usually follows the natural history of the disease in addition to specific problems associated with progressive curves in this age group.
- Regardless of the etiology, progression of scoliosis during the first 5 years of life adversely affects growth as well as pulmonary function. Scoliosis inhibits the growth of both the alveoli and the pulmonary arterioles, causing ventilation defects. The scoliotic spine does not distort the architecture of the alveoli; rather, the total number is decreased significantly and is directly proportional to the age of onset. The earlier the onset of scoliosis, the more hypoplastic the lung is, with a diminution of alveoli greater than would be expected from just a lack of space.
- Patients with EOS also may suffer from a restrictive pattern of pulmonary dysfunction. Lung compliance is reduced, with an associated decrease in total lung capacity as well as vital capacity. In contrast to patients with LOS, the severity of scoliosis in EOS is proportional to the severity of restrictive disease. The restrictive lung disease causes hypoventilation and vasoconstriction of the pulmonary tree and leads to pulmonary hypertension. EOS is associated with a higher risk of cardiopulmonary decompensation in middle-aged patients, which can lead to disabling and even fatal respiratory failure.

PATIENT HISTORY AND PHYSICAL FINDINGS

- Evaluation of the patient with EOS includes a complete history, including the family history, prenatal history, birth history, and developmental history. IIS has been associated with breech presentation and, in boys, with premature birth. Curve progression also has been correlated with cognitive delay, so it is important to ask parents about the achievement of developmental milestones.
- The physical examination of EOS heavily relies on the perceptive capabilities of the clinician and is the same examination that is performed on all scoliosis patients. After a careful history has already been obtained, a thorough physical examination, including inspection, palpation, motor testing, sensory testing, and reflex testing is necessary.
- Inspection includes observation of gait, respiration, truncal and pelvic balance in the coronal and sagittal planes, cutaneous lesions, and any prominence on forward bending. Any deficits in

motor, sensory, or reflex function, including abdominal reflexes, may indicate central nervous system pathology and should be thoroughly evaluated with advanced diagnostic studies.

- Flexibility of the curve can be assessed either by the manual application of traction through the cervical spine or by applying a three-point bending force at the apex of the curve. Examination techniques unique for early-onset scoliosis include the thumb excursion test for thoracic expansion and sitting height measurement.

IMAGING AND OTHER DIAGNOSTIC STUDIES

- All patients should have full-length standing anteroposterior (AP) and lateral radiographs (**FIG 1A,B**) covering the cervical spine to the pelvis, including the entire thorax. For patients who are unable to stand, supine radiographs encompassing the same area should be taken.
  - The cervical spine, lumbosacral spine, pelvis, and hips all may need to be studied to elicit whether or not developmental hip dysplasia or other vertebral anomalies are contributing to the scoliosis.
  - Side-bending or traction radiographs are necessary to help delineate the degree of flexibility of the curves.
  - Similar to LOS evaluation, the Cobb technique is used to measure any curve by measuring the angle created by a line through the superior endplate of the most cranial vertebra and a line through the inferiormost point of the most caudal endplate. This should be done in both the coronal and sagittal planes and compared to normal values. These angles can be used to measure progression of the curve with successive visits but are subject to a small amount of user error variability between 5 to 6 degrees.
  - Spinal height is obtained by measuring the distance from the top of T1 to the top of S1 on the AP view of the spine (**FIG 1C**).

- Coronal balance is measured by the distance from the center of C7 to a line drawn up from S1.
- The sagittal balance is measured from the posterior-cranial corner of S1 to a line drawn down from the center of C7.
- All of these measurements should be recorded and compared on successive visits to document any change in curve magnitude or growth of the spine.

- The rib-vertebral angle difference of Mehta (RVAD; **FIG 2**), first described in 1972, measures the amount of rotation at the apex vertebra and has some prognostic value.[6]
  - The angles formed by a line perpendicular to the vertebra and a line drawn down the center of the rib is compared between the convex and concave side. If the difference calculated by subtracting the convex angle to the concave angle is 20 degrees or less, there is an 85% to 90% chance the curve will resolve; when there is a difference of 21 degrees or more it will likely progress.
  - The phase of the rib head also is described by ascertaining whether the head of the convex rib overlaps the vertebral body.
    - If there is no overlap (phase 1), then the RVAD is calculated as previously mentioned.
    - If there is overlap (phase 2), the risk of progression is high, regardless of RVAD.

- Another method of evaluating rotation is the Nash-Moe method (**FIG 3**). Evaluating the pedicles of the apical vertebra at the convexity, the distance of the pedicle on the convex side is measured.
  - Zero: the pedicles are equidistant from the sides
  - Grade 1: the concave pedicle is partially obscured, and the convex pedicle moves away from the edge toward the center
  - Grade 3: the convex pedicle is in the midline of the vertebral body.
  - Grade 2: between grades 1 and 3
  - Grade 4: the convex pedicle lies past the midline.

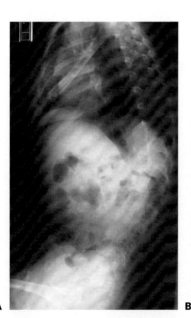 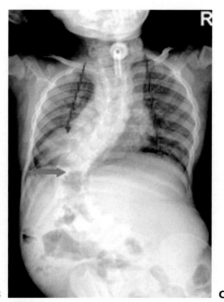 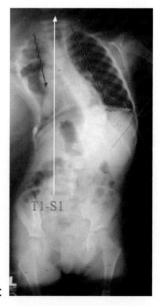

FIG 1 • **A.** Lateral radiograph of a neuromuscular patient with early-onset scoliosis. **B.** AP radiograph with space available for the lung (SAL) of a patient with early-onset scoliosis. **C.** Measurement of vertebral height from T1 to S1.

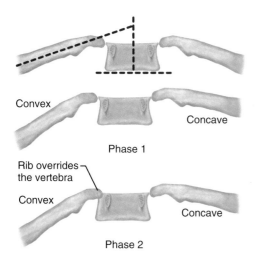

Convex

Concave

Phase 1

Rib overrides
the vertebra

Convex

Concave

Phase 2

FIG 2 • The rib-vertebral angle difference (RVAD) measures the angle of a line drawn perpendicular to the apical thoracic vertebra endplate and a line drawn down the center of the concave and convex ribs. The difference is calculated by subtracting the convex from the concave angle. An RVAD of 20 degrees or less indicates a curve that is likely to resolve; an RVAD of 21 degrees or greater often is associated with curves that will progress. The phase of the rib head notes the position of the convex rib head on the apical vertebra. A "phase 1" relationship indicates no overlap of the rib head or neck on the apical vertebra. In cases that have a phase 1 relationship, the RVAD may be calculated and used to determine the likelihood of progression. In a phase 2 relationship, the head of the rib on the convex side of the apical vertebra overlaps with the vertebra, and the curve is likely to progress. (Adapted from Mehta MH. The rib-vertebra angle in the early diagnosis between resolving and progressive infantile scoliosis. J Bone Joint Surg Br 1972;54B:230–243.)

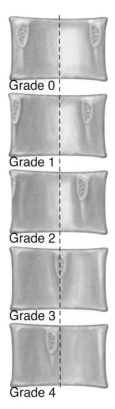

Grade 0

Grade 1

Grade 2

Grade 3

Grade 4

FIG 3 • Measurements performed on apical vertebra. If the pedicles are equidistant from the sides, rotation is classified as zero. If the concave pedicle is partially obscured and the convex pedicle moves away from the edge toward the center, that is considered grade 1. Grade 3 is defined as the convex pedicle in the midline of the vertebral body. Grade 2 lies between grades 1 and 3. Grade 4 indicates that the convex pedicle lies past midline. (Adapted from Nash CL Jr, Moe JH. A study of vertebral rotation. J Bone Joint Surg Am 1969;51A:223–229.)

- The space available for the lung (SAL) is calculated by taking the ratio of the distance from the apex of the most cephalad rib to the highest point of the hemidiaphragm of the concave side divided by the convex side (see Fig 1B).
  - Any decrease in the SAL points toward a poorer prognosis for lung function.
- MRI allows the best visualization of the central nervous system and is indicated in EOS associated with neurologic abnormalities or curve greater than 20 degrees.
- CT scanning with 3-D reconstructions is helpful to delineate bony architecture and is warranted when plain radiographs do not provide enough information and for preoperative planning for patients who have vertebral abnormalities (eg, dysplastic pedicles or hemivertebrae).
  - The CT scan or MRI is also used to measure lung volume and assess thoracic architecture when thoracic insufficiency is an issue. It often is difficult to assess these parameters with plain radiographs, but CT allows better visualization of each hemithorax and measurement of the lung volume.
  - In severe congenital deformity, the ribs may spiral around the vertebrae, causing the thoracic volume on one side to be severely diminished while the other is larger, creating what Campbell calls a "windswept thorax" (**FIG 4**).

DIFFERENTIAL DIAGNOSIS

- Congenital vertebral or spinal anomalies
  - Vertebral bars
  - Hemivertebrae
  - Syrinx
  - Tethered cord

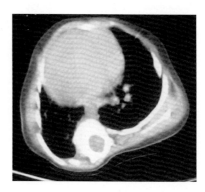

FIG 4 • CT scan of the chest showing decreased lung volumes due to scoliosis.

- Neuromuscular diseases
  - Cerebral palsy
  - Myelodysplasia
  - Muscular dystrophy
- Syndromes associated with scoliosis
  - Beel syndrome
  - Trisomies
- Infantile idiopathic scoliosis

NONOPERATIVE MANAGEMENT

- Nonoperative treatment for EOS is indicated in curves that are not expected to progress or that are expected to progress only mildly, taking into consideration the etiology of the curve and the radiographic parameters described by Mehta[6] in cases with IIS.
  - Patients with a curve less than 25 degrees and RVAD less than 20 degrees may be followed with serial radiographs every 4 to 6 months to document any progression.
  - Active treatment is warranted in:
    - Progression greater than 10 degrees; treatment starts with casting and bracing.
    - Phase 2 rib-vertebral relationship, RVAD greater than 20 degrees, or a Cobb angle greater than 20 degrees in any skeletally immature patient
    - Progression of more than 5 degrees in a patient with a Cobb angle greater than 35 degrees
  - Casting usually is done under anesthesia. The cast is changed every 6 to 12 weeks until the ultimate correction is achieved.
  - After casting, a Milwaukee brace (**FIG 5**) is used for 23 hours a day to help maintain the correction. Fully circumferential braces may distort the rib cage and adversely affect pulmonary status, because the immature thoracic wall may deform before any correction of the spine occurs.
  - Bracing is continued for a minimum of 2 years until the Cobb angle and RVAD are stable.
  - The goal is to correct the deformity completely before the prepubertal growth spurt.

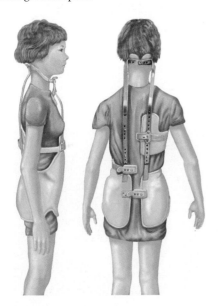

FIG 5 • The Milwaukee brace consists of metal rods attached to pads at the hips, rib cage, and neck.

- Nonoperative treatment for neuromuscular or congenital scoliosis can be attempted for curves of lesser magnitudes. Treatment options available include casting and bracing.
  - Bracing is less effective for these types of deformities than for idiopathic scoliosis, but can be used in long flexible curves.
  - Deformities with large sagittal components are not amenable to brace treatment.
  - Brace treatment for congenital or neuromuscular scoliosis should be abandoned when unacceptable curve magnitude or progression is seen.

SURGICAL MANAGEMENT

- Surgical treatment of EOS attempts to stop progression of the scoliosis, allowing improvements in growth of the spine, thorax, and lungs.
- Surgery is recommended for progressive curves greater than 45 degrees.
- The age of the patient helps to decide the type of surgery needed.
  - Adolescents and more skeletally mature patients may do well with spine fusions, which stabilize the spine but also stop growth.
  - Younger patients with substantial growth potential suffer from the "crankshaft" phenomenon if fusion is performed early in life from an isolated posterior approach. They suffer from severe growth retardation in height and thorax volume if fusion is performed using a combined anterior and posterior technique.
- The growing rod technique for EOS was developed to correct spinal deformity while allowing spinal growth to continue or even enhancing that growth.

Preoperative Planning

- Careful evaluation of radiographic studies allows planning of surgical levels. Typically, the cranial level of the construct includes T2 and extends two or three levels caudal to the end vertebra of the curve.
- Either pedicle screws or hooks can be used in the construct. Review of the pedicle structure using radiographs and CT scans is necessary to be sure the desired implants are selected.
- Medical and subspecialty consultations should be obtained before operation if the patient has any history of medical comorbidities.
  - Cardiopulmonary, renal, skeletal, and other neuromuscular defects often are associated with scoliosis.
  - Pulmonary function tests may be obtained in children who are able to cooperate if thoracic insufficiency is suspected.

Positioning

- The patient is placed under general anesthesia on the stretcher and then placed on the operating room table in the prone position on two longitudinal chest rolls or tightly rolled blankets.
- Neural monitoring is used during the procedure for neurologically intact patients. Leads should be placed before prone positioning, as should a Foley catheter.
- Care must be taken to be sure all bony prominences and compressible nerves are well padded.

Approach

- The growing rod technique is performed posteriorly through either a single long midline incision or two smaller incisions cranially and caudally.

GROWING ROD INSTRUMENTATION FOR EARLY-ONSET SCOLIOSIS

Single-Incision Technique
Exposing the Foundations

- The single-incision technique consists of a long superficial posterior incision beginning 2 to 3 cm cranial to the planned levels and ending caudal to the lowest vertebra by 2 to 3 cm. Infiltration of epinephrine may be used before subcutaneous incision.
- The spinous processes of the cranial and caudal foundations are exposed and marked with a metallic object such as a Kocher clamp, and a lateral radiograph is then used to confirm the levels.
  - The foundations are critical to the construct in the dual growing rod technique.
    - They are composed of at least two pair of anchors and usually span two or three vertebral levels.
    - The foundations consist of the vertebral segments at either ends of the constructs, which are internally fixed with anchors.
  - Because the corrective loads are applied to these foundations, it is imperative that strong and stable constructs be achieved to decrease the incidence of implant or fixation failure.
- Limited fusions of the foundation levels often are performed using local bone graft or allograft extenders to provide more stability.
- The posterior elements of the cranial and caudal foundations are exposed subperiosteally out to the level of the transverse processes.
  - Vertebral levels not involved in a foundation should not be exposed, to decrease the chance of unwanted fusion.

Placing the Anchors

- Once exposure has been obtained, the anchors are placed.
- The foundations may be anchored using either pedicle screws or hooks.
- If hooks are used, the superior edges of the most cranial lamina or transverse processes (TP) on either side are exposed, and supralaminar hooks or TP hooks are placed in a downgoing manner on both sides.
  - Contralateral supralaminar hooks may be staggered over two levels if canal stenosis is a concern.
  - Next, upgoing hooks are placed, usually under the facet articulations of the same vertebra but sometimes in a staggered arrangement.
  - Foundations using supralaminar hooks generally consist of three vertebral levels with supralaminar hooks placed on either side of the cranial two vertebra and the facet hooks placed on the most caudal one.
  - If TP hooks are used, only two vertebral levels are used, with the TP hooks placed on either side of the cranial vertebra and the facet hooks placed on the same cranial vertebra.
  - For more stability, additional facet hooks can be used to extend the foundation to three levels. It is important to achieve adequate stability at initial surgery.

- Pedicle screws also may be used, usually with four screws spanning two vertebral levels. Pedicle screws may offer increased stability to the construct and are preferred for both foundations as long as the anatomy allows their safe placement.
  - Multiple methods for thoracic pedicle screw placement have been popularized. In general, the thoracic pedicle starting point is located at the intersection of the lateral border of the superior articular facet and the cranial aspect of the transverse process.
  - The trajectory of the thoracic pedicle screw generally travels lateral to medial about 30 degrees and from cranial to caudal 10 degrees, but varies by level (**TECH FIG 1A–C**).
  - Lumbar pedicle screws start at the junction of the pars interarticularis, the midpoint of the transverse process, and the base of the superior articular process.
  - Lumbar screw trajectory also varies, from about 10 degrees at L1 to 30 degrees at L5 from lateral to medial, and varies in the sagittal direction approximately 10 degrees from L1 to L5, depending on lordosis (**TECH FIG 1D**).
  - Fluoroscopy and neural monitoring are helpful in aiding pedicle screw placement, especially in patients with deformity. If needed, a combination of hooks and screws can be used.

Adding the Rods

- The dual rod technique employs two rods, each made up of a cranial foundation rod and a caudal foundation rod joined by a connector, for a total of four rods for the entire construct.
- Either of two types of connectors may be used: a tandem connector, which houses the cranial and caudal rods inside a rectangular box so the ends meet end to end, or side-to-side connectors, which allow the rods to overlap.
  - Tandem connectors usually are favored. Because they are straight and cannot be contoured, the rods are measured so that they meet inside the tandem connector in the relatively straight thoracolumbar region.
- The ends of the rods that fit inside the connector also must be straight. If any contouring is necessary in the region where the cranial and caudal rods meet, closed dual connectors must be used, with an overlap of 2 to 4 inches to allow future lengthening.
- Bilateral rods are prepared for each foundation by measuring the length of the spine in the corrected position and carefully contouring the rod. The concave side usually is constructed first to gain maximal correction.
- The rods can be placed either subcutaneously or subfascially. Subfascial placement involves a much deeper dissection, both initially and with each lengthening, however, and may increase the risk of premature fusion. Subcutaneous placement may be associated with a higher incidence of skin problems and wound infection.

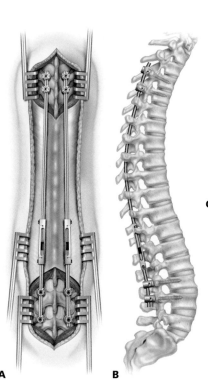

A

B

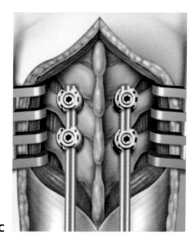

C

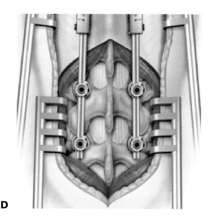

D

TECH FIG 1 • A. A single skin incision may be used with subperiosteal exposure of the cranial and caudal foundation sites. The rods and tandem connectors are placed above the fascia in this picture. Pedicle screws have been used as anchors. **B.** The lateral view shows the straight tandem connector placed in the thoracolumbar region. The trajectory of the pedicle screws can also be seen and varies between patients. **C.** Close-up of the cranial foundation shows four pedicle screws spanning two levels in the thoracic region. **D.** Close-up of the caudal foundation shows four pedicle screws spanning two levels in the lumbar spine. Hooks may also be used for either foundation. (From Akbarnia BA. Growing rod technique for the treatment of progressive early onset scoliosis in fusionless surgery for spine deformity. In: Kim DH, Betz R, Huhn SL, Newton PO, eds. Surgery of the Pediatric Spine. New York, Thieme, 2007:814.)

- After the rods are placed in the hooks or screws of each foundation, transverse connectors are placed between the two cranial rods and the two caudal rods, preferably between the points of fixation on each foundation.
- If the transverse connectors are close-holed, it may be necessary to preload them onto the rods before they are placed in the anchors, and the spinous processes may be removed to allow proper seating.
  - These transverse connectors increase the stability of the construct, especially when hooks have been used. There is less need for transverse connectors when screws are used.
- The tandem connector is held with a rod holder and slid onto the cranial rod; once the caudal rod is cleared, it is slid onto the caudal rod.
- The cranial anchors and transverse connector are tightened first, followed by the caudal anchors and transverse connectors. Cranial and caudal set screws are located on the side of the tandem connector that correlates to the most prominent side.
- To create distraction, the caudal set screw is tightened, a distractor is implemented in the slot of the tandem connector between the two rods, and the cranial set screw is tightened (**TECH FIG 2A**).
  - Similarly, a rod clamp can be used to distract against if a closed dual connector is used or even on a tandem connector (**TECH FIG 2B**).
- Next, the rod construct on the convex side of the curve is created similarly and tightened. The surgical area is then irrigated, followed by a limited arthrodesis applying autograft bone or other graft extenders between the vertebrae making up each foundation.

- Before final closure, anteroposterior and lateral radiographs are taken to confirm alignment and proper position of the implants (**TECH FIG 2C,D**).
- The wound is then closed in standard fashion.

Dual-Incision Technique

- The dual-incision technique differs from the single-incision technique in a few ways.
- The incisions are centered over the foundation sites with a long skin bridge between them (**TECH FIG 3**).
- The subperiosteal dissection is the same, as are placement strategies of either hooks or pedicle screws for anchors.
- In placing the rods, however, subcutaneous or subfascial dissection must be performed carefully and bluntly with either a finger or blunt clamp to facilitate rod passage.
  - Careless dissection or poor control of the rod during passage can lead to pleural violation.
  - The rods must be placed beneath the skin bridge and the tandem connector placed on the caudal rod before they are fitted into the anchors.
- The rest of the procedure is similar to the single-incision technique.

Lengthening and Exchange

- Lengthening of the dual rod construct may be performed as either an in- or outpatient procedure with neural monitoring for patients with normal neurologic function.
- The connector is located through palpation or fluoroscopy, and a small incision is made over that area where the lengthening is planned.

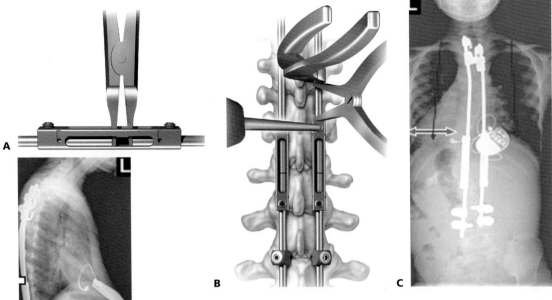

TECH FIG 2 • **A.** Lengthening may be performed by inserting the distractor between the rods through the slot of the tandem connector. One set screw is loosened, distraction is performed, and the set screw secured. **B.** Alternatively, a rod clamp can be placed on the rod a few centimeters from the connector and the distractor placed between the rod clamp and the end of the connector. The set screw nearest the rod clamp is then loosened, the distractor employed, and the screw retightened. **C.** AP radiograph after the dual growing rod procedure was performed on the patient shown in Figure 1B and C. **D.** Lateral radiograph after the dual growing rod procedure was performed on the same patient. (**A,B:** Bagheri R, Akbarnia BA. Pediatric Isola instrumentation. In: Kim DH, Vaccaro AR, Fessler RG, eds. Spinal Instrumentation: Surgical Techniques. New York: Thieme, 2005:640,642.)

- After dissection of the connector is performed, lengthening similar to that performed during the index procedure is carried out by loosening the set screw (mostly cranial), distracting between the two rods, and then tightening the set screw again.
- Lengthening is performed every 6 months.
- Once further distraction is no longer achievable, final correction and arthrodesis are performed.

Changing the Connector or Rod

- Exchange of the tandem connector or the rod may be needed if the amount of lengthening exceeds the initial length of the tandem connector.

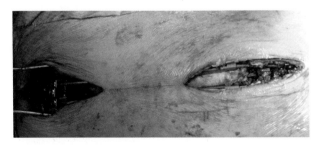

TECH FIG 3 • The dual-incision technique employs two separate incisions centered over the foundations and separated by a skin bridge.

- In such a case, both set screws should be loosened and the tandem connector slid cephalad until full clearance of the caudal rod is achieved.
- The connector can then be removed off the cranial rod, replaced by a longer connector, and slid onto the caudal rod again.
- Longer than 70 mm connector is rarely used, to minimize the adverse effect on sagittal balance.
- If the needed length exceeds the longest connector or if the longest connector is too long, it is necessary to fashion new rods and remove the old ones.
  - This entails exposing and removing the tandem connectors, exposing the foundation, and removing the rods and replacing them with longer rods, creating a construct similar to the initial procedure.
  - Replacement of the cephalad rods is most common.

Final Fusion

- Final fusion is performed near the end of the adolescent growth spurt or when the rods can no longer be lengthened.
- The first step entails removing the dual growing rod implants, including the anchors and exploring foundations for solid fusions. One should be careful to cause the least trauma to the soft tissues.
- For most patients, the fusion should extend from the cranial foundation to the cephalad foundation.

- Either hooks or pedicle screws can be used in the foundations and at the apices of the curves.
- Rods are then contoured to the desired shape, keeping in mind that the goal is to achieve global balance rather than a totally straight spinal segment. Thus, upper and lower curves should be considered together when contouring the rods.
  - A consideration when performing the final fusion is that posterior osteotomies may be required, especially if a subfascial technique is employed, because the posterior elements may become stiff after repeated exposures.
    - This usually can be done safely by finding the neural canal and then osteotomizing the pars on either side.

- Another consideration is that the areas around the anchor sites often are overgrown with bone, and taking the implants out often entails osteotomizing the bone around the anchors.
  - Care should be taken to point away from the spinal canal to avoid neural injury.
  - Although pedicle screws offer three-column support in the foundations, replacing hooks in the fusion mass provides sufficient strength if placed properly, and hooks are easier to place, especially if they were used initially for the growing rods.
  - Sublaminar wires also offer an attractive option and are useful if lateral translation of the spine is required.

PEARLS AND PITFALLS

Exposure	▪ Avoid subperiosteal dissection anywhere except the foundation to avoid premature fusion. ▪ Use careful blunt dissection beneath the skin bridge to avoid pleural violation.
Implants	▪ Perform a careful radiographic examination if pedicle screws are desired. ▪ Use proper rod contouring to correct both coronal and sagittal deformity. ▪ Tandem connectors are straight and should be placed at the thoracolumbar region, which also is straight.
Lengthening	▪ Do not be too aggressive with lengthenings, especially at the index procedure and first lengthening, to avoid implant issues.
Indications	▪ May not be indicated in very stiff curves, poor bone quality, older children with limited growth potential, or children too young to allow internal fixation.

POSTOPERATIVE CARE

- Patients are braced postoperatively with a thoracolumbosacral orthosis, beginning when they have been upright for up to 6 months and continuing until fusion of the foundations. Rehabilitation proceeds according to the patient's tolerance and ability.

OUTCOMES

- Documented outcomes are short-term, and no level I studies are currently available.
- One study showed Cobb angle correction from an average of 82 degrees to 36 degrees at last visit or final fusion.
- Spine growth is almost equal to normal, averaging 1.21 cm/year.
- Some patients averaged almost 12 cm of growth.
- SAL increased from 0.87 to 1.
- Better balance and cosmesis

COMPLICATIONS

- Wound breakdown
- Infection
- Junctional kyphosis
- Crankshaft phenomenon
- Curve progression
- Implant failure

- Patients with more frequent lengthenings have fewer implant problems but more wound problems, whereas patients with less frequent lengthenings have more implant problems and fewer wound complications. Implant complications often can be treated during scheduled lengthenings, but wound infections should be treated urgently.

REFERENCES

1. Akbarnia B. Management themes in early onset scoliosis. J Bone Joint Surg Am 2007;89 (Suppl 1):42–54.
2. Akbarnia BA, Marks DS. Instrumentation with limited arthrodesis for the treatment of progressive early-onset scoliosis. Spine 2000;14: 181–189.
3. Akbarnia B, Marks DS, Boachie-Adjei O, et al. Dual growing rod technique for the treatment of progressive early-onset scoliosis: a multicenter study. Spine 2005;30:46–57.
4. Bagheri R, Akbarnia B. Pediatric isola instrumentation. In: Kim DH, Vaccaro AR, Fessler RG, eds. Spinal Instrumentation: Surgical Techniques. New York: Thieme, 2004:636–643.
5. Gillingham B, et al. Early onset idiopathic scoliosis. J Am Acad Orthop Surg 2006;14:101–112.
6. Mehta MH. The rib-vertebra angle in the early diagnosis between resolving and progressive infantile scoliosis. J Bone Joint Surg Br 1972;54B:230–243.
7. Thomspson G, Akbarnia BA, Kostial P, et al. Comparison of single and dual growing rod techniques followed through definitive surgery: a preliminary study. Spine 2005;30:2039–2044.

Daniel J. Hedequist and John B. Emans

DEFINITION

■ A hemivertebra is a congenital anomaly of the spine that forms during the 8th to 12th weeks of embryologic development. It is characterized by the formation of half of a vertebral body, a corresponding pedicle, and a corresponding hemilamina.

■ Hemivertebra are classified as a congenital failure of formation.

■ A hemivertebra may be classified as fully segmented (ie, separated from the bodies above and below by discs); partially segmented (ie, separated from one adjacent body by a disc and fused to the other adjacent body); or unsegmented (ie, fused to the body above and below; **FIG 1**).[3]

■ Progressive curvatures of the spine caused by a hemivertebra result from unbalanced growth. Full-segmented hemivertebra have a much higher rate of progression, because the presence of an intact disc space above and below signifies the presence of growth plates and potential asymmetrical spinal growth.

ANATOMY

■ The hemivertebra has a partial vertebral body, a pedicle, and a hemilamina.

■ Anatomically, it may be joined to the level above or below at either the body, the hemilamina, or both. If the hemivertebra is not fused to either adjacent segment, the potential for asymmetric spinal growth is high.

■ A local kyphotic or lordotic deformity may occur with hemivertebra if the associated failure of formation is greater anteriorly or posteriorly.

PATHOGENESIS

■ Progressive spinal curvatures due to hemivertebra are a result of disordered growth.

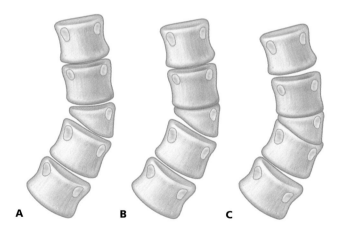

FIG 1 • Schematic of a hemivertebra. **A.** Fully segmented hemivertebra. **B.** Partially segmented hemivertebra. **C.** Unsegmented hemivertebra.

■ The hemivertebra is a wedge on the convex side of a curve. In the presence of healthy growth plates above and below (ie, a fully segmented hemivertebra) convex growth is faster than contralateral concave growth, causing a progressive scoliosis.

■ In cases of hemivertebra, if the vertebral body lies in the posterolateral quadrant, a progressive kyphosis may arise with the scoliosis.

■ The disordered growth eventually may cause curvature to such a degree that normally segmented areas of the spine become involved in the curve, causing deformity and spinal imbalance.

NATURAL HISTORY

■ The natural history of a hemivertebra depends on its location and the potential for growth and curve progression.

■ Hemivertebrae that are fully segmented progress at approximately 2 degrees a year and can exceed over 45 degrees at maturity.[5] These require treatment to prevent deformity and also to prevent adjacent spinal curvature.

■ Partially segmented hemivertebrae have much less growth potential (less than 1 degree per year), rarely exceeding 40 degrees at maturity. They usually do not require treatment. Unsegmented hemivertebrae require no treatment.

■ Hemivertebra at the lumbosacral junction almost always require treatment, because the lumbar spine takes off obliquely from the sacrum, causing a long compensatory curve in normally segmented regions of the lumbar spine, with resultant cosmetic deformity and spinal imbalance.

PATIENT HISTORY AND PHYSICAL FINDINGS

■ Embryologic development of the spine occurs between the 8th and 12th weeks of gestation; hence, other organ systems developing at the same time also may have a congenital anomaly.

■ A complete musculoskeletal examination looking for diagnoses such as clubfoot, developmental dysplasia of the hip, and limb anomalies is warranted.

■ A complete neurologic examination should be performed, because as many as 40% of patients with congenital scoliosis have a corresponding spinal dysraphism. This examination includes sensory, motor, and reflex testing.

■ Occult signs of spinal dysraphism include cutaneous manifestations such as midline spinal hemangiomas, penetrating sacral dimples, or midline hairy patches. Foot anomalies such as vertical talus or asymmetric cavus feet can signify spinal dysraphism.

■ Cardiac auscultation should be done, because 20% of patients with congenital scoliosis have congenital heart anomalies.

■ Observe shoulder position, trunk position, and waist symmetry. Truncal imbalance is an indicator of curvature.

■ Observe the flexibility of the patient's spine.

■ Rotation of the spine during the Adams forward bend test is indicative of deformity and points to its location.

IMAGING AND OTHER DIAGNOSTIC STUDIES

■ Standing 36-inch posteroanterior (PA) and lateral radiographs are mandatory to define the deformity and assess the Cobb measurement. Apparent progression may be seen from supine radiographs to standing radiographs (**FIG 2A**).
   ■ Bending radiographs, in which the patient is directed to bend in a concave and then in a convex direction, are necessary to assess the flexibility of curves above and below the hemivertebra.
■ MRI scanning of the brainstem and spinal cord is mandatory before any surgical intervention, given the height rate (30% to 40%) of congenital scoliosis with spinal dysraphism.[3]
■ CT scans with three-dimensional (3D) reconstructions should be obtained to delineate the anatomy of the anterior and posterior elements as an aid in planning the operation and to avoid intraoperative problems such as unexpected posterior element deficiencies or fusions (**FIG 2B**).[4]
   ■ A pediatric protocol should be used for CT scans to avoid the significant radiation exposure that results when adult protocols are used for children.
■ Preoperative evaluation of the genitourinary system with a screening ultrasound and evaluation of the cardiac system with an echocardiogram are necessary if these have not been performed, given the rate of anomalies associated with congenital scoliosis.

DIFFERENTIAL DIAGNOSIS

■ Failure of vertebral formation
■ Failure of vertebral segmentation
■ Sequela of infection causing partial vertebral body destruction
■ Tumor

NONOPERATIVE MANAGEMENT

■ Nonoperative management is reserved for nonprogressive curves caused by hemivertebra.
■ Hemivertebra associated with little or no curve progression (unsegmented or partially segmented) may be followed during growth with radiographs every 6 to 12 months, depending on the degree of deformity and age of the basis.
■ Bracing has no role in the management of a hemivertebra.

SURGICAL MANAGEMENT

■ The classic indication for a hemivertebra resection is a patient with a progressive curve secondary to a fully segmented hemivertebra in the thoracolumbar, lumbar, or lumbosacral regions with a resultant deformity.
■ We have found that excision is best performed between the ages of 18 months and 4 years.
   ■ Patients younger than this may be more difficult to instrument, and waiting until this age rarely has caused irrevocable deformity.
   ■ Excision in older patients is feasible; we have found, however, that if diagnosed early there is no reason to wait past the age of 4 years given the progression of curvature and its effect on normally segmented regions of the spine.
   ■ Instrumentation at these ages is technically feasible.

Preoperative Planning

■ Review of the preoperative MRI of the spine
   ■ If spinal dysraphism is present, referral to a neurosurgeon is mandatory.
   ■ If the patient requires neurosurgical intervention for dysraphism, that procedure should precede the hemivertebra excision, either at the same setting or in a staged setting, at the discretion of the spine surgeon and neurosurgeon.
■ Review of the 3D CT scans
   ■ A complete understanding of the anatomy of the hemivertebra is crucial to avoid intraoperative confusion, especially because associated posterior element fusions or absences can make identifying levels difficult.
   ■ Studying the pedicle anatomy (ie, length and diameter) of the levels above and below is efficacious given the smaller size of these patients.
■ Neurologic monitoring is important and should be done using somatosensory evoked potentials and motor evoked potentials.
   ■ Communication between the monitoring and anesthesia teams should be facilitated to prevent any change in neurologic function brought on by anesthetics, hypotension, or low blood volume.

Positioning

■ We perform hemivertebra excisions with the patient in the prone position.
   ■ This is done on a radiolucent operating frame with chest and pelvic support, which leaves the abdomen free.
   ■ We also have found it useful to slightly "airplane" the table or bolster the patient so that the convex side is slightly higher than the concave side. This helps with visualization anteriorly, control of bleeding, and retraction of the dura and its contents (**FIG 3**).
■ Before draping the patient, we place a marker over the hemivertebra region and obtain a radiograph.
   ■ This both confirms the side of the hemivertebra and helps limit excessive incisions and dissections.
■ In the past we recommended that hemivertebra excision be performed as a simultaneous anterior-posterior procedure.[4]
   ■ If the surgeon elects to do this, the patient is placed in the lateral decubitus position with the anterior and posterior fields being prepped into the fields. The patient should be

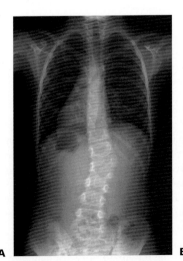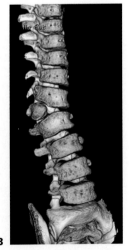

FIG 2 • A. Standing PA radiograph of a 5-year-old patient with a fully segmented hemivertebra at the thoracolumbar junction. **B.** A three-dimensional reconstructed CT scan of a fully segmented hemivertebra in a different patient.

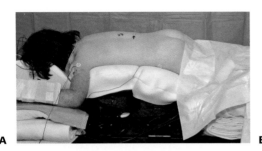
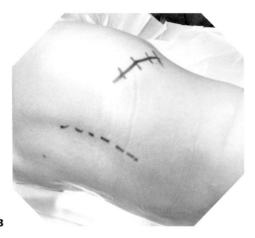

FIG 3 • Positioning for a hemivertebra resection. **A.** Prone positioning. Observe the paper clip placed for radiographic marking before incision. **B.** Positioning for simultaneous AP excision.

placed at the edge of the bed to facilitate retractor placement in the posterior field.

- The anterior approach is on the convex side and should be marked before the patient goes to the operating room.
- We still recommend considering an anterior–posterior procedure when medical conditions (eg, congenital heart disease) caution against excessive bleeding, when a lordotic component renders access to the vertebral body difficult, and when the surgeon is unfamiliar with posterior-only approaches to circumferential surgery.

Approach

- If an anterior–posterior procedure is being performed, the anterior procedure should be a standard transthoracic, transthoracic-retroperitoneal, or retroperitoneal approach, depending on the location of the hemivertebra. The anterior

approach often can be a limited one, because the only exposure needed is of the hemivertebra and the discs above and below.

- The posterior approach is a standard posterior midline incision with subperiosteal dissection out to the tips of the transverse processes.
  - Diathermy aids in keeping blood loss to a minimum during dissection.
  - Preoperative review of the CT scan should forewarn the surgeon of posterior element fusions and, more importantly, posterior element deficiencies.
  - Dissection should proceed with caution over areas of laminar deficiency.
  - Once completely dissected, a spot radiograph or fluoroscopic view should be obtained to confirm the appropriate level.

HEMIVERTEBRA EXCISION

Pedicle Screw Placement

- Implant anchors should be placed before excision, because blood loss at this point should be at a minimum.
  - Where possible, we prefer bilateral pedicle screws as a basis for fixation. Pedicle screws may be placed in patients as young as 1 year of age.
  - Preoperative CT scans can help assess the feasibility of screw placement.
- Implants should be titanium, and either 3.5- or 4.5-mm rod systems should be used in younger patients.
  - Screw diameter and length can be at least estimated based on the preoperative CT scan.
- Screws should be placed in a stepwise manner, beginning with obtaining a cancellous blush with a burr at the appropriate starting position.
  - Starting positions in normally segmented areas of the spine are well documented.

- A pedicle awl can then be used to obtain access down the pedicle into the vertebral body.
- Once the pedicle has been accessed, probing of the four walls of the pedicle and floor of the body is necessary to confirm accurate position. We then use the probe as a depth gauge to determine screw length.
  - The hole is then tapped 0.5 mm under the expected screw diameter, and the pedicle walls and floor are reprobed.
  - A fixed-angle screw of the appropriate diameter and length is then placed (**TECH FIG 1A**).
- Appropriate screw position is confirmed using triggered EMG stimulation of all screws (**TECH FIG 1B**) and then checking PA and lateral radiographs and fluoroscopic views (**TECH FIG 1C**).

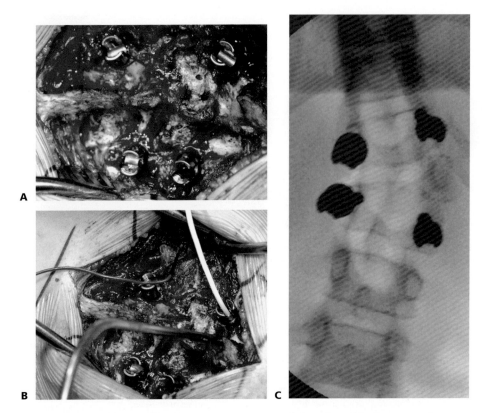

TECH FIG 1 • Pedicle screw placement. **A.** Exposure of the spine with placement of screws. **B.** Triggered EMG stimulation of the pedicle screws. **C.** Fluoroscopic view confirming correct screw placement.

Hemivertebra Excision

- The first step in excision is dissecting over the edge of the transverse process and down the lateral wall of the body using a Cobb elevator and curved-tip device, followed by curved retractor placement (**TECH FIG 2A**).
  - This step aids in protection of structures lateral and anterior to the wall on the hemivertebra. If the hemivertebra is in the thoracic region, it will be necessary to resect the rib head first to obtain access.
- The cartilaginous surfaces of the concave facet should be resected to encourage fusion.
- Resection then begins in the midline with the ligamentum flavum using a Kerrison rongeur (**TECH FIG 2B,C**), followed by resection of the hemilamina.
  - Resection should extend over to the facet, while the exiting nerve roots above and below the hemivertebra are identified and protected.
  - The transverse process and dorsal cortical bone over the pedicle can be resected in similar fashion until the cancellous bone of the pedicle and cortical outlines of its wall are visualized (**TECH FIG 2D,E**).
    - Care should be taken to avoid nerve roots, which are present rostral and caudal to the pedicle walls of the hemivertebra.
  - Gelfoam (Pfizer Inc, New York, NY) and cottonoids should be used judiciously to protect the dura and create a space between dura and bone to be resected.
- The subperiosteal plane down the lateral wall of the pedicle and body is then developed, with a Cobb elevator

used to facilitate retraction and protection. The dural contents can be protected by a nerve root retractor.
  - Bipolar sealing of epidural vessels that lie on the medial aspect of the pedicle and down on the inner wall of the body will aid in controlling blood loss and improving visualization.
  - Continued resection down the pedicle and into the hemivertebra body can be done by a diamond-tipped burr, which helps protect against unwanted injury to soft tissue structures.
- Working stepwise within the walls of the pedicle and down within the confines of the body helps protect surrounding vital structures and makes removal of the cortical shells easier (**TECH FIG 2F**). The walls of the pedicle can then be easily resected with a curette or pituitary rongeur, as can the remaining walls of the body of the hemivertebra.
  - Protection lateral and anterior to the confines of the hemivertebra wall is necessary to avoid injury to vital structures such as the aorta. Generally, the dorsal cortex of the vertebral body is removed last (**TECH FIG 2G**).
- This resection is a wedge resection, which includes the discs above and below as well as the concave area of the disc.
  - The disc material should be removed with a pituitary rongeur and curettes; the dura and its contents are protected with a nerve root retractor.
  - If the disc material above and below is not removed, correction will be limited, and anterior fusion will be less reliable.

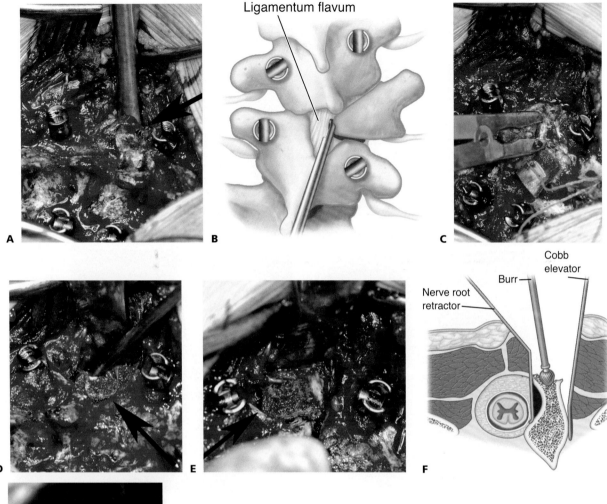

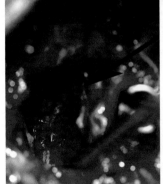

TECH FIG 2 • Hemivertebra excision. **A.** Placement of Cobb elevator at lateral border of hemivertebra (*arrow*). **B.** Resection of the posterior hemilamina using a Kerrison rongeur. **C.** Rongeur resecting down the pedicle with Gelfoam protecting the dura. **D.** Further resection down the pedicle (*arrow*), with lateral structures protected. **E.** Complete visualization of the vertebral body (*arrow*) with anterolateral protection. **F.** Axial schematic illustration of working down the pedicle with medial and lateral protection. **G.** Arrow points to the area of complete resection.

Closure of Wedge Resection

- We place resected vertebral cancellous bone as well as allograft clips into the wedge resection site anteriorly.
- We have found that it is beneficial to compress and close the resection site with laminar hooks and by external three-point pressure on the body (**TECH FIG 3A**).
  - We place a downgoing supralaminar hook at the superior level and an upgoing infralaminar hook on the inferior level.
  - We place a rod and compress with closure of the resection site and correction of the deformity. Using this rod avoids having to place large compression forces across pedicle screws. This allows the screws to maintain correction without possible plowing of the screws into the immature bone or pedicles.
- The compression should be slow and controlled, with the dura under visualization so that it is not caught in the closure of the posterior elements (**TECH FIG 3B,C**).
  - If insufficient correction is achieved or if the adjacent laminae abut prematurely, it may be necessary to resect further along the edges of the laminae.
- Two additional rods are then placed, one on either side of the spine, connected to the corresponding screws. A crosslink should be applied if at all possible (**TECH FIG 3D**).
- The spine is then decorticated. We prefer to place corticocancellous allograft, because it is effective and avoids harvesting the iliac crest.

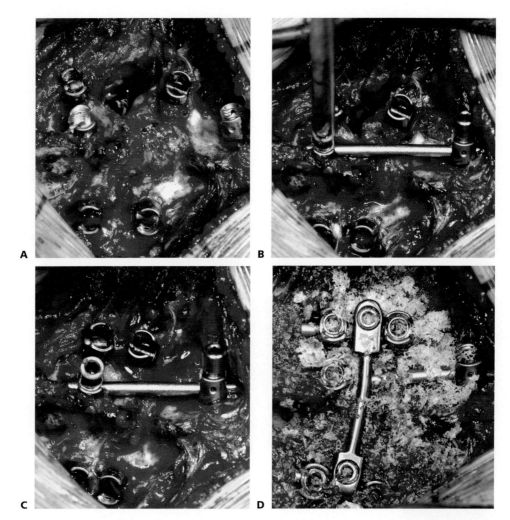

TECH FIG 3 • Closure of wedge resection. **A.** Laminar hooks in place. Note the spacing between pedicle screws. **B.** Compression of laminar hooks with closure of the excision site. **C.** Complete closure of the excision site. The convex screws have now come together, representing wedge closure. **D.** The three-rod system in place, plus the crosslink that should be applied if technically feasible.

Anteroposterior Excision

- We routinely place our posterior implant anchors before performing any resection. Once complete exposure (both anterior and posterior) has been performed (**TECH FIG 4A**), posterior screws are placed.
- Anterior resection begins by creating a full-thickness subperiosteal flap over the hemivertebra after localization is confirmed (**TECH FIG 4B**).
- Starting at the inferior endplate of the adjacent superior body and the superior endplate of the adjacent inferior body, we create longitudinal full-thickness cuts in the periosteum.
    - At the endplate region, we make anteroposterior cuts in the periosteum and start a full-thickness periosteal flap, working anteriorly to the contralateral side.
    - We move posteriorly until we can visualize the hemivertebra pedicle.
- The discs above and below the hemivertebra are resected all the way posteriorly to the posterior longitudinal ligament.

- We then start resection of the hemivertebra vertebral body back to the posterior cortical wall of the body with rongeurs and a diamond-tipped burr.
    - The posterior wall can be resected and peeled off the posterior longitudinal ligament with a rongeur, obtaining access by starting at the level of the disc resections.
    - Part of the visualized pedicle can be resected.
- Posterior resection can then begin, starting with the hemilamina and proceeding to the pedicle (**TECH FIG 4C**).
- With both incisions open and fields exposed, resection of the pedicle can be done by working through both regions (**TECH FIG 4D**). This allows complete visualization and maximum control of the surgical field.
- Once the hemivertebra has been resected, correction of the deformity is the same as described earlier, using a three-rod technique if possible (**TECH FIG 4E**).
    - With this technique, correction is aided by unbreaking the table (or removing any lateral bolster) and pushing down on the convex spine to facilitate closure of the wedge resection.

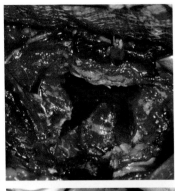
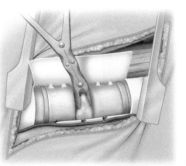
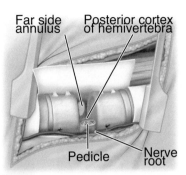

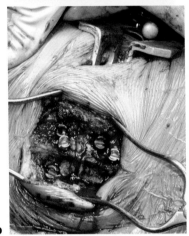
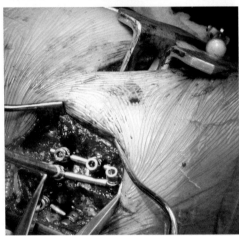

TECH FIG 4 • AP excision. **A.** Hemivertebra isolated anteriorly with removal of discs above and below. **B.** Anterior resection. **C.** Resection back to the pedicle. **D.** Photograph of surgeon working through both operative sites simultaneously. **E.** Compression to close wedge resection site.

PEARLS AND PITFALLS

Localization of the hemivertebra	■ The intraoperative anatomy can be confusing. A thorough understanding of the patient's anatomy can be gained by studying the preoperative 3D CT scans.
Implant placement	■ It is useful to place implant anchors first, because the resection may make this difficult owing to blood loss and possible instability of the spine following resection.
Blood loss	■ Blood loss may be minimized by sealing the epidural veins on the inner aspect of the hemivertebral wall and pedicle with a bipolar cautery before resecting these areas.
Inadequate correction	■ Can be avoided by resection of the far-side concave disc and complete resection of the hemivertebra.

POSTOPERATIVE CARE

■ The immediate postoperative hospitalization and care are similar to that for most patients being treated for spinal deformity.

■ When fixation is adequate, we place the patients in a custom-molded thoracolumbosacral orthosis for 3 months.

■ In patients who are younger than 2 years of age, or in cases where fixation is not adequate, we recommend a Risser-type cast, to include a shoulder or both thighs for 2 months, followed by a brace for up to a total of 6 months postoperatively.

■ The removal of spinal implants is not mandatory; however, given the young age of the patients and individual body habitus, occasionally it is necessary to remove the implants after a year secondary to prominence.

OUTCOMES

■ Hemivertebra excision may be performed as a posterior-only technique or as a combined anterior–posterior technique, with excellent curve correction of approximately 70% (**FIG 4**).[6]

■ The rate of union for this procedure is near 100% in pediatric patients.

■ The procedure may be performed safely using either technique with no neurologic complications.

COMPLICATIONS

■ Inadequate correction
■ Dural injury
■ Neurologic injury

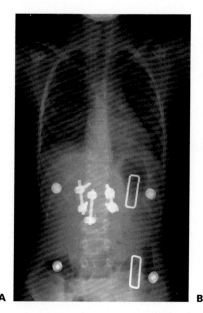
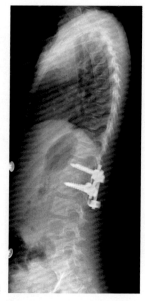

FIG 4 • Correction of deformity. **A.** Postoperative standing radiograph after excision and curve correction of patient shown in Figure 2A. **B.** Standing lateral radiograph of the same patient showing excellent sagittal balance after excision.

- Loss of fixation
- Implant failure
- Excessive blood loss
- Nonunion
- Infection

REFERENCES

1. Belmont P, Kuklo T, et al. Intraspinal anomalies associated with isolated congenital hemivertebra; the role of routine magnetic resonance imaging. J Bone Joint Surg Am 2004;86A:1704–1710.
2. Hedequist DJ, Emans JB. The correlation of preoperative three-dimensional computed tomography reconstructions with operative findings in congenital scoliosis. Spine 2003;28:2531–2544.
3. Hedequist D, Emans J. Congenital scoliosis. J Am Acad Orthop Surg 2004;12:266–275.
4. Hedequist DJ, Hall JE, et al. Hemivertebra excision in children via simultaneous anterior and posterior exposures. J Pediatr Orthop 2005;25:60–63.
5. McMaster MJ, David CV. Hemivertebra as a cause of scoliosis: A study of 104 patients. J Bone Joint Surg Br 1986;68B:588–595.
6. Ruf M, Harms J. Hemivertebra excision by a posterior approach: innovative operative technique and first results. Spine 2002;27:1116–1123.

Chapter 41

Decompression, Posterolateral, and Interbody Fusion for High-Grade Spondylolisthesis

Gilbert Chan and John P. Dormans

DEFINITION

- *Spondylolisthesis* is the forward displacement of a vertebra over the next adjacent segment.
- In children and adolescents, this most commonly occurs in the presence of a spondylolytic defect or a nonunion of the pars interarticularis. It also may occur in the presence of inherent spinal anomalies such as deficient or maloriented lumbar and lumbosacral facets.
- Spondylolisthesis has been grouped into five different types under the Wiltse-Newman classification: dysplastic, isthmic, degenerative, traumatic, and pathologic.[25]
  - Ordinarily, the dysplastic and isthmic types apply to children (**FIG 1A**).
- The Meyerding classification is used to grade the degree of slippage (**FIG 1B**). The classification is divided into five grades:
  - Grade I: 0 to 25% slip
  - Grade II: 26% to 50% slip
  - Grade III: 51% to 75% slip
  - Grade IV: 76% to 100%
  - Grade V: corresponds to spondyloptosis

- Anterior slippage of 50% or more (Meyerding grade III or IV) of the transverse width of the caudal segment is termed a *high-grade slip*.

ANATOMY

- The vertebral bodies have a tendency to increase in size with progression caudally. This increase is believed to be related to the demands of increased stress and weight bearing placed on the lumbosacral spine.
- The lumbar vertebrae are widest in transverse diameter than in the anterior-posterior plane. The lumbar foramina appear trefoil-like. The spinous processes are large and have an oblong appearance. Its transverse processes are long and slender and project directly lateral. The facet joints of the lumbar spine are oriented more toward the sagittal plane, allowing for more flexion and extension motion.
- The neurovascular structures in the lumbar spine run a similar course when compared to the thoracic spine. The segmental vasculature arises directly from the aorta and run dorsally around the lateral aspect of each vertebral body. Branching occurs near the pedicles, where one branch supplies the spinal

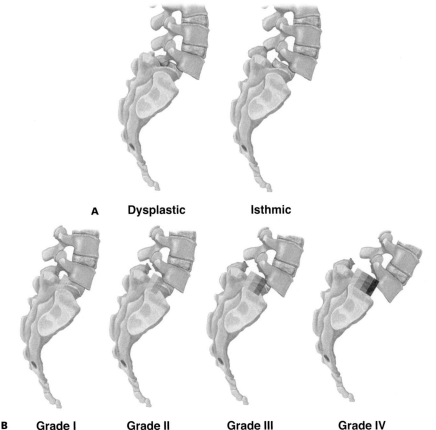

A   **Dysplastic**   **Isthmic**

B   **Grade I**   **Grade II**   **Grade III**   **Grade IV**

FIG 1 • **A.** The dysplastic and isthmic types of spondylolisthesis. **B.** The Meyerding classification is based on degrees of slippage: grade I, 0 to 25%; grade II, 26% to 50%; grade III, 51% to 75%; grade IV, 76% to 100%.

canal and the other supplies the paraspinal musculature. These vessels run between the transverse processes, where they may be susceptible to injury in more lateral exposures.

■ The spinal cord ends most commonly at the level of L1–2. The conus medullaris extends from the most distal portion and goes on to innervate the bowel and bladder. Beneath the conus, the lumbar and sacral nerve roots are arranged to form the cauda equina. Each of these roots exits segmentally below the pedicle of the corresponding vertebrae.

■ The pedicles are cylindrical structures that bridge the posterior elements of the spine with the vertebral body. The height and diameter of the pedicles increases from the thoracic to the lumbar spine. The transverse diameter of the pedicle gradually increases from L1 to L5. The transverse angulation of the pedicles is directed medially, increasing gradually from L1 to L5. The sagittal plane orientation of the lumbar spine pedicles is neutral.[4,18,20,26,27]

■ The spinal cord and the dural sac lie medial to the pedicles. Corresponding nerve roots are found both superior and inferior to each pedicle, with the inferior nerve root in closer proximity to the pedicle.[5,20]

■ The orientation of the facet joints in the lumbar and lumbosacral spine is related to function. In the upper part of the lumbar spine, the orientation of the joints allows for multidirectional stabilization. This is in contrast to the lumbosacral facet joint, which is flat and more coronally oriented and acts to resist shearing forces through the joint.[7]

PATHOGENESIS

■ Spondylolisthesis is a disorder related to upright posture, increasing the forces acting upon the lower segments of the spine, and is never seen in the nonambulatory individual.

■ The lumbar spine is subject to high shear forces and compressive loads. The "bony hook," consisting of the pedicle, the pars interarticularis, and the inferior facets, provides stability by resisting these shear forces and preventing forward slippage or sliding over the inferior endplates.

■ In the setting of congenital or dysplastic spondylolisthesis, the spine begins to slip even if the posterior elements are intact. This is brought about by the structural abnormality's inability to resist the load and shear forces seen in the lumbosacral spine.

■ In the isthmic type of spondylolisthesis, secondary to a pars defect, the high shear and compressive forces occurring through the lumbar spine and lumbosacral joint are less well resisted. This is due to the loss of posterior restraint, allowing forward displacement of one vertebral segment over the next more caudal level.[9]

NATURAL HISTORY

■ Harris and Weinstein[10] reviewed 38 cases with high-grade spondylolisthesis treated nonoperatively and with in situ fusion with a mean follow-up of 24 years and showed that 36% of patients treated nonoperatively were asymptomatic, 55% had back pain, and 45% had neurologic symptoms.

■ Beutler et al,[1] in a 45-year follow-up study of 30 patients diagnosed with spondylolysis, screened in the 1950s from a pool of 500 first-grade children, showed that no patients with unilateral pars defects developed spondylolisthesis. They also showed that cases with bilateral pars defects and low-grade slips follow a course similar to that seen in the general populace. Slowing of slip progression was observed with each decade.

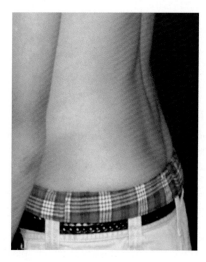

FIG 2 • A 14-year-old boy diagnosed with spondylolisthesis with flattening of the lumbar lordosis.

■ In a comparison of the progression of the slip between isthmic and dysplastic types of spondylolisthesis, dysplastic types showed increased progression.[15]

PATIENT HISTORY AND PHYSICAL FINDINGS

■ In symptomatic patients, the most common clinical manifestation is low back pain, with or without radicular pain radiating through the L5 or S1 dermatome. Onset of pain is usually chronic and insidious, but acute episodes do occur.

■ In patients with radicular symptoms, unilateral involvement is more common.

■ Flattening of the lumbar lordosis is commonly seen on physical examination (**FIG 2**).

■ Abnormal gait exemplified by a hip-flexed, knee-flexed gait pattern may be present.

■ Hamstring tightness, which also may be present, is tested by measuring the popliteal angle. Many patients with high-grade slips will have a tendency to develop tight hamstrings owing to the development of abnormal biomechanics in the lumbar spine.

■ Straight leg raise should be done to test for nerve root compression or hamstring tightness. A positive examination with radicular pain denotes either an L5 or S1 nerve root compression. Radicular pain elicited before 70 degrees is indicative of root compression, whereas that elicited above 70 degrees might denote extraspinal compression of the sciatic nerve. Pain in the posterior thigh denotes hamstring tightness.

■ A rectal examination should be done in the presence of bladder and bowel dysfunction.

■ Examination should also include the Lasgues test. If the pain is exacerbated, that finding supports the diagnosis of a nerve root compression. Posterior thigh pain secondary to tight hamstrings will not be aggravated.

IMAGING AND OTHER DIAGNOSTIC STUDIES

■ Initial imaging includes standing posteroanterior and lateral radiographs of the spine as well as oblique views (**FIG 3A–C**).

■ Plain radiographs are used to establish the overall alignment of the spine in both the coronal and sagittal planes. The

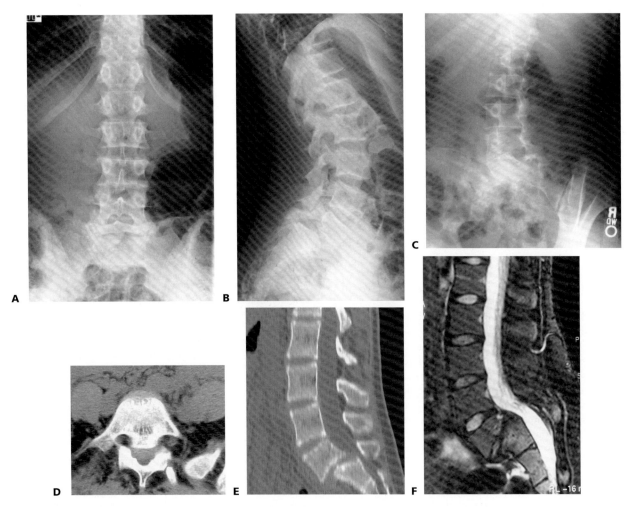

FIG 3 • PA (**A**), lateral (**B**), and left and right oblique (**C**) radiographs demonstrating high-grade spondylolisthesis. Axial (**D**) and sagittal (**E**) CT scan sections demonstrating bony deformity. **F.** MRI demonstrating high-grade spondylolisthesis.

sagittal alignment should be noted, particularly the degree of lumbar lordosis above the lumbosacral kyphosis. Any structural abnormalities in the spine aside from the slip should be noted. These abnormalities include the presence of spina bifida occulta, scoliosis, or sagittal plane abnormalities. Other spinal problems should be treated as separate entities.
▪ CT scans are valuable in defining the exact bony abnormality and will help in preoperative planning (**FIG 3D,E**).
▪ MRI studies are indicated when there is evidence of neurologic compromise. MRI provides good visualization of nerve root or cauda equina compression (**FIG 3F**).

DIFFERENTIAL DIAGNOSIS

▪ Mechanical disorders: trauma, overuse syndromes, herniated disc, slipped vertebral apophysis
▪ Developmental disorders: Scheuermann's kyphosis
▪ Inflammatory disorders: discitis, vertebral osteomyelitis, calcific discitis, rheumatologic conditions
▪ Neoplastic disorders

NONOPERATIVE MANAGEMENT

▪ The treatment of high-grade spondylolisthesis is surgical. Even in asymptomatic cases, the risk of progression or the development of cauda equina syndrome warrants surgical intervention.

SURGICAL MANAGEMENT

▪ The first goal of surgical management is to avoid complications ("first do no harm").
▪ Surgical management is indicated in high-grade slips, with or without the presence of neurologic compromise, or in refractory symptomatic patients.
▪ Selecting the appropriate surgical intervention for each patient requires:
   ▪ A thorough evaluation of the deformity
   ▪ An in-depth understanding of the nature of the pathology
   ▪ An understanding of the indications for treatment
   ▪ Awareness of the limitations of each procedure and its possible complications

Preoperative Planning

- A detailed assessment of the history and physical and neurologic examinations should be performed.
- All imaging studies must be carefully reviewed and analyzed with attention to trying to correlate physical and neurologic findings with those found in special examinations.
- The degree of the slip as seen on the lateral standing spine radiographs is assessed and graded according to the Meyerding classification.
  - Slippage of 50% or more is considered a high-grade slip.
- The *slip angle* measures the degree of lumbosacral kyphosis.
  - A slip angle greater than 50 degrees is associated with progression, instability, and pseudoarthrosis (**FIG 4A**).
- *Pelvic incidence* (PI) is a fixed anatomic parameter that estimates the position of the sacral endplates and overall pelvic morphology. It helps determine the overall sagittal profile of the spine.[3,12]
  - The PI increases with age and stabilizes in adulthood.[14]
  - The mean PI is 47 degrees in children and 57 degrees in adults.
  - Increased PI is indicative of increased lumbar lordosis and increased shear forces (**FIG 4B**). Increased PI may predispose to the development of spondylolisthesis.[3,11,12]
  - In the presence of spondylolisthesis, an increased PI may be indicative of an unbalanced pelvis and is a risk factor for slip progression. Slip reduction is required in these cases to restore proper spinopelvic biomechanics and stabilize the spine. In those cases, where the spine is balanced and PI is low, a fusion in situ may be all that is required for treatment.

Positioning

- The patient is positioned prone on the operative frame.
- Two operative positions are commonly used for posterior approaches to the spine.
  - The first is the knee-chest position, where both the hips and knees are flexed.
  - The second position is with the use of a four-poster frame, where the lower extremities are fairly parallel to the trunk. In this position, the patient is supported under the anterior superior iliac spines and pectoral muscles bilaterally.

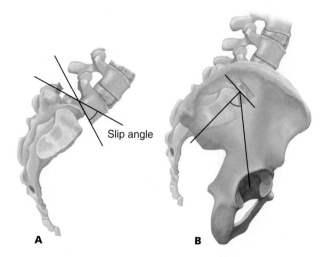

FIG 4 • A. Slip angle is a measure of lumbosacral kyphosis. A slip angle greater than 50% is associated with progression, instability, and pseudoarthrosis. **B.** Pelvic incidence is the angle formed between a line perpendicular to the center of the sacral endplate and a line connecting this point to the center of the femoral heads. It is a good indicator of pelvic shape and morphology. Increased pelvic incidence has been associated with increased shear forces and the development of spondylolisthesis.

Slip angle

- Our preference is to place the patient in the Jackson spinal table with the hips and knee in the flexed position, allowing for easier access to the lumbar spine.
- The position of the face and arms is important. The face should be adequately supported, making sure that no excessive pressure is applied, especially around the orbits. The neck should be in neutral position. The upper extremities should also be in 90–90 position, in which the arms are in 90 degrees of abduction and the elbows are in 90 degrees of flexion. The upper extremities should be adequately padded to allow for venous and arterial access. Adequate padding, support, positioning, and monitoring of the upper extremities likewise prevents undue neurologic injury due to stretch or excessive pressure.[19]

TECHNIQUES

ROUTINE REVISION WITHOUT DIAPHYSEAL DEFECT

Bohlman Technique

- In the Bohlman technique,[22] the procedure starts with a standard posterior midline approach extending from the second lumbar vertebra to the level of S2.
- The spine is exposed subperiosteally, revealing all the posterior elements.
- The posterior elements of L5 and S1 are removed (the posterior elements of L4 are removed if needed).
- A wide foraminotomy is performed to decompress the L5 and S1 nerve roots.
- The dura is gently freed and retracted.
- A curved osteotome is used to make a ventral trough through the sacrum to remove pressure from the dura (**TECH FIG 1A**).
- The dura is retracted, and a ⅛-inch guide pin is placed in the midline of the sacrum toward the body of L5. This is

- done under fluoroscopic guidance to ensure proper placement.
- A ½-inch cannulated drill bit is used to drill over the guide pin, taking extra care not to violate the anterior cortex of L5. The depth is approximately 5 cm.
- A mid-diaphyseal fibular graft is trimmed to fit into the drill hole and inserted (**TECH FIG 1B**). The position of the graft is confirmed fluoroscopically.
- Alternatively, a split fibular graft can be inserted as described by Bohlman in 1982.[2]
  - This is performed by inserting a guide pin through the posterior prominence of the sacrum approximately one cm from the midline to the body of L5, avoiding the first sacral nerve root. The position of the guide pin is confirmed radiographically. This process is done bilaterally.

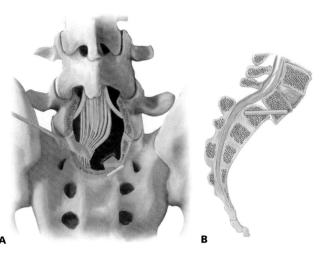

TECH FIG 1 • A. A wide laminectomy is performed removing the posterior elements of L5 and S1. The dura is retracted gently, and a curved osteotome is inserted to perform a sacroplasty to take pressure off the dura. **B.** A fibular strut graft is fashioned and inserted into the sacrum to the body of L5. The procedure is then completed by performing bilateral posterolateral fusion.

- A ⅜-inch cannulated drill bit is used to drill over each guide pin, taking extra care not to violate the anterior cortex of L5. The depth is approximately 5 cm on both sides.
- A fibular graft is split in half and trimmed. It is then inserted and countersunk 2 mm into each hole.
- A standard posterolateral transverse process fusion is done, extending from the sacral alae to L4, to complete the procedure.

Children's Hospital of Philadelphia (CHOP) Technique

Incision and Dissection

- The lumbar spine is approached posteriorly through a direct midline incision extending from L2 to S2 (**TECH FIG 2A**).
- The dissection is done using loupes for magnification and head lamps for illumination.
- The midline incision is carried down to the fascia through sharp dissection of the skin and subcutaneous tissue.
- The midline dissection is carried down subperiosteally, exposing the posterior elements of the spine, with care taken to protect the most proximal intact facets (**TECH FIG 2B,C**).

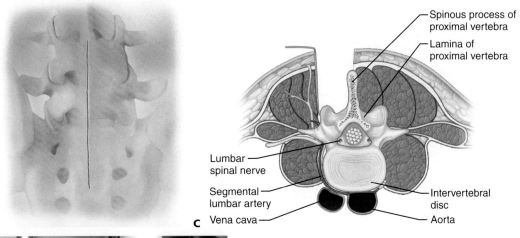

Labels: Spinous process of proximal vertebra; Lamina of proximal vertebra; Lumbar spinal nerve; Segmental lumbar artery; Vena cava; Intervertebral disc; Aorta

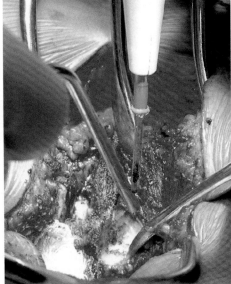

TECH FIG 2 • A. A direct midline posterior skin incision along the spine is made, extending from L4 to S2. **B,C.** The fascia is incised along with the skin incision, and the paraspinal muscles are dissected off of the posterior elements subperiosteally.

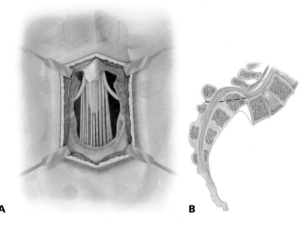

TECH FIG 3 • **A.** A wide laminectomy and adequate decompression of the nerve roots are performed. **B.** A sacroplasty is then performed to take pressure off of the dura.

- In isthmic spondylolisthesis, removal of loose bodies and the posterior elements of L5 is done.

Decompression

- The nerve roots of L5 and S1 are identified, and a wide decompression of the L5/S1 roots is carried out bilaterally (**TECH FIG 3A**).
- The dura and neural elements over the sacrum are gently retracted, and a sacroplasty is done using an osteotome or a high-speed diamond burr (**TECH FIG 3B**).

Reduction and Fusion

- Pedicle screws are placed into the L4, L5, S1, and S2 pedicles (**TECH FIG 4A**).
- The anesthetic and spinal monitoring team is informed before any corrective maneuvers are performed.
- The reduction is performed under fluoroscopic guidance, avoiding overcorrection. With the use of reduction tools

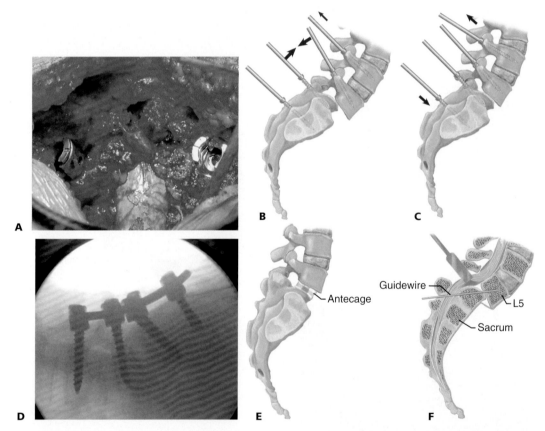

TECH FIG 4 • **A.** Pedicle screws are placed from L4 to S2. Once all of the pedicle screws have been placed, a gentle reduction is performed, aimed at correcting the slip angle. **B.** Using reduction tools attached to the pedicle screws, a dorsal extension force is applied to the lumbar spine while a counterforce is applied to the sacrum. This maneuver gently corrects the slip angle and restores lumbar lordosis. Attention to spinal cord monitoring is crucial at this point in the operation to avoid undue neurologic injury. **C.** Following correction of the slip angle, gradual correction of the slip is performed by applying pressure on the sacrum while the lumbar spine is held and a gentle force is applied in the opposite direction, affording reduction. Overcorrection of the slip should be avoided. **D.** The entire construct is checked after reduction under fluoroscopy to ensure proper implant placement and adequate correction of the spondylolisthesis, and final tightening is done. **E.** The dura is gently retracted, and a cage is placed to add anterior column support. **F.** Alternatively, fibular strut grafting may be used to provide anterior column support. This is done by inserting a guide pin through the sacrum to the body of L5. *(continued)*

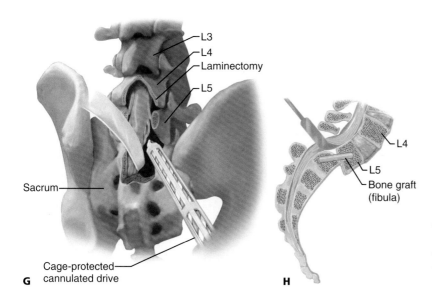

G Cage-protected cannulated drive

H

Labels in figure: L3, L4, Laminectomy, L5, Sacrum, Cage-protected cannulated drive, L4, L5, Bone graft (fibula)

TECH FIG 4 • *(continued)* **G.** A. cannulated drill bit is used to ream through to the body of L5. **H.** A split fibular graft is fashioned and countersunk into each drill hole bilaterally.

attached to the pedicle screws, the slip angle is gradually reduced under fluoroscopic guidance by applying a dorsal extension maneuver to the lumbar pedicle screws (**TECH FIG 4B**). The key points are to correct slowly, pay close attention to the spinal cord monitoring, and focus on the reduction of the slip angle rather than the slip itself.

- The reduction is performed slowly and maintained over time to allow for stretch of the soft tissue. Once a satisfactory correction of the slip angle has been achieved, gradual reduction of the slip is performed by applying force to the sacrum, while a counterforce is applied to the lumbar spine (**TECH FIG 4C**).
- Reduction of the slip angle is much more important than reduction of the slip itself. Close attention to spinal cord monitoring is crucial during the entire reduction maneuver.
- The rods are templated, cut, and contoured, and then attached to the construct while reduction is maintained.
- Final tightening of the entire construct is done and checked with fluoroscopy or plain radiographs (**TECH FIG 4D**).

- The L5–S1 disc is identified and removed, a fusion is performed, and the L5–S1 disc space is filled with cancellous autograft or allograft.
- An anterior cage is placed to provide adequate anterior column support (**TECH FIG 4E**).
- As an alternative, a double split fibular strut graft (modified Bohlman technique) can be inserted from the sacrum to the body of L5 to add anterior column support. The dura is gently retracted to one side, and a guide pin is inserted from the sacrum to the body of L5 (**TECH FIG 4F**).
  - A 6-mm cannulated reamer is then used to ream this channel (**TECH FIG 4G**).
- A fibular auto- or allograft is then placed through the channel and countersunk (**TECH FIG 4H**).
  - The same procedure is repeated on the contralateral side.
- The procedure is completed by placing bone graft lateral to the implants along the transverse processes from L4 to the sacrum.
- Meticulous hemostasis is carried out, and a layer-by-layer closure of the operative site is performed.

PEARLS AND PITFALLS

Indications	■ A complete history and physical and neurologic examination must be performed before surgery. ■ All needed and appropriate imaging studies must be evaluated carefully to identify all aspects of the deformity—including the degree of the deformity and the type (eg, isthmic vs congenital)—as well as any other spinal deformity that may be present (eg, spina bifida occulta).
Surgical exposure	■ Careful and meticulous technique must be observed. Care should be taken, especially when pathologies such as spina bifida occulta are present, to prevent iatrogenic neurologic injury. ■ Decompression of at-risk nerve roots is a key component to exposure and operation.
Instrumentation	■ Careful preparation should be undertaken before performing instrumentation and reduction. ■ Adequate decompression of all neurologic structures at risk should be ensured to prevent iatrogenic injury. ■ Close attention must be paid to neurophysiologic monitoring during both instrumentation and reduction.
Reduction	■ Slow, gentle force is applied during the reduction maneuver. This procedure should be done over time to allow for relaxation of the soft tissue structures. ■ Avoid excessive reduction. Reduction of the slip angle is more important than complete reduction of the slip. Excessive reduction may result in neurologic compromise.

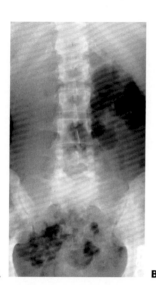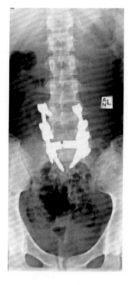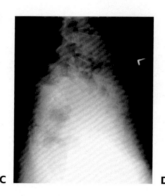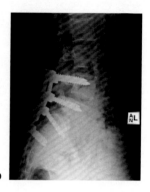

FIG 5 • Radiographs from a 17-year-old girl with high-grade isthmic spondylolisthesis who underwent decompression, reduction, and instrumented fusion. **A,B.** Initial PA and lateral radiographs showing the preoperative deformity. **C,D.** PA and lateral films showing postoperative correction using the CHOP technique.

POSTOPERATIVE CARE

▪ High-quality radiographs are taken immediately postoperatively to ensure proper graft and instrumentation placement before the patient is taken out of the operative suite (**FIG 5**).
▪ In the immediate postoperative period, the hips and knees are flexed and elevated using pillows to alleviate pain.
▪ Pain control is instituted (eg, intrathecal analgesia and IV patient-controlled analgesia), and the patient is fitted with a thoracolumbosacral orthosis (TLSO) for comfort. The patient is then encouraged to stand and ambulate as tolerated. Postoperative anteroposterior and lateral standing spine radiographs are taken before discharge.
▪ Activity restriction (ie, avoidance of bending and rotational motion) is carried out until fusion has occurred.
▪ The patient may return to sports and strenuous physical activity after 1 year as long as spinal fusion has been confirmed. Adequate precautionary measures should be taken before engaging in any contact sport.
▪ Full-contact sports, which may entail collision, should still be avoided.

OUTCOMES

▪ In high-grade spondylolisthesis treated with in situ fusion techniques, clinical improvement in back pain symptoms has been reported in 74% to 100% of cases. Solid fusion rates have also been reported to be 71% to 100%.[6,8,13,23,24]
▪ A study on 18 adolescents with high-grade spondylolisthesis treated with instrumented reduction and fusion reports complete resolution of preoperative neurologic symptoms with 100% fusion rates. No loss of fixation or instrument-related failures were reported at a minimum of 2 years' follow-up.[21]
▪ Another series[16] comparing in situ fusion, decompression, reduction and instrumented posterior fusion, and circumferential fusion techniques in treating high-grade spondylolisthesis reports a 45% (5 of 11 patients) pseudoarthrosis rate in patients treated with in situ fusion and a 29% (2 of 7 patients) pseudoarthrosis rate in cases treated with posterior decompression, instrumentation, and fusion. All of these cases had small transverse processes (less than 2 cm²). Circumferential techniques achieved the highest fusion rates. Excellent functional outcomes were observed in those cases where a solid fusion was achieved. Final outcomes, however, did not differ among the three groups.
▪ Another study comparing posterior fusion and reduction with posterior fusion and reduction augmented by anterior column support reported a 39% pseudoarthrosis rate in posterior fusion alone. In the cases augmented with anterior column support, 100% fusion rates were achieved.[16]

COMPLICATIONS

▪ Pseudoarthrosis
  ▪ Pseudoarthrosis is the most common complication.
  ▪ Signs include lucency around implants, implant breakage, and slip progression.
  ▪ Pseudoarthrosis may be minimized by using meticulous technique and proper preparation of the graft site.
▪ Neurologic complications
  ▪ Root lesions (L5 root)
  ▪ From direct trauma, manipulation of nerve roots, epidural hematoma formation (compression)
  ▪ Cauda equina syndrome
  ▪ Autonomic dysfunction
  ▪ Chronic pain
  ▪ Immediate release of the correction should be done when necessary.
  ▪ Must be thoroughly evaluated with proper imaging techniques
  ▪ May be minimized by good preoperative planning and meticulous surgical technique and by using multimodality spinal cord monitoring
▪ Transition syndromes
  ▪ Spondylolisthesis acquisita
  ▪ Adjacent segment degeneration
  ▪ S1–S2 deformity
▪ Instrument-related complications

REFERENCES

1. Beutler WJ, Fredrickson BE, Murtland A, et al. The natural history of spondylolysis and spondylolisthesis: 45-year follow-up evaluation. Spine 2003;28:1027–1035.
2. Bohlman HH, Cook SS. One-stage decompression and posterolateral and interbody fusion for lumbosacral spondyloptosis through a posterior approach. Report of two cases. J Bone Joint Surg Am 1982;64: 415–418.
3. Duval-Beaupere G, et al. Sagittal profile of the spine prominent part of the pelvis. Stud Health Technol Inform 2002;88:47–64.
4. Ebraheim NA, Rollins JR Jr, et al. Projection of the lumbar pedicle and its morphometric analysis. Spine 1996;21:1296–1300.
5. Ebraheim NA, Xu R, Darwich M, et al. Anatomic relations between the lumbar pedicle and the adjacent neural structures. Spine 1997;22:2338–2241.
6. Frennered AK, Danielson BI, Nachemson AL, et al. Midterm follow-up of young patients fused in situ for spondylolisthesis. Spine 1991;16:409–416.
7. Grobler LJ, Robertson PA, Novotny JE, et al. Etiology of spondylolisthesis. Assessment of the role played by lumbar facet joint morphology. Spine 1993;18:80–91.
8. Grzegorzewski A, Kumar SJ. In situ posterolateral spine arthrodesis for grades III, IV, and V spondylolisthesis in children and adolescents. J Pediatr Orthop 2000;20:506–511.
9. Hammerberg KW. New concepts on the pathogenesis and classification of spondylolisthesis. Spine 2005;30(6 Suppl):S4–11.
10. Harris IE, Weinstein SL. Long-term follow-up of patients with grade III and IV spondylolisthesis. Treatment with and without posterior fusion. J Bone Joint Surg Am 1987;69:960–969.
11. Labelle H, Roussouly P, Berthonnaud E, et al. Spondylolisthesis, pelvic incidence, and spinopelvic balance: a correlation study. Spine 2004;29:2049–2054.
12. Legaye J, Duval-Beaupere G, Hecquet J, et al. Pelvic incidence: A fundamental pelvic parameter for three-dimensional regulation of spinal sagittal curves. Eur Spine J 1998;7:99–103.
13. Lenke LG, Bridwell KH, Bullis D, et al. Results of in situ fusion for isthmic spondylolisthesis. J Spinal Disord 1992;5:433–442.
14. Mac-Thiong JM, Berthonnaud E, Dimar JR III, et al. Sagittal alignment of the spine and pelvis during growth. Spine 2004;29:1642–1647.
15. McPhee IB, O'Brien JP, McCall IW, et al. Progression of lumbosacral spondylolisthesis. Australas Radiov1981;25:91–95.
16. Molinari RW, Bridwell KH, Lenke LG, et al. Anterior column support in surgery for high-grade, isthmic spondylolisthesis. Clin Orthop Relat Res 2002;(394):109–120.
17. Molinari RW, Bridwell KH, Lenke LG, et al. Complications in the surgical treatment of pediatric high-grade, isthmic dysplastic spondylolisthesis: a comparison of three surgical approaches. Spine 1999;24: 1701–1711.
18. Roy-Camille R, Saillant G, Mazel C. Plating of thoracic, thoracolumbar, and lumbar injuries with pedicle screw plates. Orthop Clin North Am 1986;17:147–159.
19. Schwartz DM, Drummond DS, Hahn M, et al. Prevention of positional brachial plexopathy during surgical correction of scoliosis. J Spinal Disord 2000;13:178–182.
20. Senaran H, Yazici M, Karcaaltincaba M, et al. Lumbar pedicle morphology in the immature spine: a three-dimensional study using spiral computed tomography. Spine 2002;27:2472–2476.
21. Shufflebarger HL, Geck MJ. High-grade isthmic dysplastic spondylolisthesis: Monosegmental surgical treatment. Spine 2005; 30(6 Suppl):S42–48.
22. Smith MD, Bohlman HH. Spondylolisthesis treated by a single-stage operation combining decompression with in situ posterolateral and anterior fusion: An analysis of eleven patients who had long-term follow-up. J Bone Joint Surg Am 1990;72:415–421.
23. Velikas EP, Blackburne JS. Surgical treatment of spondylolisthesis in children and adolescents. J Bone Joint Surg Br 1981;63B:67–70.
24. Wiltse LL. The paraspinal sacrospinalis-splitting approach to the lumbar spine. Clin Orthop Relat Res 1973;91:48–57.
25. Wiltse LL. Newman PH, Macnab I. Classification of spondylolysis and spondylolisthesis. Clin Orthop Relat Res 1976;117:23–29.
26. Zindrick MR, Knight GW, Sartori MJ, et al. Pedicle morphology of the immature thoracolumbar spine. Spine 2000;25:2726–2735.
27. Zindrick MR, Wiltse LL, Doornik A, et al. Analysis of the morphometric characteristics of the thoracic and lumbar pedicles. Spine 1987;12:160–166.

Richard E. McCarthy

DEFINITION

- The treatment of neuromuscular spinal deformities frequently requires fusion to the pelvis with firm fixation. This can be accomplished with a number of devices that allow for correction of pelvic obliquity and pelvic rotation while allowing for a solid base on which to attach rods for correction of curves above.
- One of the most reliable structures in the formation of the spine, even in the dysplastic setting of myelomeningocele, is the sacral ala.
  - The S-rods are contoured to press-fit over the sacral ala.[1,3,4]
  - Historically the elongated Harrington hooks were used in a similar manner.

ANATOMY

- The sacral ala in children is a structure 1.5 to 2 cm in depth (front to back) and 2 to 3 cm wide.
- The L5 nerve root traverses anterior to the ala in an oblique direction progressing from posterior to anterior and superior to inferior obliquely from the neural foramina.
- Immediately inferior to the pedicle of L5 the nerve transgresses anterior to the sacral ala, separated by a distance of 1.5 cm.
- Besides the L5 root, the tissue anterior to the sacral ala is retroperitoneal fat.

- Of key importance is identification and release of the ileotransverse ligament traversing between the iliac wing and the L5 transverse process.
  - To ensure clear access to the sacral ala, this ligament must be released from its attachment to the transverse process (**FIG 1**).
- The dissection of the soft tissues around the sacral ala is done posteriorly with a curette; the surgeon must use caution against inserting tools anterior to the sacral ala for fear of injuring the L5 nerve root or plunging into the retroperitoneal space.

PATHOGENESIS

- The multiple types of neuromuscular scoliosis requiring fixation to the pelvis include cerebral palsy, dystrophic muscle conditions, spina bifida, and many others.
- The types of pelvic abnormalities associated with spinal deformities include pelvic obliquity, pelvic rotation, and flexion and extension of the sacrum.

NATURAL HISTORY

- The natural history is one of progression and worsening of these deformities.

IMAGING AND OTHER DIAGNOSTIC STUDIES

- Special imaging and other diagnostic studies are only occasionally necessary.
- The sacral ala can usually be clearly visualized as a horseshoe-shaped outline on upright or supine lateral radiographic films.
- The Ferguson view (45-degree angle) in the frontal plane provides the clearest view of the width.
- If there is doubt, a CT scan can better elucidate the exact configuration.

SURGICAL MANAGEMENT

- The surgical management, in terms of preoperative planning, positioning, and approach, is the same as for neuromuscular scoliosis.
- The techniques include cleaning of the soft tissues from the sacral ala with release of the ileotransverse ligament.
- The sizing of the hook to the size of the sacral ala in its front-to-back diameter can be done at surgery.
  - Small and medium sizes are available, and it is important to use the appropriate size rod or hook (right or left) so the rod lies medial to the ala (**FIG 2**).

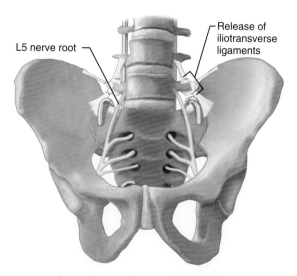

L5 nerve root

Release of iliotransverse ligaments

FIG 1 • Anterior view showing position of S-rod or S-hook with reference to L5 nerve root.

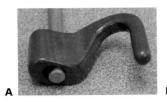 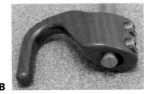 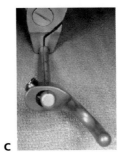 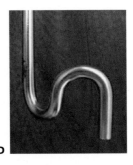

FIG 2 • **A.** Left-sided S-hook, anterior view. **B.** Left-sided S-hook, posterior view. **C.** With a rod clamp positioned to demonstrate the posterior plane, a right-sided S-hook is shown in its correct position. **D.** Right-sided S-rod, side view.

S-ROD PLACEMENT

- Proper alignment of the S-rod necessitates placement of the sagittal bends in the appropriate plane with reference to the best fit of the S-portion on the ala (**TECH FIG 1A**).
  - This can be aided by placement of a vise grip on the rod in the plane of the lordosis once the S-portion of the rod is positioned over the sacral ala.
- The rod is removed from the wound and the three-point bender applied to produce the proper sagittal contours.

- If the S-hook is used instead, the sagittal contours can be made in the rod independent of the hook position.
- It is best to leave 1 cm protruding from the lower end of the hook when it is first placed on the ala (**TECH FIG 1B**).
- The S-hook is temporarily tightened to the rod and spread between the L4 pedicle screw and the S-hook by tightening one Allen set screw on the hook (**TECH FIG 1C,D**).
  - The correction of the spinal deformity can then occur above this area.

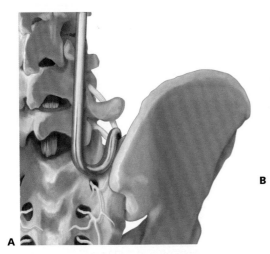 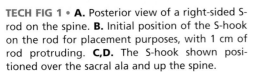

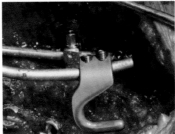

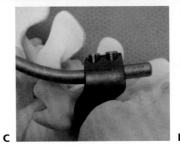

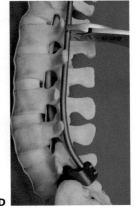

TECH FIG 1 • **A.** Posterior view of a right-sided S-rod on the spine. **B.** Initial position of the S-hook on the rod for placement purposes, with 1 cm of rod protruding. **C,D.** The S-hook shown positioned over the sacral ala and up the spine.

TECHNIQUES

FINAL FIXATION

- Once the final correction has been achieved, the final tightening of the S-hook occurs by distracting once again between the L4 pedicle screw and the concave side S-hook, then the convex side rod, distracting the hooks to the end of the rod (**TECH FIG 2**).
  - Both Allen set screws are firmly tightened.
- A strong cantilever force can be created to correct pelvic obliquity by using two sagittally contoured rods fixed to S-hooks positioned against the sacral ala distracted against the L4 pedicle screws.
  - A transverse rod connector above the S-hooks will supply further stability.
- The pelvis can then be pivoted by grasping the rods above and correcting the pelvic deformity in one maneuver.
- The final fixation of the S-hook is completed with both set screws firmly tightened.[2]

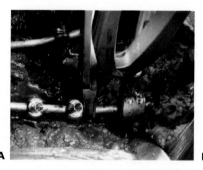

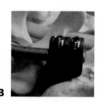

TECH FIG 2 • A. The final seating of the S-hook, distracting it against the L4 pedicle screw. **B.** Final position of the S-hook on the rod.

PEARLS AND PITFALLS

The surgeon must avoid the pitfall of thinking the transverse process of L5 is the ala and positioning the S-hook or S-rod against this structure.	■ This can happen if the ileotransverse ligament is not completely released and the sacral ala clearly visualized (**FIG 3**).
The surgeon should avoid using an L5 pedicle screw.	■ An L4 polyaxial pedicle screw works well to ensure proper pressure and fixation between the L4 screw and the sacral ala.

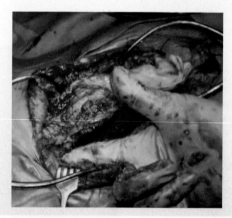

FIG 3 • The sacral ala clearly demonstrated during a myelokyphectomy with only the surgeon's finger inserted anterior to the ala.

POSTOPERATIVE CARE

- It is important to maintain hip flexion at 45 degrees or greater for the first 6 months to avoid levering on the pelvis with physical therapy.
  - No physical therapy is done about the hips for the first 6 months.

OUTCOMES

- This technique has been used in more than 200 cases since 1984. Outcomes are generally solid fusions, ease of caregiving, and attainment of level pelvis for sitting (**FIG 4**).

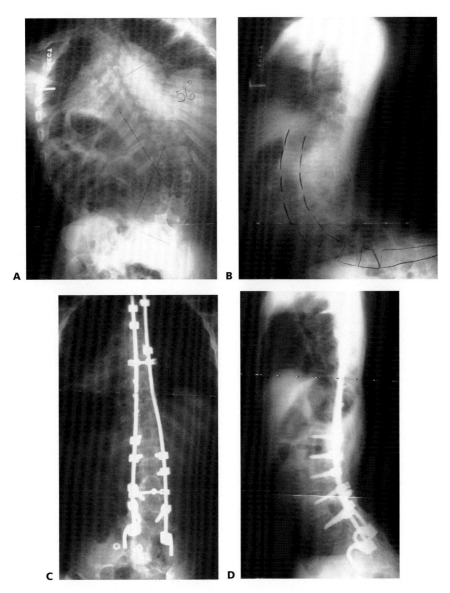

FIG 4 • Neuromuscular spinal deformity: spastic lordoscoliosis with S-hooks.

COMPLICATIONS

▪ Rod migration into myelo pelvis with a growth rod
▪ I have not experienced any neurologic impairment of the L5 root.

REFERENCES

1. McCarthy RE. Sacral pelvic fixation in neuromuscular deformities. Semin Spine Surg 2004;16:126–133.

2. McCarthy RE. S-rod technique. In: Spinal Instrumentation Techniques Manual, ed 2. Scoliosis Research Society, 1998.
3. McCarthy RE, Bruffett WL, McCullough FL. S-rod fixation to the sacrum in patients with neuromuscular spinal deformities. Clin Orthop Relat Res 1999;364:26–31.
4. McCarthy RE, Dunn H, McCullough FL. Luque fixation to the sacral ala with the Dunn modification. Spine 1989;14:281–283.

Chapter 43 Anterior Cervical Approaches

John Heflin and John M. Rhee

GENERAL CONSIDERATIONS

Anterior Approach (Smith-Robinson)

- The approach chosen depends on a number of factors, including the spinal segments that must be exposed, the nature of the procedure to be performed, and the patient's body habitus.
- In general, the Smith-Robinson approach allows access from C2 down to T1 in most patients. However, local variations in patient morphology may either limit or increase the extent of available exposure.
- Ease of access to the C2-3 disc depends on the location of the mandible and can be assessed on the preoperative lateral radiograph.
- Nasal intubation is preferable when approaching this level as it allows the mandible to be maximally closed, away from the line of sight of the disc.
    - Depending on the location of the mandible with respect to C3-4, nasal intubation may be preferable in certain instances of C3-4 access as well.
- For pathology at C7-T1 or distal, careful scrutiny of the disc space with respect to the sternal notch on lateral radiographs will help to assess whether a sternal-splitting approach may be necessary.
    - In some patients with long necks, access to T2 or even T3 may be possible with a standard Smith-Robinson approach.
    - In those with short or stocky necks, even getting to C7 may be a challenge (**FIG 1**).
- Imaging studies should be evaluated for anatomic variations such as medial aberrancy of the vertebral artery.

- Considerable debate exists as to whether the "sidedness" of approach affects the rate of postoperative superior laryngeal nerve palsy. The literature is not conclusive but suggests higher rates with right-sided approaches.
    - If a patient has had prior neck surgery and it is desirable to approach the spine from the opposite side to avoid scar, a preoperative indirect laryngoscopy should be performed by ear, nose, and throat (ENT) consultation to rule out a recurrent laryngeal nerve palsy.
    - If one exists, the spine must be approached from the side of the injury to avoid the possibility of bilateral vocal cord palsy. If one does not exist, the spine can be approached from either side.

Lateral Retropharyngeal Approach (Whitesides)

- This approach can be used for anterior access to the upper cervical spine but not the basiocciput.
- It is often used for high cervical bony lesions, including tumors or infections for which a posterior approach is not possible, unstable fractures or dislocations with deficient or incompetent posterior elements, or posterior nonunions (particularly for fusions of C1 to C2).
- It is also useful for access to high cervical ventral or ventrolateral intradural lesions such as neurofibromas or meningiomas.
- It allows unilateral access to C1 to C3. Access to the far contralateral side requires a second approach.
- Potential complications include injury to the spinal accessory nerve and the vertebral artery. The jugular vein also lies within the operative field and can be a site of significant bleeding if inadvertently injured.
- Significant retropharyngeal swelling has occurred and can result in prolongation of intubation if the patient's airway becomes obstructed.

Anterior Approach to the Cervicothoracic Junction (Transmanubrial-Transclavicular Approach)

- There are several different approaches for exposing the cervicothoracic junction, including the transmanubrial-transclavicular and the sternal-splitting (median sternotomy) approaches.
    - The sternal-splitting (median sternotomy) approach may be useful in providing improved distal access to the upper thoracic spine.
- Deep dissection is essentially the same for the two approaches.
    - Cranial to caudal dissection is recommended to avoid injury to the major crossing vessels distally (eg, the left brachiocephalic vein).
- With a left-sided approach, the thoracic duct is at greater risk. It passes into the left venous angle between the subclavian artery and the common carotid artery.

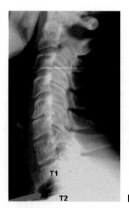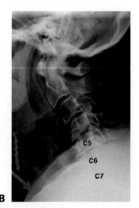

FIG 1 • Long versus short necks. **A.** In patients with long necks, anterior exposure through a standard Smith-Robinson approach readily provides far distal access (eg, down to T1-2 disc space [*arrow*]). **B.** In those with short necks, however, even getting to C6-7 may be difficult if the sternum blocks the necessary trajectory to the disc space (*arrow*), although it can almost always be done.

■ With a right-sided approach, the recurrent laryngeal nerve is at greater risk because of its greater variability versus the left side, where the nerve is more constant in its location in the tracheoesophageal groove.

POSITIONING

Anterior Approach (Smith-Robinson)

■ The patient is positioned supine with the neck slightly extended.
■ The amount of extension tolerated by the patient without developing neurologic symptoms should be assessed preoperatively and not exceeded during positioning (**FIG 2**).
■ A bump (eg, rolled sheets) under the shoulders facilitates gentle extension of the spine.
■ A halter or Garner-Wells tong is optional but not routinely necessary for anterior cervical discectomy and fusion (ACDF) surgery.

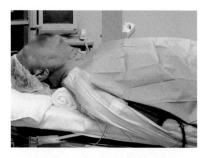

FIG 2 • Positioning. Especially in patients with myelopathy, the amount of preoperative extension tolerated without worsening of neurologic symptoms should be assessed and never exceeded during positioning. A rolled sheet is placed under the scapulae to help gently extend the neck.

■ A foam doughnut is placed behind the occiput to prevent pressure necrosis.
■ The head is placed in neutral rotation. Doing so provides landmarks (the nose and the sternal notch) that are in line with the longitudinal axis of the spine for orientation during decompression and instrumentation.
■ Depending on the relationship of the mandible to the upper cervical spine, proximal approaches to C2-3 may be easier if the head is gently rotated away from the side of the approach.
  ■ The amount of rotation should be kept in mind to prevent disorientation during surgery.
■ The shoulders are gently taped down to facilitate intraoperative radiographic visualization.
  ■ Excessive force should be avoided when taping down the shoulders to avoid brachial plexus injuries.
■ Spinal cord monitoring (eg, somatosensory evoked potentials [SSEP] and motor evoked potentials [MEP]) can be used to help prevent positioning-related nerve injuries, but it is not completely sensitive in detecting injury.

Lateral Retropharyngeal Approach (Whitesides)

■ The patient is placed supine with the head turned away from the side from which the approach will be performed unless the patient is constrained in a halo for instability reasons.
  ■ If this is the case, the exposure will be more challenging but still possible.
■ Nasotracheal intubation opposite the side of the approach is desirable as it allows the jaw to be fully closed, offering the least inhibited exposure.
■ The pinna (earlobe) can be retracted forward and sewn anteriorly to allow better access to the styloid process and posterior ear area.
■ The entire cervical region and lower face is prepared and draped.

ANTERIOR APPROACH (SMITH-ROBINSON)

TECHNIQUES

Incision and Superficial Dissection

■ A transverse incision placed in a skin crease is more cosmetic and suffices for accessing up to three disc levels in most instances.
  ■ A longitudinal incision, although less cosmetic, allows for a more extensile approach (C2-thoracic spine) and should be considered when three or more discs require access, or if the patient has a very thick, muscular neck.
■ The incision is made using palpable anterior structures as a guide (ie, C3 hyoid bone, C4-5 thyroid cartilage, C6 carotid tubercle, C7 cricoid cartilage) (**TECH FIG 1A**).
  ■ The preoperative lateral radiograph can also be used to determine roughly where to make the incision to allow optimal access to the desired disc(s).
  ■ The surgeon should try to make the incision such that it will be in line with the "line of sight" of the intended disc space (**TECH FIG 1B**).
  ■ Transverse incisions may extend from the anterior two thirds of the sternocleidomastoid (SCM) to beyond the midline.

■ Longer incisions and greater tissue mobilization facilitate multilevel procedures and will heal with a nearly imperceptible scar if placed within a natural skin crease.
■ Vertical incisions, if used, are placed along the medial border of the SCM.
■ The incision is continued through the subcutaneous fat to the platysma (**TECH FIG 1C**).
■ The platysma is divided in line with the skin incision using electrocautery.
■ Blunt dissection with scissors undermines the edges of the platysma.
  ■ This allows for greater mobilization of the soft tissues, which is helpful in accessing multiple disc levels and getting enough exposure to place plates and screws.
■ Superficial veins crossing the field of dissection may need to be ligated to facilitate exposure (**TECH FIG 1D**).

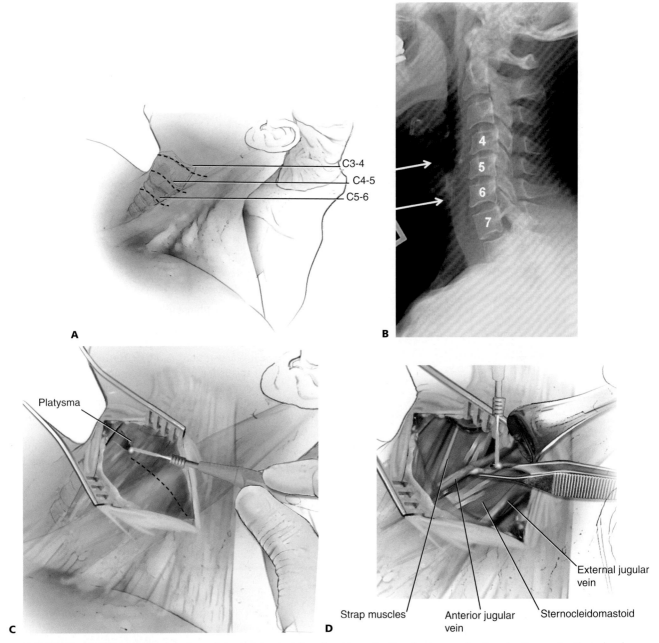

TECH FIG 1 • Incision. **A.** The location of the incision is determined by palpating for known landmarks. Generally, these landmarks overlie specific vertebrae or disc spaces, such as the hyoid bone (C3), thyroid cartilage (C4-5), cricoid cartilage (C7), and carotid tubercle (C6). **B.** Alternatively, by looking at the preoperative lateral radiograph, one can estimate the optimal location for the skin incision. (*Top arrow* indicates the C4-5 approach, *bottom arrow* the C5–7 approach.) **C.** The incision is continued through the subcutaneous fat to the platysma. Platysma fibers are cut in line with the incision. **D.** The surgeon should avoid injuring crossing structures when possible. Superficial veins crossing the field of dissection may need to be ligated to facilitate exposure, however.

Deep Dissection

- The anterior border of the SCM is identified.
- Blunt dissection is then carried through the deep cervical fascia directly medial to the SCM.
- The SCM is retracted laterally to allow palpation and identification of the carotid artery (**TECH FIG 2A**).
    - The carotid artery should be visualized and will form the lateral border of the approach; the esophagus will define the medial border of the approach.

- Once the carotid is identified, a plane through the pretracheal fascia lying between the carotid sheath and the medial structures (thyroid gland, trachea, and esophagus) is created (**TECH FIG 2B**).
    - Finger dissection in this plane is useful in allowing extensile exposure.

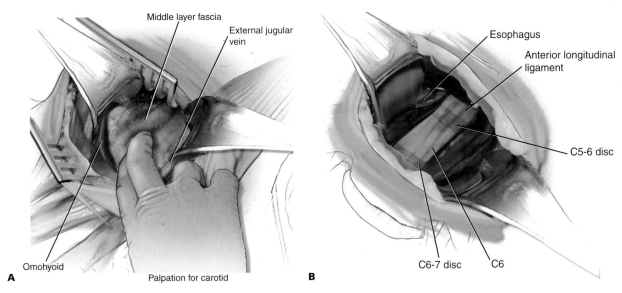

TECH FIG 2 • A. The sternocleidomastoid is retracted laterally using blunt retractors. This will allow palpation and identification of the carotid artery. **B.** After the carotid artery is identified, a plane is created between the carotid sheath and the medial structures (thyroid gland, trachea, and esophagus). Blunt dissection techniques are most effective in developing this plane.

Extending the Exposure

- If surgery involves one level, minimal mobilization may be necessary. If the surgery involves multiple levels or the skin incision is not collinear with the desired disc space, greater mobilization is helpful.
- In general, crossing structures should be preserved if possible to avoid potential injury to neural structures (eg, laryngeal nerves). Blunt dissection with scissors, Kittners, or fingers works best.
  - The superior thyroid vessels typically overlie C3-4, and the inferior thyroid vessels generally overlie C6-7.
- The omohyoid is encountered crossing distal-lateral to cephalad-medial in the interval medial to the sternomastoid at roughly the C6 level. It can be divided with electrocautery or left intact.
- Dividing the omohyoid will allow for a more extensile cephalad-caudal exposure and less tension on the wound for easier placement of plates and screws in multilevel or very distal constructs.

Elevation of Longus Colli and Identification of Levels

- Using bipolar electrocautery, subperiosteal elevation of the longus colli should be done to the level of the uncinate processes bilaterally, and at least from the midportion of the vertebral body above to the midportion of the body below the level for which discectomy is planned (TECH FIG 3A).
- Time and care spent on carefully elevating the longus colli facilitates proper, stable placement of self-retaining retractors, which in turn facilitates decompression and accurate placement of hardware.

- Retractor blades are then placed beneath the elevated longus colli (TECH FIG 3B).
  - Careful placement of retractors will help avoid injury to the esophagus and sympathetic chain (which runs along the ventral surface of the longus colli).
- TECHNIQUES FIGURE 3C represents a cross-sectional view at the C5 level demonstrating the plane of dissection for the Smith-Robinson approach.
- Location of the appropriate level should be ensured by intraoperative radiographs before disruption of the disc.

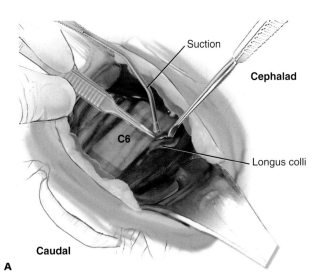

TECH FIG 3 • A. Bipolar electrocautery is used to elevate the longus colli in a subperiosteal fashion to the level of the uncinate processes bilaterally. *(continued)*

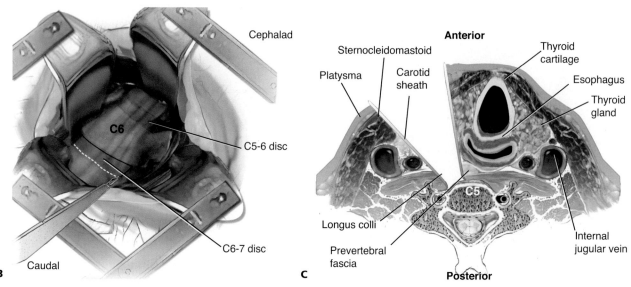

TECH FIG 3 • *(continued)* **B.** Self-retaining retractors can be placed beneath the elevated longus colli to allow an unimpeded view of the anterior spine. Care should be taken to avoid injuring the esophagus and sympathetic chain during placement of the retractors. The use of cephalad/caudal retractors is optimal but not necessary in most cases. **C.** A cross-sectional view through the neck at C5 demonstrating the plane of dissection.

LATERAL RETROPHARYNGEAL APPROACH (WHITESIDES)

Incision and Superficial Dissection

- A transverse incision is extended from the mastoid tip, posterior to the ear, and is carried along the inferior border of the mandible, preferably in a natural skin crease.
- The incision is then directed caudally along the anterior border of the SCM (**TECH FIG 4A**).
- This incision can be extended as needed according to the amount of distal cervical spine exposure required. It can be carried as far as the sternal notch.

- The incision is then carried through the subcutaneous tissues and platysma muscle using electrocautery.
- Dissection is carried out using blunt dissection techniques in the subplatysmal plane, allowing the creation of superior-anterior and inferior-posterior musculocutaneous flaps (**TECH FIG 4B**).
- The superior-anterior flap is elevated to the inferior border of the parotid gland.
- The greater auricular nerve is identified and dissected out of the subcutaneous tissue both caudally

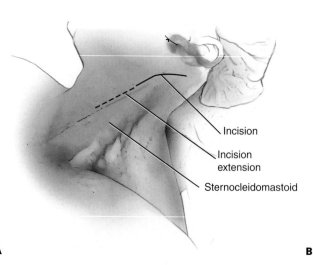

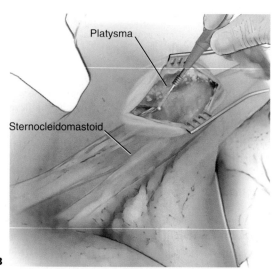

TECH FIG 4 • A. A transverse incision is extended from the mastoid tip and is carried along the inferior border of the mandible, turning caudally and continuing along the anterior border of the sternocleidomastoid muscle. **B.** The incision is carried through the subcutaneous tissues and platysma muscle using electrocautery in line with the incision. Subplatysmal flaps are developed with blunt dissection techniques to allow adequate mobilization of tissue. *(continued)*

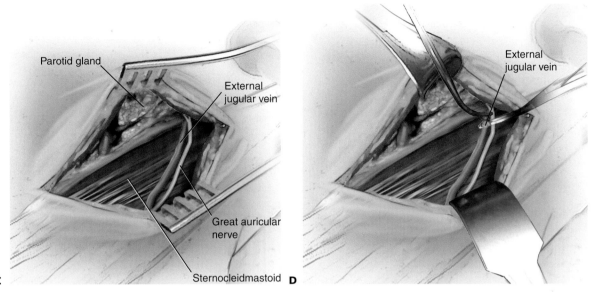

C   **D**

TECH FIG 4 • *(continued)* **C.** The greater auricular nerve is identified and mobilized from the subcutaneous tissues to allow adequate retraction. It is sometimes necessary to sacrifice the greater auricular nerve. This will result in a small area of insensate skin but otherwise has no functional significance. **D.** The external jugular vein and collaterals are mobilized or ligated as needed. The sternocleidomastoid is mobilized anteriorly with the carotid sheath. For additional exposure the sternocleidomastoid can be taken down from the mastoid prominence by sectioning through the tendinous insertion.

and cephalad to allow adequate retraction (**TECH FIG 4C**).

- It is occasionally necessary to sacrifice the greater auricular nerve; this will leave the patient with a small insensate patch of skin but no long-term functional deficit.
- The external jugular vein is identified and then mobilized or ligated as needed (**TECH FIG 4D**).
- The SCM is mobilized and retracted medially and anteriorly with the carotid sheath.

Mobilization of Sternocleidomastoid

- Depending on the amount of exposure required, the SCM may be detached partially or entirely from its tendinous insertion at the mastoid prominence.
  - Be sure to leave enough tissue cuff to allow reapproximation of the muscle on closure.
- Take care to identify and protect the spinal accessory nerve, which enters the SCM about 3 cm distal to the tip of the mastoid process.
  - For limited exposure, the spinal accessory nerve can be retracted anteromedially with the SCM (**TECH FIG 5**).
  - For more extensive exposure, it can be dissected off the jugular foramen in a cephalad direction and retracted posterolaterally while the SCM is everted.

Deep Dissection

- Lymph nodes found in the field of dissection and around the spinal accessory nerve can be excised.
- The lateral process of C1 is now easily palpable about 1 cm distal to the mastoid process.
- The interval between the jugular vein and the longus capitis muscles is then created, allowing access to the retropharyngeal space.
- The retropharyngeal space can be opened further with blunt dissection techniques employing scissors, Kittners, or fingers.

- A sharp elevator or bipolar electrocautery can then be used to elevate the longus capitis and longus colli muscles from the transverse processes and lateral masses of C1 and C2 (**TECH FIG 6A**).
- Retraction is best accomplished by bending a malleable retractor so that it can be used as a lever against the contralateral transverse process, thus elevating the soft tissues anteriorly and medially (**TECH FIG 6B**).

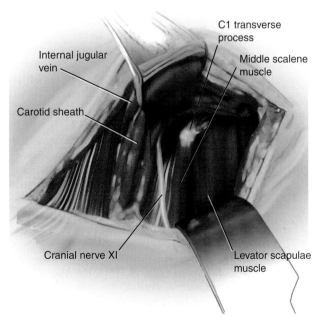

TECH FIG 5 • The spinal accessory nerve is identified as it enters the sternocleidomastoid about 3 cm distal to the tip of the mastoid process and retracted anteriorly with the sternocleidomastoid. The lateral process of C1 will lie essentially in the middle of the field of dissection, about 1 cm distal to the mastoid process.

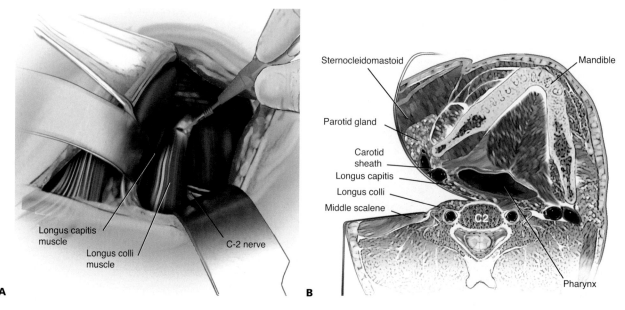

TECH FIG 6 • **A.** Bipolar electrocautery can be used to elevate the longus capitis and longus colli muscles subperiosteally from the transverse processes and lateral masses of C1 and C2. **B.** Plane of dissection for the retropharyngeal approach. For deep retraction, a malleable retractor can be used as a lever against the contralateral transverse process, allowing elevation of the soft tissues anteriorly and medially.

ANTERIOR APPROACH TO THE CERVICOTHORACIC JUNCTION (TRANSMANUBRIAL-TRANSCLAVICULAR APPROACH)

Incision and Superficial Dissection

- A standard Smith-Robinson approach is taken, with the incision extended distally over the manubrium (**TECH FIG 7A**).
- The sternal and clavicular heads of the SCM are released at the tendinous attachments and retracted proximally and laterally. Be sure to leave enough tissue cuff to allow reapproximation of the muscle on closure.
- Likewise, the sternohyoid and sternothyroid are sectioned and retracted proximally and medially (**TECH FIG 7B**).
  - The omohyoid is also generally sectioned for better exposure. It does not need to be repaired.

Mobilization of Clavicle

- The medial third of the clavicle and the left side of the manubrium is then cleared of any remaining soft tissue.
- The clavicle is then divided (typically with a Gigli saw) at the junction of the medial and middle thirds (**TECH FIG 8A**).
  - Care must be taken to avoid injuring the left subclavian vein, which is normally closely apposed to the undersurface of the clavicle.
- At this point, the medial third of the clavicle can be disarticulated from the manubrium (**TECH FIG 8B**).
  - If more exposure is needed, the left side of the manubrium can be removed in a piecemeal fashion by a rongeur.
  - Alternatively, the medial third of the clavicle and a section of the manubrium can be removed together by careful sectioning. This will allow plate or wire reconstruction of the clavicle and manubrium if desired.

- If the manubrium and medial third of the clavicle are removed in this manner, the sternal head of the SCM can be left in continuity with the manubrium and reflected en bloc (**TECH FIG 8C**).

Deep Dissection

- The inferior thyroid vein and artery are often encountered with deeper dissection and may need to be ligated for better exposure.
- Careful blunt dissection proceeds in the same interval as for the standard Smith-Robinson approach (ie, between the carotid sheath laterally and the trachea and esophagus medially).
  - The recurrent laryngeal nerve is almost always found between the esophagus and trachea on the left side of the neck within this plane.
- Blunt retractors are then placed and the carotid sheath, left brachiocephalic artery, and innominate vein are retracted inferolaterally (**TECH FIG 9A**).
- Likewise, a blunt retractor is used to retract the trachea, esophagus, left recurrent laryngeal nerve, and right brachiocephalic vessels inferolaterally to the patient's right.
- The prevertebral fascia is then identified and incised to expose the vertebral bodies. Once adequately dissected, the surgeon can visualize and access as far distally as T3 or T4.
- **TECHNIQUES FIGURE 9B** represents a cross-sectional view at the cervicothoracic junction demonstrating the plane of dissection for the transmanubrial-transclavicular approach.
- At the completion of the procedure, the clavicle is replaced and plated.

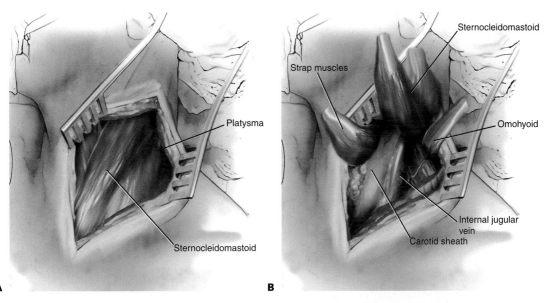

A   **B**

TECH FIG 7 • A. The incision for a low Smith-Robinson approach can be extended along the anterior border of the sternocleidomastoid to the midsagittal plane at roughly the sternal notch and then extended vertically to just beyond the manubrial–sternal junction. **B.** The sternal and clavicular heads of the sternocleidomastoid are released and reflected laterally while the sternohyoid and sternothyroid muscles are sectioned and reflected medially. The omohyoid is usually released during the exposure. It does not need to be repaired.

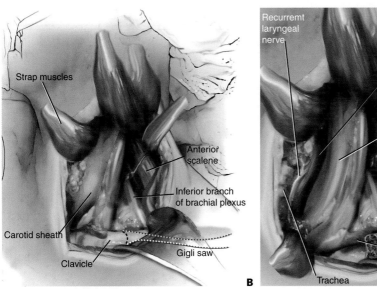

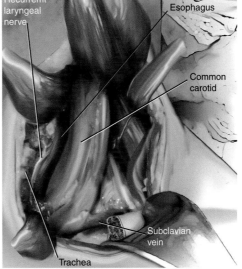

A   **B**

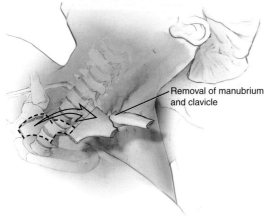

C

TECH FIG 8 • A. The clavicle is divided at the junction of the medial and middle thirds, taking care to avoid injuring the left subclavian vein, which is normally closely apposed to the undersurface of the clavicle. **B.** The medial third of the clavicle can be disarticulated from the manubrium at the manubrioclavicular joint. This will generally provide adequate exposure to the C7-T1 level. **C.** For additional exposure, the left side of the manubrium can be removed piecemeal using a rongeur. A second option involves careful sectioning of the manubrium, which will allow lateral reflection of both the manubrium and medial third of the clavicle without disarticulation of the manubrioclavicular joint.

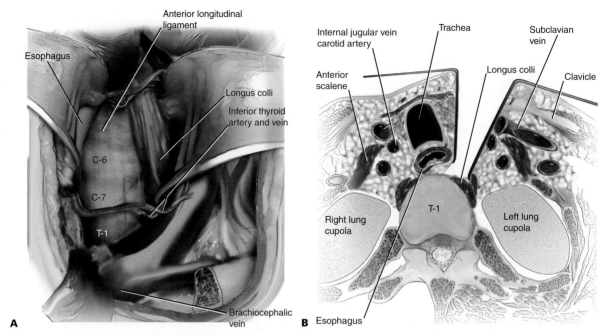

TECH FIG 9 • A. Blunt retractors are used to carefully retract the carotid sheath, left brachiocephalic artery, and innominate vein inferolaterally, while the trachea, esophagus, left recurrent laryngeal nerve, and right brachiocephalic vessels are retracted inferomedially. **B.** Cross-sectional view through the cervicothoracic junction demonstrating the plane of dissection for the transmanubrial-transclavicular approach.

Chapter 44

Posterior Cervical Approach

Raj Rao and Satyajit V. Marawar

ANATOMY

Posterior Cervical Musculature

- The muscles covering the posterior aspect of the cervical spine are arranged in three layers (**FIG 1**).
- Superficial layer: The trapezius muscle originates from the superior nuchal line of the occiput, the ligamentum nuchae, and the spinous processes of the upper thoracic spine. It inserts into the spine of the scapula and the acromion.
- Intermediate layer: The splenius capitis arises from the lower half of the ligamentum nuchae and upper six thoracic vertebrae, inserting onto the mastoid process and the lateral half of the superficial nuchal line under the sternocleidomastoid.
- The deep layer consists of the semispinalis capitis, the semispinalis cervicis, the multifidus, and the rotators, arranged from superficial to deep layers respectively.
  - The semispinalis capitis arises from the transverse processes of the upper six thoracic vertebrae and the articular processes of the midcervical vertebrae and inserts onto the occiput between the superior and inferior nuchal lines.
  - The semispinalis cervicis arises from the transverse processes of the upper six thoracic vertebrae and inserts onto the spinous processes of C2 to C5.
  - The multifidus muscle lies deep to the semispinalis cervicis. It originates from the articular processes of the lower cervical vertebrae and inserts onto the spinous processes of the upper cervical vertebrae.
  - The rotators lie deep to the multifidus. They originate from the transverse process of one vertebra and ascend obliquely to insert on the spinous process of the vertebra one or two levels cranial to their origin.

Suboccipital Musculature

- The rectus capitis posterior minor originates from the posterior tubercle of the atlas and inserts onto the medial half of the inferior nuchal line.
- The rectus capitis posterior major originates from the spinous process of the axis and inserts onto the lateral half of the inferior nuchal line.
- The obliquus capitis superior originates from the transverse process of the atlas and inserts onto the occiput laterally between the superior and inferior nuchal lines.
- The obliquus capitis inferior muscle originates from the spinous process of the axis and inserts onto the transverse process of the atlas.
- The suboccipital triangle lies between the rectus capitis posterior major and the superior and the inferior obliques.
  - The greater occipital nerve is the medial branch of the posterior division of the second cervical nerve at the medial angle of the suboccipital triangle. It runs cephalad between the semispinalis capitis and the obliquus inferior, toward the occiput, where it pierces the semispinalis capitis and the trapezius. It is responsible for cutaneous innervation of the back of the scalp (**FIG 2**).

Osteoligamentous Anatomy

- The external occipital protuberance or inion is an easily palpable bony landmark in the midportion of the occiput. The superior nuchal line extends as a bony ridge on either side of this prominence. A small ridge or crest, called the median nuchal line, descends in the medial plane from the external occipital protuberance to the foramen magnum. The inferior nuchal line runs parallel to the superior nuchal line, midway between the inion and foramen magnum (**FIG 3**).
- The atlas does not have a spinous process but has a posterior tubercle marking the center of the posterior arch.
- The spinous process of the axis is tall, bifid, and broadest in the cervical spine.
- A broad sheet of thick fibrous tissue called the posterior atlanto-occipital membrane extends from the posterior border of the foramen magnum to the superior border of the posterior arch of the atlas.
- The posterior atlantoaxial membrane is a broad, thin membrane extending from the inferior border of the posterior arch of the atlas to the superior border of the lamina of the axis.
- The tectorial membrane is the cranial extension of the posterior longitudinal ligament, running posterior to the transverse ligament to attach onto the anterior border of the foramen magnum.
- The anterior atlantoaxial ligament is the continuation of the anterior longitudinal ligament, extending from the inferior border of the anterior arch of the atlas to the front of the body of the axis (**FIG 4**).
- The pars interarticularis or isthmus of C2 is the waist of the posterior arch of C2, connecting the superior and inferior articular processes. The medial margin of the pars interarticularis along the superior border of the C2 lamina is a guide to the medial margin of the C2 pedicle.
- The C1–2 facet joint is oriented largely in the axial plane, while the C2–3 and remaining subaxial cervical facet joints are coronally oriented 45 degrees to the plane of the spine.
- The spinous processes from C3 to C6 are small and bifid. The C7 spinous process tends to be straight and long and terminates in a single tubercle. It is usually the longest of the cervical spinous processes.
- The lateral mass of the cervical spine refers to the lateral column of each vertebral body that includes the superior and inferior articular processes and the transverse foramen on either side.
  - It offers a secure fixation anchor for screw insertion from C3 to C6, particularly when the spinous process and lamina are fractured or removed.
  - A faint longitudinal groove marks the separation between the laminae and lateral masses.
  - The exiting nerve root and posterior portion of the transverse process lie anterior to the lateral mass.
  - The anteroposterior depth of the lateral mass reduces gradually from C3 (about 8.9 mm) to C7 (about 6.4 mm).[3]

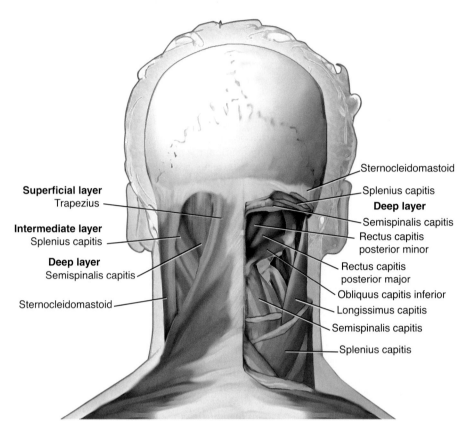

Superficial layer
Trapezius

Intermediate layer
Splenius capitis

Deep layer
Semispinalis capitis

Sternocleidomastoid

Sternocleidomastoid
Splenius capitis
Deep layer
Semispinalis capitis
Rectus capitis posterior minor
Rectus capitis posterior major
Obliquus capitis inferior
Longissimus capitis
Semispinalis capitis
Splenius capitis

FIG 1 • Superficial, intermediate, and deep layers of the posterior cervical musculature are shown on the left. The suboccipital muscles lie deep to these muscles and are shown on the right.

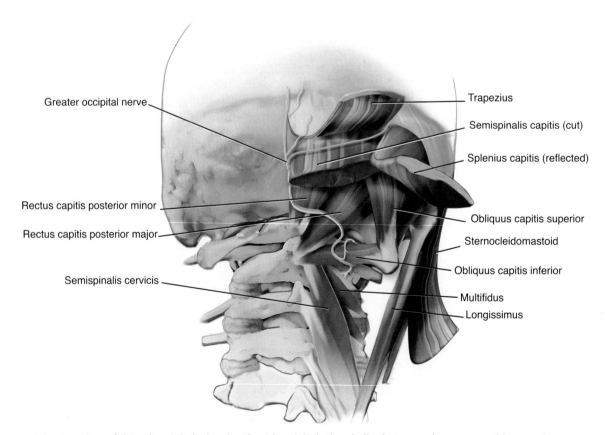

Greater occipital nerve

Rectus capitis posterior minor

Rectus capitis posterior major

Semispinalis cervicis

Trapezius
Semispinalis capitis (cut)
Splenius capitis (reflected)
Obliquus capitis superior
Sternocleidomastoid
Obliquus capitis inferior
Multifidus
Longissimus

FIG 2 • Anatomy of the suboccipital triangle. The suboccipital triangle lies between the rectus capitis posterior major, the obliquus superior, and the obliquus inferior. The greater occipital nerve is seen crossing the suboccipital triangle along its medial angle. The posterior arch of the atlas with the vertebral artery is seen in the floor of the suboccipital triangle.

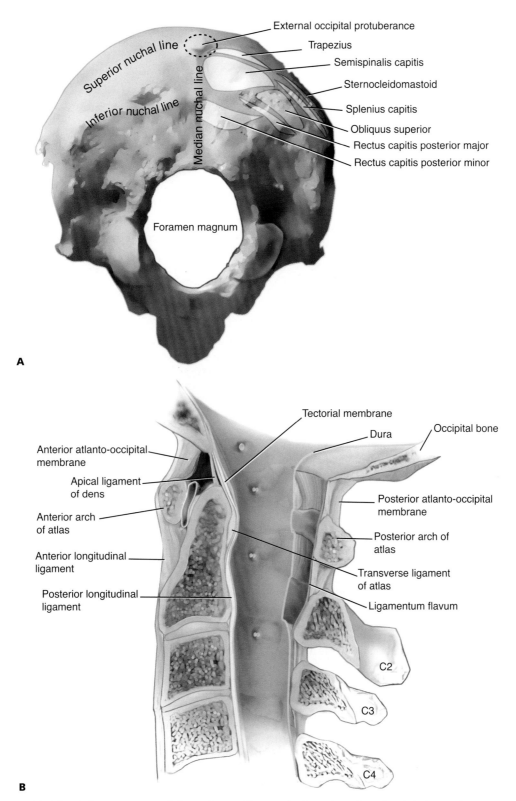

FIG 3 • A. Bony anatomy of the occiput with muscular insertions. Superior, inferior, and median nuchal lines are the prominent bony ridges on the posterior occipital surface. The major posterior cervical muscles and muscles of the suboccipital triangle insert on these bony ridges and on the posterior occipital surface between these ridges. **B.** Sagittal cross-section showing the ligamentous architecture of the proximal cervical spine. Anterior and posterior atlanto-occipital as well as atlantoaxial ligaments and the ligaments stabilizing the odontoid process are depicted: the apical ligament of the dens and the transverse ligament of the atlas.

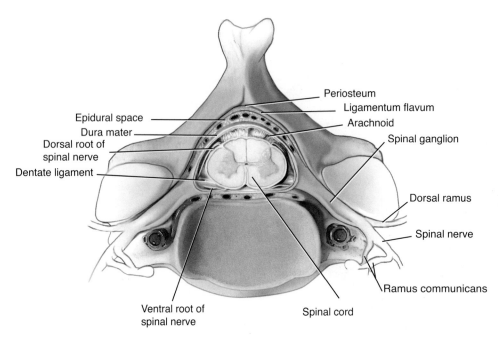

FIG 4 • Axial section showing nerve root anatomy. The spinal rootlets join to form the ventral and the dorsal roots of the spinal nerve. The dorsal root ganglion is seen as the enlargement of the dorsal root lying between the facet joint and the vertebral artery. The roots merge outside the intervertebral foramen to form the spinal nerve.

- The lateral mass of C7 is elongated superoinferiorly but is thinner in the anterior posterior plane than the other cervical vertebrae.
- The pedicles of the cervical vertebrae are smaller than those in the lumbar spine. The dimensions are generally appropriate for pedicle screw insertion at C2 and C7.
  - Computed tomography should be obtained in all patients before screw fixation to verify pedicle width and morphology, particularly between C3 and C6.

Nerve Root Anatomy

- The dorsal and ventral nerve roots formed from the respective rootlets enter a common sleeve of the arachnoid and dura mater.
- The nerve root runs 45 degrees anterolaterally and 10 degrees inferiorly to enter the intervertebral foramen by passing over the top of the corresponding pedicle.
- The dorsal nerve root lies anterior to the superior articular process, positioned at the tip of the superior articular facet medially and then coursing inferiorly to lie on top of the pedicle laterally.
- The ventral root lies anteroinferiorly adjacent to the uncovertebral joint.
- The cervical nerve roots occupy the lower third of the intervertebral foramen, while the upper two thirds of the foramen is filled with fat.
- In the lateral part of the intervertebral foramen, the dorsal nerve root is enlarged to form the dorsal root ganglion, which lies between the vertebral artery and a groove on the anterolateral aspect of the superior articular process (Fig 4).
- The dorsal and the ventral nerve roots join distal to the dorsal root ganglion outside the intervertebral foramen to form the spinal nerve.

Vertebral Artery

- The vertebral artery is a branch of the first part of the subclavian artery, lying anterior to the transverse process of the seventh cervical vertebra at its origin.
- The vertebral artery courses medially and posteriorly through the subaxial cervical spine within the transverse foramina of the sixth through the first cervical vertebra.

- It is at risk of injury where it lies unprotected between the transverse foramina and during anterior procedures lateral to the disc space, particularly at the upper cervical levels (**FIG 5**).
- Anatomic variations in the course of the vertebral artery are not infrequent. Following its origin off the subclavian artery, the vertebral artery typically enters the C6 transverse foramen. Bruneau et al reported entry into the C3, C4, C5, or C7 transverse foramina in 0.2%, 1.0%, 5.0%, and 0.8% of patients, respectively.[1]
  - A 2% incidence of tortuosity of the vertebral artery has been reported, leading to a potentially dangerous medial course of the vessel within the vertebral body.[1,2]
- More cephalad, after emerging from the transverse foramen of C2, the artery lies lateral to the C1–2 facet joint before it enters the transverse foramen of the atlas.
- The artery exits the transverse foramen of the atlas and continues posteromedially in a groove on the superior surface of the posterior arch of the atlas.
- It enters the foramen magnum by piercing the atlanto-occipital membrane about 10 mm from the midline.[1]
- In approaches to the posterior cervical spine, the vertebral artery is at risk of injury during exposure of the posterior arch of the atlas and in the transverse foramina of C1 and C2 during screw insertion for occipitocervical or atlantoaxial fusion procedures.
  - To protect the vertebral artery during these procedures, dissection should be limited to within 12 mm of the midline on the posterior aspect of C1 and within 8 mm of the midline on the superior surface of the posterior arch of the atlas.[1] Further lateral dissection can be performed on the inferior surface of the C1 arch versus the superior surface because the vertebral artery runs on the superior surface of the C1 arch.
- The width of the lateral mass of the atlas averages 11.6 ± 1.4 mm. The height of the portion of the lateral mass of the atlas inferior to its posterior arch averages 4.1 ± 0.7 mm.[2] The lateral mass of C1 thus can generally safely accommodate a 3.5-mm screw below its attachment to the posterior arch.

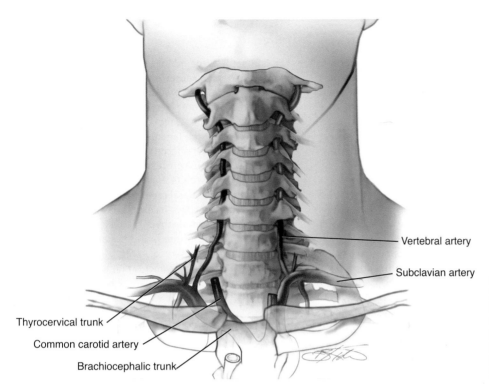

FIG 5 • Origin and course of the vertebral artery. The vertebral artery branches out from the first part of the subclavian artery. It passes through the transverse foramina of the upper six cervical vertebrae and has a significantly tortuous course in the proximal cervical spine.

SURGICAL MANAGEMENT

- Indications
  - Posterior spinal cord decompression via laminoplasty or laminectomy
  - Nerve root decompression via foraminotomy
  - Occipitocervical or atlantoaxial decompression, fusion, and instrumentation
  - Posterior cervical fusion
  - Cervical pedicle or lateral mass instrumentation

Positioning

- The patient's cervical spine should be ranged in flexion and extension in the preoperative area to determine a safe range that does not produce symptoms. Movements of the neck during intubation should be minimized, particularly in myelopathic patients.
- Awake intubation and positioning should be considered in myelopathic patients with markedly reduced canal dimensions.
- In patients undergoing occipitocervical and atlantoaxial procedures, the chin should be tucked to facilitate exposure of the occipitocervical region. For subaxial procedures, slight flexion of the neck reduces overlap of the laminae and facet joints, making deep dissection easier and facilitating decompression of the central and lateral canal. The neck should be brought back into neutral position for fusion or instrumentation procedures.
- Hyperextended or hyperflexed positions under anesthesia, particularly when held for prolonged periods of time, may contribute to spinal cord injury.
- We recommend use of the Mayfield three-point clamp to hold the cranium during posterior occipitocervical and posterior cervical surgery. The clamp is secured to the operating table with an adaptor.
- We infrequently use intraoperative tong traction because we believe the amount of traction transmitted to the operative site is variable.

- The shoulders are pulled down and taped to the distal end of the bed to facilitate intraoperative radiographic visualization (**FIG 6**). Excessive traction on the shoulders should be avoided to minimize the risk of brachial plexus injury.
- The reverse Trendelenburg position reduces epidural venous congestion and intraoperative bleeding. We avoid the sitting position to minimize the risk of intraoperative air embolism.
- Bony prominences and peripheral nerves in the upper and lower extremities should be well padded to protect against intraoperative decubiti or neurapraxia.
- Allowing the abdomen to hang free facilitates venous return to the heart, maintains cardiac output, and decreases the required peak inspiratory pressure.
- Radiographs are obtained after positioning to verify cervical alignment. Placement of a radiopaque marker before obtaining these radiographs facilitates planning of the incision.

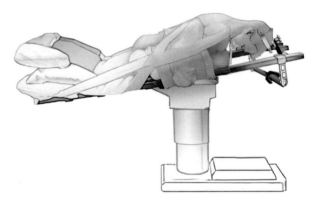

FIG 6 • Positioning of the patient for posterior cervical surgery. In the prone position, the patient's head is stabilized with a Mayfield three-point clamp while traction is applied through the shoulders by taping them down. The patient is in the reverse Trendelenburg position with the abdomen allowed to hang free.

POSTERIOR APPROACH TO SUBAXIAL SPINE

- A midline skin incision is used for most surgical procedures to the subaxial spine. Palpation of the prominent spinous processes of C2 and C7 beneath the skin or the use of intraoperative radiographs can help restrict the incision to the area that requires exposure.
- The incision is deepened through the relatively avascular median raphe, which is a condensation of the deep fascia. This appears as a "white line" in the midline.
- Electrocautery is then used to incise the ligamentum nuchae.
  - Troublesome bleeding from the paraspinal muscles can be minimized by staying within the avascular median raphe.
  - Intermittent palpation of the spinous processes helps the surgeon stay oriented to the midline. The posterior cervical paraspinal musculature generally originates laterally and caudally, passing obliquely cephalad.
  - Reduction of intraoperative bleeding is facilitated by dissecting caudal to cephalad in a subperiosteal fashion.

- For laminoplasty or multilevel laminectomy, the interspinous tissues are cauterized to minimize bleeding and then stripped off the spinous processes.
  - Deep retractors are inserted beneath the fascial layers directly on bone. Deep dissection is carried further laterally along the laminae.
- Localization of level is facilitated by identifying the large C2 and C7 spinous processes and the bifid spinous processes from C2 to C6.
- An intraoperative lateral radiograph should be obtained to confirm the operative levels.
- If facet fusion is not planned, the dissection should stop at the medial third of the facet joint and the facet joint capsule should be preserved.
  - If facet fusion or instrumentation is required, the dissection is extended to the lateral border of the lateral mass.

POSTERIOR APPROACH TO OCCIPITOCERVICAL REGION

- The external occipital protuberance and the prominent bifid C2 spinous process can be palpated in most patients beneath the skin. A midline skin incision is made extending from just above the occipital protuberance to the cervical level required.
- The incision on the scalp is deepened down to bone, and the occiput is exposed in subperiosteal fashion from the inion down to the foramen magnum.
  - The dissection is carried laterally for a distance of 2.5 cm on either side of the median occipital crest. Excessive lateral dissection or retraction can injure the greater occipital nerve.
- The incision is extended caudally through the ligamentum nuchae in the midline. Staying in the midline reduces blood loss.
  - Self-retaining retractors are applied at both ends of the incision.
- The large bifid spinous process of C2 is easily identified. It is exposed subperiosteally by dissecting the attachments of the rectus capitis posterior major and obliquus capitis inferior from these structures.
  - The greater occipital nerve exits posteriorly along the inferior border of the obliquus capitis inferior muscle and can be preserved by keeping the dissection on the C2 posterior arch.
  - Preserving the soft tissue attachments to the distal and lateral aspects of C2 and the C2–facet joint helps maintain subaxial stability postoperatively.
- The C1 ring lies deep in the space between the occiput and C2. The posterior arch of C1 has no muscular attachments.

- Soft tissue from the posterior arch of C1 is dissected subperiosteally, taking care to stay within 12 mm of the midline on the posterior aspect of the posterior ring of C1 and within 8 mm of the midline on the superior aspect of the posterior ring of C1 to avoid vertebral artery injury (**TECH FIG 1**).

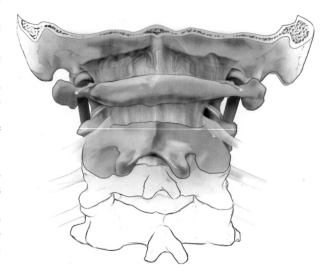

TECH FIG 1 • The vertebral artery emerges from the transverse foramen of the atlas and courses medially in the groove on the superior surface of the posterior arch of the atlas. At the medial end of the groove it turns anteriorly and pierces the atlanto-occipital membrane about 10 mm from the midline.

EXPOSURE OF C1–2 FACET JOINT

- Exposure of the articulation between the lateral mass of C1 and the superior articular process of C2 is occasionally required for screw fixation of the lateral mass of C1 and fusion of this joint.
- After dissection and retraction of the muscles off the posterior aspects of C1 and C2 of the upper cervical spine, the lamina of C2 is identified.
- Soft tissue is carefully dissected off the lamina of C2 using a Freer elevator or dissector.
- Tracing the lamina of C2 proximally exposes the pars interarticularis of C2 and the superior medial corner of the C2 pedicle.

- Exposure of the C1 lateral mass can be obtained by following the inferior arch of C1 laterally until the lateral border of the spinal canal is identified by visualizing its corresponding location on C2.
  - From this point on C1, ventral dissection with a Penfield or Freer will allow palpation of the C1 lateral mass. The greater occipital nerve is encountered and swept distally. A large venous plexus is present and must be controlled with Gelfoam and bipolar cautery.

PEARLS AND PITFALLS

Posterior vertebral arch fragments	▪ Unstable or fractured fragments should be stabilized with a clamp during dissection to avoid inadvertent contusion of the spinal cord.
Stenotic canal	▪ Excessive manipulation of the posterior elements in a patient with a stenotic canal should be avoided as it may inadvertently result in spinal cord injury.
Excessive bleeding	▪ Venous bleeding from epidural veins can occasionally be profuse. The patient should be positioned in reverse Trendelenburg position to decrease the blood loss. Hemostatic agents and bipolar cautery are used to control bleeding from these veins.
Vertebral artery	▪ The vertebral artery is endangered at lower cervical levels (C3 to C6) only if the transverse processes at these levels are destroyed by tumor or infection.
Spina bifida	▪ Cervical spina bifida is a rare condition that can lead to cord damage during dissection if not recognized.

REFERENCES

1. Bruneau M, Cornelius JF, Marneffe V, et al. Anatomical variations of the V2 segment of the vertebral artery. Neurosurgery 2006;59:20–24.
2. Curylo LJ, Mason HC, Bohlman HH, et al. Tortuous course of the vertebral artery and anterior cervical decompression: a cadaveric and clinical case study. Spine 2000;25:2860–2864.
3. Ebraheim NA, An HS, Xu R, et al. The quantitative anatomy of the cervical nerve root groove and the intervertebral foramen. Spine 1996;21:1619–1623.
4. Ebraheim NA, Xu R, Ahmad M, et al. The quantitative anatomy of the vertebral artery groove of the atlas and its relation to the posterior atlantoaxial approach. Spine 1998;23:320–323.
5. Hong X, Dong Y, Yunbing C, et al. Posterior screw placement on the lateral mass of atlas: an anatomic study. Spine 2004;29:500–503.

Chapter 45

Anterior Thoracic Approach

Morgan N. Chen, Sheeraz A. Qureshi, and Andrew Hecht

DEFINITION

■ The anterior approach can be used to access the thoracic spine for decompression, deformity correction, and stabilization. This approach allows for access to treat conditions such as intervertebral disc herniation, infection, tumor, and trauma.

ANATOMY

■ The thoracic spinal cord may have a tenuous blood supply, particularly in patients with congenital anomalies and kyphosis.
■ The midthoracic cord represents a watershed zone for vascularity. The artery of Adamkiewicz supplies the thoracic cord but can have a variable origin. Its origin is usually (80%) from the left side at the T10 level but can vary from T5 to L5.[1]

SURGICAL MANAGEMENT

Preoperative Planning

■ Radiographs of the thoracic spine and chest should be obtained to determine the level of surgery and help in "rib counting."
  ■ It is often helpful to obtain lumbar radiographs also to determine the number of lumbar segments below the most distal thoracic rib. Knowing this information preoperatively helps in counting "up" from the sacrum intraoperatively if needed.
  ■ In the absence of obvious bony pathology such as fractures, infections, or tumors, it is very easy to inadvertently localize the wrong level in the thoracic spine. The surgeon should be sure to have a strategy for intraoperative level identification based on careful scrutiny of radiographs and MRI or CT scans before surgery, understanding that the quality of portable films obtained intraoperatively may not be optimal.
  ■ When obtaining an MRI to better understand the nature of the pathology in relation to the thoracic spinal cord, the surgeon should ask for a topogram to be performed so that there is no question as to the level or levels of involvement.
  ■ On CT scan or MRI, the surgeon should pay close attention to the position of the aorta and inferior vena cava, especially on the axial cuts, as this may affect the side from which the spine is approached, especially if a corpectomy will be performed.
■ Anesthesia considerations include the use of an oral gastric tube and double-lumen endotracheal tube, which allows for collapse of the ipsilateral lung.
  ■ If the surgical site is T10 or distal, selective deflation of the ipsilateral lung is usually not necessary.
  ■ If the surgical site is proximal to T10, selective deflation is helpful in keeping the lung out of the field, but it may lead to more postoperative issues with atelectasis.
■ Neurologic monitoring is frequently used when performing thoracic operations.

Positioning

■ The patient should be in the lateral decubitus position with the arms in prayer position.
■ The thorax vertex should be positioned over the break of the bed, all pressure points should be padded, pillows should be placed between legs and arms, and an axillary roll should be used to prevent compression of the axillary vessels (**FIG 1**).
■ The operating surgeon typically stands behind the patient during the exposure. However, it may be helpful to stand in front of the patient when performing the decompression, as the line of sight into the spinal canal is better from that vantage point.

Approach (Right Versus Left)

■ Considerations for thoracic approaches include:
  ■ Approach from the side of herniation in cases of posterolateral or lateral herniation.
  ■ Look at the axial CT or MRI scans to determine the location of the heart and great vessels. In most thoracic cases, these structures are either on the left or central. Thus, all other factors being equal, a right-sided approach is favored in most cases.
  ■ In the distal thoracic spine (eg, T10–12), the liver may be in the way of a right-sided approach. Because it is a bit more difficult to retract the liver than the kidney or spleen, a left-sided approach may be favorable.
■ Considerations for thoracolumbar approaches include:
  ■ The left-sided approach is generally favored, as it is easier to mobilize the great arteries (aorta, iliacs) from their left-central position to the right, rather than mobilizing the great veins (which tend to be further to the right) toward the left.

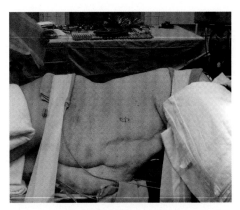

FIG 1 • Patient placed in the lateral decubitus position. It is important to ensure that all bony prominences are well padded.

ANTERIOR THORACIC APPROACH FROM T1 TO T4

- For upper thoracic exposures a right-sided approach is preferred to avoid the heart.
- The surgeon makes a curved skin incision below the tip of the scapula (**TECH FIG 1A**).
- This incision is carried down to the latissimus dorsi muscle and then the latissimus is incised, leaving a cuff of the muscle on the scapula for later closure (**TECH FIG 1B**).
- A large retractor (ie, Richardson retractor) can then be held by the assistant while the surgeon incises the periosteum over the appropriate rib and then resects the rib as far anteriorly and posteriorly as possible (**TECH FIG 1C**).

- At this point, the chest is entered through the rib bed and a Finochietto or Omni retractor can be placed, with one of the blades holding the scapula up and out of the way.
  - Now the lung can be deflated and retracted anteriorly and inferiorly (**TECH FIG 1D**).
- The pleura overlying the spine is now sharply incised. Placing suture into the edges of the pleura makes subsequent closure easier.
- Segmental vessels are identified and ligated as needed and the vertebral bodies (the "valleys") and disc spaces (the "hills") are identified.

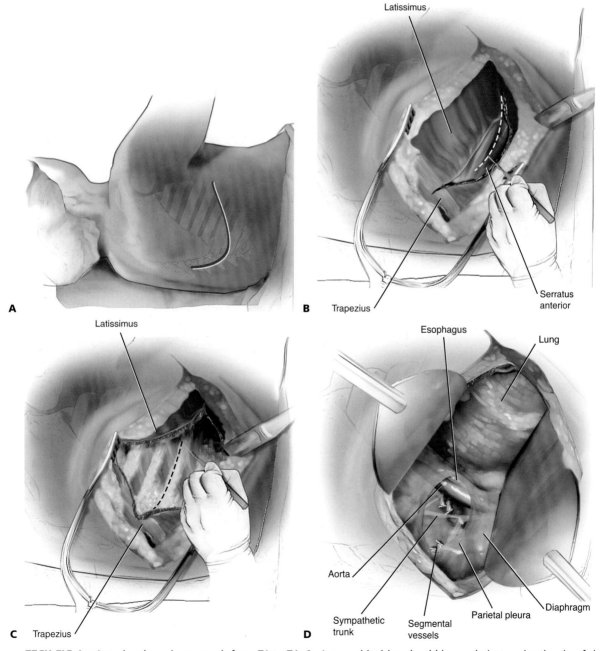

TECH FIG 1 • Anterior thoracic approach from T1 to T4. **A.** A curved incision should be made just under the tip of the scapula. **B.** The incision is carried down to the latissimus dorsi. A cuff of muscle is left attached to the scapula for repair upon closure. **C.** The surgeon incises the periosteum over the rib. **D.** The deflated lung is retracted anteriorly and inferiorly while protecting the esophagus and great vessels.

TECHNIQUES

ANTERIOR THORACIC APPROACH FROM T5 TO T12

- The surgeon should plan the incision directly over the desired rib (ie, 10th rib for T9-10 disc). A curvilinear skin incision is made along the path of the rib from the anterior border of the latissimus dorsi to the costochondral junction anteriorly (TECH FIG 2A).
  - Due to the downslope of the ribs, it is generally preferable to make an incision that is more proximal rather than distal. If the incision is too distal, the ribs may impede access to the more proximal segment, necessitating a second thoracotomy. In contrast, it is easier to access levels that are distal to the rib that is resected. Thus, if in doubt as to the exact rib to be resected, the incision should be made more proximal.
- Skin and subcutaneous fat are incised to expose the trapezius and latissimus dorsi.
- The trapezius and latissimus dorsi are divided in line with the incision using electrocautery. The rhomboids may need to be split to gain more exposure cephalad.

- Once the correct rib is identified, the surgeon divides the periosteum over the upper border of the rib to avoid injury to the intercostal nerve and vessels (TECH FIG 2B).
- The rib is stripped subperiosteally anteriorly to the costochondral angle and as far posteriorly as possible (TECH FIG 2C).
- The rib is removed with a rib cutter and passed off the field. The rib is cut at the midaxillary line anteriorly and as far posteriorly as possible. The rib can be used as a strut graft or autologous bone graft.
- The periosteal rib sleeve and parietal pleura are incised to enter the thorax. A rib spreader is placed to hold the ribs apart (TECH FIG 2D).
- The ipsilateral lung is deflated and retracted medially to expose the parietal pleura overlying the spine.
- The parietal pleura overlying the spine is incised and retracted medially. Stitches can be placed in the parietal

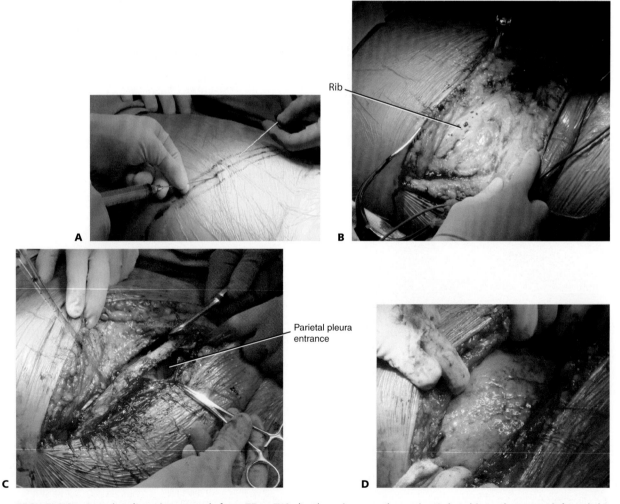

Rib

Parietal pleura entrance

TECH FIG 2 • Anterior thoracic approach from T5 to T12. (In these images, the patient's head is to the upper left and the patient's back is toward the surgeon.) **A.** The incision in planned directly over the rib. Injecting the subcutaneous tissues with a combination of anesthetic and epinephrine aids in hemostasis. **B.** The skin and subcutaneous tissues have been divided, exposing the desired rib. **C.** Subperiosteal exposure of the rib before excision. Note the thin parietal pleura beneath the rib bed. **D.** After excision of the rib the parietal pleura is entered, exposing the ipsilateral lung. *(continued)*

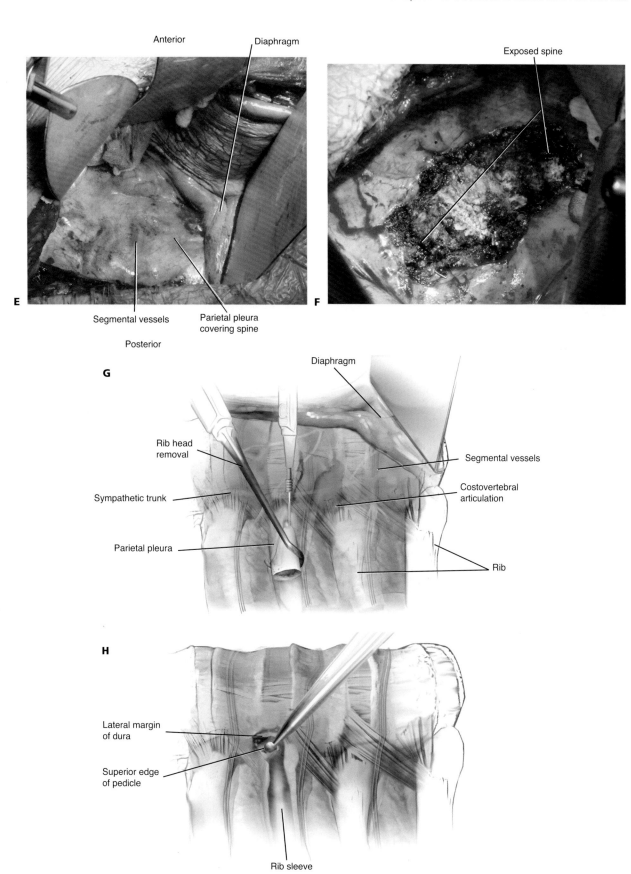

Anterior

Diaphragm

E

Segmental vessels

Parietal pleura
covering spine

Posterior

Exposed spine

F

G

Diaphragm

Rib head
removal

Segmental vessels

Costovertebral
articulation

Sympathetic trunk

Parietal pleura

Rib

H

Lateral margin
of dura

Superior edge
of pedicle

Rib sleeve

TECH FIG 2 • *(continued)* **E.** The parietal pleura and the underlying segmental vessels. **F.** The vertebral bodies and intervertebral discs are exposed after segmental arteries are ligated and the overlying soft tissues are removed. Once the costotransverse and costovertebral articulations are excised (**G**), the rib head can be removed with a high-speed burr (**H**).

pleura to make closure easier. The underlying segmental vessels are visualized (**TECH FIG 2E**).

- The segmental arteries arising from the aorta can run in an ascending, recurrent, horizontal, or descending direction depending on the level of involvement.
- The surgeon carefully ligates as few segmental vessels as possible to gain adequate exposure to the spine. Ligating more segmental vessels than necessary places the spinal cord at increased risk for ischemia because the thoracic spinal cord has a tenuous blood supply (**TECH FIG 2F**).
  - In cases of suspected vascular anomalies, such as congenital kyphosis, the surgeon should consider temporary occlusion of the segmental vessels and check evoked potentials before vessel ligation. If a patient has had a prior spine exposure on one side, the surgeon should be wary of ligating the contralateral segmental vessels. Instead, the surgery should be performed through the previously exposed side, or a preoperative angiogram should be obtained to identify the important arterial feeders to the spinal cord.
- The intrathoracic vertebral bodies and intervertebral discs are now exposed. To gain access to the posterior intervertebral disc, the rib head may need to be removed.
- The costotransverse and costovertebral articulations are removed to excise the rib head (**TECH FIG 2G**).
- The soft tissues overlying the transverse process, pedicle, and vertebral body are removed.
- The superior edge of the pedicle is identified and followed back to the intervertebral space.
- The superior edge of pedicle is burred to expose the posterior intervertebral disc and lateral margin of the dura (**TECH FIG 2H**).

Detaching the Diaphragm

- Exposure of T12-L1 may require detaching the diaphragm.
  - The diaphragm inserts and originates from the xiphoid and the inferior six ribs.
  - The lateral arcuate ligament arises from the transverse process of L1.
  - The crura extend more distally on the right.
  - The diaphragm is innervated centrally by the phrenic nerves.

- The surgeon starts at the costal angle and incises the costodiaphragmatic reflection until extraperitoneal fat is visualized.
- The diaphragm is divided off the anterior chest wall (**TECH FIG 3**). The surgeon should leave a 1- to 2-cm cuff of diaphragm on the anterior chest wall to allow for diaphragm repair at closure. To avoid diaphragm denervation, the diaphragm should be incised only at its periphery. The diaphragm is split up to the lateral arcuate ligament.
- The medial and lateral crura are detached, exposing the underlying peritoneum.
- The peritoneum is swept medially until the retroperitoneal space is visualized.
- The surgeon bluntly dissects and sweeps the fascia of Gerota medially to expose the spine and the overlying parietal pleura.
- The aorta and vena cava are identified.
- The surgeon can elevate the psoas muscle if needed.
- The parietal pleura is incised to expose the spine.

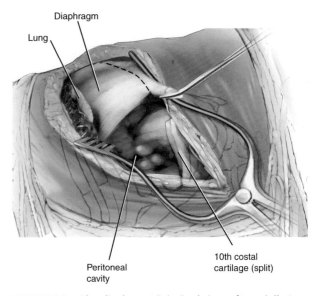

TECH FIG 3 • The diaphragm is incised circumferentially 2 cm from its peripheral attachment to the chest wall. Marker stitches should be placed for resuturing upon closure.

THORACOABDOMINAL RETROPERITONEAL LUMBAR SPINE APPROACH FROM T10 TO L3

- The patient is positioned in the lateral decubitus position with the right side down. The approach should be made from the left side to avoid the liver and inferior vena cava.
- The crura of the diaphragm are detached as described above.
- An oblique incision is made from the quadratus lumborum to the lateral border of the rectus abdominis (**TECH FIG 4**).
  - This approach can be extended to L5 in most patients and even to S1 in those with low-riding iliac crests.
- The subcutaneous tissue is incised and the fascia of the external oblique is divided.
- The external and internal obliques, transverse abdominis, and transversalis fascia are incised.

- The peritoneum is exposed and bluntly reflected anteriorly.
- The ureter is identified and reflected anteriorly with retroperitoneal fat.
- The vertebral bodies, psoas, and great vessels are identified.
- The genitofemoral nerve lies on anterior psoas muscle, and excessive traction should be avoided.
- The segmental vessels that lie over the middle of the vertebral bodies are identified and ligated.
- The psoas is bluntly dissected off the vertebrae and retracted laterally.
- The vertebral body, pedicle, and neuroforamen can be visualized.

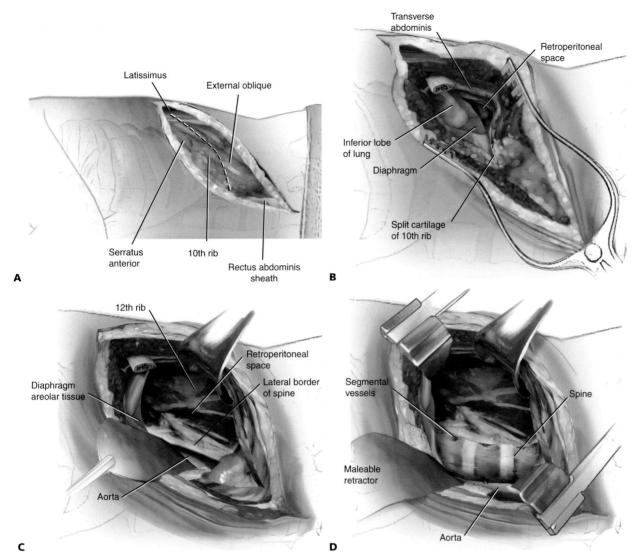

TECH FIG 4 • Thoracoabdominal approach. **A.** A curvilinear incision is made over the 10th rib and the muscle layers are identified. **B.** The retroperitoneal space is entered through the costal cartilage after removing the 10th rib. **C.** The light areolar tissue that signifies the retroperitoneal space is identified, and the peritoneum is mobilized from the undersurface of the diaphragm and abdominal wall as well as the aorta. **D.** Exposure of the spine is done after ligation of segmental vessels.

PEARLS AND PITFALLS

Neurologic compromise	■ The surgeon should consider preoperative angiography before left-sided approaches between T8 and T12 to identify the artery of Adamkiewicz and prevent spinal cord infarction. ■ The surgeon should consider temporarily clamping the segmental arteries before ligation and assessing for changes in evoked potentials to avoid vascular catastrophe, because blood supply to the spinal cord is tenuous in the thoracic region, especially in the "critical zone" from T4 to T9.
Avoiding wrong-level surgery	■ The surgeon should place a hand under the scapula and count rib spaces. The first rib is often difficult to feel, but the second rib space is the largest. ■ Preoperative anteroposterior and lateral chest radiographs can aid in rib counting, especially in kyphotic patients.
Exposure	■ Using a double-lumen endotracheal tube will allow deflation of the ipsilateral lung and improve exposure. ■ Detaching the psoas muscle off the transverse processes can improve exposure of the intervertebral disc space and neuroforamen. The transverse processes can also be removed to further increase exposure. ■ Flexing the patient's hips can decrease tension on the psoas and improve visualization of the lumbar spine. ■ More ribs may need to be excised to gain better exposure, especially in older patients, in whom the ribs may not be as compliant to the rib spreader. ■ From T2 to T5 it may help to detach the serratus anterior muscle from the anterior chest wall and reflect it cephalad to gain better exposure. The surgeon should avoid cutting the long thoracic nerve at this level. ■ If scapular manipulation is needed to gain better exposure, the rhomboids, trapezius, and dorsal scapular muscles can be divided, allowing the scapula to be mobilized laterally.
Visceral injury	■ When approaching from the right side, the surgeon should dissect the soft tissues away from the spine as close as possible to the bone with a blunt gauze or finger to prevent injury to the cisterna chyli and thoracic duct.

POSTOPERATIVE CARE

▪ Chest tubes are left in place until output is less than 150 mL over 24 hours.

COMPLICATIONS

▪ The exiting nerve root can be injured while removing the pedicle.
▪ Vascular injury
▪ Intercostal neuralgia
▪ Atelectasis
▪ Neurologic injury
▪ Wrong-level surgery
▪ Significant bleeding can be encountered when entering the epidural space.
▪ Visceral injury

REFERENCE

1. Grace RR, Mattox KL. Anterior spinal artery syndrome following abdominal aortic aneurysmectomy: case report and review of the literature. Arch Surg 1977;112:813–815.

P. Justin Tortolani, Samer Saiedy, and Ira L. Fedder

DEFINITION

▪ The anterior lumbar approach provides excellent access to the lumbar spine extending from the L2–3 disc to first segment of the sacrum (S1).

ANATOMY

▪ The anterior abdominal wall has a layered configuration that changes depending on whether the approach is proximal or distal to the arcuate line.
▪ Above the arcuate line, the layers in order are skin, subcutaneous fat (containing fascia of Camper and Scarpa), anterior rectus sheath (aponeurosis of the external and internal oblique muscles), rectus muscle, posterior rectus sheath (aponeurosis of the internal oblique and transversus abdominis muscles), transversalis fascia, and peritoneum (**FIG 1**).
▪ Below the arcuate line, the posterior rectus sheath is not present, and thus the rectus muscle lies directly on the transversalis fascia.
▪ For retroperitoneal exposures, the approach goes through the abdominal wall to the layer of the transversalis fascia and then progresses laterally until this fascia ends, exposing the retroperitoneal fat.
▪ For transperitoneal exposures, the transversalis fascia is divided in the midline, as is the peritoneum, and the exposure proceeds directly posteriorly to the level of the sacral prominence.
▪ The abdominal contents are retracted to expose the great vessels overlying the anterior lumbar spine.
▪ Key anatomic structures with relationship to the spine are shown in **FIGURE 2**.
▪ Vascular
  ▪ The abdominal aorta and the bifurcation into the left and right common iliac arteries lies anterior to the venous system, and the left iliac artery is typically encountered first (L4–5). In most people, the bifurcation occurs at L4–5.
    ▪ Preoperative scrutiny of MRI or CT scans can help identify the location of the bifurcation, which can be important in planning.
  ▪ The left renal artery and vein (L2) restrict exposure proximal to L2.
  ▪ The inferior vena cava (IVC) lies posterior and to the right of the aorta. Because of this deep, right-sided position, the IVC should not be mobilized to the left.
  ▪ The L5–S1 disc occupies a position between the bifurcation of the aorta and the IVC in most patients, so mobilization of the large vessels is rarely required for access. The middle sacral artery and vein branch off the left common iliac and should be ligated or cauterized if small.
  ▪ Exposures above L5–S1, however, require mobilization of the great vessels to the right. To do this, the iliolumbar vein, which branches off the left common iliac, must be identified and ligated (see Techniques section).

▪ Genitourinary
  ▪ Left kidney: rarely visualized, surrounded by perinephric fat (L1–2)
  ▪ Left ureter: easily retracted anteriorly with peritoneal contents and can be identified by stimulated peristalsis
▪ Muscular
  ▪ Psoas (paraspinal, L1–L5)
▪ Neurologic
  ▪ Sympathetic chain (paraspinal, anterior and medial to psoas)
  ▪ Presacral plexus (directly over sacrum)
  ▪ Lumbosacral plexus (posteromedial to and within psoas muscle)
  ▪ Genitofemoral nerve (lies on anterior aspect of psoas)
▪ Lymphatic
  ▪ Paraspinal lymphatics and lymph nodes
  ▪ Lymphatic drainage will appear as a milky white fluid, which is rarely of clinical consequence.

PATIENT HISTORY AND PHYSICAL FINDINGS

▪ Previous abdominal surgery (eg, hysterectomy, hernia repair) can create challenges during this exposure. The presence of midline abdominal mesh, cellulitis or abscess, and a colostomy are relative contraindications to the anterior approach.
▪ Previous exposure of the anterior lumbar spine, particularly if it involved mobilization of the great veins, makes revision approaches much more risky due to the greater likelihood of vascular injury.
▪ Obesity (body mass index above 40) is a relative contraindication to anterior exposure of the lumbar spine due to the depth of the operative field.

IMAGING AND OTHER DIAGNOSTIC STUDIES

▪ Plain radiographs are used to assess the degree of aortic calcification and lumbopelvic deformity.
▪ Preoperative axial MRI or CT allows for estimation of the level of the bifurcation of the aorta and IVC (**FIG 3**).
▪ Routine angiography, CT-angiography, or MR-angiography is not necessary unless there is a concern for aberrant anatomy (eg, history of situs inversus).
▪ Preoperative arteriograms, venograms, and prophylactic IVC filters should be considered before any revision approaches to the anterior lumbar spine. Preoperative ureteral stents can also help prevent ureteral injury during revision exposure.

SURGICAL MANAGEMENT

▪ Indications for the anterior lumbar approach are as follows:
  ▪ Anterior discectomy for interbody fusion, total disc replacement, disc débridement in cases of discitis and vertebral osteomyelitis, radical discectomy for deformity correction

411

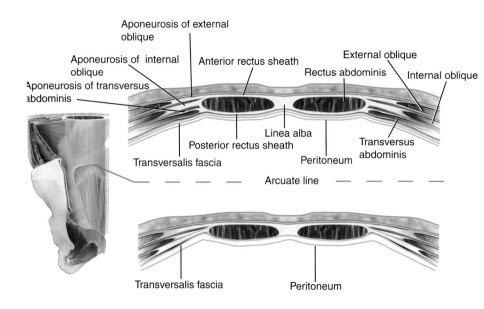

Aponeurosis of external oblique

Aponeurosis of internal oblique

Aponeurosis of transversus abdominis

Anterior rectus sheath

Rectus abdominis

External oblique

Internal oblique

Transversalis fascia

Posterior rectus sheath

Linea alba

Peritoneum

Transversus abdominis

Arcuate line

Transversalis fascia

Peritoneum

FIG 1 • Above (proximal to) the arcuate line, the posterior rectus sheath is present and contains fibers from the internal oblique and transversus abdominis aponeuroses. Below (distal to) the arcuate line, the posterior rectus sheath is no longer present. Exposures to the L4–5 disc space generally require identification and incision of the posterior rectus sheath.

- Anterior corpectomy for tumor resection, radical deformity correction, and vertebral body osteomyelitis

Preoperative Planning

- When exposure of the L5–S1 disc is required, the direct anterior lumbar approach should be used in most cases, as the ilium blocks satisfactory access from a lateral approach.
- The direct anterior approach is less morbid than the lateral approach to the lumbar spine because the latter involves greater division of the abdominal wall musculature.[3]

- For these reasons, we prefer the direct anterior approach (versus the lateral approach) even in cases of multilevel disc exposures (eg, lumbar scoliosis correction) unless the L1–2 disc or L2 vertebra requires exposure, or if anterior instrumentation in the form of screw–rod constructs is needed. Anterior plates can be used from a direct anterior approach at L5–S1 and in some cases L4–5, depending on the vascular anatomy.
- However, greater mobilization of the great vessels at the level of the bifurcation is needed from a direct anterior versus lateral approach. Thus, a lateral approach may provide better

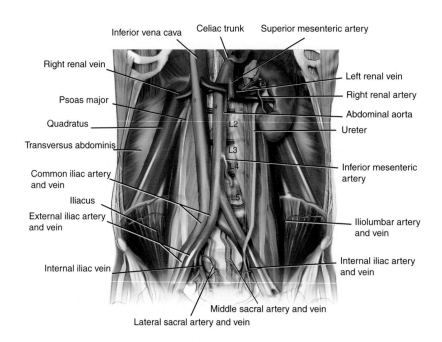

Inferior vena cava

Celiac trunk

Superior mesenteric artery

Right renal vein

Psoas major

Quadratus

Transversus abdominis

Common iliac artery and vein

Iliacus

External iliac artery and vein

Internal iliac vein

Left renal vein

Right renal artery

Abdominal aorta

Ureter

Inferior mesenteric artery

Iliolumbar artery and vein

Internal iliac artery and vein

L2

L3

L4

L5

Middle sacral artery and vein

Lateral sacral artery and vein

FIG 2 • **A.** Vascular and genitourinary anatomy of the retroperitoneal space. **B.** Neurologic, muscular, and lymphatic anatomy of the retroperitoneal space.

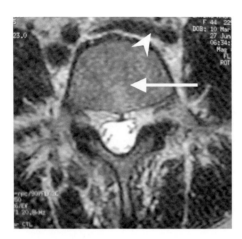

FIG 3 • T2-weighted axial MRI image demonstrates the bifurcation of the inferior vena cava (*arrowhead*). In this case the bifurcation occurs at the level of the L5 vertebra rather than the L4–5 disc space. This configuration may make access easier at the L4–5 disc but harder at the L5–S1 disc, as the left iliac vein may obliquely cross over it (*arrow*).

exposure to the spine if the great vessels are anticipated to be difficult to mobilize.

Positioning

▪ The patient is positioned supine over an inflatable pillow (**FIG 4A**).
▪ The operating room table should allow for free passage of the fluoroscopic C-arm (**FIG 4B**).
▪ Care should be taken to ensure that the pelvis is level so that true anteroposterior and lateral fluoroscopic images can be easily obtained.
▪ The patient's arms can be tucked at the side, placed into a "cross" position, or crossed over the chest but must not restrict appropriate fluoroscopic imaging (**FIG 4C**).

Approach

▪ Various skin incisions can be used.
  ▪ The Pfannenstiel can be used for L5–S1 exposures but is less extensile if additional proximal exposure is necessary.
  ▪ The direct midline and paramedian incisions are useful for multilevel exposures as they are easily extended proximally or distally (**FIG 5A–D**).
▪ Palpation of the sacral promontory allows more accurate placement of the skin incision (**FIG 5E**). Alternatively, a lateral C-arm view can be taken to mark the location of the incision, keeping in mind that the trajectory needed to access the disc, especially at L5–S1, may require that the incision be placed where the path of this trajectory meets the skin rather than directly over the disc space itself.
▪ Retroperitoneal versus transperitoneal
  ▪ The transperitoneal approach carries a higher risk of retrograde ejaculation due to the theoretically greater likelihood of injury to the presacral sympathetic nerve fibers.
  ▪ This approach is useful, however, in revision approaches to L5–S1 in which the retroperitoneal exposure was used at the index procedure.
  ▪ Transperitoneal approaches likely increase the risk of adhesion formation and possible small bowel obstruction. In addition, small or large bowel perforation and postoperative

ileus are relatively more likely when the peritoneum is entered. Finally, extra time and care are required to retract the small intestines; this generally requires more retractors and large sponges to prevent interference during the remainder of the procedure.
▪ Right versus left retroperitoneal
▪ With certain failures of lumbar disc replacement, revision exposures of the lumbar spine are necessary. To preserve the left retroperitoneal exposure for a potential revision exposure, some surgeons advocate performing a right-sided retroperitoneal incision at the index surgery.
  ▪ Because optimal placement of a lumbar disc correlates with improved functional outcomes for the patient, we advocate performing the exposure that provides the ideal set of circumstances for accurate device placement at the outset.[5]
  ▪ Because the right common iliac artery and vein lie more vertical, crossing the L5–S1 disc space, whereas the left common iliac artery and vein traverse the disc diagonally, access to L5–S1 is easier and provides a more expansive exposure when performed from the left retroperitoneal approach.

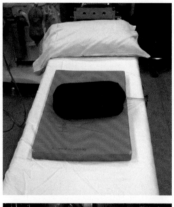
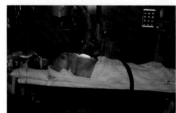
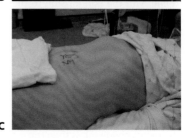

FIG 4 • **A.** An inflatable pillow can be modulated during the case to allow increased or decreased lordosis. The pillow is placed over a thick foam pad (blue), which allows the patient's arms to be tucked along the side and thus out of the lateral fluoroscopic image beam. **B.** The operating room table is radiolucent and open underneath, allowing the fluoroscopic C-arm (in the distance) to pass under the table. **C.** The patient's arms are tucked to the side with a draw sheet after padding the elbows.

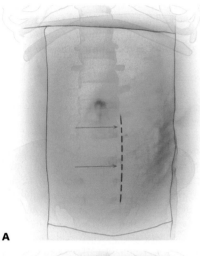

A

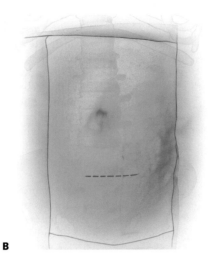

B

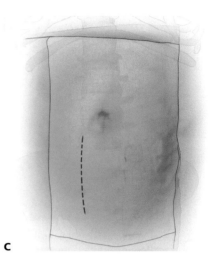

C

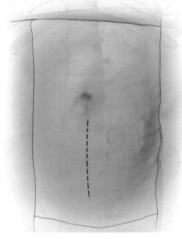

D

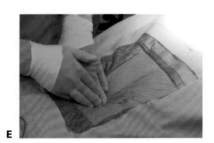

E

FIG 5 • **A.** A left vertical paramedian incision allows excellent exposure of the anterior rectus sheath and not only facilitates closure but also provides easy access to the left retroperitoneal space. The arrows indicate the expected spinal levels (L4–5 *upper arrow*, L5–S1 *lower arrow*). Other skin incision options are Pfannenstiel (**B**), right paramedian (**C**), and midline (**D**). **E.** Palpating the sacral promontory allows the surgeon to tailor the skin incision to the appropriate spinal level.

ANTERIOR EXPOSURE OF LUMBAR SPINE (LEFT PARAMEDIAN INCISION AND RETROPERITONEAL APPROACH)

Dissection

- Once the skin is incised, the subcutaneous fat is divided in line with the skin incision to the level of the anterior rectus sheath.
- The anterior rectus sheath is identified and stripped clean of all fat to assist in identification of the fascial edges at the time of wound closure (**TECH FIG 1A**).
- The anterior rectus sheath is incised in line with the skin incision—centered over the disc of interest—and then retracted laterally, exposing the underlying rectus abdominis muscle (**TECH FIG 1B**).
- The rectus abdominis is then retracted laterally, exposing the underlying transversalis fascia (**TECH FIG 1C**).
- With the rectus abdominis retracted, the transversalis fascia is followed laterally to its insertion on the abdominal wall. A sponge on a stick can be used to gently strip the transversalis fascia off this insertion (**TECH FIG 1D**).
- Handheld retractors are then used to sweep the peritoneum and left ureter to the midline and beyond, to the patient's right.

Further Exposure

- If exposure of L4–5 is required, the arcuate line is identified and a small, 1-inch incision is created to allow more freedom in mobilization of the peritoneum (**TECH FIG 2A,B**).
- For exposure of the L4–5 disc or above, the lateral border of the left common iliac artery and vein are first identified using blunt dissection. These vessels are then retracted toward the midline to expose the iliolumbar veins coursing posteriorly (**TECH FIG 2C**).
  - There is often more than one iliolumbar vein, and retracting the common iliac too forcefully can result in avulsion and significant bleeding that can be difficult to control, especially if the wound is deep or the distal end of the vein retracts behind the psoas after avulsion.
- At L5–S1, blunt dissection with a Kittner exposes the disc space and defines the vascular anatomy. Palpation of the sacral promontory helps guide the blunt dissection.

TECHNIQUES

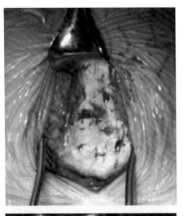

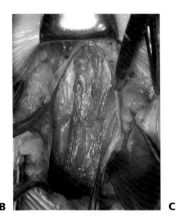

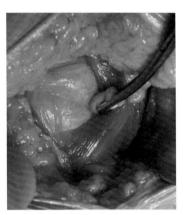

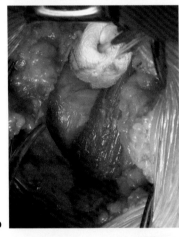

TECH FIG 1 • A. The anterior rectus sheath can be clearly visualized. A small Richardson retractor has been placed at the top of the incision and a cerebellar retractor has been placed inferiorly. The *blue arrow* marks the center of the planned vertical fascial incision. **B.** The vertical fibers of the rectus abdominis muscle are visualized as the anterior rectus sheath is held to the patient's left with two Kocher clamps. **C.** The rectus abdominis muscle is retracted laterally with a Kittner, exposing the underlying transversalis fascia. **D.** A sponge on a stick is used to bluntly dissect the transversalis fascia off the undersurface of the rectus.

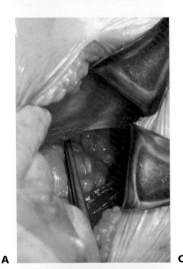

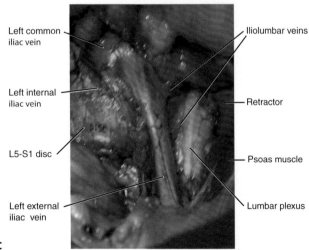

Left common iliac vein

Iliolumbar veins

Left internal iliac vein

Retractor

L5-S1 disc

Psoas muscle

Left external iliac vein

Lumbar plexus

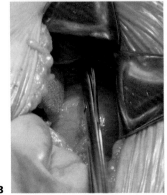

TECH FIG 2 • A. For exposures at L4–5, the posterior rectus sheath (arcuate line) is identified and the peritoneum is retracted away. **B.** Once the arcuate line is identified, it can be cut vertically; this enables the surgeon to safely retract the abdominal contents to the patient's right. **C.** In this cadaveric dissection, the iliolumbar veins can be visualized branching off the left common iliac vein, coursing posteriorly and laterally. By retracting the vein toward the midline and the psoas muscle laterally, the vein takes on a more transverse orientation and is easier to ligate. One of the lumbar nerve roots can be seen directly lateral to the iliolumbar vein. Excessive retraction pressure can injure these nerve roots. The arterial system has been removed.

Retractor Placement

- While a vascular surgeon or assistant retracts the great vessels with handheld retractors, sharp, narrow Hohmann retractors are placed directly into the vertebrae.
  - Alternatively, blunt radiolucent retractors can be used. These retractors can be held by hand, can be fixed with transfixion pins, or can be clipped to an external frame (Omni) or ring (Endo-ring) for the remainder of the procedure.
- The optimal configuration of retractors for L5–S1 and L4–5 exposures is depicted in **TECHNIQUES FIGURE 3A,B.**
  - At L5–S1, placing a malleable retractor against the sacrum keeps the peritoneal contents and bladder out of the operative field and also provides a safety barrier to inadvertent movements of surgical instruments.
  - For L5–S1 exposures, we prefer to use a sharp Hohmann retractor, which penetrates the bone on the (patient's) left side of the inferior vertebral body of L5. This ensures that the left common iliac vein will not slip under the retractor. Since this retractor is embedded in bone, there is no retraction on the lumbar nerve plexus.
  - For L4–5 exposures, since there are no vascular structures to retract on the (patient's) left side, a handheld retractor can be used to gently retract the psoas muscle. With a handheld retractor, it is critical that the blade does not extend too deep along the lateral edge of the vertebra, where it can impinge on the lumbar plexus. Surgical assistants need to pay attention to the force and location of their retraction effort.
- At L5–S1, retractors are positioned to retract the right and left common iliac artery and veins lateral to the superior margin of the disc.
- Before incising the disc, lateral fluoroscopic imaging should confirm the operative level and ensure that the retractors have not pierced the endplate (**TECH FIG 3C**).

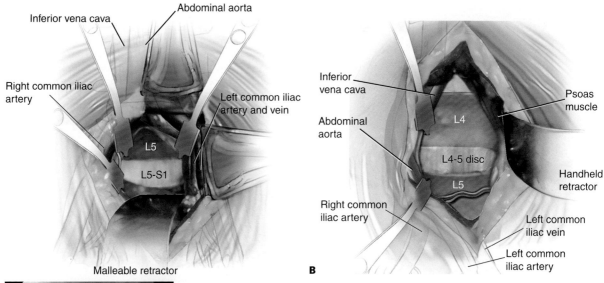

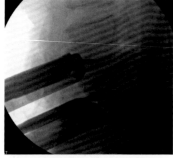

TECH FIG 3 • A. Optimal configuration of retractors for exposure of the L5–S1 disc. **B.** Optimal configuration of retractors for exposure of the L4–5 disc. Thin Hohmann retractors with sharp tips can be used to pierce the vertebral body and keep the great vessels out of the operative field. Handheld radiolucent blade retractors can also be used to retract the great vessels. Some retractors are cannulated, allowing them to be fixed with a transfixion pin into the vertebral body. **C.** The lateral fluoroscopic image confirms that the teeth of the Hohmann retractors are not in the disc space and that they are surrounding the disc of interest.

PEARLS AND PITFALLS

Cleaning the prerectus sheath of fat aids in finding this fascial edge at the end of the case.

Use of bipolar and blunt dissection theoretically reduces the risk of presacral plexus injury and retrograde ejaculation.

If the sympathetic chain is injured in the approach, the ipsilateral leg will feel warmer postoperatively; this is not to be confused with a cold contralateral leg.

When ligating the iliolumbar veins, the surgeon should tie or clip each side of the vein twice to prevent loss of ligature.

POSTOPERATIVE CARE

- The patient is given 24 hours of antibiotics for wound infection prophylaxis.
- A perioperative nasogastric tube is used to reduce the incidence of postoperative ileus.
- The patient is mobilized on postoperative day 1 with a lumbar corset.
- Incentive spirometry is used.
- Skin staples are removed on postoperative day 10 to 14.
- Stood softeners and laxatives are used as needed to avoid fecal impaction.

OUTCOMES

- The prevalence of major vein lacerations was 1.4% and the prevalence of left iliac artery thrombosis was 0.45% in a series of 1315 consecutive retroperitoneal exposures.[2]
- Ureteral and nerve injuries (lumbosacral nerve root or sympathetics) occur less frequently than major vascular injuries.[4]
- Mortality after anterior lumbar exposures is less than 1%.[4]
- Anterior approaches to the spine likely result in reduced patient satisfaction in terms of self-image and appearance.[3]
- The possibility of retrograde ejaculation should be discussed preoperatively with all male patients, as the prevalence ranges from 0.1% to 13.3%.[1,6] To preclude the need to harvest sperm from the bladder in affected men, donation before surgery is a viable option.

COMPLICATIONS

- Retrograde ejaculation
- Ureteral injury
- Abdominal or umbilical hernia
- Wound infection and dehiscence
- Bowel injury
- Bladder injury
- Lumbosacral plexus injury
- Deep venous thrombosis and pulmonary embolism
- Major vessel injury and massive blood loss
- Reflex sympathetic dystrophy

REFERENCES

1. Brau SA. Mini-open approach to the spine for anterior lumbar interbody fusion: description of the procedure, results, and complications. Spine J 2002;2:216–223.
2. Brau SA, Delamarter RB, Schiffman ML, et al. Vascular injury during anterior lumbar surgery. Spine 2004;4:409–412.
3. Horton WC, Bridwell KH, Glassman SD, et al. The morbidity of anterior exposure for spinal deformity in adults: an analysis of patient-based outcomes and complications in 112 consecutive cases. Proceedings from the Scoliosis Research Society Annual Meeting, October 2005.
4. Ikard RW. Methods and complications of anterior exposure of the thoracic and lumbar spine. Arch Surg 2006;141:1025–1034.
5. McAfee PC, Cunningham BW, Holtsapple G, et al. A prospective, randomized, multi-center FDA IDE study of lumbar total disc replacement with the CHARITE™ Artificial Disc vs. lumbar fusion: Part II. Evaluation of radiographic outcomes and correlation of surgical technique accuracy with clinical outcomes. Spine 2005;30: 1576–1583.
6. Sasso RC, Burkus KJ, LeHuec JC. Retrograde ejaculation after anterior lumbar interbody fusion: transperitoneal versus retroperitoneal exposure. Spine 2003;28:1023–1026.

Chapter 47

Posterior Thoracic and Lumbar Approaches

Thomas Stanley, Michael J. Lee, Mark Dumonski, and Kern Singh

ANATOMY

- Superficial landmarks allow for gross determination of anatomic level. Proximally, C7 and T1 are the largest spinous processes and act as landmarks for determining anatomic level. Distally, the intercrestal line approximates the L4–5 interspace.
- There are three layers to the posterior musculature of the spine (**FIG 1**, Table 1):
  - Superficial layer: trapezius, latissimus dorsi, rhomboid major and minor, and levator scapulae
  - Intermediate layer: serratus posterior superior and inferior, and levatores costarum
  - Deep layer: erector spinae, transversospinalis, interspinalis, and intertransversarii
- The superficial and intermediate layers receive their nervous supply from peripheral nerves, which are not encountered through the posterior approach (**FIG 2**). The deep layer receives its nervous supply segmentally from the posterior dorsal rami. There is a large amount of redundancy in the innervation of the deep layer.
  - The midline approach is a true internervous plane, and nerve injury occurs only with excessive lateral dissection.
- The vascular supply to the deep layer is from segmental branches of the aorta. These vessels enter the operative field at the level of the intertransverse ligament and can be a source of significant bleeding.
- The facet joint capsules have a shiny white appearance and the individual fibers can be seen inserting onto the lateral edge of the laminar trough. Care should be taken to avoid violating the capsular fibers unless that segment is being fused.
- The ligamentum flavum has a yellow appearance, with the fibers running in a cephalad–caudad direction. The cephalad end of the ligament has a broad insertion from the base of the spinous process to between 50 and 70 percent of the anterior surface of the lamina. The caudad end of the ligament inserts from the superior edge of the lamina to between 2 and 6 mm of the anterior surface of the lamina.[4]
- Particularly at the L5–S1 level, the interspace may be widened or the posterior bony anatomy only partly formed. Care should be exercised when exposing this level as inadvertent plunging into the canal may occur.
- Laterally, the intertransverse membrane overlies the iliopsoas and protects the neural structures that lie beneath.
- In children, the spinous process apophysis has not fused. During dissection, the apophysis is split down to the bone and then elevated with the paraspinal musculature.

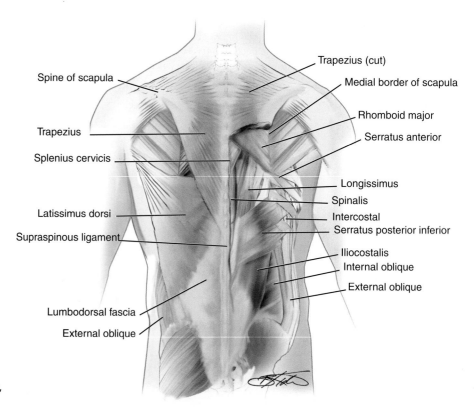

FIG 1 • The superficial, intermediate, and deep musculature of the back.

Table 1	Musculature of the Back			
Muscle	**Origin**	**Insertion**	**Innervation**	**Blood Supply**
Superficial layer				
Trapezius	Medial third of superior nuchal line of occiput, external occipital protuberance, and ligamentum nuchae; spinous processes of C7–T12	Lateral third of clavicle, acromion, spine of scapula	Motor supply from spinal accessory nerve, sensory fibers from C3 and C4	Transverse cervical artery
Latissimus dorsi	Spinous processes of T7—sacrum, medial third of iliac crest, ribs 9–12, inferior angle of scapula	Floor of bicipital groove	Thoracodorsal nerve (C7, C8)	Thoracodorsal artery
Levator scapulae	Transverse processes of C1–C4	Medial border of scapula	Dorsal scapular nerve (C5), with branches of C3–C4 innervating upper part of muscle	Dorsal scapular artery
Rhomboid major	Spinous processes of T2–T5	Medial border of scapula	Dorsal scapular nerve (C5)	Dorsal scapular artery
Rhomboid minor	Caudad end of ligamentum nuchae, spinous processes of C7–T1	Medial border of scapula	Dorsal scapular nerve (C5)	Dorsal scapular artery
Intermediate layer				
Serratus posterior superior	Spinous processes of C7–T3	Ribs 1–4	Intercostal nerves	Posterior intercostals arteries of T1–T4
Serratus posterior inferior	Thoracolumbar fascia, spinous processes of T11–L2	Ribs 9–12	Intercostal nerves	Posterior intercostal arteries, subcostal artery, and L1–L2 lumbar arteries
Levatores costarum	Tip of transverse process of C7–T11 vertebrae	Rib below level of origin	Posterior rami of thoracic spinal nerves	Dorsal intercostal arteries
Deep layer				
Erector spinae (vertically oriented and superficial)				
Iliocostalis	Iliac crest, sacrum, transverse and spinous processes of vertebrae and supraspinal ligament	Ribs, transverse and spinous processes of vertebrae, posterior aspect of skull	Segmental innervation by dorsal primary rami of spinal nerves C1–S5	Segmental supply by deep cervical arteries, posterior intercostal arteries, subcostal artery, and lumbar arteries
Longissimus				
Spinalis				
Transversospinalis (obliquely oriented and intermediate)				
Semispinalis	Transverse processes T1–T12	Spinous processes of C2–T5	Dorsal rami of spinal nerves	Segmental arteries from aorta
Multifidus	Articular processes of cervical vertebrae, transverse processes of thoracic vertebrae, mammillary processes of lumbar vertebrae, posterior superior iliac spine	Spinous processes of C2–L5	Dorsal rami of spinal nerves	Segmental branches from aorta
Rotatores	Transverse processes	Base of spinous processes above. Long skip one level; short attach at level above.	Dorsal rami of spinal nerves	Segmental branches from aorta
Deepest muscle				
Interspinales	Spinous processes	Spinous processes one level above	Dorsal rami of spinal nerves	Segmental branches from aorta
Intertransversarii	Anterior and posterior transverse processes of cervical vertebrae, transverse and mammillary processes of lumbar vertebrae	Anterior and posterior processes of cervical vertebrae one level above, transverse and accessory processes of lumber vertebrae one level above	Dorsal rami of spinal nerves	Segmental branches from aorta

SURGICAL MANAGEMENT

Positioning

- Patients should be placed in the prone position on a radiolucent table (**FIG 3A**).
- Care is taken to ensure that the neck is in a neutral position with no hyperextension.

- The arms are positioned at 90 degrees or less of abduction to minimize the likelihood of rotator cuff impingement. The arms are allowed to slightly hang down in a forward-flexed position about 10 degrees. The axilla should be clear from any padding to prevent brachial plexus palsy.
- Elbow pads are placed along the medial epicondyle to protect the ulnar nerve.

Thoracic Region

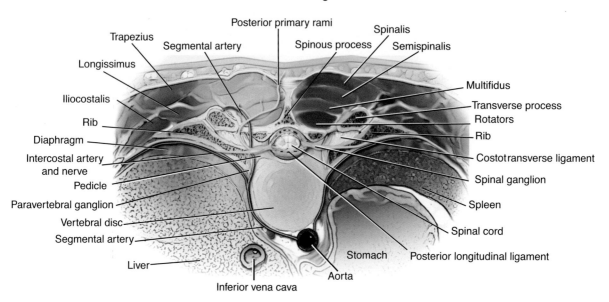

Lumbar Region

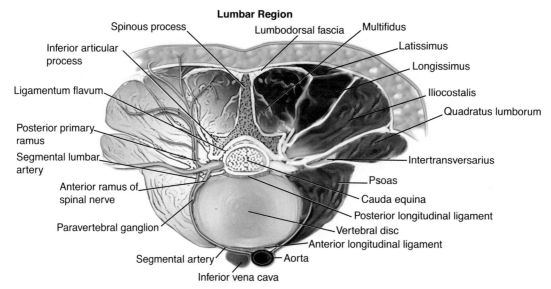

FIG 2 • Cross-sectional anatomy of the thoracic and lumbar spine.

- Pads are placed at the chest and iliac crests.
- The chest pad is placed just proximal to the level of the xiphoid process and distal to the axilla. In women, care is taken to tuck the breasts and ensure that the nipples are pressure-free.
- The iliac pads are placed two fingerbreadths distal to the anterior superior iliac spine, allowing the abdomen to hang free and reducing any unnecessary epidural bleeding.
- Proper placement of the chest and iliac pads allows for restoration of normal sagittal alignment via gravity.
- Alternatively, for lumbar decompressive procedures alone, the knees are positioned in a sling, allowing the hips to flex and eliminating lumbar lordosis and widening the laminar interspaces (**FIG 3B**). This position improves access to the lum-

bar spinal canal but should be avoided when instrumenting as lumbar lordosis is decreased.

Approach

- Two approaches are used: midline and paraspinal.
- The midline approach is used for most spinal procedures as it allows direct access to the spinal canal.
- The paraspinal approach, also known as the Wiltse approach, was initially described for spondylolisthesis but is now being used during far-lateral discectomies and minimally invasive muscle-sparing techniques.
  - There is increased interest in the paraspinal approach, particularly in conjunction with transforaminal lumbar interbody fusion procedures.

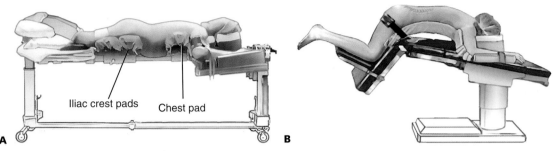

FIG 3 • **A.** Prone position on a radiolucent table. The abdomen is not compressed. **B.** The knee–chest position is obtained using a Wilson frame.

MIDLINE POSTERIOR APPROACH

Incision and Dissection

- Anatomic landmarks are identified to center the skin incision appropriately (**TECH FIG 1A**).
- A midline incision is made over the spinous processes down to the level of the fascia.
- A Cobb elevator is used to create 2-mm full-thickness skin flaps with subcutaneous fat. This allows for better visualization of the fascia during closure (**TECH FIG 1B,C**).
- The location of the spinous processes is again verified, and electrocautery is used to reflect the fascia from the tips of the spinous processes.
- Electrocautery is used to subperiosteally elevate the paraspinal musculature laterally to the trough of the lamina. The surgeon should avoid going beyond this point to protect the insertion of the facet joint capsule.

- A sponge and Cobb are then used to gently dissect the paraspinal musculature off the facet joint capsule.

Cautery

- Two venous bleeders are encountered that require electrocautery (**TECH FIG 2A**).
  - The first is located adjacent to the pars interarticularis (**TECH FIG 2B,C**).
  - The second is located just lateral to the facet joint.
- Electrocautery is used to elevate the paraspinal musculature off the transverse processes. Care should be taken to stay on the transverse process and not to violate the intertransverse membrane.
- Bipolar cautery should be used at the intertransverse ligament to avoid damage to the spinal nerves.

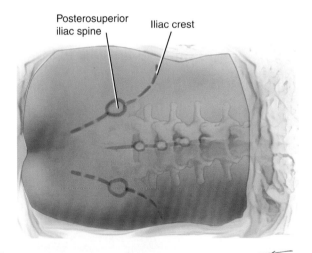

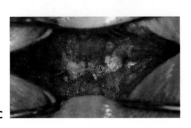

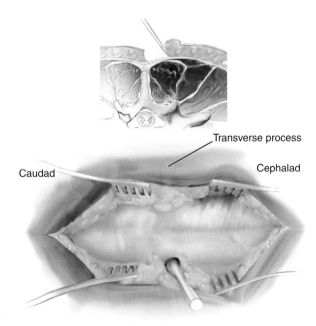

TECH FIG 1 • **A.** Anatomic landmarks. **B,C.** The fascia is exposed with full-thickness skin flaps.

TECHNIQUES

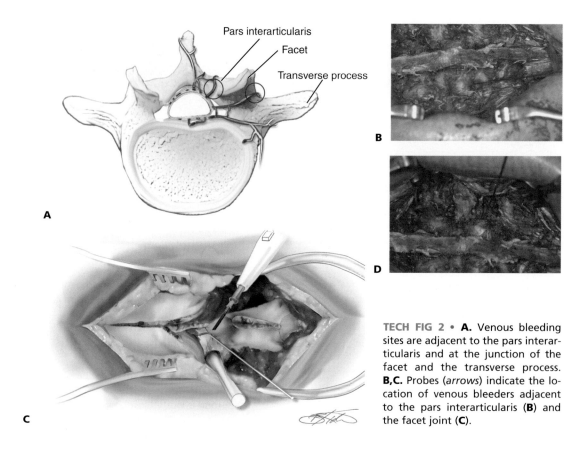

TECH FIG 2 • **A.** Venous bleeding sites are adjacent to the pars interarticularis and at the junction of the facet and the transverse process. **B,C.** Probes (*arrows*) indicate the location of venous bleeders adjacent to the pars interarticularis (**B**) and the facet joint (**C**).

Paraspinal Resection

■ In large and muscular patients, often it is necessary to excise a portion of the paraspinal muscles overlying the transverse processes to be fused.

■ The muscle is resected beginning underneath the fascia and extending toward the lateral edge of the transverse processes. This creates a pocket over the transverse processes that serves as a bone graft cavity (**TECH FIG 3**).

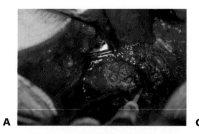

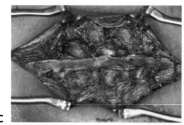

TECH FIG 3 • **A,B.** Electrocautery is used to excavate a muscular pocket for the fusion mass. **C,D.** Complete posterior exposure.

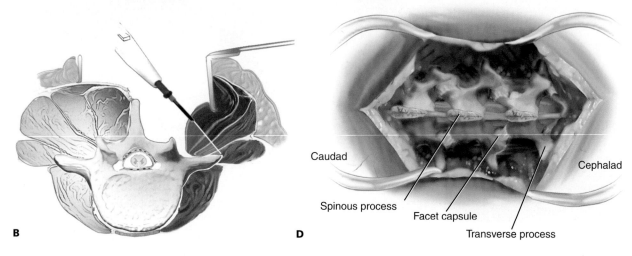

PARASPINAL APPROACH

- The approach is typically performed two fingerbreadths lateral to the spinous process.
- After the fascia has been exposed, the paraspinal muscles are palpated and the interval between the multifidus medially and longissimus laterally is identified.
- A sharp incision through the fascia is made at this interval (**TECH FIG 4**).
- The interval is defined with blunt dissection down to the lateral edge of the facet joint and transverse process junction.

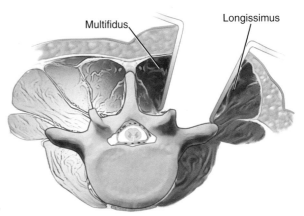

TECH FIG 4 • Cross-section of spine showing Wiltse interval.

PEARLS AND PITFALLS

Pars interarticularis bleeder	■ Lateral to the pars; can be prophylactically identified and cauterized
Lateral facet bleeder	■ A ball-tipped probe can be placed along the undersurface of the lateral edge of the superior articular process where the facet bleeder originates. Electrocautery can then be used to coagulate this vessel, which hinders intertransverse exposures.
Facet capsule preservation	■ A sponge can be placed over the facet. Muscle stripping is then performed with a Cobb elevator as the sponge protects the capsular fibers from being disrupted and accidentally incised.
Widened lower lumbar interspace	■ An anteroposterior radiograph should be evaluated preoperatively to assess for spina bifida occulta and widened interlaminar windows. Extra caution should be employed when working in these areas to avoid inadvertent injury to the thecal sac.

Table 2	**Complications Associated with the Posterior Approach[2,3]**	
Complications		**Occurrence**
Major		
Wound infection		1–10%
Pneumonia		5%
Renal failure		5%
Myocardial infarction		3%
Respiratory distress		2%
Neurologic deficit		2%
Congestive heart failure		2%
Cerebrovascular accident		1%
Minor		
Urinary tract infections		34%
Anemia requiring transfusion		27%
Confusion		27%
Ileus		22%
Arrhythmia		7%
Transient hypoxia		7%
Wound seroma		5%
Leg dysesthesia		2%

COMPLICATIONS

- Major and minor complication rates of up to 80% have been reported in some series (Table 2).[2]
- Risk factors for complications include patient age, length of surgery, levels exposed, blood loss, and postoperative urinary incontinence. Diabetes and other medical comorbidities have not been shown to be independent risk factors for the development of postoperative complications.[1–3]

REFERENCES

1. Benz RJ, et al. Predicting complications in elderly patients undergoing lumbar decompression. Clin Orthop Relat Res 2001;384:116–121.
2. Carreon LY, et al. Perioperative complications of posterior lumbar decompression and fusion in adults. J Bone Joint Surg Am 2003;85A:2089–2092.
3. Olson MA, et al. Risk factors for surgical site infection in spinal surgery. J Neurosurg 2003;98:149–155.
4. Olszewski AD, et al. The anatomy of the human lumbar ligamentum flavum: new observations and their surgical importance. Spine 1996;21:2307–2312.

INDEX

Page numbers followed by *f* and *t* indicated figures and tables, respectively.